# Developing Practical Skills for Nursing Children and Young People

# Developing Practical Skills for Nursing Children and Young People

## Edited by

### Alan Glasper
**Professor of Children's and Young People's Nursing**
School of Nursing & Midwifery, University of Southampton, Southampton

### Marion Aylott
**Lecturer in Child Health Nursing**
School of Nursing & Midwifery, University of Southampton, Southampton

### Cath Battrick
**Matron**
Southampton Children's Hospital, Southampton

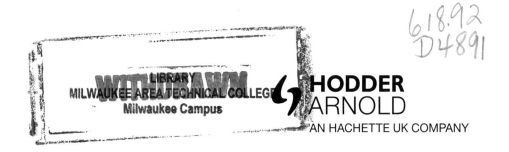

**HODDER
ARNOLD**
AN HACHETTE UK COMPANY

First published in Great Britain in 2010 by
Hodder Arnold, an imprint of Hodder Education, an Hachette UK Company
338 Euston Road, London NW1 3BH
http://www.hoddereducation.com

Hachette UK's Hodder Headline's policy is to use papers that are natural, renewable and recyclable products and made from wood grown in sustainable forests. The logging and manufacturing processes are expected to conform to the environmental regulations of the country of origin.

Whilst the advice and information in this book are believed to be true and accurate at the date of going to press, neither the authors nor the publisher can accept any legal responsibility or liability for any errors or omissions that may be made. In particular (but without limiting the generality of the preceding disclaimer) every effort has been made to check drug dosages; however, it is still possible that errors have been missed. Furthermore, dosage schedules are constantly being revised and new side-effects recognized. For these reasons the reader is strongly urged to consult the drug companies' printed instructions before administering any of the drugs recommended in this book.

*British Library Cataloguing in Publication Data*
A catalogue record for this book is available from the British Library

*Library of Congress Cataloging-in-Publication Data*
A catalog record for this book is available from the Library of Congress

ISBN   9780340974193

1 2 3 4 5 6 7 8 9 10

Commissioning Editor:      Naomi Wilkinson
Project Editors:           Clare Patterson and Joanna Silman
Production Controller:     Rachel Manguel
Cover Designer:            Lynda King
Indexer:                   Jan Ross

Typeset in 9.5 point Berling Roman by Transet Limited, Coventry, England
Printed and bound in Malta

What do you think about this book? Or any other Hodder Arnold title?
Please visit our website: www.hoddereducation.com

# Contents

# Contributors

**Diana Agacy-Cowell** RGN AdvDip (Psychiatry and Psychology) AdvDip(Child Branch) BSc
Specialist Practitioner of Transfusion, Blood Transfusion Department, Southampton University Hospitals NHS Trust, Southampton

**Palo Almond** RGN RM HV(Dip) RNT BSc PgD(Ed) AHCP MSc
School of Nursing and Midwifery, University of Southampton, Southampton

**Diane Atwill** RGN
Team Leader, Children's Continence Service, Bitterne Health Centre, Southampton

**Marion Aylott** MA BSc(Hons) RGN RM RSCN
Senior Lecturer in Child Health Nursing, Faculty of Health and Life Sciences, University of the West of England, Bristol

**Colleen MD Baker** BN RNC
Hampshire Primary Care Trust

**Cath Battrick** RGN RSCN PGDip MSc
Matron, Paediatrics, Southampton Children's Hospital, Southampton

**Helen Bennett** RGN RSCN BA(Hons) CTHE MSc
Care Manager, Naomi House, Stockbridge Road, Sutton Scotney , Winchester

**Mary Booy** RGN RSCN SCM Diploma in Nursing Studies
School Nurse, Southampton City Primary Care Trust, Southampton

**Maria Brenner** RGN BSc MSc
Head of Children's Nursing, School of Nursing, Midwifery and Health Systems, University College Dublin, Belfield, Dublin, Ireland

**Sylvia Buckingham** RSCN DipNursing BEd(Hons) RNT MSc
Senior Lecturer, School of Health Sciences, University of Southampton, Southampton

**Naomi Campbell** BNChild
Sister, Paediatric High Dependency Unit, Southampton General Hospital, Southampton

**Desmond Cawley** RGN RCN HDip(Dist) MSc(Hons) Doctoral Candidate
Lecturer in Nursing Studies, Department of Nursing and Health Science, Athlone Institute of Technology, Athlone, Ireland

**Sarah Chalk**
Lead Paediatric Phlebotomist, Children's Outpatients Department, Southampton General Hospital, Southampton

**Lizzie Dickin** RGN RSCN
Clinical Nurse Specialist (Paediatric Pain Management), Southampton Hospital, Southampton

**Lubna Ezad** MBBS MRCP
Associate Specialist in Community Paediatrics, Bitterne Health Centre, Southampton

**Margaret Fergus** BSc(Hons) SRN RHV PGCE(A)
Southampton, University, School of Nursing and Midwifery, Southampton

**Donna Forbes** BN RNC
Southampton City PCT, Southampton

**Alan Glasper** BA(Hons) PhD RGN RSCN DN(Lond) ONC Cert Ed RNT
Professor of Children's and Young People's Nursing, School of Nursing & Midwifery, University of Southampton, Southampton,

**Liz Gormley-Fleming** MA PGDip(HE) BSc(Hons) RNT, RGN, RSCN
Senior Lecturer, Children's Nursing, University of Hertfordshire, Hatfield

**Diane Gow** RGN, RSCN, RCNT, RNT, BA (Hons), MSc
School of Health Sciences, University of Southampton

**Helen Green** BN(Hons) Child
Sister Children's Orthopaedics, Southampton General Hospital, Southampton

**Joanna Groves** NNEB BTEC Diploma (Hospital Play Specialism)
Hospital Play Specialist, Wessex Cardiothoracic Unit, Southampton General Hospital, Southampton

**Carol Hall** RGN RSCN DipN(Lond) Bsc(Hons) PGDip(AdEd) RNT PGDip(ResM) PhD FHEA
Associate Professor, School Of Nursing Midwifery and Physiotherapy, University of Nottingham, Queens Medical Centre, Nottingham

**Joanne Harvey** RGN RSCN DipNursing
Paediatric Immunology Nurse Specialist,
Southampton General Hospital, Southampton

**Jan Heath** RGN CertEd BA Ed (Hons)
Skills for Practice Lead, Southampton University
Hospital Trust, Southampton

**Joanna Himsworth** BN
Sister, Paediatric Assessment Unit, Southampton
General Hospital, Southampton

**Liz Hopper** RN RM DipCouns
Family Support Coordinator, Naomi House,
Stockbridge Road, Sutton Scotney , Winchester

**Rachel Howe** RGN RCN HDip Nursing Studies(Sick
Children's) PGDip(Clinical Practice) MSc(Nursing) CNM2
Clinical Facilitator – Children's Hospital, The
Adelaide & Meath Hospital incorporating The
National Children's Hospital (AMNCH), Dublin,
Ireland

**Di Keeton** RSCN PgDip(Allergic disease)
Paediatric Dermatology Nurse Specialist,
Southampton University Hospitals NHS Trust,
Southampton

**Deidre Kelleher** RGN RNT BNS(Hons) MScNursing
Lecturer, School of Nursing Midwifery and Health
Systems, University College Dublin, Dublin, Ireland

**Janet Kelse** RGN RSCN BSc(Hons) AdvDip(Ed) PGCE RNT MSc
Academic Lead for Child Health Nursing, Faculty of
Health & Social Work, University of Plymouth,
Plymouth

**Rosie King** RGN RN(Child) PGCert in Allergy
Paediatric Allergy Nurse Specialist, Southampton
University Hospitals NHS Trust, Southampton

**Sue Laker** RGN RN(Child) MSc(Nursing)
Staff Nurse, Paediatric Intensive Care Unit,
Southampton General Hospital, Southampton

**Caroline Langford** RN(Child) BSc MSc
Oncology Department, Alder Hey Children's NHS
Foundation Trust, Liverpool

**John Larkin** RGN RCN BSc(Nursing) MSc(Health Service
Management) GradCert(Nursing Education)
Lecturer in Nursing Studies, Department of Nursing
and Health Science, Athlone Institute of Technology,
Athlone, Ireland

**Jane McConochie** SRN RSCN BSc(Hons)Nursing Studies
ENB Higher Award
Senior Staff Nurse Orthopaedic/Surgical Paediatric
ward, Queen Alexandra Hospital, Portsmouth

**Gill McEwing** RGN RSCN RNT DipNursing CertED MSc
Lecturer in Child Health, Faculty of Health and
Social Work, University of Plymouth, Plymouth

**Colman Noctor** MSc GradDip HDip RPN
School of Nursing, Midwifery and Health Systems,
University College Dublin, Dublin, Ireland

**Karen O'Donnell** RGN DipHE RNChild CM.
Ward Manager, National Spinal Injuries Centre, Stoke
Mandeville Hospital, Aylesbury, Buckinghamshire

**Shirin Pomeroy** RN(Child) BA(Hons)
Clinical Nurse Practitioner, Paediatric Burns, Barbara
Russell Children's Unit, Frenchay Hospital, Bristol

**Sue Robson** RSCN Bsc(Hons) Nursing
Staff Nurse Paediatric Intensive Care, Southampton
General Hospital, Southampton

**Jane Shelswell** RGN RN(Child) BSc(Hons) Nursing
Sister, Paediatric Intensive Care, Southampton
General Hospital, Southampton

**Sandie Skinner** RGN RSCN ANNP BN MSc
Neonatal Unit, Royal Hampshire County Hospital,
Winchester

**Sue Slater-Smith** RGN RSCN DN Dip
Specialist Encopresis Sister, Children's Continence
Team, Bitterne Health Centre, Southampton

**Jill Thistlethwaite** RGN RSCN BSc(Hons) Nursing(PICU)
Senior Sister Paediatric Intensive Care, Southampton
General Hospital, Southampton

**Naomi Watson** NNEB RGN RSCN BSC(Hons)
Paediatric Oncology Outreach Nurse Specialist,
Southampton General Hospital, Southampton

**Katy Weaver** Dip Childhood Studies (Nursery Nursing) BTEC
Professional Development Cert (Hospital Play Specialism)
Hospital Play Specialist, Southampton General
Hospital, Southampton

**Jane Willock** RGN RSCN BSc(Hons) PGDE MSc
Senior Lecturer in Child Health, University of
Glamorgan, Pontypridd, Paediatric Nurse
Practitioner, University Hospital of Wales, Cardiff

**Lyn Wilson** BSc PGCE MSc
Lecturer, Public Health, School of Health Sciences,
University of Southampton, Southampton

**Michelle Wright** RN(Child Branch) BSc MSc
Advanced Nurse Practitioner, Oncology Unit, Alder
Hey Children's NHS Trust, Liverpool

# Foreword

I am delighted to write the foreword to this excellent book. I know that nurses caring for children and young people everywhere will welcome this text book. I am sure that it will be a standard reference for nursing students, as well as qualified nurses in practice, management and as an *aide memoire* for those in education.

Children and young people are very different to adults. For this reason, nurses need special skills when planning their care. In this book, the chapters begin with learning outcomes, an overview of the topic area and then provide very practical advice on the nursing care required for the disease or condition. The skills are set out in a way that is easy to follow, and can be used as a reference in the clinical setting. There are also helpful further suggested reading lists. The authors have given a wealth of tips and ideas that can only come from their extensive experience. The book addresses the particular needs of children and young people at all stages of their development, from baby to young adult.

I am also pleased to see the emphasis on the contribution of the family which is rightly seen as central to the well being of the child.

Congratulations to all the chapter authors and contributors, the editors and the publishers.

Nurses at all academic and professional levels will find this a useful tool when working with children and young people.

*Angela Horsley*
*Chair, Association Chief Children's Nurses (ACCN)*
*Clinical Lead, The Nottingham Children's Hospital*

# Preface

This book and its companion website has been written and developed by experienced children's and young people's nurses specifically to assist readers in developing the practical skills necessary to care for children and their carers in a variety of acute care settings. Practical nursing skills, carried out with competence and compassion, are highly valued by children, young people and their families. These skills promote health, recovery and comfort, making an essential contribution to positive healthcare experiences. The Nursing and Midwifery Council (NMC) highlights the importance of fundamental skills by explicitly identifying them in their Essential Skills Clusters for pre-registration nursing students. This information related to specific skills detailed within this book has been mapped against the NMC skills clusters and other healthcare competencies. The early chapters in the book discuss fundamental skills for caring, skills expected of any nurse entering the first part of the NMC register for the child field of practice. Later chapters provide details of more specialist skills for caring for children and young people with more specific healthcare problems. To achieve this we have recruited a number of senior nurses from specialist clinical areas in differing parts of the British Isles to contribute to the book. We hope you will be inspired to learn from all our contributors who have endeavoured to give you an insight into the real world of children's and young people's nursing where the emphasis is on the delivery of safe and evidence-based care.

In some care environments nurses are more likely to supervise or support children and their carers than directly carry out these practical skills themselves. It is important to stress that to supervise others in providing quality fundamental care requires a sound knowledge and understanding of these skills, and a commitment to their value.

The book's first three chapters explain the caring context for the undertaking of skills with children and young people, emphasising the importance of the nurses underpinning knowledge and attitudes as well as the practical component of skills. Many chapters cite individual procedural policies from different healthcare institutions. It is important to stress that, although the procedures detailed within this book are based on best evidence, some healthcare institutions will have differing procedural policies, and readers are therefore strongly advised to read their own polices before attempting to implement any of these procedures in practice.

The book and the accompanying website are interactive, evidence-based and promote theory–practice links and reflective practice.

While this book is particularly applicable to recently qualified nurses and pre-registration child field of practice nursing students, it is also relevant to care assistants who are studying qualifications in care, students on a range of assistant practitioner (foundation degree) healthcare-related programmes, and to all those involved in the teaching of practical skills, including university and college lecturers, and practitioners.

Children's and young people's nurses care for children and their families across the age continuum in a wide range of healthcare settings in different circumstances.

We hope that this book will be essential reading for those who practice or aspire to become practitioners, in which the cardinal tenet is to 'first do the child no harm'.

*Alan Glasper*
*Marion Aylott*
*Cath Battrick*
*June 2009*

# How to use this book and website

This textbook has an accompanying website **www.hodderplus.com/childnursingskills**
For each chapter you will find PowerPoint slides giving more information, interactive Multiple Choice Questions to test your knowledge and links to further sources of information. There is also an image bank which includes full colour photographs.

To access these resources, please register on the website using the following serial number:
152GHK91WER

You will see the following symbol throughout the book

This indicates when you can go to the website for further information, colour illustrations and further reading on that topic.

# Key concepts in undertaking clinical procedures with children and young people:

## A) Elements to consider before performing clinical nursing procedures

### Alan Glasper and Diane Gow

### LEARNING OUTCOMES

*Upon completion of this chapter, the reader should be able to accomplish the following:*

1 Recognise the importance of adhering to the NMC Code when delivering procedural care to sick children, young people and their families
2 Understand the importance of ensuring privacy and dignity when performing nursing procedures on children and young people following the prevailing philosophy of family-centred care
3 Recognise the importance of confidentiality when working with children, young people and their families
4 Acknowledge the complexity of obtaining consent in the world of children's nursing
5 Appreciate aspects of risk when performing nursing procedures
6 Demonstrate the importance of delivering care based on best evidence only

all aspects of the Nursing and Midwifery Council (NMC) Code which constitutes standards of conduct, performance and ethics for nurses and midwives.[1]

Although all the NMC standards are pertinent to your practice, this chapter will discuss only those aspects of the code which directly pertain to the carrying out of procedures on children and young people (Box 1).

---

**Box 1 The NMC Code**

1 Make the care of people (i.e. children and young people and their families/carers) your first concern, treating them as individuals and respecting their dignity.
2 Work with others to protect and promote the health and wellbeing of those in your care, their families and carers, and the wider community.
3 Provide a high standard of practice and care at all times.
4 Be open and honest, act with integrity and uphold the reputation of your profession.

---

## CHAPTER OVERVIEW

This introductory chapter identifies elements of your practice that you must think about before you undertake any procedure to guarantee that the children and their families you are caring for receive the best evidence-based care by a competent children's nurse. These procedural elements of the care you deliver are supported by

## MAKE THE CARE OF PEOPLE YOUR FIRST CONCERN, TREATING THEM AS INDIVIDUALS AND RESPECTING THEIR DIGNITY

The NMC Code instructs all nurses to treat people as individuals. It is therefore crucial that you must treat all children, young people and their families or carers as individuals and respect their dignity. The concept of the maintenance of dignity is now pivotal to the practice of good nursing practice.[2,3]

A report by the chief nursing officer for England[4] has highlighted some problems with the provision of single-sex accommodation in some hospitals.[5] This primarily applies to adult patients, because following guidance from the *National service framework for children, young people and maternity services*[6] segregation by age is a more important issue than segregation by gender, especially for young people. However, it is important to stress that some young people and indeed children may also want to be able to choose between being in a single- or a mixed-sex environment.

To achieve the NMC code related to dignity, the children's nurse must always consider aspects of dignity which are sometimes difficult to achieve in some older hospitals. For example, in order to maintain child patient dignity, consider the provision of toilet and bathroom facilities (for children and carers). This is especially pertinent for carers who may be rooming in with their sick children. Good children's units have appointed family care coordinators to help manage such aspects of the family admission. Undoubtedly the care of children and young people and their families is improved by respecting their wishes and dignity. Importantly, children's nurses should reflect on the work of Rylance,[7] who interviewed the parents of 300 hospitalised children and ascertained that dignity, privacy and, significantly, confidentiality were badly valued on children's wards As far as the NMC code is concerned children, young people and their carers should have the same rights to these principles of dignity as adult patients. The Code states that you must not discriminate in any way against those in your care. Remember children have enshrined rights! Reed *et al.*[8] have highlighted the complex issue of promoting child dignity, comparing it with that of the older adult where the nurse has to care for the patient who may, in the case of the head-injured or older patient, no longer be the same person they once were, versus the sick child who is developing into a person who is yet to reach their full potential. The healthcare professionals who deliver care to children and young people in healthcare environments including the home therefore need to act in such a way that they respect the dignity of the child throughout their temporal lifespan for both the present and future human being.

*Essence of care,*[9] which importantly also applies to children's nursing, identifies nine key areas of care that have been identified by patients as needing attention, including privacy and dignity, which are now firmly re-established at the forefront of nursing. Importantly, if your own unit has no specific age-related divisions, close attention must be paid to privacy and dignity in the wider context of gender, ethnicity and developmental age and with due regard to that aspect of the code which instructs you not to discriminate in any way against those in your care.

Importantly the NMC Code also asks that nurses treat all people kindly and considerately and the NMC Code significantly asks you to act as an advocate for those families in your care. The advocacy role of children's and young people's nurses should be manifest by adhering to the NMC Code, which asks nurses to help families' access to relevant information and support. In Chapter 38 Battrick and Glasper outline how children's nurses can harness a variety of media formats to support the spoken word. Helping families navigate the labyrinth of information in the real and virtual world is a skill all children's nurses must harness.

The NMC Code asks each children's nurse to respect children's, young people's and families' right to confidentiality. Importantly the NMC Code states that you must ensure that people are informed about how and why information is shared by those who will be providing their care. Only in safeguarding situations can a children's nurse not promise confidentiality (see Chapter 3). Hence the NMC Code states that you must disclose information if you believe someone (a child) may be at risk of harm. Significantly, student nurses are monitored and cautioned by their universities not to disclose information about a child or a family inadvertently in, for example, case study or other assignments. Additionally, any conversations or discussions about families must remain within the clinical domain and never disclosed in a public forum of any description (for example discussions about particular family cases by students on the bus to class). In small communities this could be catastrophic for some families.

The growth of web-based networking sites such

as 'Facebook' can place children's nurses in a difficult and potentially compromising position as photographs of them, for example in a clinical domain, may inadvertently show other children in the clinical domain, thus breaching their right to confidentiality. The Association of Chief Children's Nurses (accnuk.org) is specifically advising children's nurses to politely decline any invitation to join a family's Facebook pages. Furthermore children's nurses are asked to monitor how mobile phones are used by families in clinical domains, not because of the telephone usage but rather because of the photographic cameras they contain. Photographs taken with mobile phone digital cameras may inadvertently show other children and again may breach their right to confidentiality, exacerbated if placed on a networking web site

### Practice tip

Using ward funds buy some cheap pay as you go mobile phones without cameras and allow children and their families to use these in safe mobile phone havens

The NMC Code asks each nurse to work in collaboration with children, young people and their carers. Furthermore, the NMC Code asks each nurse to listen to children and families in their care and respond to their concerns and preferences. This involves listening to their needs at each stage in the healthcare journey and responding to their concerns and preferences. The NMC Code specifically asks (children's) nurses to support families in self-caring activities to improve and maintain their health. In contemporary society where a range of emerging health issues such as type 2 diabetes linked to rising levels of childhood obesity are prevalent, this aspect of the code is of paramount importance. Thus the health promotion and advocacy role of the children's nurse is enshrined in regulatory protocol. In light of this the NMC Code asks that the nurse recognise the contribution that people (children and their families) make to their own care and wellbeing. The overarching principle of family-centered care, which is the mantra of children's nursing, is entirely congruent with this aspect of the code. Additionally, the NMC Code emphasises the need for nurses to make arrangements to meet families' language and communication needs, highly

pertinent in contemporary children's settings where nurses may come into contact with many for whom English is not their native tongue. In light of this the NMC Code states that you must share with children and their families in a way that they can understand the information they want or need to know about their health.

The NMC Code asks each nurse to ensure that consent is gained before any treatment or procedure is started.

The *NHS plan*[10] formulated in the wake of the events at Bristol Royal Infirmary and Alder Hey Children's Hospital in Liverpool, where consent procedures were later deemed to be less than optimum,[9,11] acknowledged the need for changes in the way that patients and their families are asked to give their consent. This is because there is a prima facia need to make certain that the procedure of gaining consent is actually focused on the rights of the child.[12]

The primary purpose of gaining consent is to ensure that the patient's autonomy of choice is fully protected, hence the term informed consent. Importantly, gaining consent allows and facilitates meaningful decision-making.[1,11,13–16] The NMC Code is quite specific when it states you must uphold people's rights to be fully involved in decisions about their care

It is important to recognise that children and young people are different not in the fundamental right of being able to give consent but in how children's nurses apply the principles in actual practice settings. It is worthy of note that the issues surrounding consent and young people under 16 years old was not addressed in the Family Law Reform Act of 1969. However, the subsequent Gillick case,[17] in which the rights of parents to make null and void the consent of their children, which was subject to the ruling of the House of Lords, ultimately recognised that a minor under 16 years of age could give their own consent to medical treatment unfettered by that of their parents or guardians if they had the capacity and capability of doing so. In this context, capacity simply means that the child can show that they have enough comprehension and intellect to recognise the value of what is being proposed. This capacity of the child to understand what is being proposed by a healthcare practitioner is now commonly referred to as being 'Gillick competent'.

Some professionals use the term interchangeably with 'Fraser guidelines' in recognition of the law lord who ruled on the case. However, it should be stressed that Fraser guidelines specifically relate only to girls who may consent to contraception and not the more complex and more comprehensive consent-related elements of caring for children and young people, which are now linked to the term Gillick competence.[18]

Of crucial importance to any children's nurse are the criteria which are used when they are ascertaining if an individual child achieves the notion of being Gillick competent. In this context the child or young person should be able to demonstrate they:

- Understand simple terms, nature, purpose and necessity for proposed treatment
- Believe the information applies to them
- Can retain the information long enough to make a choice
- Can make a choice free from pressure (after Larcher)[19].

The NMC Code states that you must respect and support people's rights to accept or decline treatment and care but children's nurses have to consider other elements of the consent paradigm. This means according to the NMC Code that you must be aware of the legislation regarding mental capacity, ensuring that people (children and their families) remain at the centre of decision-making and are fully safeguarded.

Apart from Scotland, young people in the UK aged 16–18 can give consent, but cannot automatically refuse treatment that is anticipated to preserve their lives or thwart serious harm or deterioration in their medical status.

This has important ramifications for children's nurses, especially when dealing with children with specific types of illnesses, for example anorexia nervosa and other eating disorders where the risk of premature death is high. The British Medical Association[20] guidelines relating to consent underpin the reality that children and young people now have an established right to give consent. However, the BMA also confirm the uncertainty about a young person's right to not give consent and refuse treatment. Therefore, in some situations a competent young person's refusal to give consent could be superseded and overturned,

i.e. in circumstances where the child's negative response to consent means that they could potentially suffer 'grave and irreversible mental or physical harm'.[21] In such situations where the case cannot be reconciled through negotiation and mediation, and best avoided, it may be necessary to instigate some legal intervention. Courts of law have for example overruled a young person's refusal to take medication for certain mental health disorders and transfusions necessary for treating childhood leukaemia or heart disease.

When this happens and the child's refusal to give consent is overruled, the children's nurse must consider the detrimental psychological sequelae that will ensue in the wake of this. This sequence of events should be carefully considered before overturning the child's refusal to give consent. Having to make children and young people accept procedures or treatments against their will may perpetrate psychological trauma, and exacerbate problems with any future encounter or procedure in the future. The inconsistency of allowing young people to consent to treatment, but denying their rights to refuse treatment remains controversial.[20]

### Case study

Children's nurses become very skilled at negotiating with children and young people the consent issues involved with procedures.

In one well-known case a young girl refused point blank to accept chemotherapy treatment for her newly diagnosed acute lymphoblastic leukaemia, stating vociferously that she preferred to die. Despite many efforts by the parents and doctors the girl continued to refuse to give consent for the first dose of medication.

One of the children's nurses caring for the girl spent some time with her and helped her comb her long blonde hair, which had become matted during the previous night's sleep. The nurse remarked to the girl what lovely hair she had and it was at this point that she confided in the nurse that it was neither the chemotherapy she was frightened of nor the insertion of the central venous line but rather the loss of her hair. The children's nurse was able to contact a local hairdresser, who prior to the commencement of the treatment came to the hospital and cut the child's hair, which was subsequently made into a beautiful wig! Sometimes immovable roadblocks to communication can be overcome with a little considerate thought of an alternative strategy. Similarly, children who have debilitating fears such as needle phobia can often be managed through appropriate distraction provided by a qualified hospital specialist (see Chapter 7).

Although children under 16 years may legally consent if they meet the criteria of competence and voluntariness and are deemed Gillick competent, in contrast in Scotland such children and young people may consent to treatment irrespective of age. It should be highlighted that competence is situation dependent and may fluctuate depending on the context. The child's current psychological status, the presence or absence of pain or the state of the care environment may positively or negatively impact on a child's competence. For example, a child being asked for consent in an adult emergency department full of hostile sounds and sights may react very differently in a specific child-orientated environment. Similarly, a child's past experience of illness may increase or decrease competence.

The law demands that doctor's take responsibility for the assessment of competence, although Larcher[19] states that other professionals with appropriate skills may be delegated to assist with the process. Children's nurses acknowledge that some complex procedures will present more challenging consent issues for those caring for certain groups of children.

Subtle or overt coercion of children and young people to give consent must be avoided but are not uncommon in some clinical environments. Time is especially important as children need adequate time to ponder on the information they have given. In addition, children used to living in hierarchal worlds may perceive that they have to show subservience to the decisions made on their behalf by authoritarian figures such as doctors and nurses. In light of this, many child healthcare professionals adopt casual dress/uniform to detract from this.

In the world of children's nursing, obtaining the consent of the individual child is fundamental to their practice, perhaps ratified by the mission statement of London's Great Ormond Street's Hospital 'The child first and always'. The NMC Code is quite specific about the need to obtain consent and any nurse who does not obtain valid consent may be liable to legal action by the child and family. Children's nurses would also find themselves having to account for their actions to the regulatory body the NMC.[21]

Before you undertake any of the procedures in this book, you must acquire the knowledge and understanding of the subject of consent. This will help ensure that a valid and meaningful consent has been obtained from the child and family before continuing with the procedure. Please note that consent is an ongoing process and not a one-off event. It is required whenever a nurse wishes to undertake a procedure on a sick child or young person, unless it is an emergency situation. However, remember that the NMC Code states that you must be able to demonstrate that you have acted in someone's (i.e. a child's) best interests if you have to provide care in an emergency.

## Performing care without consent

Glasper et al.[12] state that in such emergencies where treatment is necessary to preserve life or where the capacity of the patient is permanent or likely to be long-standing, *and in the absence of a legal guardian, it is lawful to carry out procedures that are in the best interest of the child*.[11,15,16,22–24]

## Types of consent

Consent may be expressed by the child explicitly or implied, and may be given verbally or in writing. (This will depend upon the circumstances.)

### Implied consent

Implied consent is a generally accepted notion that is attributed to the behaviour of the child or legal guardian that lets the children's nurse know that there is agreement to the procedure. Thus, implied consent is acceptable for simple care procedures such as aspects of personal hygiene or nutrition delivery. However, children' nurses should take heed of Aveyard,[25] who is cautious about an over-reliance on implied consent before undertaking a nursing procedure where compliance may be mistaken for consent. When in doubt the children's nurse should ascertain express consent instead. Despite this, implied consent can be interpreted from the child's actions, e.g. when the child readily reaches out to blow in the peak flow meter.

### Express consent

Express consent encompasses both written and verbal consent, and is used prior to carrying out any procedures that might carry a risk element. Importantly the law does not denote when consent should be obtained through the written word as opposed to the spoken word.[22,24] Written consent is usually obtained through the use of specially designed consent forms and brings to the child's/guardian's attention that they are consenting to a clinical procedure, one in which there may be risks and consequences. It is important to remember that the filling in of the form does not in itself convey that the process of obtaining consent has taken place.[26] A signature on a piece of hospital paper will not make the consent valid.[21] Perhaps the most important factor to appreciate is the validity of the consent process.[11,16,22,24]

## Validity of consent

A voluntary and uncoerced decision must be made by a competent or autonomous person on the basis of adequate information and deliberation to accept rather than reject some proposed course of action that will affect them.[27]

For consent to be valid, certain conditions must apply.

It must be given voluntarily without coercion and it must be given by a mentally competent individual who has been given adequate information.[11,22–25]

### Assent

Assent is when agreement is given by a child who is not competent to give legally binding consent under current legislation.[12] Obtaining assent from children is a fundamental component of children's nursing, as only through this process can a nurse ascertain that a child has indicated that they are compliant to participate in a procedure, even when they are considered in law to be insufficiently mature give informed consent.[28] All children should be provided with information about procedures, and this is discussed in Chapter 38 in more depth. Prior to and during any procedure, children's nurses must make an effort to gain the child's assent and any sustained dissent must be heeded and acted upon.[29] Good practice suggests that the use of special assent forms for younger children written and couched in terms they will understand should become universal. Does your own unit have such an assent form? Furthermore, a signed assent form in addition to the consent form signed by the child's legal

guardian will assist in ratifying the family-centred care philosophy much espoused by children's nurses.

### Information

For consent to be legally valid, the child and legal guardian needs to understand in broad terms the nature and purpose of the procedure.[11] With reference to the procedures detailed in this book, the information given to the child and family member must actually impart knowledge about the procedure, be individualised for each patient and given in a format that is understood by the readers or listeners (see Chapter 38).

Kennedy[30] believes that any information must be based on current evidence, and in a format that is comprehensible to the child and their guardians. Hence when a nursing procedure is undertaken, the information should be given to the child (and family) on all aspects of the procedure, i.e. the why's and the risks involved. The children first for health website (www.childrenfirst.nhs.uk/kids/), which is now part of many children's units websites, is designed to help children and their families learn about illnesses, tests and treatments.

## Who should obtain consent?

In most instances this is obtained by the individual performing the procedure. This is of relevance to the procedures discussed in this book, where verbal oral consent is most likely to be obtained prior to the point of the procedure being implemented.

## When should consent be sought?

The Department of Health[23] describes the process of gaining consent as either single-stage consent or as a process of two or more stages. The latter is particularly pertinent to elective daycare surgery, for example where the family make a preliminary decision and later confirm the decision when they have had time to fully appreciate the ramifications of the information they have been given.

Single-stage consent is the usual process for obtaining consent for the procedures detailed within this book. In this situation the procedure is undertaken immediately after the child and family have been given the relevant information and after ensuring that the required competence and lack of coercion are present.

## Withdrawal of consent during a procedure

A child with capacity is entitled to withdraw their consent at any time, including during the performance of a procedure. If this happens, it is good practice, if safe to do so, to stop the procedure and find out what their concerns are (good practice suggests that this also applies to children who have given assent). The child should also be given a frank explanation of the consequences of stopping the procedure. It is important at this stage of the events to empower the child by giving back control. This can be invaluable as they may be finding it difficult to cope with what seems to be an overwhelming situation. The hospital play specialist armed with a Starlight Distraction box and with expertise in distraction techniques, such as guided imagery, plays a useful role in such situations. Note, however, if it is deemed to be life threatening to stop the procedure, the individual carrying out the procedure may carry on until the imminent danger has passed.

The NMC Code is clear about maintaining clear professional boundaries. The NMC Code states that you must refuse any gifts, favours or hospitality that might be interpreted as an attempt to gain preferential treatment. Clearly this does not apply to the families who bring in a box of chocolates to the ward on their child's discharge. In addition, the NMC Code states that you must not ask for or accept loans from anyone in your care or anyone close to them. Likewise the NMC Code clearly indicates that you must establish and actively maintain clear sexual boundaries at all times with children and young people in your care, their families and carers. This ruling is particularly pertinent to the care of young people, where the age differences between for example the student nurse and the teenage patient may be minimal.

## WORK WITH OTHERS TO PROTECT AND PROMOTE THE HEALTH AND WELLBEING OF THOSE IN YOUR CARE, THEIR FAMILIES AND CARERS AND THE WIDER COMMUNITY

This aspect of the code details a number of criteria which all nurses must abide by but, in particular, several pertain specifically to the carrying out of procedures. The NMC Code asks each nurse to work with colleagues to monitor the quality of their work and to maintain the safety of those in their care. Crucially the NMC Code mandates each nurse to work effectively as part of a team and to share skills and experience for the benefit of colleagues. Additionally the NMC Code asks nurses to consult with and take advice from colleagues when appropriate and treat colleagues fairly and without discrimination. In addition, the NMC Code is quite clear in stating that you must make a referral to another practitioner when it is in the best interest of someone in your care. This is particularly pertinent to novice practitioners who may still be developing their skills. Similarly, the NMC Code in asking you to delegate effectively states that you must establish that anyone you delegate to is able to carry out your care instructions. This would be particularly pertinent with students and untrained members of staff when asking them to undertake specific procedures. Furthermore, it is your responsibility under the NMC Code to confirm the outcome of any delegated task and to ensure that the required standards are met; hence the NMC Code is actually very supportive in reminding you that everyone (students, heathcare assistants, etc.) you are responsible for is supervised and supported (for additional information on mentoring see Chapter 37 by Buckingham and Glasper).

The NMC Code is emphatic that nurses should manage risk and therefore child patient safety.

Reason[31] has indicated that 1 in 10 hospitalised patients suffer from an adverse event during the course of their treatment. Children are especially vulnerable, and children's nurses must address the context in which they work and deliver care. In acute hospitals, patient accidents (especially falls) treatment and procedures, medication, clinical assessment (including diagnosis) and documentation incidents constitute a greater proportion of reported incidents. The NMC Code therefore asks each nurse to act without delay if they believe that they or a colleague or anyone else has put someone at risk. Given the high incidence of procedures leading to an adverse incident, children's nurses need to be vigilant and follow strict procedures and guidelines. Therefore the NMC Code states that you must inform someone in authority if you experience problems that prevent you working with the code or other nationally agreed standards. All procedural guidelines therefore must be evidence based and updated regularly. Staff performing procedural skills must be trained to do so and their competency monitored through their personal development plans. Annual updating must be recorded. An adverse incident can be defined as any healthcare occurrence that has led to an unintended or unexplained harm to a child. A near miss is defined as an occurrence which may have led to a child being harmed, but either the mistake was aborted before harm occurred or no harm actually resulted by chance alone.

Harm may befall a child in a healthcare setting because of:

- medication delivery;
- mismatching patients and their treatment;
- equipment error;
- working beyond competency;
- failure or delay to make an accurate diagnosis;
- sub-optimal handover;
- sub-optimal continuity of care;
- failure to ensure follow-up of investigations;
- lack of awareness of local procedures and policies.

The NMC Code explicitly states that you must report your concerns in writing if problems in the environment of care are putting your children and their families at risk. Prior to undertaking any procedure a nurse must always ensure that health and safety, infection control, and local and, if applicable, national policies and procedures are adhered to.

### What should children's nurses do in their working environment to protect children?

- Governance forum where risk issues pertinent to children are debated regularly
- Local lead for risk management activities
- Identification of specialty triggers
- Regular review of your adverse event reporting
- Full investigation (Root Cause Analysis) of all 'red' National Patient Safety Agency graded incidents
- Evidence of lessons learnt/practice change, e.g. nasogastric tube checking, cannula dressings

- Link to audit programme

All children's nurses should adhere to the guiding philosophy of children's nursing: *first do the child no harm*.

### Family-centred care in partnership

In addition to preserving the child's dignity the fundamental aspects of caring for sick children and young people are embedded within the concept of family centered-care in partnership.

## PROVIDE A HIGH STANDARD OF PRACTICE AND CARE AT ALL TIMES

To do this the NMC Code insists that nurses use the best available evidence. In examining the evidence related to family-centred care, Smith *et al*.[32] reinforce family-centred care as one of the most significant concepts to have evolved from the realms of children's nursing over the last 50 years, where the child and family are perceived as an indivisible unit and in which the family occupies a central tenet in the sick child's life. Family-centred care has been defined as 'the professional support of the child and family through a process of involvement, participation and partnership underpinned by empowerment and negotiation'.[33,p.22]

This has important ramifications for children's nurses who may not actually perform the skills themselves but may undertake this through a third party in the guise of parents or guardians or the child patients themselves. Hence the role of the children's nurse will encompass both skills tuition and delivery. Importantly the NMC code asks each nurse to ensure that any advice they give is evidence based, especially if they are recommending to families particular healthcare products or services. Note that the NMC Code is emphatic in asking you to ensure that the use of complementary or alternative therapies is safe and in the best interests of those in your care.

When guardians/children are taught skills, this must follow a training schedule where competency is assessed and recorded within the patient record. Casey,[34] the architect of the concept of partnership in care with families in hospital, in a survey of 243 children found that 85 per cent of the children were receiving some or all of their nursing care from a member of the family, usually the mother.

Furthermore, the NMC Code states that you must keep secure, clear and accurate records. Therefore, all procedures must be accompanied by accurate documentation to demonstrate that the duty of care has been fulfilled, to enable continuity of care and to show the nurse's professionalism.

## BE OPEN AND HONEST, ACT WITH INTEGRITY AND UPHOLD THE REPUTATION OF YOUR PROFESSION

There are 14 criteria related to this NMC standard, but the most import one pertinent to the delivery of procedures to sick children is the NMC Code element which states that you must inform any employers you work for if your fitness to practice is called into question (a full copy of the NMC Code can be accessed via the companion website which accompanies this book).

### Safeguarding

Although safeguarding is covered in Chapter 3 by Kelleher with regard to safeguarding children during procedures, children's nurses need to understand the risk factors and recognise children in need/in need of support.

#### Safeguarding children: overarching principles

- Be familiar with your organisation's policies and procedures for safeguarding and promoting the welfare of children within the area you practice.

- Know the signs and symptoms and indicators of potential abuse or neglect in children and young people; be alert and observe for indicators of abuse. This may include parental conditions that might have an impact upon the child or young person.
- Ensure the referral of concerns to social services or police (after discussion with a senior colleague/designated nurse).
- Document concerns and issues relating to the procedure.
- Do not promise confidentiality.

*The NMC Code states that you must provide a high standard of practice and care at all times.* This is especially pertinent in the quest of preventing infection in children in your care, one of the cardinal roles of nursing since the days of Florence Nightingale.

## CONCLUSION

This introduction has identified many fundamental key concepts that must be considered before commencing any clinical procedure discussed in this book. In addition, the chapter has endeavoured to link actions commonly undertaken by children's nurses with certain aspects of the NMC Code. Crucially this chapter has outlined some of the elements that you must consider and implement prior to the undertaking of any procedures with children and their families

 Go to the website to find the PowerPoint presentation for this chapter and MCQs to test your knowledge. **www.hodderplus.com/childnursingskills**

# REFERENCES

1  Nursing and Midwifery Council (2008) The Code. Standards of conduct, performance and ethics for nurses and midwives. London: NMC.

2  Haddock J (1996) Towards further clarification of the concept 'dignity'. *Journal of Advanced Nursing* **24**: 924–931.

3  Walsh K, Kowanko L(2002) Nurses' and patients' perceptions of dignity. *International Journal of Nursing Practice* **8**: 143–145.

4  DH (2007) Privacy and dignity. A report by the Chief Nursing Officer into mixed sex accommodation in hospital Family Law Reform Act 1969 S8 Age of Majority Act (NI).

5  NT( 2007) Improving patients' privacy and dignity on mixed-sex wards. *Nursing Times* **103**: 23.

6  Department of Health (2004) The national service framework for children, young people and maternity services (www.dh.gov.uk).

7  Rylance G (1999) Privacy, dignity and confidentiality: interview study with structured questionnaire. *British Medical Journal* **318**: 301.

8  Reed P, Smith P, Fletcher M, Bradding A (2003) Promoting the dignity of the child in hospital. *Nursing Ethics* **10**(1): 67–76.

9  Department of Health (2001) *The report of the public inquiry into children's heart surgery at the Bristol Royal Infirmary 1984–1995. Learning from Bristol*. London: DH.

10  Department of Health (2000) *The NHS plan*. London: DH.

11  Department of Health (2001) *The Royal Liverpool children's inquiry: summary and recommendations*. London: The Stationery Office.

12  Glasper A, Gow D, Ireland L, Prudhoe G (2007) Fundamental aspects of undertaking nursing procedures with children ,young people and their families. In: Glasper A, Aylott M, Prudhoe G (eds) *Fundamental aspects of children's and young peoples nursing procedures*. Salisbury: Quay Books, Chapter 1, pp. 1–21.

13  Aveyard H (2001) The requirements for informed consent prior to nursing care procedures. *Journal of Advanced Nursing* **37**: 243–249.

14  Beauchamp TL, Childress JF (2001) *Principles of biomedical ethics*, 5th edition. Oxford: Oxford University Press.

15  Cable S, Lumsdaine I, Semple M (2003) Informed consent. *Nursing Standard* **18**(12): 47–53.

16  Dimond B (2003) *Legal aspects of consent*. Salisbury: Quay Books.

17  Gillick v West Norfolk and Wisbech Area Health Authority [1985] 3 All ER 402 (HL).

18  BMJ editorial (2006) Gillick or Fraser? A plea for consistency over competence in children. *British Medical Journal* **332**: 807.

19  Larcher V (2005) Consent, competence and confidentiality. *British Medical Journal* **330**: 353–356

20  BMA (2001) *Consent, rights and choices in health care for children and young people*. London: BMJ Books.

21  Department of Health (2001) *Reference guide to informed consent for examination or treatment*. London: DH.

22  Kennedy I, Grubb A (2000) *Medical law*, 3rd edition. London: Butterworth.

23  Department of Health (2002) *Model policy for consent to examination or treatment*. London: DH.

24  Montgomery J (2003) *Health care law*, 2nd edition. Oxford: Oxford University Press.

25  Aveyard H (2002) Implied consent prior to nursing care procedures. *Journal of Advanced Nursing* **39**: 201–207.

26  Dyer C (1992) *Doctor patients and the law*. London: Blackwell Science.

27  Gillon R (1986) *Philosophical medical ethics*. Chichester: Wiley.

28  Callery P, Neill S, Feasey S (2006) The evidence base for children's nursing practice. In: Glasper EA, Richardson J (eds) *A text book of children's and young peoples nursing*. Edinburgh: Churchill Livingstone, Chapter 14.

29  Harrison C, Kenny NP, Sidareous M, Rowell M (1997) Bioethics for clinicians. 9. Involving children in medical decisions. *Canadian Medical Association Journal* **156**: 825–828.

30  Kennedy I (2001) *Bristol Royal Infirmary Inquiry. Learning from Bristol: the Report of the Public Inquiry into Children's Heart Surgery at the Bristol Royal Infirmary 1984–1995*. London: Stationery Office.

31  Reason J (1990) *Human error*. Cambridge: Cambridge University Press.

32  Smith L, Coleman V, Bradshaw M (2006) Family-centred care. In: Glasper EA, Richardson J (eds) *A text book of children's and young people's nursing*. Edinburgh: Churchill Livingstone, Chapter 6.

33  Smith L, Colman V, Bradshaw M (Eds) (2002) Family-centred care: concept, theory and practice. Basingstoke: Palgrave.

34  Casey A (1995) Partnership nursing: influences on involvement of informal carers. *Journal of Advanced Nursing* **22**: 1058–1062.

## FURTHER READING

Alderson P, Goodey C (1998) Theories of consent. *British Medical Journal* **317**: 1313–1315.

Beckett C (2007) *Child protection: an introduction*, 2nd edition. London: Sage Publications.

Corby B (2005) *Child abuse: towards a knowledge base*, 3rd edition. Maidenhead: Open University Press.

Department of Health, Home Office, Department for Education and Skills, Department for Culture, Media and Sport, Office of the Deputy Prime Minister, Lord Chancellor (2003) *What to do if you're worried a child is being abused*. London: Department of Health.

Department of Health (2001) *Reference guide to consent for examination or treatment*. London: Department of Health.

Department of Health (2003) *Every child matters*. London: The Stationery Office

Department for Education and Skills (2004) *Every child matters: next steps* London: DES

Department for Education and Skills (2004) *Every child matters: change for children*. London: DES

Department of Health, Home Office, Department for Education and Employment (2006) *Working together to safeguard children*. London: The Stationery Office

Department of Health (1997) *The Caldicott Committee: report on the review of patient identifiable information*. London: DH

Department of Health (2001) *Essence of care*. London: DH.

Department of Health (2000) Final report of the Bristol Royal Infirmary inquiry. www.bristol-inquiry.org.uk/final_report/index.htm (accessed 1 May 2009).

Kolcaba K (1992) Holistic comfort: operationalising the construct as a nurse sensitive outcome. *Advanced Nursing Science* **15**(1): 1–10.

Kolcaba K, Wilson L (2002) Comfort care: a framework for perianesthesia nursing. *Journal of Perianesthesia Nursing* **17**(2): 102–114.

Mains ED (1994) Concept clarification in professional practice: dignity. *Journal of Advanced Nursing* **19**: 947–953.

Malinowski A, Leeseberg Stamler L (2002) Comfort: exploration of the concept in nursing. *Journal of Advanced Nursing* **39**: 599–609.

Robinson S (2002) Warmed blankets: an intervention to promote comfort for elderly hospitalized patients. *Geriatric Nursing* **23**: 321–323.

Royal College of Nursing (2003) *Restraining, holding still and containing children and young people. Guidance for nursing staff*. London: RCN.

Royal Australasian College of Physicians Paediatrics and Child Health Division (2005) *Guideline statement: management of procedure related pain in children and adolescents*. Sydney.

Siefert ML (2002) Concept analysis of comfort. *Nursing Forum* **37**(4): 16–23.

Tutton E, Seers K (2003) An exploration of the concept of comfort. *Journal of Clinical Nursing* **12**: 689–696.

Walker AC (2001) Safety and comfort work of nurses glimpsed through patient narratives. *International Journal of Nursing Practice* **8**: 42–48.

Wurzbach ME (1996) Comfort and nurses' moral choices. *Journal of Advanced Nursing* **24**: 260–264.

# Key concepts in undertaking clinical procedures with children and young people:

## B) Fundamental infection control techniques required for all clinical procedures: using aseptic non-touch technique (ANTT)

Naomi Watson

## LEARNING OUTCOMES

*Upon completion of this chapter, the reader should be able to accomplish the following:*
1 Define aseptic non-touch technique (ANTT)
2 Describe the process of ANTT
3 List the equipment required to perform ANTT
4 Explain possible outcomes if ANTT is not followed
5 Effectively carry out the procedure

## CHAPTER OVERVIEW

Each year as many as 5000 patients die of nosocomial infection within the NHS. Failed aseptic technique and poor hand washing are believed to contribute to the number of deaths.[1,2] Over the years studies within a number of healthcare trusts have demonstrated that aseptic technique within the NHS is poor and variable, thus demonstrating that failures in hand washing, poor hand-washing technique, poor choice of aseptic field, failed management of the aseptic technique and contamination when using a non-touch technique all contribute to poor patient outcomes and death.

Rowley[3] believed that a tendency in nursing to place ritual ahead of logic led to inconsistencies in practice, which contributed to poor techniques. Stephen Rowley thus devised ANTT in 1996 as a safe and efficient technique for intravenous therapy. Today a large number of paediatric health care environments are using ANTT in one form or another for peripheral and central intravenous therapy. ANTT is the accepted policy for intravenous care within the paediatric unit here at Southampton; it is estimated that another 150 NHS hospitals have adopted ANTT. It is likely that more will follow suit as ANTT is now recommended as an aseptic technique that promotes best practice by both the Department of Health and EPIC2.

### KEY WORDS

Nosocomial    Asepsis    Aseptic technique
Key parts    Sterile

## WHAT IS ANTT

ANTT is the foundation for *all* aseptic procedures.

### Why ANTT

- Provides a framework for aseptic technique
- Standardises practice
- Has a part in reducing hospital nosocomial infection

### Principles of the aseptic technique

To reduce the risk of introducing infection it is important that the practitioner

| Definitions | |
|---|---|
| **Nosocomial:** relates to something that was not present or incubating before the patient was admitted to hospital, therefore Nosocomial infection is an infection acquired within a hospital or healthcare environment. | **Key parts:** parts or sites which, if contaminated by micro-organisms, will increase the risk of infection, i.e. injectable bung, syringe tip, needle, intravenous connections, liquid infusion, etc. |
| **Asepsis:** free from infection or infectious material. | **Sterile:** free from micro-organisms that could cause infection. Owing to organisms in the air it is impossible to achieve in the true sense, therefore sterile precautions must also be applied. |
| **Aseptic technique:** procedure or practice used to prevent the introduction of pathogens, i.e. bacteria, viruses, micro-organisms, etc. | |

- recognises effective hand washing is prerequisite to all procedures;
- recognises and protects key parts;
- recognises potential sources of contamination and acts accordingly.

The main principle of ANTT is that, if a key part is not touched, it cannot therefore be infected. The aim is such that key parts, i.e. the injectable port, should contact only with other aseptic key parts or aseptic key sites. Rowley[3] gives credence to the idea that practitioners should touch non-key parts with confidence, as long as at a later stage this will not impact negatively on other key parts.

## When is ANTT suitable?

ANTT is the core technique and the principles of ANTT apply to *all* aseptic procedures.

## Level of precautions

The ANTT technique remains unchanged and aseptic precautions must always be 'strict'.

However, the level of aseptic precaution required is dependent on potential risk factors for the procedure. Every clinical procedure must be risk assessed for the likelihood of introducing infection. Practitioners need to determine whether they can perform the procedure without directly or indirectly touching key parts.

## ANTT

ANTT is suitable when the intended procedure can be performed without the practitioner touching key parts and when key parts can be protected from touching anything that is not a key part. For the majority of intravenous (IV) procedures this will be possible and therefore ANTT (non-sterile gloves) should be adhered to, e.g. IV therapy, simple wound care.

## ANTT sterile precautions+

This is applicable to procedures where the practitioner considers the protection of key parts difficult and/or where the procedure cannot be performed without touching key parts directly; in such instances extra infective precautions such as sterile gloves should be used. However, the ANTT technique continues to apply and key parts should still not be touched unless essential, e.g. switch changing, central venous catheter (CVC) repairs, bung changing on CVCs, needle insertion for IVADs (indwelling venous access devices), wounds that require cleaning.

## ANTT full barrier precautions

Invasive procedures such as PICC line insertion involve multiple key parts. This is a complex procedure requiring the maintenance of a large aseptic field. The core principles of the ANTT technique remain consistent but it is necessary to implement full barrier precautions in addition.

## PROCEDURE: For aseptic non-touch technique (ANTT)

| Procedural steps | Evidence-based rationale |
|---|---|
| **1** With clean hands wash tray with soap and water. Dry thoroughly with a paper towel | Prevention of infection |
| **2** Collect all the equipment you will need and place outside your tray. Check expiry dates | To ensure procedure runs smoothly |
| **3** Wash and dry hands or apply alcohol gel | Prevention of infection |
| **4** Put on non-sterile gloves | Prevention of infection |
| **5** Prepare drugs and equipment, taking care not to touch 'key parts' (end of line, blue connector, infusion spike, needle, interlink, infusion fluid, etc.). Use a non-touch technique. Do not place anything in your tray that does not need to be there | To prevent infection and avoid cross-contamination |
| **6** Remove gloves and wash or gel hands | To prevent spread of infection |
| **7** Take the tray of equipment to the patient. Prepare the patient to gain free access to the IV line | To ensure the procedure runs smoothly with minimal risk of introducing infection |
| **8** Wash or gel hands and apply new non-sterile gloves | Prevention of infection |
| **9** Clean the access port (bung 'key part') by scrubbing the tip for 5 seconds. Repeat another four times using different parts of the same wipe. Then clean the sides of the port working away from the tip. Allow to air dry for 30 seconds and then access the IV line taking care not to contaminate the bung or any key parts | Sani-cloth wipes comply with NICE guidance and EPIC2. They contain 2 per cent chlorhexidine and 70 per cent isopropyl alcohol and therefore are the most effective cleaning agent for the prevention of infection. Using different parts of the tissue removes any contaminates |
| **10** Administer medication using non-touch technique (see procedure for administration of fluids). Re-clean bung with sani-cloth wipe | Reduces risk of infection |
| **11** Dispose of all equipment safely and as per hospital policy | Safe disposal of clinical waste |
| **12** Remove gloves and wash and dry hands | Prevention of cross-infection |
| **13** Wash and dry tray and put away | Prevention of cross-infection |

1 **With clean hands wash tray with soap and water. Dry thoroughly with a paper towel.**

Presuming your hands have been recently washed and are socially clean you can begin by washing your tray with soap and water. Dry with clean paper towels. The tray can be cleaned with an alcohol-based cleaner but then must be allowed to air dry. Clean the tray starting on the inside of the tray, working out to the sides and finishing on the outside.

Plastic trays are ideal as the field needs to be robust, easy to clean and portable; furthermore high sides prevent equipment falling out as well as helping to contain any spillages.

Remember: clean hands/effective hand washing is a prerequisite to all procedures!

2 **Collect all the equipment you will need and place outside your tray. Check expiry dates.**

Gather all the required equipment and place around aseptic field close to hand. Check the expiry dates of any equipment that you will be using.

Remember: you should put nothing in your tray that isn't required for the procedure!

3 **Wash and dry hands or apply alcohol gel.**

An effective hand-washing technique involves three stages: preparation, washing and rinsing, and drying. Preparation involves wetting your hands under tepid running water before applying the soap. The soap must come into contact with all surfaces of the hands and when washing you need to pay particular attention to the tips of your fingers, the thumbs and the areas between the fingers. Hands should be rinsed thoroughly before drying with paper towels.

If your hands are visibly clean you can use the alcohol-based gel. The seven-stage hand-washing technique should be used both for hand washing and when applying the alcohol gel.

Remember: hand washing is the single most important thing that healthcare professionals can do to reduce the risk of cross-infection within the hospital environment.

4 **Put on non-sterile gloves.**

Sterile gloves are not required to maintain asepsis and therefore non-sterile gloves can be used safely for most peripheral and central procedures as long as the procedure can be performed without key parts being touched directly.[3]

Through regular hand washing, the practitioner's hands at times will be moist or damaged; this may result in the shredding of skin and the spread of bacteria[4,5] and therefore gloves are bacteriologically cleaner than skin.

Remember: gloves also protect us from exposure to drugs like antibiotics in accordance with COSHH regulations!

5 **Prepare drugs and equipment, taking care not to touch 'key parts' (end of line, blue connector, infusion spike, needle, interlink, infusion fluid, etc.). Use a non-touch technique. Do not place anything in your tray that does not need to be there.**

Assemble equipment using non-touch technique taking care not to touch key parts (i.e. infusion bag port and giving set spike).

Part of the non-touch technique is to protect key parts when they are not being used (such as syringe tip and needle). Being able to identify and then protect the key part is the most fundamental aspect of ANTT.[3]

In IV therapy key parts are those which come into direct or indirect contact with the liquid infusion and also parts of equipment that if contaminated could infect the patient (i.e. needle or injectable bung).

IV infusion key parts: antibiotic bottle top, needle, port on bag, IV line spike, syringe tip, patient bung – these must remain untouched at all times!

Remember: ANTT focuses on getting the basics right; it is suitable for all patients irrespective of age, diagnosis, drug given or the route of intravenous access; standards of care should be equally high for peripheral and central intravenous access!

6 **Remove gloves and wash or gel hands.**

When you've prepared the drug you need to remove your gloves and then wash or gel your hands. The warm damp environment under gloves means that bacteria reproduce at an alarming rate[5].

Remember: gloves create a greenhouse effect for organisms on the hands; it is therefore imperative to clean hands immediately after gloves are removed.

7 **Take the tray of equipment to the patient. Prepare the patient to gain free access to the IV line.**

Take the tray of equipment straight to the patient to minimise any environmental contact. Prepare the patient to get clean access to the IV device.

Remember: when preparing the patient identify the key parts for the procedure!

8 **Wash or gel hands and apply new non-sterile gloves.**

If your hands have become contaminated/dirty while preparing the patient you will need to wash them again. If they are still socially clean you can use the alcohol gel instead. Put on new non-sterile gloves; these act as a barrier to prevent the de-scaling of skin on to key parts.

Maintaining the asepsis of key parts in intravenous therapy is achieved by preventing them from coming into contact with harmful organisms. This is a difficult as our hands are covered in bacteria (it's estimated that as many as 3 million bacteria are present per square centimetre of normal skin).[5] Non-sterile gloves are bacteriologically cleaner than skin.

Remember: Gloves provide us with protection and reduce or prevent the incidence of antibiotic-resistant organisms surviving on the practitioners skin![9] Clean the access port (bung 'key part') for 30 seconds using several different parts of the sani-cloth wipe. Allow to air dry for 30 seconds and then access the IV line taking care not to contaminate the bung or any key parts.

9 **Using gentle friction, clean the injectable port on the IV access device with your sani-cloth wipe for 30 seconds.** It's essential to clean vigorously: the injectable port may look clean but microbiologically it will be very dirty.

Clean the access port (bung 'key part') by scrubbing the tip for 5 seconds. Repeat another four times using different parts of the same wipe (you will need to use different parts of the sani-cloth wipe just to prevent moving dirt around). Then clean the sides of the port working away from the tip. It is very important to allow the key part to dry before using (approximately 30 seconds).

Remember: if it's still wet then it's not aseptic and you will be placing the patient at risk!

10 **Administer medication using non-touch technique (see procedure for administration of fluids). Re-clean bung with sani-cloth wipe.**

Once this is dry access the IV line taking care not to contaminate the bung or any key parts, and administer the drugs using a non-touch technique.

A non-touch method when it comes to the practitioner's hands is not letting key parts come into contact with anything apart from, of course, the equipment it is supposed to connect to, which is another key part, i.e. interlink connected to a syringe tip.

Remember: if you accidentally contaminate a key part, re-clean or change it!

11 **Dispose of all equipment safely and as per hospital policy.**

Dispose of all your equipment both safely and appropriately; consider what should go in the sharps bin and the yellow clinical waste bags for incineration. Do you have any waste that can go in the black domestic waste bags?

Remember: if you have used a needle never re-sheath it!

12 **Remove gloves and wash and dry hands.**

After removing your gloves wash your hands straight away; the most frequent breakdown in universal precautions has been identified as a lack of hand washing after glove removal.

Remember: every year between 5000 and 10 000 patients die from hospital-acquired infections; what you do does make a difference!

13 **Wash and dry tray and put away.**

Finally wash your tray, dry it and put it away. If you have given chemotherapy or taken blood, you may wish to wash your tray before removing your gloves.

Remember: the three principles of ANTT
1 Effective hand cleaning
2 Appropriate aseptic field
3 Key part protection by a non-touch technique.[3]

---

Go to the website to find the PowerPoint presentation for this chapter and MCQs to test your knowledge. **www.hodderplus.com/childnursingskills**

## ACKNOWLEDGEMENT

The author would like to thank Stephen Rowley for his support and advice whilst writing this chapter.

## REFERENCES

1 Jones PM (1987) Indwelling central venous catheter related infections and two different procedures of catheter care. *Cancer Nursing* **10**(3): 123–130.

2 Pritchard P, David J (2006) *The Royal Marsden Hospital manual of clinical nursing procedures*, 6th edition. Oxford: Blackwell Science.

3 Rowley S, Laird H (2006) Aseptic non-touch technique: In: Trigg E, Mohammed TA (eds) *Practices in children's nursing: guidelines for hospital and community*, 2nd edition. Edinburgh: Churchill Livingstone.

4 Ojajarvi J (1990) Effectiveness of hand washing and disinfection methods in removing transient bacteria after patient nursing. *Journal of Hygiene* **85**: 193–203.

5 Gould D (1991) Skin bacteria. What is normal? *Nursing Standard* **18**(5): 25–28.

## FURTHER READING

Crow S (1994) Asepsis: a prophylactic technique. *Perioperative Nurse* **3**(2): 93–100.

EPIC (2007) *National evidence based guidelines for preventing hospital-acquired infections in England*. London: EPIC.

Kaler W, Chinn R (2007) Successful disinfection of needleless access ports: A matter of time and friction. *Journal of the Association for Vascular Access* **12**(3): 140–142.

Maki DG, Goldman DA, Rhame FS (1973) Infection control in IV THERAPY. *Annals of Internal Medicine* **79**: 867–887.

Pratt RJ, Pellowe, CM, Wilson JA, *et al.* (2007) EPIC2: National evidence-based guidelines for preventing healthcare-associated infections in NHS Hospitals in England. *Journal of Hospital Infection*. S1–S64.

## CHAPTER 2

# Clinical holding of children and young people

## Maria Brenner and Colman Noctor

*To deprive a child of mobility is to take away his best avenue of coping with the inevitable frustration of hospitalization.[1]*

### LEARNING OUTCOMES

*Upon completion of this chapter, the reader should be able to accomplish the following:*
1 Understand the complexity of clinical holding and its potential impact on the child
2 Appreciate the communication and emotional needs of children undergoing invasive procedures
3 Understand the role of the children's nurse in the process

## CHAPTER OVERVIEW

In an ideal world every child in hospital would lie quietly and not attempt to obstruct any nursing or medical procedures that may need to be performed. Unfortunately there is no such utopia.[2] As children's nurses there are times when it is necessary to hold or restrain a child for a nursing/medical procedure, and it is generally considered acceptable to do so.[3] However, this can be a very stressful event for everyone involved,[4–6] and it is suggested that some children may find the experience of being restrained more distressing than the pain involved in treatment or procedures,[6] although there is little research on this area of nursing practice. Discussing how we hold, or even acknowledging that we do hold, may be perceived as a negative endeavour that focuses on, and highlights, poor care. However, the real neglect would be to disregard the impact of restraint or holding on all those involved.

Children's nurses find many types of procedures stressful and sometimes traumatic, and often have questions around when and how such procedures should be initiated. The chapter will begin by examining the complex issues around clinical holding. This chapter will aim to outline the importance of communication and psychological nourishment of children undergoing invasive procedures. This will be followed by a clear plan for decision-making.

## DEFINING HOLDING

In children's nursing the terms restraint, clinical holding, immobilisation and holding are often used interchangeably, and it is imperative to outline the nuances between these concepts. It is suggested that restraint includes the use of force.[7,8] This is further elucidated by Jeffery,[9] who suggests an operational definition of restraint as '… used to administer medication or carry out a procedure to which the child objects, and is carried out in what is considered to be the child's best interest'. This implies that agreement is not always sought and

### KEY WORDS

Clinical holding    Consent    Emotional development    Correct positioning    Empathising

this concurs with Lambrenos and McArthur,[10] who suggested the use of the term 'clinical holding', which refers to 'positioning a child so that a medical procedure can be carried out in a safe and controlled manner', but not always with the consent of the child/parent. In contrast, the terms immobilisation and holding imply a greater partnership between the healthcare team and the child/parents, with agreement and with all parties appreciating the need for absolute stillness for the success of particular procedures.

## COMPLEXITIES OF HOLDING

It is well documented that specific procedural safety requirements and specialist training needs to be adhered to when one is required to physically hold a child for treatment purposes. However, there are also important interpersonal dimensions to consider during clinical holding procedures.

The child's ability to regulate emotion is now identified as a distinctive feature of the child from toddlerhood onwards, though it must be stressed here that the majority of studies on emotional research focus on the younger child. Similarly, as an emerging focus of research in children's nursing, there is a noticeable gap in research to address the complexities of clinical holding in the older child and adolescent.

Emotional regulation in children is a relatively new area of interest in child development and refers to the child's ability to inhibit, enhance and balance their emotions.[11] It is also defined as a mechanism inherent in maintaining the child's physical and psychological integrity.[12,13] Two studies were found which explored emotional regulation in infants,[14,15] and both found that infants significantly increased their reactivity to restraint during the second 6 months of their first year. The results support the work of Sroufe,[16] who found that infants at 2–3 months are beginning to differentiate between emotions, but by 6 months they can experience disappointment. The studies also demonstrate the infant's ability at 6–10 months to seek a distraction, perhaps to try to regulate their emotions. As a new area of research interest there is a need to cautiously interpret the results; nonetheless, it supports an increasing emphasis on acknowledging the emotional needs of the child in hospital.

Furthermore, distress in childhood can have a negative impact on the emotional development of the child, and may lead to physical and psychological problems in later life.[17] This highlights the responsibility of the children's nurse to ensure the best possible care is provided to address emotional needs and to minimise distress. In child psychiatry the emphasis is on modifying the use of physical restraint, although much of the current discussion in this area focuses on the merits of chemical restraint and rapid tranquillisation.[18–20] Aversive interventions such as restraint have been observed in intellectual disability nursing to control or change behaviour.[21] However, the use of restraints for these purposes are increasingly linked to the inappropriate trigger of traumatic responses, which in turn may affect the development of trusting relationships and the child's developmental progression.[22]

In acute clinical practice children's nurses cite preventing treatment interference as their main reason to restrain a child.[4,5] Selekman and Snyder[4] examined the use of restraint in four different paediatric settings in the United States and found that children's nurses take developmental needs and the specific individual's situation into account prior to deciding to use restraints. These findings are supported by Collier and Robinson[5] in a UK study of 394 children's nurses. This study highlighted that the factors, which influenced the decision to hold a child, included the necessity of the procedure, the child's safety, the type of procedure, the child's level of agitation, the child's age, the parent's opinion, the child's consent and staff safety. The age profile of children requiring restraint was also examined by Selekman and Snyder,[4] and they found that the need for restraints decreased with the child's age, with the greatest need for restraint in the 1- to 6-year-old age group. This finding is supported by Graham and Hardy,[8] who found that 93 per cent of radiographers undertook restraining children as part of their current practice. The majority of radiographers restrain all children under 1 year, fewer under 2–3 years and progressively fewer as age increases. There is a dearth of studies that explore the impact of child restraint; however, it is acknowledged to be a stressful event, and thereby requires nurses to ensure they are providing specific safeguards for children to protect them from physical or mental injury. It is a good practice that your area of children's nursing should have, or be in the process of, developing guidelines for holding children still for the delivery of nursing care. There should also be education available on restraint and seclusion, and on optimum positions for care in each area of care in the hospital. However, it is acknowledged that there is very little research available to guide nurses on best positioning for procedures. In the absence of local guidelines or specific education you should assess your scope of practice to identify if you have the nursing skills and knowledge to carefully hold a child still. You should also be aware of national policy pertaining to holding. As outlined by the RCN[7] this involves understanding that holding the child still for a procedure is a last resort, that the nurse should make every effort to prevent the need for holding still, and if necessary then it should involve consent for holding with parental presence (if parents agree and wish to be involved). Sedation is used as a last resort, and guidance for this is provided in the Scottish Intercollegiate Guideline Network,[30] though it is not discussed in this chapter as the focus is on encouraging a therapeutic relationship which may prevent medical intervention. The nurse has a duty of care to protect the child in hospital from any undue distress, and this can only happen when the children's nurse appreciates and is equipped with relevant communication skills, and these are now discussed.

---

**KEY POINTS**

Important interpersonal dimensions to consider:

- acknowledgement of emotional needs of the child in hospital
- development of trusting relationships

---

## COMMUNICATION

The literature suggests that a variety of alternatives such as distraction, play therapies, parents, improved pain relief and behavioural interventions can lead to less restraint in practice.[3,23,24] Many recommendations have been made pertaining to the application, monitoring and care of a child in restraints.[6,7,9,25] Folkes[6] developed a comprehensive

decision-making algorithm, which highlights the importance of consent and explanations or alternatives to restraint. This tool also offers a pathway in an emergency situation, whereby restraint may be required. The final part of the tool highlights the importance and necessity of documentation. Documentation is also a key focus of Jeffrey,[9] who offers a broader framework for nurses who are considering the use of restraint. According to Jeffrey,[9] the key to decision-making and restraint is reliant on two areas – thorough assessment of the child's current needs, and appraisal of the documentation regarding any previous immobilisation or restraint of this child. This should include methods required, consent sought, duration, child's experience and the outcome of the event. Valler-Jones and Shinnick[25] also highlighted the need for evidence-based practice, and suggested that student nurses should be encouraged to discuss restraint in order to appreciate the complexities of dealing with a variety of situations.

In working with children it is a fundamental assumption that we all strive to relate in a caring, open and sensitive way. This task is often made easier when the child is compliant, likeable and amenable. However, human nature and life being what it is, this is not always the case. There are incidences where children's nurses will come upon considerably more resistance than they would ideally anticipate. This section of the chapter will explore the interpersonal dynamics that can often take place during these episodes of resistance and explain ways in which children's nurses can be effective in managing these difficult situations.

### Preparation

Before we enter into a situation where a child is distressed, it is imperative that we acknowledge that our actions and reactions can strongly influence subsequent behaviour in the person we are interacting with.[26] This is never more pronounced then in times of crisis and upset. It is therefore paramount that we attend to updating our skills, knowledge and professional judgement that prove critical to help children cope with feelings of fear, frustration and anger. In order to do this effectively one must develop a framework in which to respond adaptively to the crisis situation.

The essential factors to consider include:

- the importance of assessing and positively manipulating the environment where the child is upset;
- the value of self-awareness and cognisance of our own feelings when relating to the distressed child;
- the centrality of the therapeutic relationship with the child and how this can be used to understand the child's needs and respond appropriately;
- practical interpersonal skills that will optimise the response of the nurse to the child's distress.[6]

It is crucial before embarking on any relational issue to attempt first to understand the developmental capacity of the child in question.[27] There may be cases where these cognitive capacities can vary significantly between two children and often the chronological age of the child can be misleading. Communication must be first and foremost understandable to both parties; therefore, the manner in which children's nurses relate to their patients will vary from child to child and will certainly differ from child to adolescent. It is important that the information given to the child is appropriate to their developmental capacity and is not too complicated or simplistic.

Some of the periods of distress that children experience in hospital can be triggered by the need to carry out a simple procedure. However, although this is the perception of the nurse, the child may not share your relaxed confidence. As children's nurses we may feel that taking a child's blood pressure, for example, is a simple procedure and we may have full confidence in our ability to administer it. However, this is not the same for the child who is new to this experience and may therefore have a significant fear of the unknown. Children's nurses need to be cognisant of this possibility and adequately prepare all child patients for any interventions. This also involves awareness that the assigned nurse may not be the most appropriate person to communicate with the child, and to this end it is imperative that the nurse is mindful of the child's relationships within the hospital to identify who they are most relaxed/trusting with.

Some nurses feel that it is improper to make a 'big deal' out of a simple procedure and may assume that minimising the intervention is the most effective way of proceeding. However, much of human anxiety is a fear of the unknown and therefore being forewarned can help alleviate such worries. Also, if someone is anxious they can often become more acutely anxious if they feel that their concerns are not being acknowledged; therefore, it is often best to explore the degree or cause of the child's anxiety while all the time offering containing reassurance.

It is a common misunderstanding of adults to associate the size of the person with the size of the problem. This is a gross misjudgement. With comments like 'she's only a child, don't worry' we reinforce this delusion. The fact is that young people and children can experience really intense emotions, many of which are felt with the same veracity as adults, thus endorsing their claim to be listened to and their worries acknowledged.

**KEY POINTS**

- Assess environment
- Understand the value of self-awareness
- Explore degree or cause of child's anxiety

## Identifying possible resistance

Although the majority of research on emotional development of children currently focuses on the younger child, there are often symptoms of anxiety or worry that are expressed by children or adolescents and it is often at this point that the response is required. Children of all ages may have difficulty expressing themselves when emotionally distressed. The limited emotional vocabulary of the youngest child and the developing self-awareness skills of the older child mean that a heightened sense of awareness must exist in those around them, some time before an episode reaches crisis. This may be a series of uncharacteristic behaviours such as misbehaviour, or anger, or withdrawals.

Often the busy nature of the hospital ward environment means that the time and space to consider these expressions of anxiety is not often there or at least the time to respond to them is inconvenient. However, it would seem that some time allocated to explore this unusual indicative behaviour may be a worthwhile investment in the longer term. These behaviours may be expressions of something underlying that often a response from a reassuring individual if skilfully carried out can be enough to avert further upset.

### De-escalation

The dynamics of a crisis situation can change rapidly and drastically. When involved in such incidences the nurse must try to continually make judgements and attempt to de-escalate the situation. It is also important to evaluate the impact of our behaviour on the child and the situation.

De-escalation involves attempts to avert a crisis or potentially difficult situation. In the *Strategies for crisis intervention procedures, Cornick et al.*[28], page 27 suggest six calming techniques.

### The six steps to calming

- *Identify*: Correctly connect with the child's feeling state. The child may appear angry but it may be primarily fear that has converted to anger. Ask questions if you are unsure of how the child is feeling but avoid labelling at all if you are uncertain.
- *Reflect*: Tell the child the name of the emotion and help them to differentiate how he/she is feeling. Labelling feelings helps to reduce frustration and hence the child is less likely to act out the emotion just to let the world know how badly they are feeling.
- *Empathise*: This keeps the child from feeling alone; however, your empathy must be on target otherwise tension may mount as opposed to diminishing.
- *Reassure*: Let the child know that you are there to help, which can help contain overwhelming feelings.
- *Redirect*: Discuss possible activities for after the procedure, which can instil hope in the child of an end to their fear and a confidence that things will be better soon.
- *Praise*: Reward the child for constructive actions and encourage them to repeat this good display of self-control the next time they are feeling upset.

### The 'don't' rules of de-escalation

- Don't plant suggestions of misbehaviour, e.g. 'Don't even think about throwing that'.
- Don't threaten consequences of misbehaviour,

e.g. 'If you don't behave I'll remove the TV.'.
- Don't present commands as a question, e.g. 'Are you going to sit quietly for me?'.
- Don't have more than one staff member give directions to an individual simultaneously.
- Don't rehash a past incident in front of the individual: 'I don't want to see another episode like at lunch yesterday'.[28]

## MANAGEMENT OF THE CLINICAL HOLDING SITUATION

Despite reassurance and preparing a child for an intervention, the anxiety may continue to escalate into a crisis.

### Assessing the situation

There are a variety of skills to use when intervening with an upset or distressed child. These skills are neither intuitive nor natural and do not necessarily evolve from experience.[26 p.10] There are four key questions that one must ask oneself at the outset of a potential crisis situation.

1  *What am I feeling now?*
   We communicate our feelings often even through silence. Children are astute observers of non-verbal behaviour and have often learned to anticipate angry outbursts. Being aware of our own feelings is the first step to controlling our behaviour and what we intentionally or otherwise communicate to the child.

2  *What does this child feel, need or want?*
   In a crisis situation it is important to try and establish what the child's motivation for their behaviour is? This can lead to greater empathy towards the child because it may reveal the child's behaviour represents an attempt – however dysfunctional – to meet a need.

3  *How is this environment affecting this child?*
   Many crisis situations can be diverted by modifying the conditions of the environment. It is important to be mindful of these triggers and ameliorate them where possible.

4  *How can I best respond?*
   It is always helpful to try and be conscious of the need to respond to the child's distress in a timely, helpful and therapeutic manner. In order to safely contain the crisis we must firstly contain ourselves.

## Psychological considerations for emotive situations

- Know yourself
- Keep yourself calm
- Be competent and self-assured
- Listen
- Be sensitive to the child's self-esteem
- Identify and acknowledge the child's feelings
- Do not create a power struggle
- Be supportive[28, page 17]

## Importance of the nurse–patient relationship

Childhood is very different from adulthood. Most children have relatively few life experiences to draw from and are still in the process of developing skills needed for communicating. Therefore all communication must be cognisant of the developmental framework.[29] Because of the developmental gap that exists, communication between the adult and the child is compromised from the outset. If one considers the added factors of limited understanding of subtle nuances, facial expression, inflection and word meanings coupled with the stressors of illness, and unfamiliar environment, then situational crises are a high probability.

Hospitalisation is always stressful.[29] The child not only has to contend with the physical challenges of illness but also the possible separation from their family as well as a strange, frightening and probably hurtful environment. A severe illness can also cause a child's behaviour to be reminiscent of an earlier stage of development and a certain amount of this regression is normal. Common behaviours indicative of regression include uncustomary whining, teasing other children, demanding attention or having toileting accidents. In most cases this abnormal behaviour can be explained as an expression of powerlessness and the child's maladaptive attempt to cope with the sense of potential threat.[29]

Given all of these developmental and environmental factors the nurse must always be mindful of the experience of the distressed child. Many of the interventions required in a time of crisis are best introduced before the crisis has occurred.[26] With the contributory factors outlined

in this chapter the nurse must ensure that the impact of such experiences is minimised wherever possible for the child and their family. Therefore the nurse–child patient relationship should include an awareness of the child's developmental level and preventative strategies being implemented in accordance with it. This may be something as obvious as providing appropriate stimulation for the child albeit through talking, listening or playing.

---

**Pre-holding – STOP**
What am I feeling now?
Why does this child need to be held still?
Is this procedure urgent/necessary?
Are there any alternatives to clinical holding that could be considered distraction/imagery/sedation?
Are you educated/experienced to competently hold this child?
Are the parent(s) present?
Have you considered what their input can be?
Have you explained the rationale and proposed positioning to the child and parent(s)?

↓

**During holding – CONSIDER**
Is the child held for the shortest time necessary?
Are the child's and parent's physical and emotional needs being met?

↓

**Post holding – REFLECT**
Was there an appropriate rationale for clinical holding?
Was the method/length of holding suitable in this situation?
Are there any potential effects for the child/parents?
Were they addressed and how can this be addressed in future?
Document.

---

**Figure 2.1** Considerations pre-, during and post holding.

A large proportion of anxiety can be relayed by discussing one's fears and getting support and explanation in return. It is important that nurses are creative in how they approach such interactions with children of different ages. This begins on admission by carefully listening to the child (and parents), and by identifying and documenting the child/young persons interests to enable more individual communication with them through the course of their hospital stay. For the younger child discussing fears may need to take place over a game of scrabble or a short discussion between puppets or dolls, which will creatively provide the dialogue of reassurance that the anxious child may need. For the older child it may be through discussion of their hobbies or music tastes. It is perhaps helpful to consider these approaches for all of our interactions with young children and not reduce this creative form of communicating to just those exhibiting overt behaviours indicative of anxiety (Figure 2.1).

Go to the website to find the PowerPoint presentation for this chapter and MCQs to test your knowledge. **www.hodderplus.com/childnursingskills**

## REFERENCES

1 Dowd E, Novak J, Ray E (1977) Releasing the hospitalized child from restraints. *The American Journal of Maternal Child Nursing* 370–373.

2 Thomas J (2005) Brute force or gentle persuasion. Editorial. *Paediatric Anaesthesia* **15**: 355–357.

3 Tomlinson D (2004) Physical restraint during procedures: issues and implications for practice. *Journal of Pediatric Oncology Nursing* **21**(5): 258–263.

4 Selekman J, Snyder B (1995) Nursing perceptions of using physical restraints on children. *Pediatric Nursing* **21**: 460–464.

5 Collier J, Pattison H (1997) Attitudes to children's pain: exploring the myth. *Paediatric Nursing* **9**(10): 15–18.

6 Folkes K (2005) Is restraint a form of abuse? *Paediatric Nursing* **17**(6): 41–44.

7 Royal College of Nursing (2003) *Restraining, holding still and containing children; guidance for good practice*. RCN: London.

8 Graham P, Hardy M (2004) The immobilisation and restraint of paediatric patients during plain film radiographic examinations. *Radiography* **10**: 23–31.

9 Jeffrey K (2002) Therapeutic restraint of children. *Paediatric Nursing* **14**(9): 20–22.

10 Lambrenos K, McArthur E (2001) Introducing a clinical holding policy. *Paediatric Nursing* **15**(4): 30–33.

11 Eisenberg N, Champion, C, Ma, Y (2004). Emotion-related regulation: an emerging construct. The maturing of the human developmental sciences: appraising past, present, and prospective agendas. *Merrill-Palmer Quarterly* (special issue) **50**(3): 236–259 (www.csa.com).

12 Damaiso A, Grabowski T, Bechara A, *et al.* (2000) Subcortical and cortical brain activity during the feeling of self generated emotions. *Nature*

*Neuroscience* **3**: 1949–1056.

14 Stifter C, Spinrad T (2002) The effect of excessive crying on the development of emotion regulation. *Infancy* **2**: 133–152.

15 Moscardino U, Azia G (2005) Infants' responses to arm restraint at 2 and 6 months: a longitudinal study. *Infant Behaviour and Development* **29**: 59–69.

16 Sroufe I (1996) *Emotional development: the organization of emotional life in the early years*. Cambridge: Cambridge University Press.

17 Heim C, Nemeroff C (2001) The role of childhood trauma in the neurobiology of mood and anxiety disorders: preclinical and clinical studies. *Biological Psychiatry* **49**: 1023–1039.

18 National Institute of Clinical Excellence (2005) *Clinical practice guidelines for violence: the short-term management of disturbed/violent behaviour in psychiatric in-patient settings and emergency departments*. London: NICE.

19 Whitington R, Lancaser G, Meehan C, et al. (2006) Physical restraint of patients in acute mental care settings: patient, staff, and environmental factors associated with the use of a horizontal restraint position. *J Forensic Psychiatric Psychology* **17**(2): 253–265.

20 Winship G (2006) Further thoughts on the process of restraint. *Journal of Psychiatric and Mental health nursing* **13**: 55–60.

21 Carr E, Dunlap G, Horner R, *et al* (2002) Positive behaviour support: evolution of an applied science. *Journal of Positive Behaviour Intervention* **4**(4): 16–20

22 Amos P (2004) New considerations in the prevention of aversives, restraint, and seclusion: incorporating the role of relationships into an ecological perspective. *Research and Practice for Persons with Severe Disabilities* **29**(4): 263–272.

23 Willock J (2004) Peripheral venepuncture in infants

and children. *Nursing Standard* 18(27): 43–50.

24 Piira T, Sugiura T, Champion GD, *et al.* (2005) The role of parental presence in the context of children's medical procedures: a systematic review. *Child: Care, Health and Development* 31(2): 233–243.

25 Valler-Jones T, Shinnick A (2005) Holding children for invasive procedures: preparing student nurses. *Paediatric Nursing* 17(5): 20–22.

26 Family Development Center (2001) *Therapeutic crisis intervention*, 5th edition. New York: Family Development Center, Cornell University.

27 Geary DC (2005) *The origin of mind, evolution of brain, cognition and general intelligence*. Washington, DC: American Psychological Association.

28 Cornick M, Holt L, Bromley J (1996) *Strategies for crisis intervention and prevention SCIPr-UK*. New York: The Loddon School.

29 Arnold E, Boggs K (2003) *Interpersonal relationships, professional communication skills for nurses*, 4th edition. Philadelphia: W.B. Saunders.

30 Scottish Intercollegiate Guideline Network (2002) *Safe Sedation of children undergoing diagnostic and therapeutic procedures*. Edinburgh: SIGN.

## FURTHER READING

Prince GS (1963). *Prevention of mental disorders in children*. New York: Basic Books.

Schneider W, Schumann-Hengsteler R, Sodian B (eds) *Young children's cognitive development: interrelationships among executive functioning, working memory, verbal ability, and theory of mind*. New York: Routeledge.

## CHAPTER 3

# Safeguarding children and young people

Deirdre Kelleher

## LEARNING OUTCOMES

*Upon completion of this chapter, the reader should be able to accomplish the following:*

1 Define the four categories of abuse that can affect the child or young person
2 Discuss the key legislative provisions that govern child protection
3 Recognise the risk factors that may give rise to a concern or a suspicion about child maltreatment
4 Analyse the role and responsibilities of the nurse in safeguarding children

## CHAPTER OVERVIEW

This chapter examines the role of the children's nurse in protecting children from maltreatment. The chapter aims to prepare student nurses who care for children to recognise children who may be at risk of abuse or who are being maltreated. It also provides guidance on how to gain access to support and referral to the appropriate authorities and follow through. Emphasis is placed on not only guidance, but also on the provision of training and support in child protection practice.

The chapter opens with an overview of key legislation in this area that has emerged following key cases such as the Victoria Climbié Inquiry, which have far reaching implications for nursing practice and professional responsibility. The theories relating to this area will be briefly discussed, including the correlation between child poverty and child abuse.

The role of children's rights and how it impacts on the area of child maltreatment will be considered. The role of the children's nurse in the promotion of positive parenting skills to prevent the maltreatment of the child is highlighted. The subject of child protection is an emotive and difficult subject that has far-reaching consequences for society as a whole as well as the individual child and family. Suggestions for accessing further information, help and support are provided.

## KEY WORDS

Child abuse    Maltreatment    Child protection
Safeguarding    Children's nursing

## INTRODUCTION

*Child Protection cases do not always come labelled as such…Good communication, checking with partner agencies at the point of referral, and talking to the child as appropriate, must be the main way to decide how best to safeguard and promote a child's welfare.*[1]

The terms 'child protection' or 'safeguarding children' rather than 'child abuse' are now used to emphasise the proactive approach undertaken in the protection of children from maltreatment.[2] Maltreatment is an umbrella term used to encompass all forms of intentional harm to children by caregivers.[3] Child protection is a part of safeguarding and promoting welfare and refers to any activity that is undertaken to protect specific children who are suffering or are at risk of suffering significant harm. The document *Working together to safeguard children*[2] emphasises the key role that healthcare professionals and organisations have to play in the safeguarding and promoting the welfare of children.

The general principles that should apply are:

1 aiming to ensure that all affected children receive appropriate and timely therapeutic interventions;

2 professionals working directly with children should ensure that safeguarding and promoting their welfare form an integral part of all stages of care they offer;

3 professionals who come into contact with children, parents and carers in the course of their work also need to be aware of their safeguarding responsibilities;

4 ensuring that all heath professionals can recognise factors and contribute to reviews, enquiries and child protection plans, as well as planning support for children and providing ongoing promotional and preventative support through proactive work.[2,p.11]

Child protection emphasises prevention through early identification of children thought to be 'at risk' of maltreatment. Nurses have a key role in the protection and care of children and are often are well situated to identify children and young people who may be at risk and act to safeguard their welfare.[4-6]

In more recent times major child abuse inquiries reported situations where children have continued to be seriously harmed after presentation to hospital services and/or admission to hospitals. Particularly harrowing cases were that of Victoria Climbié in 2000 and more recently the Baby P case in 2008. When Baby P died aged 17 months he had suffered 50 injuries at the hand of his abusers, including a broken back, fractured ribs and missing fingernails. He had been on the child protection register for 9 months before he died and was visited 60 times by care workers. He died at the hands of his stepfather, mother, and a lodger (see http://www.guardian.co.uk/society/2008/nov/11/baby-p-death).

At the time of writing this chapter a report on this case is being compiled by Ofsted, the office for standards in education, children services and skills, whose remit is to inspect and regulate care for children and young people and inspect education and learning for children of all ages. The work of Ofsted can be read online at http://www.ofsted.gov.uk. The Victoria Climbié Inquiry Report can be read online (http://www.victoria-climbie-inquiry.org.uk/finreport/finreport.htm)

The Climbié report made 43 recommendations to be implemented by the UK NHS over 2 years and set in motion Governmental action in the UK on safeguarding children. While many lessons have emerged from these inquiry reports and some have already been implemented into hospital practices, reviews and inquiries into cases such as these, as well as others where children have not been supported by child services, often identify the same issues:

- poor communication and information sharing between professionals and agencies;[5]
- administrative and management failings;[6]
- difficulties in locating and collating case notes;[6]
- lack of audit training;[6]
- revalidation of staff;[6]
- lack of funding;[6]
- inadequate training and support for staff;[5]
- failure to listen to children.[5]

Studies has shown that one important aspect is the psychological defence mechanism that professionals develop that make them unable or unwilling to identify child abuse.[6,8-10]

There may be a perception that reporting suspicions of child abuse may do more harm than good and working with the family may be preferable. A reluctance by staff in asking questions may be due to fear of litigation and a tendency towards optimism when assessing the circumstances surrounding a harm or injury.[6,8-10]

## KEY DEFINITIONS AND CONCEPTS

This section examines the views of childhood, children's rights and child maltreatment. A critical understanding of these concepts can enhance understanding of contextual issues of how children are treated and current approaches to the welfare of children.

### Children

In this chapter as in the Children's Acts of 1989 and 2004 *a child* is anyone who has not yet reached their eighteenth birthday. 'Children' therefore mean children and young people. Even if a child is living independently, in further education or in the armed forces, is in hospital, in prison or in a Young Offenders' Institution, this does not change their legal status or entitlements to services or protection under the Children's Act 1989.[2,p.34]

## Historical perspectives on childhood abuse

There are two commonly held beliefs about the early history of child abuse: first is the idea that children were treated worse the further one goes back into history, and the second is that it is only in more recent times that societies have sought to make better provision for the welfare of children who are maltreated.[11] While there is no comparison between the severe existence for children in the past to today's child population who enjoy better health and welfare and are more likely to survive infancy, evidence by historians such as Boswell[12] suggests that children in every era have been cared for. It would seem that every society has taken some steps to deal with the issue of the care of its young and has devised some means of intervention into family life to ensure this.[11] By analysing the history of child abuse, current problems in this area can be put into perspective and enhance our understanding of current approaches to the problem.[11]

## Contemporary childhood

In order to understand the concept of child protection, it is necessary to understand the notion of childhood.

Childhood is largely socially constructed and influenced by social historical and cultural change.[2,13] Some writers suggest that the notion of childhood is a recent phenomena while others believe that the separation of childhood and adulthood has always existed.[4,11,13]

One aspect on the concept of childhood is that children need to be protected. Children however remain largely understood as dependent individuals who develop primarily within a family structure.[12]

It has been suggested that the position of children in society is a key contributory factor in the problem of child maltreatment.[3] Childhood tends to last longer in rich industrialised countries to enable the development of a highly technological workforce, while poorer countries demonstrate the visible presence of street children and may have a reliance on child labour.[11] Although most people now relate childhood to having not reached a certain chronological age, the meaning of childhood may be different depending on our cultural and historical backgrounds.[14]

Any person under the age of 18 years of age is considered to be a child in the eyes of the law both in the UK and other jurisdictions. While childhood is usually recognised as the reaching of a chronological age, there are developmental aspects of the child to consider as well. The child's cognitive, physical, emotional and social attributes are maturing and require nurturing, optimal health and social care at this susceptible time. Recent findings provide neurophysiological evidence that social inequalities are associated with alterations in prefrontal cortex function in low socioeconomic status children. Researchers found that prefrontal-dependent electrophysiological measures of attention were reduced in low socioeconomic status children compared with children from a higher socioeconomic level in a pattern similar to that observed in patients with lateral prefrontal cortex (PFC) damage.[37]

Safeguarding children recognises the vulnerability of the child in this period of their lives with particular reference to the child who has a learning or physical disability.[2]

## Children's rights

The children's rights movement may be seen as a positive sign, a sign of progress rather than evidence of the decline of childhood and family life.[13] The children's rights movement received a boost with the government's signing and ratifying the United Nations Convention on the Rights of the Child (UNCRC) in the early 1990s. Many organisations that work with children now routinely refer to the UNCRC in their campaigning and draw on particular provisions of the UNCRC to support their claims.

Children's rights organisations are increasingly concerned to promote policies that empower children. They argue that while childcare policies are promoting child protection they do not represent a departure from a more traditional view of children as recipients of adult help and benevolence (Roberts).[13, pp52–64] A more radical change in social attitudes and government policies to implement Article 12 of the Convention, *which embodies the principle that children have the right to express their views on matters of concern to them and to have those view taken seriously in accordance with their age and maturity)*, is required (Landsdown)[13, pp87-97].

There must be recognition that children are not simply recipients but participants in the running of institutions and the making of decisions that most closely affect them. We need to ensure that all services to children and their families are firmly centred on the carefully elicited needs and wishes of the children themselves.[15]

Listening to children and taking them seriously is an important element in their protection (Lansdown)[13 pp87-97; 41].

There is continuing resistance to the concept of children's rights reflected in a strong cultural tradition that children are 'owned' by their parents and that the state should play a minimal role as possible in their care.[42] In addition, many organisations such as parenting groups have fears that their own role will be eroded. Children's rights is about moving away from the outdated belief that adults alone can determine what happens in children's lives without regard for children's own views, ideas and aspirations. It means that even very small children have an entitlement to be listened to and taken seriously. It means acknowledging that, as children grow older, they can take greater responsibility for exercising their own rights. Finally a commitment to respecting children's rights does not mean abandoning their welfare: it means promoting their welfare by an adherence to the human rights standards defined by international law.[36]

---

**ACTIVITY**

**Seminar discussion topic**

Part of the contention around children's rights is the idea that children can own these rights as possessions in the same way that adults own rights. In what way can we implement this concept? Do you agree with this argument?

---

## Legislative framework

### United Nations Convention on the Rights of the Child

The Convention on the Rights of the Child was unanimously adopted by the United Nations General Assembly on 20 November 1989.[16] The Convention is in essence 'a bill of rights' for all children, including the right to survival, development, protection and participation.[17] This legal document was subsequently ratified in most of the world's countries including the UK in 1991 and Ireland in 1992, making themselves legally bound to comply with its provisions and obligations. If the USA and Somalia were to ratify, the Convention on the Rights of the Child would become the first universal law of humankind.[16,p.1]

- Article 3 emphasises that the best interests of the child shall be a primary consideration when action is taken concerning children.
- Article 9 states that children should not be separated from their parents unless absolutely necessary.
- Article 19 outlines the appropriate measure that should be taken to protect the child from abuse and neglect.
- Article 37 discusses the use of torture, and other cruel treatment and punishment, and the deprivation of the child's liberty either unlawfully or arbitrarily.
- Article 39 discusses the appropriate measures to be taken to promote the physical and psychological recovery and social reintegration of a child victim of any form of neglect or abuse.

Further information can be obtained from www.everychildmatters.gov.uk/uncrc/

### The Children Act 2004

The Children Act 2004 is a UK act that was passed on 15 November 2004. The Act was an amendment of the Children Act 1989, largely as a consequence of the Victoria Climbié inquiry. It provides the legislative basis for dealing with children in need of care and protection and brings all government funtions for the child's welfare and education under the statutory authority of local directors of children's services. These and similar acts in other jurisdictions have seen a major attitude shift away from children being seen as the belongings of their parents. The emphasis now is towards parental responsibilities away from parental rights. This has significant repercussions for children's nursing, especially when the family unit is complex. Acts and guidelines such as these embody the principles contained in the UN Convention on the Rights of the Child.[18]

## Definition and recognition of child abuse

Powell[15] notes specifically the comments by Dr Chris Hobbs, a Reading UK paediatrician that maltreatment is now the single biggest cause of morbidity in children and that children who present with possible indicators of harm should be subject to the same systematic and rigour approach of management as children who present with other potential fatal conditions (Hobbs cited in Ref. 15). However, for nurses to identify abuse they need to be aware of related issues such as indications of abuse and disclosure. The term abuse is open to many interpretations but for the aim of this chapter constitutes any form of behaviour that disregards the dignity of the child or young person.

For the purposes of clarity, child abuse is commonly divided into four categories: physical abuse, emotional abuse, sexual abuse and neglect. However, experienced healthcare professionals working in the field are aware that this is an artificial classification. In reality, child abuse rarely manifests itself in one type alone, simple cause and effect is inadequate and it has to be seen in the context of the child's developmental stage.[6] The forms of abuse and neglect are defined in *Working Together to Safeguard Children*[2] (as well as similar documents in the other countries of the UK and Ireland). In England and Wales section 17 of the Children Act 1989 advances the notion that a child in need is unlikely to have the opportunity to attain or maintain a good standard of health and development, or one whose health and development is likely to be significantly impaired or further impaired without services, or is disabled.[7] A similar provision is set out in the Scottish Children's Act 1995 section 93. Although the child in need might become a child who suffers from harm, use of this approach when making a referral to a social services department could help deflect some parents' deeply held, even unsubstantiated, feelings of persecution.[7]

### Physical abuse

Physical abuse is any form of non-accidental injury or injury from wilful or neglectful failure to protect a child.[6] Even before they are born some children are exposed to damaging levels of alcohol or drugs. All aggression by others causes those who are attacked to feel threatened, aroused and distressed.[19] A particularly distressing condition is Munchausen's syndrome by proxy, now more commonly known as fabricated or induced illness, where physical harm may be caused to a child when a parent or carer fabricates the symptoms of, or deliberately induces, illness in a child.[5,6]

Common indicators of physical abuse are listed in Table 3.1 (p. 31).

### Sexual abuse

Sexual abuse involves forcing or enticing the child or young person to take part in sexual activities, including prostitution, whether or not the child is aware of what is happening. It may include the following:

- sexual intercourse with child, whether oral, vaginal or anal;
- non-penetrative acts;
- non-contact activities, such as involving children in looking at, or in the production of, sexual online images, watching sexual activities or encouraging children to behave in sexually inappropriate ways;
- exposure of the sexual organs or any sexual act intentionally performed in the presence of a child;
- intentional touching or molesting of the body of a child whether by a person or object for the purpose of sexual arousal or gratification;
- masturbation in the presence of a child or involvement of the child in the act of masturbation.

Sexual abuse may not always be identified by physical examination. It is characterised by fear, secrecy and shame, all of which make it difficult for a child to disclose. Adult inhibitions and embarrassment tend to compound this reluctance, and fear of asking leading questions can make staff reticent to investigate.[6,19]

In relation to child sexual abuse consensual sexual activity between an adult and a child under 17 years is a criminal act and can lead to prosecution (Table 3.2), p. 31.

### Emotional abuse

Emotional abuse has been described by Riddell-Heaney and Allott[20] as the persistent emotional ill-treatment of a child such as to cause severe and persistent effects on the child's emotional development. It is not normally manifested in

**Table 3.1** Physical abuse

| Physical indicators | Behavioural indicators |
| --- | --- |
| Shaking | Self-mutilation tendencies |
| Use of excessive force in handling | Poor concentration/learning |
| Suffocation | Chronic runaway |
| *Munchausen's syndrome by proxy* (where parents fabricate stories of illness about their child or cause physical signs of illness, now known as fabricated or induced illness) | Aggressive or withdrawn |
| Allowing or creating a substantial risk of significant harm to a child | Fear of returning home |
| Scratches, bite marks or welts | Undue fear of adults |
| Bruises in places difficult to mark, e.g. behind ears, buttocks, groin and thighs. *Bruising as a result of falls are usually over bony prominence and rarely over soft tissue*[36] | Bullying/being a victim |
| Burns, especially cigarette burns | |
| Under nourishment: severe childhood obesity may also be considered with many parallels between the treatment of severely obese children and the treatment of children who have non-organic causes of their failure to thrive. This remains very controversial and requires new guidelines. For severe childhood obesity to become a child protection issue it must be specific to the individual child and his or her circumstances[40] | |
| Untreated injuries | |
| Deliberate poisoning | |

Department of Health and Children.[36]

**Table 3.2** Sexual abuse

| Physical indicators | Behavioural indicators |
| --- | --- |
| Soreness, bleeding, itching in the genital or anal area | Inappropriate language or sexual knowledge for age group |
| Sexual transmitted infections | Chronic depression/low self-esteem |
| Pregnancy | Inappropriate sexual behaviour |
| Genital injury | Substance/drug abuse |
| Eating disorders | Self-harm |
| Stomach pains or headaches | |
| Pain on urination | |
| Bruises on inner thighs or buttocks | |

Department of Health and Children.[36]

terms of physical signs; it spans all social classes and cultures, and exists within the caregiver–child relationship[6] and can take the form of total rejection of the child to lack of praise, encouragement, comfort and love. Serious bullying and the instigation of fear, danger exploitation and corruption of children can occur. There may also be lack of attachment and proper stimulation of, for example, play and learning. Children can be emotionally abused unintentionally if, for example, a parent/carer suffers from a mental illness that affects their ability to relate to children.[6] Like child neglect, its long-term impact is detrimental and negatively affects the child's emotional and psychological development.[6] Finally it is important to recognise that some level of emotional abuse occurs in all types of maltreatment of a child, although it may take place alone (Table 3.3).

Features of this type of abuse include:

- persistent criticism, sarcasm, hostility or blaming;
- conditional parenting, in which the level of care shown to a child is made contingent on his or her behaviour or actions;
- emotional unavailability by the child's parent/carer;
- unresponsiveness, inconsistent or inappropriate expectations of a child;
- premature imposition of responsibility on a child;
- unrealistic or inappropriate expectations of a child's capacity to understand something or to behave and control himself in a certain way;
- under- or overprotection of a child;
- failure to show interest in, or provide age-appropriate opportunities for, a child's cognitive and emotional development;

- use of unreasonable or over-harsh disciplinary measures;
- exposure to domestic violence.

## Neglect

Although child physical and sexual abuse have a high public profile, child neglect and emotional abuse are the most common reasons that children are placed in child protection systems,[21] and the serious cumulative harm they cause is only beginning to receive the attention it deserves.[19,22–24] Neglect is the most prevalent form of child maltreatment and is rarely dramatic, but is insidious and pervasive and can often be overlooked or difficult to identify by healthcare professionals.

Neglect has been described as usually a passive form of abuse involving omission rather than acts of commission and comprises both a lack of physical caretaking and a failure to fulfil the developmental needs of the child in terms of cognitive stimulation.[25] The persistent failure to meet a child's basic physical and/or psychological needs is likely to result in the serious impairment of the child's health or development.[5]

Neglect can occur during pregnancy as a result of maternal abuse. Parents in this scenario may fail to provide adequate food, clothing and shelter for their child. The child may not be protected from physical harm and danger while adequate access to appropriate medical care or treatment may be omitted. Neglect may also involve the unresponsiveness to a child's basic emotional needs.[5] The important point to bear in mind is that a child's development is negatively affected if their needs are unmet and the long-term physical

**Table 3.3** Emotional abuse

| Physical indicators | Behavioural indicators |
| --- | --- |
| Sudden speech disorders | Mood change, e.g. depression, failure to communicate |
| Eating disorders | Rocking, thumb sucking |
| Self-harm | Fear of change |
| Wetting and soiling | Chronic runaway |
| Signs of mutilation | Poor peer relationships/isolation |
| Attention-seeking behaviour | Truancy |
| Frequent vomiting | Delinquency |

Department of Health and Children.[36]

emotional and psychological impact of neglect of children can be more significant than that of any other form of child abuse.[6]

In 2003 there were 11.7 million children under the age of 16,[26] and while fewer children are living in poverty in more recent years, statistics suggest that 3.4 million children are still living in low-income households.[26]

Poor housing/homelessness, parents with mental health problems and the environment of drugs, alcohol and smoking can also contribute to neglect of the child, with vulnerable children often living in circumstances where they are exposed to specific forms of abuse, which may include peer abuse and bullying, domestic violence, internet pornography, child trafficking and abduction. Spiritual and religious beliefs may also pose a risk for vulnerable children.[5]

Cases of abuse linked to accusations of 'possession' and 'witchcraft' have been reported worldwide. A report published in 2006 found 74 cases of abuse in the UK clearly linked to 'possession' and 'witchcraft'. The abuse in question occurs when an attempt is made to 'exorcise' the child. This may include severe beatings, burning and isolating the child. Common features between these cases include the family structure and a child becoming a scapegoat.[38]

## Recognising child abuse

To be able to recognise child abuse requires a person's readiness to accept the possibility of its existence as it does on knowledge and information. It is important to reiterate that child abuse takes many forms and may not be a 'textbook' scenario.

## YOUR ROLE AND RESPONSIBILITIES AS A NURSE

This section regards the professional responsibilities of the nurse in safeguarding children. How nurses can support families in the care of children will be discussed.

### As a nurse

Nurses have a very important role in child protection.[5,6,24] They share responsibilities for a range of outcomes for children; therefore, any nurse who has direct or indirect contact with children

**ACTIVITY**

Consider the following and discuss with your colleagues.

Mark the following on a scale of 1–10, where 1 = non-abusive; 10 = very abusive.

- A 6-month-old baby being shaken by her mother.
- A 10-year-old Nigerian boy being made kneel for 1 hour because he misbehaved.
- A father smacking his 12-year-old daughter because she was 2 hours late getting home.
- A 16-year-old boy from the travelling community with learning difficulties sleeping in the same bed as his 12-year-old sister.
- A nurse changing the trousers and pants of a 6-year-old boy who has wet himself.
- A 4-year-old having chronic infestations of head lice.
- A 2-year-old being told daily 'I'm sick of you'.
- A 12-year-old Romanian girl minding her two younger siblings while her parents go out to work.

must be able to identify children and young people who are vulnerable and are at risk of harm or abuse, and act accordingly.[5,27]

A child's welfare is paramount in every respect; regardless of your sympathetic feelings towards parents or carers, you must always act on a child's behalf if you have concerns.[5]

This concept is enshrined in the Nursing and Midwifery (NMC) *Code of conduct*,[28] which states that all nurses have a duty and personal responsibility to act in the best interest of the child and young person, and to inform and alert appropriate personnel if they suspect a child is at risk or has been abused. This means that you need to be able to know how to identify children who are at risk, and then know how to seek expert advice and support. Your local area safeguarding children committee and Trust procedures will have local policies in place. It is up to you to gain access and read them.

You have a duty to act if you have concerns about the behaviour of a colleague or student. You should report them according to local safeguarding policies and if necessary to the authorities if there is any breach in criminal law.[24]

## Parenting and child abuse

One of the factors contributing to an increase in child neglect is parental substance dependence, especially alcohol abuse, and can be seen in substantiated child protection cases.[21] Intimate-partner violence and parental illness are further important and interrelated problems.[21] Child maltreatment may have begun during babyhood and healthcare professionals including children's nurses working in the clinical areas are in a key position to detect problems with family functions and risk factors or possibly injuries related to or associated with child abuse and maltreatment.[29] Recognising child abuse is vital not only because it may save a child from recurrence of serious harm, but it may also enable the provision of services and support to a family who are in crisis or are struggling to care for their children.[6] Child abuse is an issue for individuals and families and the stress and the emotional and psychological impact of being neglected or ill-treated are the key factors for consideration; nevertheless, intervention is almost exclusively with poor families more open to scrutiny because of reliance on state support.[30] Multiprofessional collaboration is required when caring for child-maltreating families in order to better identify maltreatment and care for children and support families. While different professionals' knowledge of child maltreatment and of client families and their living circumstances is integrated it is possible to develop care.[29] Development of family support services, and child welfare and protection services now need to focus on need or vulnerability, as opposed to child abuse. This approach allows children and families to be identified as needing support before a child protection concern develops. It should also have the effect of reducing stigma attached to child protection interventions, if they are based around supporting a family rather than investigating a child protection concern. This may make it easier for parents to admit vulnerability and to seek help, since the view has been expressed that the current system with its emphasis on investigation of potential child abuse is not conducive to parents admitting to inadequacy or inability to cope.

Parents living in poor conditions coupled with low standards of parenting can have a negative impact on the child's heath and wellbeing. Intervention programmes like the Sure Start Local Programmes (SSLPs) have demonstrated an improvement in the health and wellbeing of young children living in disadvantaged neighbourhoods by preventing transmission of inequalities in health, poverty school failure and social exclusion between generations.[31] Services to children and their families should be firmly centred on the carefully elicited needs and wishes of the children themselves.[15] The risk of negative parenting can be reduced with interventions such as these programmes, with parents providing a more stimulating home-learning environment for their children. The SSLP effects on parenting can promote positive social behaviour and greater independence than those in non-SSLP areas.[31] Parents in these areas appear to be accessing the services, and early indicators suggest that children growing up in these areas had better social development with more positive social behaviour and greater independence than those in non-SSLP areas.[31] A useful strategy to implement when working with families is to focus on those parts of a family that are working well and build on existing positive attributes.[6] It has been suggested that a focus only on preventing maltreatment is less effective than a positive approach of building childcare skills, self-esteem and financial independence.[32] Family dynamics can sometimes be perceived as 'private' and it is largely thought that the way families raise their children is their own affair.[29] It is helpful to remember that neglect is a failure to meet the child's needs and is not primarily about the parents.[33]

Finally, healthcare professionals need to be aware that child abuse and neglect are not confined to poverty, and that support and treatment facilities should be universal.[11] Effective protection of children and young people at risk or in crisis, as well as the promotion of all children's wellbeing, requires a working partnership with families.

> Nursing staff need to anticipate the challenges they are likely to face and adopt strategies for coping especially where there are suspicions of abuse.

## Interagency working

Policy documents intended to assist people in identifying and reporting child abuse emphasise the important of enhanced communication and coordination of information between disciplines, departments and the statutory agencies of child protection. They aim to clarify and promote mutual understanding among statutory and voluntary organisations about the contributions of different disciplines to child protection. They emphasise that the need of children and families must be at the centre of childcare and child protection activity and their involvement in decision-making made explicit in a collaborative way with the organisations involved. They highlight the importance of consistency between policies and procedures across trusts and other statutory and voluntary organisations. They emphasise that the welfare of children is of paramount importance. Inter- and multi-agency work is an essential feature of all training in safeguarding and promoting the welfare of children. Single-agency training, and training provided in professional settings, should always equip staff for inter-agency work. All training in this field should be consistent with the *Common core of skills and knowledge*.[2]

*The common core of skills and knowledge for the children's workforce* can be accessed at www.everychildmatters.gov.uk

The guidelines for the protection and welfare of children such as the documents *Working together to safeguard children*[2] and *Safeguarding children in whom illness is fabricated or induced*[17] demonstrate how individuals, all practitioners and organisations should work together to safeguard and promote the welfare of children. The principles underpinning this document are

- child-centred
- rooted in child development
- focused in child development
- focused on outcomes for children
- holistic in approach.

## Recording keeping and report writing

Good record keeping is always unambiguous, factual, clear, comprehensive and accessible.

You should always

- write down all observations and discussions as they happen;
- avoid writing assumptions: deal with observational facts only;
- carefully record your judgements and any actions or decisions taken;

- include details and outcomes of healthcare contacts as well as follow-up arrangements;
- use good practice from the Nursing and Midwifery Council (NMC);
- use a body map to identify specific anatomical marks or injuries;
- add the date and time of every entry to your record.[5]

> **KEY POINTS**
>
> The recognition of child abuse usually runs along three stages:
> - considering the possibility
> - observing signs of abuse
> - recording information

## Dealing with disclosure

A report of suspected child abuse is the responsibility of all healthcare professionals. This responsibility to report must be based on reasonable suspicion that abuse has taken place, and the investigation should be a *collaborative* exercise that is methodically planned and carefully recorded. Errors and and disasters could have origins in failure to follow correct procedures.[7]

This concept is enshrined in the NMC *Code of conduct*.[28] The codes states that all nurses have a personal responsibility to act in the best interests of the child. *Staff* should report to their line manager/head of department in the first instance, and the consultant paediatrician should be informed and involved in the careful evaluation of the child's presentation and history. Healthcare professionals should be aware that physical sexual and emotional abuse often coexist, and in many cases accompany other forms of domestic violence.[34] This knowledge provides opportunities for cooperation between agencies for effective intervention.[18]

Information suggesting abuse may arise from a variety of sources. It may come to light in the form of a complaint from the child, an expression of concern from a member of staff or another adult, or during a professional consultation.[5,6]

## What to do if you suspect abuse

- You have a duty of care to report the matter as soon as possible to your immediate line manager.
- Record all the details in writing in the child's notes in a factual rather than a judgemental way.

- Remember you are not responsible for deciding whether or not abuse has occurred but you are obliged to report suspicions so that appropriate action can take place.
- You stay calm, listen and never interrupt when a child or young person volunteers information that may raise the suspicion of maltreatment.
- Always accept what the child is saying.
- Resist asking the child to repeat the story unnecessarily.
- Ask questions at the end of their narrative.
- It is important to reassure them that you take them seriously.
- Avoid asking leading questions.
- Never promise to keep secrets. Keeping it a secret is not an option.
- Never start to investigate the matter yourself.[2,5,6]

Note that there is no definite sign or symptom or injury. A series of seemingly minor events can be just as damaging as any one event. Concern may be raised in the following circumstances

- Disclosure of abuse by a child.
- An injury to a child with no logical or consistent explanation. Certain injuries should always raise concern, such as bruising or fractures.[39]
- Something about the appearance or behaviour of a child that raises concern, for example 'frozen watchfulness', failure to thrive, lack of hygiene, fear in the presence of a parent/guardian/visitor.
- Repeated admissions or attendance at Emergency Departments with preventable injuries.
- Previous history of abuse or evidence of domestic violence within the family.
- Allegations made by third parties that the child is being harmed either prior to or during attendance/admission to hospital.[6]

### *Keeping an open mind*

Not all suspected cases turn out to have occurred. In 2007 Perera and Pollock[35] discussed the case of a 10-year-old boy who presented with an unusual rash on his upper back with no explanation of its cause. The possibility of undisclosed physical abuse was raised. However, following an investigation including a home visit it emerged that the marks on his back were the same as and in alignment with the water outlets in the family whirlpool bath. This demonstrates the importance of keeping an open mind when presented with unexplained signs and doing a home visit.

**ACTIVITY**

Find out:

- what services are available locally
- how to gain access to them
- what sources of further advice and expertise are available
- who to contact in what circumstance, and how
- when and how to make a referral to local authority children's social care.

## Information sharing

It is imperative that all organisations working in the area of child welfare and protection services need to be constantly vigilant and that their information practices in relation to the collection storage and exchange of information best serve the needs of children at risk. Availability of good quality IT by all relevant staff would appear to be an important element in achieving this aim.

A further crucial aspect of information in the context of child welfare and protection services is the necessity for information to be made available at the appropriate level. For example, the information necessary for a member of the public to form a reasonable concern about the welfare of a child and to make the appropriate contact with the relevant authorities is less detailed than the information necessary for a child protection social worker to discharge their duties as efficiently as possible. Another level of information is the information necessary for a parent to understand what constitutes a safe environment for their children and to make the necessary demands in relation to child protection policies and procedures of service providers where services are being provided for children.

The specific actions necessary to put this principle of information sharing into operation will depend on the individual context, but the generation, availability, exchange and storage of necessary and good-quality information should be a consideration at every stage of the child welfare and protection process.

ACTIVITY

Review the policy documents pertaining to child protection in your jurisdiction and then compare them with similar documents in another jurisdiction. How different or similar are they to each other?

## SUMMARY

This chapter has aimed to provide student nurses who care for children with a comprehensive look at the key fundamentals surrounding the issue of child protection, in order to identify and respond appropriately to children who may be at risk of abuse and maltreatment. Regular education and training in safeguarding children and young people is essential for all healthcare professionals working with children in order to assist them in understanding the dynamics involved, which include a natural tendency towards optimism when assessing the circumstances surrounding a harm or injury.[6]

Children's nurses will have the opportunity to work with many vulnerable children and their families in many settings during their career. By being vigilant in the care of children and alert to the insidious nature of abuse and maltreatment, nurses may have the opportunity to prevent or diminish the catastrophic effects for the child in their care. It is important that nurses who work with children and young people are competent to support and help vulnerable children and their families as effectively as possible. To be able to do this, nurses must have the skills to acknowledge, examine and work through their own feelings, experiences, values and beliefs regarding children, child abuse and safeguarding children.[5]

ACTIVITY

Review the following statements and decide whether they are true or false. Discuss this with a colleague.

Head lice is always a form of neglect

True        False

If a 4-year-old talks about sex, she/he has been sexually abused

True        False

Children of drug abusers should be taken into care

True        False

Parents not visiting a child is neglect

True        False

Parents arguing in the presence of a child is abuse

True        False

If a child says he/she has seen Daddy's willy this means he/she has been sexually abused

True        False

A child whose parent is constantly belittling them and being negative about them is experiencing emotional abuse

True        False

It is normal to feel anger towards a parent that has abused his/her child

True        False

If a mother constantly slaps her child on the ward she is physically abusing her child

True        False

If a Nurse makes an allegation about child abuse that is not validated, he/she can be sued

True        False

 Go to the website to find the PowerPoint presentation for this chapter and MCQs to test your knowledge. **www.hodderplus.com/childnursingskills**

# REFERENCES

1 Lord Laming (2003) The Victoria Climbié Inquiry: report of an inquiry by Lord Laming. The Victoria Climbié Inquiry. http://www.victoria-climbie-inquiry.org.uk/finreport/finreport.htm (accessed 1 June 2009).

2 HM Government (2006) *Working together to safeguard children. A guide to interagency working to safeguard and promote the welfare of children. Every Child Matters Change for Children.* Department for Children, School and Families. http://www.ecm.gov.uk/safeguarding (accessed 6 July 2009).

3 Tingberg B, Bredlöv B, Ygge B-M (2008) Nurses' experience in clinical encounters with children experiencing abuse and their parents. *Journal of Clinical Nursing* 17(20): 2718–2724.

4 Powell C. (1997) Child protection: the crucial role of the children's nurse. *Paediatric Nursing* 9(9): 13–16.

5 Royal College of Nursing (2007) *Safeguarding children and young people – every nurse's responsibility. Guidance for nursing staff.* London: RCN. www.rcn.org.uk/data/assets/pdffile/0004/78583/002045.pdf (accessed 1 June 2009).

6 Council for Children's Hospital Care (2008) *Child protection guidelines for the children's hospitals.* Dublin: Council for Children's Hospitals' Care.

7 Marcovitch H, Jones DPH (2008) Protecting abused children. *Lancet* 369(9576): 1844–1846.

8 McFarlane J, Christoffel K, Bateman L, Miller V, Bullock L (1991) Assessing for abuse: self-report versus nurse interview. *Public Health Nursing* 8(4): 245–250.

9 Lewis K, Suddaby B, Mowery B. (2002) Critical thinking in critical care. When the story doesn't match. *Paediatric Nursing* 28(5): 508–509.

10 Lagerberg D (2004) A descriptive survey of Swedish child health nurses' awareness of abuse and neglect II. Characteristics of children suspected of maltreatment risk. *Acta Paediatrica* 93(5): 692–701.

11 Corby B (2006) *Child abuse towards a knowledge base,* 3rd edition. Milton Keynes: Open University Press.

12 Boswell J. (1990) *The kindness of strangers: the abandonment of children in western Europe from late antiquity to the Renaissance.* New York: Pantheon Books.

13 Foley P, Roche J, Tucker S (eds) (2001) *Children in society: contemporary theory, policy and practice.* Basingstoke: Palgrave.

14 Wyness M (2006) *Childhood and society: an introduction to the sociology of childhood.* Basingstoke: Palgrave Macmillan.

15 Powell C (2003) Lessons to be learnt from the Victoria Climbié inquiry. *British Journal of Nursing* 12(3): 137.

16 United Nations Children's Fund (2000) *The UN Convention on the Rights of the Child.* London: UNICEF http://untreaty.un.org/English/TreatyEvent2001/pdf/03e.pdf (accessed 26 January 2009).

17 Department of Health and Children (1999) *Children first: national guidelines for the protection and welfare of children.* Dublin: Stationery Office.

18 HM Government (2008) *Safeguarding children in whom illness is fabricated or induced.* Supplementary guidance to *Working Together to Safeguard Children.* Department for Children, School and Families www.ecm.gov.uk/safeguarding.

19 Howe D (2005) *Child abuse and neglect: attachment, development and intervention.* Basingstoke: Houndmills.

20 Riddell-Heaney J, Allott M (2003) 1. The role of health and other professionals. *Professional Nurse* 18(5): 280–284.

21 Scott DA (2008) The landscape of child maltreatment. *Lancet* 373(9658): 101–102.

22 Taylor J Daniel B (eds) (2004) *Child neglect: practice issues for health and social care.* London: Jessica Kingsley.

23 Kennison P, Goodman A (2008) (eds) *Children as victims.* Exeter: Learning Matters Ltd.

24 Powell C (2007) *Safeguarding children and young people: a guide for nurses and midwives.* Milton Keynes: McGraw Hill, Open University Press.

25 Department of Health and Children (2004) *Children first. National guidelines for the protection and welfare of children* Dublin: The Stationery Office.

26 Government statistics (2003) www.statistics.gov.uk/cci (accessed 29 January 2009).

27 Theobald S (2000) Child protection: why continuing education for nurses is important. *Paediatric Nursing* 12(3): 6–7.

28 Nursing and Midwifery Council (2008) *The code: standards of conduct, performance and ethics for nurses and midwives.* London: NMC.

29 Paavilainen E, Merikanto J, Åstedt-Kurki P, *et al.* (2002) Identification of child maltreatment while caring for them in a university hospital. *International Journal of Nursing Studies* 39(3): 287–294.

30 MacMillan HL, Wathen CN, Barlow J, *et al.* (2009) Interventions to prevent child maltreatment and associated impairment. *Lancet* 373(9659): 250–266.

31  Melhuish E, Belsky J, Leyland AH, Barnes J and the National Evaluation of Sure Start Research Team (2008) Effect of fully-established Sure Start local programmes on 3-year-old children and their families living in England: a quasi-experimental observational study. *Lancet* **372**(9650): 1641–1647.

32  Aynsley-Green A, Hall D (2008) Safeguarding children: a call to action. *Lancet* **373**(9660): 280–281.

33  Schapiro, N (2008) Medical neglect of children reporting issues for nurse practitioners. *The Journal for Nurse Practitioners* **4**(7): 481–482.

34  Manly JT (2005) Advances in research definitions of child maltreatment. *Child Abuse and Neglect* **29**(5) 425–439.

35  Perera A, Pollock I (2007) Suspected non-accidental injury and whirlpool use. Images in paediatrics. *Archives of Diseases in Childhood* **92**(10) 897.

36  Department of Health and Children (2008) *National review of compliance with Children First: national guidelines for the protection and welfare of children*. Dublin: The Stationery Office.

37  Kishiyama MM, Boyce WT, Jimenez AM, *et al.* (2009) Socioeconomic disparities affect prefrontal function in children. *Journal of Cognitive Neuroscience* **21**(6): 1106–1115.

38  Stobart E ( 2006) *Child abuse linked to accusations of 'possession' and 'witchcraft'*. Nottingham: DfES

Publications. www.dfes.go.uk/research/data/uploadfiles/rr750.pdf (accessed 6 July 2009).

39  Maguire S, Mann MK, Sibert J, Kemp A (2005) Are there patterns of bruising in childhood which are diagnostic or suggestive of abuse? A systematic review. *Archives of Disease in Childhood* **90**(2): 182–186.

40  Alexander SM, Baur LA, Magnusson R, Tobin R. (2009) When does severe childhood obesity become a child protection issue? *Medical Journal of Australia* **190**(3): 136–139.

41  Riddell-Heaney J, (2003) Safeguarding children: 5. Listening as part of the child-protection process. *Professional Nurse* **18**(10): 591–595

42  Kilkelly U, Donnelly M, (2006) *The child's right to be heard in the healthcare setting: perspectives of children, parents and health professionals*. Dublin: Office of the Minister for Children Dublin: Stationery Office.

## FURTHER READING

Landsdown G (2001) Children's welfare and children's rights. In: Foley P, Roche J, Tucker S (eds) *Children in society. Contemporary theory, policy and practice*. Basingstoke: Palgrave, pp. 87–97.

## CHAPTER 4

# Communicating with children, young people and their families

Alan Glasper

## LEARNING OUTCOMES

*Upon completion of this chapter, the reader should be able to accomplish the following:*

1 Acquire an understanding of concepts, definitions and categories associated with communication with children, families and others
2 Develop an awareness of a range of communication frameworks and how they might be used in contemporary child health nursing
3 Understand aspects of professional practice that enhance or detract from effective communication with children and their families
4 Identify strategies of breaking significant news to children and their families
5 Understand the role of Heron's work and its application in child health nursing practice
6 Recognise the important role of children's nurses as child and family advocates, especially for those families who are disadvantaged
7 Appreciate the use of special communication techniques for children with disabilities
8 Understand the use of the telephone, SMS texting and email as a method of communication with children and families

## INTRODUCTION

It is important to stress that all children's nurses need significant levels of knowledge of how to communicate with children, their families, fellow healthcare professionals and each other in their day-to-day working lives. Importantly children's nurses need advanced communication skills as part of their toolkit of professional attributes that they need for professional practice when working with families. When communicating with children and young people, it is important to remember that, although the child is the patient, the parent is often the broker in any communication episode. The family in most communication scenarios is often an indivisible unit. Serious illness in children and young people can be devastating for many parents, and sometimes minor illnesses are irrationally perceived and are therefore frightening for all concerned.

## FACTORS INFLUENCING COMMUNICATION

### The age of the child

Initially an infant's only method of communication is the cry. The cry of the infant is used to indicate hunger or discomfort and all human infants use this to great effect in attracting the attention of whoever is caring for them. Bell and Salter Ainsworth[1] indicate that crying becomes the method of communication in infants and is primarily directed at the mother. Importantly, as the mother learns to recognise her infant's cry by responding to it, there is a corresponding decline by the baby in its use. This is important, as children's nurses will be in clinical situations where the mother may not be present.

As the infant develops it can begin to discriminate words spoken by the mother during the later 6 months of the first year of life.

You will appreciate therefore that dialogue with the mother during the assessment process is crucial to learning about special words and phrases.

Although normal speech development will occur in most infants, children's nurses need to understand that children admitted to hospital during infancy or factors such as postnatal depression in the mother might affect the normal speech development process. Additionally, nurses should recognise that children with hearing impairments may have delayed speech development.

## Communication noise

Communication noise is anything that can interfere with communication channels. In addition to the ambient noise and noise pollution, which families with sick children in hospital are subject to, other factors can also apply. As information giving is the key to family empowerment communication, noise reduction is vital if nurses are to fully embrace notions of family-centred care. Communication noise might include, for example, worry or anxiety or fatigue. In the child it may be associated with pain or debilitating fears such as needle phobia. Hospital admission of a child is a source of considerable stress to parents and families and adversely impacts on the retention and understanding of information. It is for this reason that verbal information giving to families is inadequate alone and has to be backed up with other types of information giving. In Chapter 38, Glasper and Battrick discuss the role of written and other methods of communicating with families.

Chant et al.[2] have highlighted the lack of communication skills teaching in nurse education programmes, and this chapter reinforces the need for better communication between children's nurses and families.

How can communication noise be reduced?

- Reduce ambient noise and noise pollution to the minimum. It should be stressed that some parents with children in hospital are resident in less than optimum sleeping conditions, which sometimes might be a put-up bed in a ward area. Nurses working night shifts need to recognise that a tired parent who has lost sleep will not be able to benefit from subsequent information-giving sessions such as discharge planning, where compliance may be a real issue.
- Recognise that verbal information given to families may need to be repeated and backed up with other types of information giving, such as written, web-based or moving image.
- Always conduct information-giving sessions in a controlled environment where recipients of information such as children and their families are in a position to give their full attention to the content of the encounter. 'Corridor briefings' to families should be avoided.
- Children with specific fears should be appropriately prepared before procedures. Chapter 7 on the role of play provides further details

## Non-verbal communication

This is especially important for children's nurses and can assist or hinder effective communication, especially with young people. Chambers[3] identifies a number of important factors that professionals need to consider when using non-verbal communication.

*Personal appearance* and what the children's nurse wears etc., is particularly important. The world of children's nursing has adopted a range of strategies to enhance communication with children and young people. One of these has been the adoption of less formal uniforms. Glasper and Miller (cited in Campbell et al. Ref. 4) have explored how children's nurses have addressed the uniform issue and while many children's hospitals and units in the UK still adopt a more relaxed uniform of cotton polo shirts with blue skirts or trousers to enhance family communication, recent concerns related to hospital-acquired infection have persuaded some units to return to a more traditional nursing uniform. The debate about the optimum uniform for children's nurses continues.

*Facial expressions* are an important aspect of non-verbal communication and the human smile is internationally shared by families in all cultures. Children's nurses know that the smile is especially important when working with children and their families, and many a frightened child can be reassured by a friendly smile.

Many children's nurses adopt the SOLER (see below) stance, which is non-threatening and helps with active listening. It is especially useful when dealing with distraught families

### Using the SOLER stance

The SOLER stance was articulated by Egan.[5] The term is an acronym for

(S)it squarely in relation to the child or family
Maintain an (O)pen body posture
(L)ean slightly forward towards the child or family member
Use and maintain appropriate (E)ye contact
Try to look (R)elaxed

Children's nurses need to be highly skilled in communication strategies when caring for sick children and their families. This is because effective communication with families is crucial in ensuring that the art and science of children's nursing is practised within an overarching philosophy of family-centred care. Readers may wish to practise using the SOLER stance with each other to develop this skill of communication.

### Encoding and decoding information

In both verbal and non-verbal communication there are two key factors which children's nurses need to acknowledge.

1 The encoding or the construction of information to be given to children and their families needs to be done in such a way that the content is received appropriately by the receiver or listener. Young people especially are prone to imagine a slight in perhaps the tone of a verbal message. Think perhaps of an occasion when you have been shopping and someone has said to you 'have a nice day'. If this message is encoded without a smile using a verbal tone that may be decoded by a listener as non-genuine or perhaps laced with sarcasm, deliberate or not, this type of encryption error may potentially ruin the whole point of the communication with the child or family member. Furthermore regional dialects and/or the use of slang may negatively affect the success of the communication encounter.

2 Children's nurses also need to understand the work of Miller,[6] who has described how some people (healthcare monitors) actively respond to health message communications as a concrete way of managing health problems. Conversely, Miller identifies some people (healthcare blunters) who fail to 'listen' to certain types of healthcare information to avoid the impending threat of ill-health. This description of families into monitors and blunters brings with it problems for the children's nurse. Hence during an encounter with a family, perhaps at discharge, the nurse who aspires to successfully deliver, in this case discharge, information highly pertinent to the child's ongoing care may face some families wanting an abundance of information. This may exceed the nurse's own knowledge. Some do not fully 'hear' the information, thus jeopardising the child's ongoing care. Children's nurses should always endeavour to investigate this phenomenon, which has the potential to undermine the communication episode and potentially harm the child through non-compliance.

## THE COMMUNICATION LOOP

The communication loop is a simple process of delivering an encoded message (verbal, written, etc.) via a medium such as speech, a tape-recorded message or a publication to a receiver (a patient/client) who receives and decodes the message and finally gives feedback to the sender. This simple process is fraught with difficulties, which in turn can lead to difficulties in the nurse/family relationship!

### Developing good communication skills

Good communication with families depends on a number of prerequisites, built primarily on respect for the individual child and family member. Importantly for all children's nurses is the recognition that communicating with those families receiving care requires time and effort, for there are no shortcuts to good communication. In certain situations, such as child safeguarding, accurate and unbiased information giving may be critical to the future welfare of the child.

- *Allow enough time.* Children's nurses are universally busy and the fast turnaround times for admissions only exacerbates this, making time a precious commodity. Importantly, Pollock and Grime[7] in a qualitative study found that clients perceived that time constraints were an important aspect of their consultations with general practitioners. They believed that this anxiety about time prevented them from fully engaging with the doctor to discuss their problems. It is because of this perception held by families that no one has any time to spare that children's nurses should understand that families do perceive time entitlement to be problematic. In any encounter with a family the nurse should endeavour at the opening of the episode to reassure the family that time is not an issue.

- *Use the open ended-question technique.* Children's nurses should always use open-ended questions at the initial stage of an encounter with a child or family. This allows the nurse to ascertain precisely what their concerns and worries are. 'Can you tell me about your pain' is more likely to elicit accurate information about a child's pain than 'Does it hurt'.
- *Develop family-centred styles of communication.* This communication strategy is individual orientated and not position centred. Munson and Wilcox[8] describe the Calgary–Cambridge model of communication, which details the six stages required for the best communication encounter with families. This includes preparing the environment, which for children is so important, and developing the relationship with the child and family, and importantly making clear the reason for the encounter. Although in many acute situations children's nurses need to elicit objective physiological and anatomical data from an individual child, it is important to gather other more holistic family information covering elements of the child's life beyond the parameters of the particular illness.
- *Building a relationship with the child and family.* All communication episodes with children and their family members should be consolidated by sharing with them summaries of what has been discussed or elicited and helping them access other sources of information, such as kite-marked internet sites, e.g. 'Children First' (available on www.childrenfirst.nhs.uk/). All children's nurses should check with families that all their concerns have been addressed.
- *Ensuring that the right type and amount of information has been given to families.* Ensure that children and families fully understand the information given to them and importantly that

the children's nurse has a shared understanding of the child's or family's problem before agreeing in partnership what the plan of action should be.
- *Closing the encounter.* This element of the communication episode with children and family members is important, especially in situations such as discharge where the children's nurse needs to establish and reach a mutual end-point culminating with some forward planning as necessary.

### Getting round communication obstacles

Children's nurses need to recognise that good communication with families involves the exchange of information between themselves and the receiver, be that a child, young person or specific family member. The information the nurse imparts will need to be communicated in such a way that any elements of the message, e.g. timbre, manner, character or pitch, or quality, must be appropriately received and fully understood by the individual receiver.

When children's nurses engage with families they must understand that any successful communication episode requires

- a message sender
- an actual message
- a method of communication, e.g. verbal, written, visual, etc.
- a beneficiary of the message.

## The benefits of active listening for children's nurses

Optimum communication with children and their family members is dependent on maintaining respect and crucially developing active listening skills. Consideration from a children's nurse who is a good listener is always appreciated from families who may have been 'pushed from pillar to post' when seeking healthcare advice about a sick child. Note that this skill is not a technique, as the children's nurse who is engaging with the family must fundamentally be genuinely sincere and give attention in such a way to indicate that they really value the child and family members they are communicating with.

### Active listening

- This reassures the child and family member that the nurse is in tune with their views, worries and concerns.

- It is important in establishing therapeutic family relationships at an early stage of the communication episode.
- Active listening establishes an honest and constructive information flow between the child and family.

Importantly active listening helps nurses to decode accurately the sometimes cryptic encoding of information by children and their families.

### Reflecting

This method of active listening is like the holding of a mirror in front of the child, young person or family member because it allows the nurse to reflect back the key words or phrases they have heard to them which in turn reassures them that they have been listened to and importantly heard in the correct context.

### The use of summarising and paraphrasing

This allows the children's nurse to evaluate and consider the clarity and the shared understanding of the words being spoken to them. In translating the words, perhaps into a simple sentence, the nurse is able to reaffirm this mutual understanding. This is especially important when giving complex information, for example when discharging a newly diagnosed diabetic child.

Reflecting feelings helps the nurse stay in tune with the emotions behind the spoken words and the non-verbal signals. In attempting to reflect these back to a family member nurses can assess the precision of their own perceptions. Importantly, Le May[9] reminds professionals that the ability to communicate by clients may be compromised, particularly in old age. Speech and language may be compromised by disease such as stroke or head injury. Likewise the ability to use facial expressions, movement of gestures, posture and body position and clothing or attire as part of a person's unique non-verbal communication strategies may be compromised by disease or learning disability; this may be seen in the child or family member. The use of praise is also a real way in which children's nurses can help children or young people articulate their needs.

The main benefits of active listening are:

- children, young people and family members feel more understood;

- families feel empowered to convey their thoughts more clearly and succinctly;
- crucially, families have a chance to rectify any misunderstandings.

### The three Rs of listening

1 Readying: this is the procedure nurse uses when preparing to actively listen to a family member who is preparing to give information (an encoder)
2 Reaching: this is the process the nurse adopts in encouraging the family member to articulate their needs
3 Reflecting: this is the process of paraphrasing what the child or family member has said to ensure shared comprehension.

## AREAS OF COMMUNICATION DIFFICULTY (AFTER QUILTER WHEELER AND WINDT)

### Perceptual

Children's nurses need to be aware of how perceptions can alter a person's feeling towards another individual. In the case of children and young people and their family members, the way they look, dress and their behaviour can all lead the nurse to perhaps make a premature judgement, which in turn can cause bias, discrimination or stereotyping. Most children's nurses know that a young person who wears a 'hoodie' is not actually a delinquent after all! Such premature judgements can lead to roadblocks in communication, but these can be overcome with forethought and by being open minded. Perceptions can work in both directions: children's nurses must adhere to hospital dress (hair colour, body piercing, etc.) and professional body behaviour codes meticulously to avoid being stereotyped themselves.

### Emotional

This is sometimes observed in complex cases where the family may lack trust in the nurses or doctors, particularly after an adverse incident such as a drug error. When this happens the atmosphere within the clinical area can become emotionally charged. Only through establishing a trusting relationship with the child and family will this barrier to communication be overcome.

## Informational

When nurses do not actively listen and ask leading rather than open questions there is a risk that the child and family may not be able to fully articulate their needs. In order to fully complete an assessment of a child, for example, it is imperative to obtain the maximum amount of pertinent information to allow optimum care planning. This can only be achieved if the nurse actively listens and uses open-ended questions to elicit the parameters of the child's health problems.

## Time constraints

Giving the family insufficient time to tell you their story or conveying to them that you are short of time and in a hurry is not beneficial to a full and useful communication encounter, and the nurse therefore risks missing vital information pertinent to a particular child. This is especially pertinent in child safeguarding situations, where coming to a premature communication closure before a child has made a disclosure may have profound consequences. Hence, in all family situations the nurse must ensure that what is conveyed to the child or family is that they have an adequate amount of time to discuss their particular issues.

## Linguistic

In this situation it is the use of medical jargon or a foreign language that may undermine the communication event. Children's nurses need to understand that the language they use in their day-to-day professional lives may be unfamiliar to a child or family member. Learning to use lay and sometimes colloquial language when appropriate is a skill all children's nurses need to learn if they are to have satisfactory communication encounters with children and their families. Additionally, if the child or family member does not use English as their first language, appropriate translators should be used. Both 'language line' and one-to-one interpreters should be used for families whose first language is not English. 'Language line' is a company used by the NHS and many children's hospitals and units to help nurses communicate with families whose use of English is limited (www.languageline.co.uk/).

All hospitals keep a directory of local interpreters. Good practice suggests that one-to-one interpreters should be booked for all communication episodes. Panesar and Sheikh[10] have suggested a number of strategies that nurses might use when talking to families from other backgrounds, in particular using language resources such as the use of language line.

## USING HERON'S SIX CATEGORY INTERVENTION ANALYSIS IN CHILDREN'S NURSING

This is a systematic training tool developed by John Heron which has been designed to help nurses and others develop useful and practical communication skills for use in therapeutic encounters. Burnard and Morrison[11] have shown that this model of therapeutic communication can be used in a range of clinical and other communication scenarios. Basically, Heron[12,13] details six basic communication intervention categories that apply in one-to-one, one-to-group and intergroup communication encounters. Intervention in this situation assumes that the nurse is offering an enabling service to the family.

### The three authoritative categories: (I tell you)

1 Prescriptive
2 Informative
3 Confronting

For these first three categories the children's nurse adopts a professional practitioner role, taking responsibility, guiding behaviour and giving instructions to the child and family.

*Prescriptive*: In this situation the children's nurse attempts to direct the behaviour of the child/young person or family member and the focus of the communication exercise is aimed at giving the family member uncomplicated information about a particular childhood health issue, for example when a mother has a simple request. This method of communication is often used by children's nurses working for NHS Direct and other national telephone help lines. Although this type of communication is formulated to persuade and signpost the behaviour of the child, it does not undermine the child's or family's competence in making their own decisions. The advice of the nurse is offered in such a away that leaves the family free to decide what is best for them, whether or not it matches the information they have been given.

*Informative*: In this situation the children's nurse attempts to offer aspects of healthcare knowledge to the child or family member, for example to enable them to self-care. This method endeavours to give new knowledge or skills to the family as a whole. This knowledge should be perceived by children and their famines as being relevant to their healthcare needs and interests. Importantly, this is about sharing knowledge and in a way that fosters independence through giving general knowledge about healthcare and specific information pertinent to families.

*Confronting*: In this situation the children's nurse endeavours to alert the child or family and give them awareness of a behaviour or sometimes an attitude which they may not be aware of and which may be impeding their progress of recovery. Confronting communication interventions can only function optimally when the child or young person or family member believe that the nurse is actually acting in their best interests.

## The three facilitative categories (you tell me)

1 Cathartic
2 Catalytic
3 Supportive

In these three the role of the children's nurse is to be empowering and encouraging the family to develop autonomy and affirming the uniqueness of the individual child. This aspect of communication is often used in conditions such as diabetes, where the nurse is helping the individual child and family member manage independently the complexities of life and therapy.

*Cathartic*: Here the nurse helps the child, young person or family member let go of built-up emotions, possibly caused by fear or anger. These therapeutic aspects of communication are orientated towards the level of upset distress that the child is sufficiently comfortable to deal with, such as in the case of having a procedure.

*Catalytic*: In this situation the nurse's mission is to promote self-discovery, self-directed living, learning or problem solving, for example in the case of a child who is learning to live life as an amputee.

*Supportive*: Here the nurse seeks to establish the importance and value of a child or family's importance, qualities, actions and attitudes. This type of communication provides a feel-good factor and is essential for successful therapeutic communication with the full range of children and their families.

All six categories are:

- fundamentally supportive of the child and family;
- have a primary aim of increasing the capacity of the child or family member for resourceful self-direction;
- value free, in that no one category is better or of lesser value than the others.

## Application

The six categories in practice are blended together and are used by the children's nurse in such a way to reflect the

- child/family/nurse relationship;
- current state and potential of the child or family member;
- creativity and insight of the nurse;
- context of the communication exercise.

Although Heron's categories can be used in their original context they are also interdependent. In the real world of the complexities of children's nursing some overlap is inevitable, e.g. a catalytic intervention with a particular child may also simultaneously have an informative element: an upset child who has just had a plaster of Paris cast applied for a fracture will still need basic information about life in a cast.

John Heron[12,13] suggests that the skilled children's nurse should be

- equally proficient in each of the six types of intervention;
- able to move seamlessly from one type of intervention to another as the communication with the child or family develops;
- cognisant during the communication encounter of what type of intervention they are using and its purpose.

Three basic values underpin the everyday use of Heron's six categories of communication in the world of children's nursing:

1 hierarchical: one person decides for another, as in a nurse for a child;
2 cooperation: decision by mutual consent involving consultation and discussion;
3 autonomy: facilitation to let children and their families make their own decisions.

## METHODS OF COMMUNICATING

### Communicating by telephone

The telephone consultation of families has developed considerably over the last decade, culminating with the establishment of NHS direct in England and other similar services elsewhere. There was initial scepticism about the use of the telephone as a healthcare communication medium, and it is interesting to note that the first recorded use of the telephone in the care of sick children was in 1879. A letter to the editor of the *Lancet* described how a telephone call had been used to discount the diagnosis of croup.[14]

Telephone consultation with families involves children's nurses making management decisions based on a verbal history. In the context of sick children this is often from fraught parents, and the nurse has to then give appropriate advice over the telephone. As in the case of NHS Direct, Glasper *et al.*[14] have shown how this advice is augmented through the use of decision-making telephone advice software. With or without software communicating with families using the telephone is burdened with anxieties and Bowing[15] has described this method of dealing with famines as communicating in the dark. Aspects of the communication encounter such as the tone of the voice plays a major part in any successful telephone conversation.

In order to make an accurate assessment of a family's concerns about a child, the initial priority of the nurse is to be able to conduct the telephone interview in such a way that the family member is happy and comfortable in giving what might be sensitive information.[9] During an acute episode a child or family member may be very worried about themselves or their child. Learning to deal effectively with family members has to be acquired, as it involves very different skills. Children's nurses have to develop telephone communication skills that reassure the family member. Nurses will be aware that efficient communication requires the use of all the senses.[15] Non-verbal communication such as the tone of voice plays a crucial aspect of telephone interactions. Nurses need to understand that when a parent rings a busy ward, for example to enquire about their child, anxiety can be communicated not only by what is said, but by how it is said. Thus the children's nurse must recognise that the words they use in a telephone conversation are integral to the success of the telephone consultation. Clearly, active listening even in the midst of a busy clinical area will help the nurse understand and successfully decode the verbal information given by the family member over the telephone. This is to ensure that the information given to the family caller is clear and importantly fully understood by them. Bowing[15] acknowledges that good communication skills even in the absence of visual cues need not be an obstacle to an accurate assessment of the caller's information needs. Children's nurses need to become adept at communicating on the telephone, more perhaps than other types of nurses, and need to recognise the strengths of this medium of communication. Good telephone conversations with anxious parents may allow them the night's sleep they deserve!

Car and Sheikh[16] have suggested a number of factors required for a successful telephone encounter with a family member:

- active listening and detailed information taking;
- frequent clarifying and paraphrasing (to ensure that the messages have been got across in both directions);
- picking up cues (such as pace, pauses, change in voice intonation);
- offering opportunities to ask questions;
- offering family health information and education.[15]

### Using the internet, text and email

The advent of the mobile phone and quick and easy access to the World Wide Web from a range of easy-to-access venues such as cyber cafés, home computers and the like is changing the way in which family members source and access health information and communicate with each other.

#### Communication alert

If Facebook and mobile phone cameras are used in clinical settings, children's nurses need to be aware that many parents and children are members of 'Facebook'. Guidance from the Association of Chief Children's Nurses (ACCN) suggests that children's nurses should politely decline to be involved in a family's Facebook activities. The danger of uploading clinically based photographs of nurses in which other peripheral children may inadvertently feature and who have not given consent is great and may compromise the individual nurse's professional integrity.

### Internet services

NHS Direct Online was launched in December 1999. The service offers families a range of databases covering health topics that are available 24 hours a day. Nurses should recognise that families using the service have access to an online encyclopaedia of some 400 conditions which also gives details of appropriate support groups.[17] Additionally, family users of NHS Direct Online can interrogate a range of databases to obtain information about health and health services pertinent to themselves and their children. Huntington et al.[18] have shown that families are increasingly using the web as a source of health information. It is believed that in doing so families often feel better prepared in their dealings with healthcare professionals such as doctors and nurses. The important aspect for children's nurses to consider is that families are now much more proactive in seeking healthcare information and may ask many erudite questions at the assessment and other stages of the sick child's journey. The government quest of empowering families to benefit from health information and promotion activities lies at the heart of services such as NHS Direct Online (www.nhsdirect.nhs.uk/), which also now has the added bonus of allowing a family member who is unable to find what they want from the website to send an email request directly to NHS Direct online, where the health question will be answered usually within 5 working days.

### Communicating through, text and email

The use of the short message service (SMS) or text messaging is a global aspect of mobile phone ownership. Texting has had a major impact on the way in which families communicate with each other, and children's nurses and their organisations are quick to see its potential in a healthcare setting.

Children's outpatient departments for example have investigated its use as a way of improving outpatient appointment compliance. Downer et al.[19] believe that the ease with which large numbers of texts can be personalised and sent suggest that its use be accelerated in healthcare.

Similarly to SMS texts, the rapid rise of email both within the workplace and in the home has paved the way for its use in healthcare settings. Importantly, however, Car and Sheikh[20] have suggested that family satisfaction with email as a method of communicating with health agencies decreases if the healthcare professional such as the children's nurse does not respond to them quickly. Similarly, Bauchner et al.[21] express caution about the use of email in healthcare, as they believe it might exacerbate workload. In addition, they identify some legal–ethical issues about the use of email, including the question 'should an email correspondence be part of the child/family record'. Additionally and worthy of note is the other perennial danger of using email: the potential for email wars between fellow professionals where conflict escalation epitomises communication going badly wrong. In the winter edition of *The write stuff*[22] email disagreements are highlighted as a common cause of communication breakdown.

- An email when it is read without visual or verbal cues from the sender can be a cause of misunderstanding, especially if the correspondence has been sent in a hurry.
- Many emails are written in busy offices and it is easy to forget the courtesy and humanness which normally accompanies a piece of correspondence.
- Emails by their very nature are often less courteous than a letter or telephone conversation and they can come across as more aggressive and less polite, thus laying the way for a potential email conflict!
- Please remember that emails can live for ever on the computer hard drive and can be read and re-read by the receiver. Individuals who receive a perceived negative email can convince themselves that the writer has thought through the message, making their indignation even larger. Thus when replies are formulated the individual becomes more entrenched in their own point of view. This potentially pours fuel on the fire and the email conflict begins to escalate.

### Avoiding email conflict: email etiquette

Cleary and Freeman[23] discuss email etiquette (or netiquette) as a tangible way of preventing email conflict, highlighting the many pitfalls professionals can fall into. Some of the criteria are listed below.

- Recognise that some perceived insulting emails may be unintended. The sender may be writing on the run during a busy clinical episode with little or no time to reflect on other meanings the message may convey. A derivation of the old adage is 'I know you believe you understand what you think I have just said to you in this email but I am not sure you realise that what you read and heard in your head is not actually what I meant to say'.
- Observe for enhanced aggressiveness and carefully reflect before you answer the email.
- It is important to stress that your own response can also be interpreted as being more aggressive than you may have intended. Where possible always re-read your email messages before you press the send button. Attempt to gauge the reaction of the colleague or other professional who will be reading it. Emails can be recalled, but it really is too late once you have clicked the send button.
- Always remind yourself of the professional or therapeutic relationship you have with the reader of your email. Always endeavour to include in your message a reminder to the reader of this relationship – A *best wishes* or *kind regards* costs nothing!

## BREAKING BAD OR SIGNIFICANT NEWS

Breaking bad or other significant news to families is very daunting for many professionals such as children's nurses who may have little experience and find it difficult. However, this is a key role for the registered children's nurse because how the news is broken will ultimately impact the way in which the family copes.

Information that adversely and seriously affects a child's or family's perception of their future has to be given by healthcare professionals on a frequent basis.

- The full impact of this news will be dependent upon the difference between the family's expectations, the knowledge and age of the child and the reality of the current situation.
- A number of religious, racial and cultural factors plus previous experiences of both family and staff will direct how the news is broken and received.
- Although it is usually the senior paediatrician/surgeon who gives the information, it may fall to the senior children's nurse on duty to do this. Ideally this should be someone who has had and will have ongoing care involvement with the family.
- The child's primary nurse should attend the interview, as this enables them to support the family after the event and feed back to fellow colleagues to ensure that they will have knowledge of what information was given to the family.
- It cannot be expected that the family will remember all the information they have been given, especially as in times of stress less information is retained. This means that the information will probably need to be reiterated. Families need to know that they can re-ask questions as often as they wish.
- Where possible family members should be given the news together so that the message they receive is the same. This helps them to support each other, especially during a stressful period.

The steps to breaking significant news are not cast in stone but children's nurses may find the following steps helpful.

### Steps for breaking bad news

1 Adequate preparation
  - Facilitate uninterrupted time in a quiet part of the clinical area that provides privacy.
  - Family communication significant news encounters should be conducted sitting down, face to face without any physical barriers using the SOLER stance (see page 41). This conveys to the family that there is time to talk and eye contact can be maintained.
  - Children's nurses should introduce themselves to the family, if they are not already acquainted. Importantly it should be ascertained how family members wish to be addressed. Over familiarity or using an

incorrect form of address in many cultures can undermine the whole communication episode.

2 Establish what the child or family already knows by asking open ended questions
- It is crucial to ascertain what information the family already knows and what their subsequent information needs are.

3 Giving an indication of the tone of the significant new item, e.g. the results of the X-ray are back and they are not as promising as we first thought
- This helps reduce the distress and allows the family to prepare themselves for what the significant news they are about to be told.

4 Breaking the news
- Avoid medical jargon.
- Take cues on how to continue the communication by observing the family's reactions.
- Most families respond better to honesty; this strengthens the relationship with the nurse.
- Reassurance should be offered to the family that everything is being done for the child, but false optimism should not be given.
- Non-verbal signals or cues will be received by families in addition to what is said.

5 Time for questions and to vent feelings
- Families will display a variety of reactions to the significant news.

- It is important that time is given for feelings to be expressed and questions to be asked.

6 Further support
- Before concluding the interview at a mutually convenient time, it is important for the nurse to ensure that the family members are aware of the plans for their child's future.
- Written or other media information advice, when available, should always be given to families and their children to support the verbal message content.

In breaking significant news many nurses use the acronym SPIKES:[24]

S is for setting
P is perception
I is for invitation
K is for knowledge
E is for emotion and empathy
S is for strategy and summary

- Ensure the patient has understood the information given.
- Summarise the information before the consultation ends, including the plans for the immediate future.
- Give the patient an opportunity to ask questions.

 Go to the website to find the PowerPoint presentation for this chapter and MCQs to test your knowledge. **www.hodderplus.com/childnursingskills**

# REFERENCES

1 Bell SM, Salter Ainsworth MD (1972) Infant crying and maternal responsiveness. *Child Development* **43**: 1171–1190.

2 Chant S, Jenkinson T, Randle J, Russell G (2002) Communication skills: some problems in nurse education and practice. *Journal of Clinical Nursing* **11**: 12–21.

3 Chambers S (2003) Use of non-verbal communication skills to improve nursing care. *British Journal of Nursing* **13**: 14874–14878.

4 Campbell S, O'Malley C, Watson D, et al. (2000) The image of the children's nurse: a study of the qualities required by families of children's nurses' uniform. *Journal of Clinical Nursing* **9**(1): 71–82.

5 Egan G (1990) *The skilled helper*, 4th edition. Pacific Grove, CA: Brooks/Cole.

6 Miller SM (1987) Monitoring and blunting: validation of a questionnaire to assess styles of information seeking under threat. *Journal of Personality and Social Psychology* **52**: 345–353.

7 Pollock K, Grime J (2002) Patients perceptions of entitlement to time in general practice consultations for depression: qualitative study. *British Medical Journal* **325**: 687.

8 Munson E, Willcox A (2007) Applying the Calgary–Cambridge model. *Practice Nursing* **18**: 464–468.

9 Le May A (2007) Communicating care. *Nursing and*

*Residential Care* **9**: 363–366.

10 Panesar SS, Sheikh S ( 2006) How to talk with people from other backgrounds. *Practice Nursing* **17** (2): 93–96.

11 Burnard P, Morrison P (2005) Nurses perceptions of their interpersonal skills: a descriptive study using six category intervention analysis. *Nurse Education Today* **25**: 612–617.

12 Heron J (1976) A six-category intervention analysis. *British Journal of Guidance and Counselling* **4920**: 143–155.

13 Heron J (1990) *Helping the client: a creative practical guide.* London: Sage publications.

14 Glasper EA, Lattimer VA, Thompson F, Wray D (2000) NHS Direct: examining the challenges for nursing practice. *British Journal of Nursing* **9**(17): 1173–1178.

15 Bowing T (2000) Communication in the dark. *Practice Nursing* **11**(8): 17–20.

16 Car J, Sheikh A (2003) Telephone consultations. *British Medical Journal* **326**: 966–969.

17 Eaton L (2002) NHS Direct Online explores partnership with other health organisations. *British Medical Journal* **324**: 568.

18 Huntington P, Williams P, Blackburn P (2001) Digital health information provision and health outcomes. *Journal of Information Science* **27**(4): 265–276.

19 Downer SR, Mears JG, Da Costa AC (2005) Use of SMS text messaging to improve outpatient attendance. *Medical Journal of Australia* **183**: 366–368.

20 Car J, Sheikh A (2004) Email consultations in healthcare. 2: acceptability and safe application. *British Medical Journal* **329**: 439–442.

21 Bauchner H, Adams W, Burstin H (2002) You've got mail: issues in communicating with patients and their families by email. *Pediatrics* **109**: 954–956.

22 Bruner Business Communication (2003) *The write stuff.* (www.brunerbiz.com/page4o.htm).

23 Cleary M, Freeman A (2005) *Email etiquette: guidelines for mental health nurses. International Journal of Mental Health Nursing* 14: 62–65.

24 Baile WF, Buckman R, Lenzi R, *et al.* (2000) SPIKES: a six-step protocol for delivering bad news: application to the patient with cancer. *The Oncologist* **5**: 302–311.

## FURTHER READING

Buckman R (1992) *How to break bad news: a guide for healthcare professionals.* London: Papermac.

Dias L, Bruce A, Lynch T, Penson R (2003) Breaking bad news: a patient's perspectives. *The Oncologist* **8**: 587–596.

Giffin J, McKenna K, Tooth L (2003) Written health education materials: making them more effective. *Australian Occupational Therapy Journal* **50**: 170–177.

Glasper A, Burge D (1992) Developing family information leaflets. *Nursing Standard* **6**(25): 24–27.

Gunning R (1968) *The technique of clear writing.* Philadelphia: McGraw Hill.

Huntington P, Nicholas D, Williams P, Gunter B (2002) Characterising the health information consumer: an examination of digital television users. *Libri* **52**: 16–2.

Jacobson TA, Thomas DM, James Morton F, *et al.* (1999) Use of a low literacy patient education tool to enhance pneumococcal vaccination rates: a randomised controlled trial. *JAMA* 282: 646–650.

Kay P (1996) *Breaking bad news: a ten step approach.* Northampton: EPL Publications.

Quilter Wheeler SQ, Windt JH (1993) *Telephone triage: theory, practice and protocol development.* Albany: Delmar publishers.

## CHAPTER 5

# Promoting family health in contemporary healthcare

Margaret Fergus, Palo Almond, Colleen Baker, Donna Forbes and Lyn Wilson

## LEARNING OUTCOMES

*Upon completion of this chapter, the reader should be able to accomplish the following:*

1 Define health using a range of definitions
2 Understand the politics of health inequalities
3 Identify the contribution government policy can play in determining the health of children
4 Describe the psychosocial determinants of health impacting on children's health
5 List a range of factors that produce, prevent or deteriorate health
6 Describe the role of the family in child health
7 Discuss models of behavioural change
8 Apply health promotion models to case studies

## KEY WORDS

Child health promotion    Policy Case studies
Health inequalities

## CHAPTER OVERVIEW

The aim of this chapter is to provide nurses with guidance on how to promote the health of children and young people. As a nurse working with children or young people you will encounter many situations that require you to promote health; you may have opportunities to encourage health behaviour change in children, young people or even parents or guardians. The methods described here are applicable to this range of patients or clients. In this chapter we will use the term 'client', as it has a wider application than the term patient; the term client includes people who are not patients but may be important influences on the patient. A client could therefore be a child, a young person, a parent or a guardian. We will use the term 'child' to denote children and young people. This chapter uses the example of children who are overweight or obese, or at risk of becoming so; however, the methods are applicable to most health behaviour change, including giving up smoking, taking more exercise and new medicine regimens.

The health of the child population in the UK, and particularly the number of children who are overweight or obese, is becoming a major concern for the government and healthcare providers. In 2006, 16 per cent of children aged 2–15 years were classified as obese; in 1995 only 11 per cent of this age range were obese.[1]

*There is ongoing debate on the definition of overweight and obesity in childhood. Body mass index (BMI) is a measure of overweight and obesity in children although it is liable to change substantially as the child is growing. The clinical definition of overweight and obesity in children is based on BMI percentile charts for boys and girls plotted at different ages from 2 to 16 years. The National Institute for Health and Clinical Excellence (NICE) in England recommends that tailored clinical intervention should be considered for children with a BMI at or above the ninety-first centile, depending on the needs of the individual child and family, and that an assessment of co-morbidity should be considered for children with a BMI at or above the ninety-eighth centile.[2]*

One of the means by which obesity can be tackled is through ensuring that children and their parents are informed of healthy behaviours and provided with the tools and skills to make changes. The children's nurse can have a key role in encouraging the adoption of healthier behaviours by children and their significant adults. It is acknowledged that healthier behaviours can have a big impact on health status.

*Interventions to change behaviour have enormous potential to alter current patterns of disease.*[3,p.6]

The document *Behaviour change at population, community and individual levels*[3] acknowledges that many attempts to change people's behaviour have been unsuccessful or, at best, partially successful. The lack of success is ascribed to a failure to take account of the theories and principles guiding health promotion in practice; however, this conclusion falls short of explaining the full complexity and reasons for the success, partial success or failure of initiatives to improve health. Health – good or bad – is determined by many more factors than individual behaviour.

Not everyone experiences the same levels of health. In childhood the factors that promote health are often determined by the child's social and economic environment, which in turn is determined by family circumstances. Children are often powerless to influence the economic environment in which they live. If a family experience socioeconomic deprivation their access to healthcare, education, employment and a safe environment can be compromised and this situation leads to inequalities in health. This chapter explains the term health inequalities and discusses the subsequent challenges for nurses who are responsible for promoting children's health and preventing ill-health. The impact of government public health policy on reducing health inequalities and guiding effective practice is outlined, and the importance of maintaining a family-centred and partnership-based style of working is debated.

There is a stark lack of knowledge about the most effective ways to encourage health behaviour change in children. Indeed most behaviour change models have been designed to promote the health of adults and are either simply assumed to apply to children or, worse still, never used with children.

No specific models have yet been designed for use in child contexts. We have appraised the literature on the theories and models of health behaviour change. Using our combined expertise in public health education and research, health promotion, health visiting and children's nursing, we have presented an adaptation of Rollnick *et al.*'s[4] 'key tasks model' (Figure 5.1) (see page 54) as a suitable framework for nurses to encourage health behaviour change in children, young people, parents or guardians. Case studies are provided online by which readers can begin to see how the theories and models of health behaviour change can be applied. Two of the authors, Forbes and Baker, have extensive experience of working with families and the case studies are very typical of the real life situations they have encountered.

## HEALTH, HEALTH INEQUALITIES AND THE ROLE OF POLICY

### What is 'health' and how can 'improved health' be achieved?

| KEY WORDS |
| --- |
| Definition of health     Determinants of health |
| World Health Organization     Levels of health |
| Ottawa Charter Equity     Equality     Health policies |
| Health inequalities |

Health has long been understood as more than the simple *absence of illness*, as people's ideas of *health* and *being healthy* vary widely and will be shaped by their culture, experiences, beliefs and knowledge. Children may have a very basic understanding of what health is such as, 'When I'm ill it stops me doing the things I want to do'. Adults will have more sophisticated understandings of health and, as health professionals working with a range of clients, children's nurses should be prepared to debate and discuss the different meanings of the word *health*.

The World Health Organization[5] extended their original definition of health, which is often used to guide professional practice:

*A concept of health is the extent to which an individual … is able on one hand to realise aspirations and to satisfy needs and on the other hand to change or cope with the environment. Health is therefore seen as a*

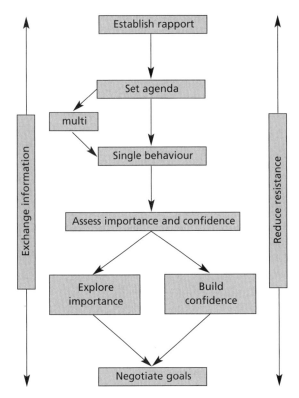

**Figure 5.1** The key tasks model (adapted with permission from Rollnick *et al.*[4]).

*resource for everyday life, not the object of living, it is a positive concept emphasising social and personal resources as well as physical capabilities.*[5,p.1]

From this definition it could be concluded that:

- health can be seen as a resource, not just a state of being;
- coping with change is an important part of being healthy;
- achievement of personal goals is important.

Seedhouse[6] argues that because the *obstacles* to health vary, *work* for health improvement will be diverse. For example, a doctor may be required to help a child overcome a biological obstacle such as an infection; a new home might provide an important motivation for a parent to make lifestyle changes; and banning smoking in public places is an example of a societal approach to improving health. A nurse might work with a family, or with individuals from a family, to discuss and resolve issues that are impacting on the health of more than one family member.

- *Health does not have a single undisputed meaning*
- *Health can be seen as a means or as an end, i.e. health can be something we want to acquire or can be seen as a way to acquire something we wish to achieve*
- *People, and their understanding of health, cannot be fully understood in isolation from what they do in their lives and what they want to achieve and, finally*
- *All theories of health help us to understand the obstacles to the achievement of human potential. The obstacles may be biological, environmental, societal, familial or personal.*[6]

Seedhouse[6] developed his own definition of health:

*A person's health is equivalent to the state of the set of conditions which fulfil or enable them to work to fulfil their realistic chosen and biological potentials.*

He argued that a person will perceive themselves as healthy if they are able to achieve personal goals – their *potential*. If health is concerned with human potential then it is important to understand the *factors* that impact on human potential. These factors can also be known as *the determinants of health* and are discussed in the next section.

## The determinants of health

From the definitions of health discussed in the previous section it can be concluded that a person will perceive themselves as healthy if they are able to achieve personal goals and to reach their potential. The *barriers* to a person's ability to reach their goals has been widely reported by many authors, including Graham,[7] Seedhouse[6] and the Department of Health publication *Saving lives: our healthier nation.*[8] The factors which determine health, i.e. the determinants of health, can be considered as layers of influence, ranging from purely individual characteristics to factors that affect society as a whole. Examples of determinants of health are given in Table 5.1. This table is more complex than it might seem, the next section explains it in more detail.

- Age, gender and genetic make-up are fixed individual characteristics which can determine a child's health. Age determines stage of development; gender and genetics will determine the diseases or conditions that a child is susceptible to, for example haemophilia is more prevalent in boys.

**Table 5.1** The determinants of health

| Layer of influence | Fixed individual characteristics | Lifestyle | Social environment | Wider environmental and cultural | Political sphere |
|---|---|---|---|---|---|
| Factors of influence | Genes | Diet | Poverty | NHS | Style of government |
| | Sex | Physical activity | Employment | Education | |
| | Age | Smoking | Quality of housing and sanitation | Social Services | |
| | | Alcohol | | Transport | |
| | | Sexual behaviour | Leisure | Food/agriculture | |
| | | Drugs | Social networks community and family | Air quality | |
| | | | | Water quality | |
| | | | | Health and safety | |
| | | | Community support services | | |

- The next layer of influence on a child's health is lifestyle factors, and here the behaviour of the child and/or the parents may be important. Lifestyle issues include whether a person smokes, the food they eat, the amount of exercise they take and the risky behaviours that they may or may not indulge in.
- Immediate environmental factors impacting on health status can include obvious environmental factors, such as the condition of housing, sanitation and access to recreational space, and also issues such as whether a parent has a job and the family social networks and support systems.
- Wider environmental and cultural determinants could include government policies to protect or maintain health, the provision of universal services such as education and health services, agriculture and food provision and the standard of living conditions – including pollution, rates of employment and health and safety at work.
- The overarching sphere of influence is that of politics and government action. A particular style of government will define decision-making and policy direction and this will impact on the provision of services and the laws of the land.

As you can see from this brief description, the determinants of health consist of a broad range of factors. It is important to understand that a child's behaviour is not the only determinant of their health status. A child's health is determined by many interacting factors, some of which are more

important at certain times in a child's life and some of which are under a child's or their parents' control but many which are not. Many determinants of health also lie beyond the control and reach of health service providers: housing, education and government policies have important effects on health but are not under the direct control of the health service. When nurses work to improve health and the focus is on health behaviour change, we need to appreciate that if the child or their parent does not change their behaviour this could be for many other reasons than our lack of skill in behaviour change technique.

## Health inequalities

Over the past 20 years the health of the population has improved; life expectancy, for example, is at its highest recorded level. Impacts have been made through improved treatments and early prevention. Improvements in health have not been consistent across different groups of the population however. For example, 5-year-olds living in the north-east and north-west of England have, on average, two decayed, missing or filled teeth. In the West Midlands, the average is one tooth.[9] This is an example of an inequality in health. Health inequality is the term used in Britain to describe the differences in health status between particular groups of the population, and these differences exist despite the provision of a universal and free health service.

Several important reports have examined health inequalities and made recommendations for action: The Black Report;[10] The Acheson Report;[11] Wanless.[12]

The term equality is not synonymous with the term equity, and they are often mistakenly used interchangeably, as are the terms inequality and inequity.[13] Inequity relates to inequalities that are avoidable, unfair and unjust.[13] Kaplan[14] suggests that improving average health is not necessarily associated with *equity*. What this means is that although *overall* the health of the population improves, the improvement is not *equal* across all groups. Factors such as poverty, unemployment, standard of housing and availability of services can contribute to poor (or good) health and are amenable to change through government and societal action.[15]

Graham[7] suggested that inequalities were inextricably linked to social position. Certainly, disease and death rates are comparatively higher in some population groups including ethnic minorities, the very old or the very young, women and those living in areas of deprivation. Children are born into families and assigned a social position dependent on the socioeconomic circumstances of the family and therefore have no control over the influences affecting their health. Social disadvantage is particularly harmful when experienced early in life,[15] so children suffer most as a result of health inequalities. When children are developing and growing the physical, psychological and social factors that impact on their personal and their family resources will affect their ability to achieve their potential both in childhood and in adulthood. Therefore we believe it is ethical and equitable that health inequalities among children should be tackled positively in order that the barriers to long-term good child health are removed. Children's nurses have an important role to play in ensuring that health inequalities are identified and addressed.

## Policy for health

The *National service framework for children, young people and maternity services*,[16] *Every child matters: change for children*[17] and The Children Act[18] all highlight that in order to be healthy children need

to be safe. The healthier children are the more likely they will be to achieve their potential in all areas of their lives and the more able they will be to make a positive contribution to society and to achieve economic well being. If one accepts that the health of children depends on the socioeconomic circumstances of their family, then steps to end child poverty is key to improving the health of children. Since 1999 the Labour government in the UK has had an aim of ending child poverty within a generation. The government has consequently placed an emphasis on collaboration and partnership working as this is key to improving health, tackling poverty and reducing health inequalities.[19] There has been an acceptance of the concept of joined-up working as the best way to tackle a wide range of health determinants.

An example of joined-up working is the use of Public Service Agreements (PSAs). PSAs have been used by the British government since 1998 to guide the work of each governmental department. Each PSA sets out an outcome to be worked towards over 3 years; for example the Department of Health PSA 18[20] aims to 'promote better health and well-being for all'. Each agreement sets out targets and outcomes to be measured and proposes a delivery plan which includes how cross-governmental links will ensure the outcomes are met. The Department for Children, Schools and Families Oversees PSA 12, 'agrees to improve the health and well-being of children and young people'.[21] PSA 12 promises a focus on prevention, early intervention and enabling of children and young people and their families to make healthy choices. There is no question that the role of nurses makes an important contribution to the aims of PSA 12, the next sections discuss in more detail how nurses can make this contribution.

## Summary

It is clear from this overview of the concept of health inequality that many factors influence a child's health, many of which are beyond their personal control. Government policy has sought to eliminate or reduce unjust and preventable inequalities as all children have the right to health. The next section focuses on what you as a nurse can do in tackling the factors that determine the child's health.

# ENCOURAGING HEALTH BEHAVIOUR CHANGE WITH CHILDREN OR YOUNG PEOPLE AND THEIR FAMILIES

## The focus of children and young people's nursing: psychosocial determinants of health

### KEY WORDS

Psychosocial determinants of health   Behaviour change   Partnership working   Family-centred care   Working with the child through parents   Case study

Psychosocial determinants are those social factors that impact on the psychology of a child, i.e. the thing that a child is doing because of the situation they find themselves in and the ways in which they understand this situation.

Psychosocial determinants are important to nurses for several reasons.

- Children's nurses have numerous opportunities to promote health with children.
- Children's nurses may be unable to directly influence economic or structural factors that could improve health for a child and family but can and should be involved in influencing policy that affects health at local and national levels.
- Children's nurses can build professional relationships with children and families. They can encourage a child and explain strategies that enable them to cope more successfully with complex situations.

As nursing has a focus on the discussion of psychosocial determinants, nurses could take the opportunity to ask questions which might prompt consideration of health behaviour change. For example, you might ask a child, 'Have you thought about how to eat more healthily?' or 'Have you considered how you might be more physically active?'

In many instances these questions may be met with resistance or a negative response and it is for these reasons that Rollnick et al.[4] suggest that health practitioners develop strategies to avoid the subject of health behaviour change. They state that practice has been

> … guided by a crude combination of common sense, direct persuasion, simple advice and fearful information.[4,p.214]

In an effort to guide child nursing practice in more positive ways, the following section discusses the evidence for effective approaches to encouraging behaviour change with children and their families.

## Family-centred care

Family-centred care has been regarded as an underpinning principle to the nursing care of children since the Platt report[22] and has subsequently been formalised in many UK policies including *The national service framework for children, young people and maternity services*.[16] The principles of the family-centred care approach have been extensively researched and described. The generally agreed principles are that the family has the greatest influence over the child's health and wellbeing, and children's nurses should work in partnership with families to achieve the best health outcomes for the child.

Partnership working at all levels, at a macro-, meso- or micro-level, is generally ill-defined[23] but in children's nursing is closely associated with concepts such as information sharing, equity, respect, negotiation and empowerment. Recent work by Lee,[24] who studied the attitudes of children's nurses and understanding of family-centred care in practice, concluded that the key principles for effective partnership were good attitudes towards the family, which led to respect for the family; good communication; and ultimately better parental understanding. Effective partnership working resulted in all parties being more satisfied with their care, and health and wellbeing was improved. Almond and Cowley[23] provide empirical findings showing that working in partnership can lead to positive health outcomes.

Partnership working with families also includes partnership working with children. The principles of child participation, involvement and collaboration were set out in the United Nations Convention, Article 12 and have been included in UK policy since the *1989 Children Act*.[18] McNeish[25] explored the meaning of working in partnership with children and concluded that practitioners working with children need to consider competency, autonomy, development, age, maturity and rights, with due regard to the issue of protection. Therefore, practitioners need to steer a clear path between paternalism and child liberation, while recognising that childhood involves biological and psychological dependencies on adults which change with age and maturity.

As family-centred care is the key principle underpinning children's nursing it is important that the methods used to encourage health behaviour change are underpinned by a theoretical model that reflects the importance of working in partnership with the child and the family. The methods described in the following sections are appropriate for use with parents or children (the 'client'). Being child or family focused involves understanding client knowledge and perception of the proposed change and supporting the client's ideas for change with well-timed information. It is not about being an expert on what changes to make – the client is in the best position to decide what will work for them – it is about supporting the client to undertake the changes. We appreciate that often nurses deal with complex care situations where health behaviour change may be very low on the agenda; however, for ease of use, in the following examples an assumption has been made that the parent or the child (the 'client') have expressed an interest in changing a particular health behaviour.

## Models of behaviour change

The pragmatic approach proposed by Rollnick *et al.*[4] helps nurses to assess the family's knowledge base, values and beliefs with respect to a potential change, explores their readiness to change and enables practitioners to work with the family to support change. The aim of Rollnick *et al's*[4] client-centred platform is

- to encourage clients to express concerns;
- to help them to be more active in the consultation;
- to allow them to articulate what information they require;
- to give them greater control over decision-making about behaviour change;
- to reach joint decisions.

Rollnick *et al.*[4,p.8] posit that 'expert knowledge has a limited role in behaviour change discussion', meaning that simple advice-giving is not enough. The key to effective behaviour change discussion lies in the methods of communicating with clients. The aim of behaviour change talk should be to

ensure that clients become active decision-makers, not complacent advice-takers.

Understanding readiness to change is fundamental to achieving success with the Rollnick *et al.*[4] approach. One of the first behaviour change models that attempted to describe readiness was Prochaska and Diclemente's[26] 'stages of change' model. The stages of change model provided a framework which explained how people think when they are making a specific behaviour change. The stages include:

- pre-contemplation (not thinking about changing a specific behaviour);
- contemplation (thinking about making a change);
- preparation (getting ready to make the change);
- action (making the change);
- maintenance (the new behaviour becomes a habit).

Also, relapse (reverting to the old behaviour) is a normal part of behaviour change and is therefore to be expected. Relapse can happen at any stage.

This was the first model to recognise that people can be at different stages with regard to making specific changes and therefore clients require individualised programmes of intervention dependent on their stage of thinking. For example, talking with a child about taking action when the child is still at the pre-contemplation stage for a change will result in resistance.

The terminology may not be appropriate to use with children (or even some parents); however, a nurse may be able to recognise when their client is at a specific stage for a specific change and may wish to comment on this;

> It sounds like you have not thought about giving up smoking – am I jumping ahead of you here? (*Pre-contemplation*)
> So you have a plan to eat at least one piece of fruit every day; that's a really positive first step. (*Preparation*)
> It's great that you are playing football twice a week; that's a really healthy habit to have. (*Action*)

An important concept regarding readiness has been described by Rollnick *et al.*[4] These authors propose that readiness to change has two components:

- the *importance* of making the change
- the *confidence* to make the change.

This is because, to be ready, a client needs to understand *why* they should make a change and *how* they will make the change. This cannot be achieved through simple advice-giving, as clients must have their own understanding of *importance* and *confidence*. The role of the nurse is to talk with the client in such way that importance and confidence to change increases. Rollnick *et al.*[4] recommend that a numerical value for importance and confidence is elicited. The children's nurse can ask:

> On a scale of 1 to 10, where 1 is low and 10 is very high, how *important* is it to you to make this change?

and

> On a scale of 1 to 10 how *confident* are you about making this change?

It has been the authors' experience that the terms importance and confident are understood by children and young people. Although it is recommended that, if young people persistently choose '5' on the scale, that the option of selecting '5' is removed!

By asking about *importance* and *confidence* the nurse can gain very useful information and insight about the client's readiness to change. For example, a child who has ill-health as a result of a certain behaviour may state that making a change is very important because they know their health will improve if they do so. At the same time the child could reveal that they lack confidence because they have tried to make the change and not succeeded. Another child may state that their confidence is high because they believe, 'I could give this up tomorrow', but won't change because it is not important to them.

Resistance will arise if the nurse talks to a client in a way that does not match their readiness to change. For example, a children's nurse may assume that a change is important and give the client lots of information about how to change. However, the outcome will be reluctance and resistance if the client does not rate the change as important. Conversely, if a client is unclear about why a change is important it may be helpful to discuss the pros and cons of making the change. Alongside the tools of health behaviour change, a variety of communication skills are required. Rollnick *et al.*[4] stress the importance of

- encouragement,
- open questions
- active listening.

Rollnick *et al.*[4] (Table 5.2, page 60), the NICE behaviour change guidance[3] and guidance for the Health Trainer Initiative[27] have all attempted to synthesise the evidence for what works when encouraging health behaviour change. Some of these ideas are briefly explained here in an attempt to provide a useful framework of methods, tools and approaches which could be helpful when discussing health behaviour change. The caveat to these suggestions has to be that very little formal research has been carried out using these methods with children or young people. Rollnick *et al.*[4] raise the issue of possible danger being caused by the use of these methods with clients. They stress that the spirit of the method, a client-centred approach, is very important. They reason that as the alternative to these methods is simply 'telling a client what to do' then any conscious and well meant attempt to understand the client's position and to listen carefully is unlikely to cause harm.

Please see website for case studies on promoting health when working with parents, a 10-year-old and a 15-year-old.

**Table 5.2** Application of the Key tasks model: to encourage healthy eating (adapted from Rollnick et al.[4])

| Key task | What to do |
| --- | --- |
| Establish the relationship | The tasks at this stage will vary according to whether this is the first meeting, a subsequent meeting or the last meeting. At a first meeting it is important to help the child and/or parents to feel at ease, to encourage them to talk and to set the parameters for the meeting |
| | At subsequent meetings you will be reviewing their action plan so an early task would be to praise their achievements, however small |
| | If this is to be their last meeting with you, you need to alert them to the imminent ending of the relationship. Overall you need to be empathetic, family centred and supportive. Depending on the age of the child questions could be targeted at the child or parent but it is important to look for confirmation from all present at the interview |
| Negotiate the agenda | Check with the client that they are clear that the agenda is to talk about a health-related behaviour change which they wish to make. Reiterate that it is neither a 'counselling session' nor 'just a chat'; the expectation is that you will help them to identify changes that they wish to make. Resist the temptation to assume that you know what change the client should discuss. A client may look overweight but their first priority may be dealing with bullying rather than eating healthily. Try asking, 'What health behaviour change would you like to talk about today?' Encourage the client to be specific and positive about the particular health behaviour change. An expectation of 'wanting to lose weight' is far too vague. A target to 'eat more healthily' is a much better start; it is positive, and manageable, specific actions can be identified at the action-planning stage. The wording of targets is important as it can impact on motivation. A target to 'eat fruit and vegetables every day' is an achievable aspiration, positive and specific. Weight loss goals have not been found to be beneficial for most obese children. Children are growing and therefore find weight loss very difficult to monitor (Scottish Intercollegiate Guidelines Network[28]) |
| Assess the importance of and the confidence in making the particular change | For example ask, 'How important is it to you to eat more healthily?' and 'How confident are you about eating more healthily?' These simple questions will provide you (and the client) with huge insight into whether they wish to change and the reasons why they might not change. You can ask the client to score their feelings using a scale of 1 to 10, where 1 = low, 10 = high |
| Explore importance | You can now use the numerical score to find out more about how important making this change is to them. If the importance is low you could ask, 'What would have to happen for it to become more important for you to make this change?' If importance is low there may be limits to what you can achieve. It may be that the client will not change until there is a crisis or something else in their life changes. Give the client information if they request it. One technique you could try is to encourage the client to look at the benefits and barriers for change; this may tip the balance towards change. Murtagh et al.[29] found that one of the greatest barriers to behaviour change in children was the parent's lack of recognition of the need for change. You may need to provide information (see later stage) to allay any fears or misconceptions |
| | If importance to change is high then acknowledge this and explain that any relapses may engender feelings of guilt |
| Build confidence | Now discuss the score for confidence. Confidence can vary in different situations so ask the client to describe situations when they would not feel confident about making or maintaining a change as this could help them to avoid relapse. If the client is fearful of relapse try, 'Let's talk through how you could deal with that situation'. Ask them to consider what has worked in the past. Resist the temptation to suggest a string of actions that they could undertake; as soon as you state 'you should …' you will encounter resistance. One method that does work is to say, |

In my experience I have found that other children/parents in your situation have tried (list ideas). What do you think?' Just changing the wording slightly ensures the emphasis is on possible options that the client could try, rather than it being a list of things they should do. Another useful technique is known as 'a look over the fence'; ask the client to describe, 'What it would be like tomorrow if you made this change tonight?'

| | |
|---|---|
| Negotiate an action plan | Encourage the client to identify actions they will take before the next meeting. Make sure the actions are specific and realistic, e.g. 'eat more fruit', measurable; 'eat one piece of fruit' and time limited, e.g. 'eat one piece of fruit each day'. Preferably these actions should be written down |
| Discuss the next steps | Tasks here may include setting a date for the next meeting or saying goodbye |

Two tasks are *ongoing* throughout the meeting

| | |
|---|---|
| Exchanging information | Provide information on the client's terms. Try asking, 'What do you need to know about healthy eating?' or 'What do you already know about exercise?' or 'What do you think about what I have told you today?' Again resist the temptation to give information that you think they should have; check out their understanding as the meeting progresses |
| Reduce resistance | The aim throughout the meeting is to not elicit any 'yes, but(s) ...' Your approach is important here; you can make your point of view clear but you must not argue with the client, for example, 'I think that (making the change) would improve your health but I hear that you do not want to, is that right?' Instead of arguing try to 'stand alongside' the client and begin to appreciate their point of view. For example, 'What I'm hearing is that it seems unfair to you that others can eat as much as they want and not put on weight. How does that make you feel?' or 'It seems that you get frustrated when people tell you that all you have to do is exercise more; somehow it seems much more complicated to you, is that right?' |

Understanding the client's point of view should help you and them to work through ambivalence. Rather than constantly discussing why they do not want to change, try finding out what it is they do want to change

If you (and the client) are clear that now is not the right time for them to change you can try the following:

• Summarise the situation as you see it and check this perception with the client

• Reassure the client that change takes time

• Let the client know that it is better to think things through rather than rush into a decision

• Reassure the client that you will be there to support them if later they decide that they do want to make the change

The term 'client' is used throughout to denote a child, young person, parent(s) or guardian(s).

 Go to the website to find the PowerPoint presentation for this chapter and MCQs to test your knowledge. **www.hodderplus.com/childnursingskills**

# REFERENCES

1  Information Centre (2008) *Statistics on obesity, physical activity and diet: England, January 2008.* The Information Centre (www.ic.nhs.uk).

2  Department of Health (2007) *Definitions of overweight and obesity* www.dh.gov.uk/en/Publichealth/Healthimprovement/Obesity/DH_4133948 (accessed 15 October 2008).

3  National Institute for Health and Clinical Excellence (2007) *Behaviour change at population, community and individual levels.* London: NICE (www.nice.org.uk).

4  Rollnick S, Mason P, Butler C (1999) *Health behaviour change: a guide for practitioners.* London: Churchill Livingstone.

5  World Health Organization (1986) *Ottawa charter for health promotion.* Canada: WHO.

6  Seedhouse D (2001) *Health: the foundations for achievement,* 2nd edition. Chichester: John Wiley & Sons.

7  Graham H (ed.) (2000) *Understanding health inequalities.* Buckingham: Open University Press.

8  Department of Health (1999) *Saving lives: our healthier nation.* London: The Stationery Office.

9  Department of Health (2007) *Health profile of England 2007.* www.dh.gov.uk/en/Publicationsandstatistics/Publications/PublicationsStatistics/DH_079716 (accessed 15 October 2008).

10  Black D, Townsend P, Davidson N (1982) *Inequalities in health: the Black report,* Harmondsworth: Penguin.

11  Department of Health (1998) *Independent inquiry into inequalities in health (The Acheson Report)* London: The Stationery Office.

12  Wanless D (2004) *Securing good health for the whole population: final report.* London: The Stationery Office (www.dh.gov.uk).

13  Almond P (2002) An analysis of the concept of equity in health services and its application to health visiting. *Journal of Advanced Nursing* 37: 598–606.

14  Kaplan GA (2002) Upstream approaches to reducing socioeconomic inequalities in health. *Revista brasileira de Epidemiology* 5(Suppl 1).

15  Starfield B (2004) Promoting equity in health through research and understanding, *Developing World Bioethics* 4(1):76–95.

16  Department of Health (2004) *National service framework for children, young people and maternity services.* London: DH.

17  Department for Education and Skills (2004) *Every child matters.* London: DfES.

18  HM Government (1989, 2004) The Children Act. London: HMSO.

19  Baggott R (2004) *Health and health care in Britain,* 3rd edition. Basingstoke: Palgrave Macmillan.

20  HM Treasury (2007) *PSA delivery agreement 18: promote better health and wellbeing for all.* London: The Stationery Office (www.hm-treasury.gov.uk).

21  HM Treasury (2008) *PSA delivery agreement 12: to improve the health and well-being of children and young people.* London: The Stationery Office (www.hm-treasury.gov.uk).

22  Platt HC (1959) *Report to the Minister for Health on the welfare of children in hospital.* HMSO: London.

23  Almond P, Cowley S (2008) Partnerships for public health: professional involvement to improve health and wellbeing. In: *Public health skills: a practical guide for nurses and public health practitioners.* Blackwell Scientific: Oxford.

24  Lee P (2007) Women and children: what does partnership in care mean for children's nurses? *Journal of Clinical Nursing.* 16: 518–526.

25  McNeish D (1999) Promoting participation for children and young people; some key questions for health and social welfare organisations. *Journal of Social Work Practice* **13**(2): 192–203.

26  Prochaska JO, DiClemente CC, Norcross JC (1992) In search of how people change: applications to addictive behaviors. *American Psychologist.* **47**: 1102–1114.

27  Michie, S, Rumsey, N, Fussell, A, et al. (2007) *Improving health: changing behaviour. NHS health trainer handbook.* London: Department of Health (www.dh.gov.uk).

28  Scottish Intercollegiate Guidelines Network (2003) *Management of obesity in children and young people: a national guideline.* www.sign.ac.uk.

29  Murtagh J, Dixey R. and Rudolf M (2006) A qualitative investigation into the levers and barriers to weight loss in children: opinions of obese children. *Archives of Diseases in Childhood* **91**: 920–923.

## FURTHER READING

Ewles L, Simnett I (2003) *Promoting health: a practical guide,* 5th edition, Edinburgh: Balliere Tindall.

## CHAPTER 6

# Planning and assessing the care of children and young people

Alan Glasper and Gill McEwing

## LEARNING OUTCOMES

*Upon completion of this chapter, the reader should be able to accomplish the following:*
1 Identify the sources of nursing theory
2 Define the nursing process and discuss its importance in the delivery of nursing care
3 Discuss the application of APIE and SOAPIE
4 Write a care plan
5 Discuss the use of different nursing models

## CHAPTER OVERVIEW

Nursing has a theoretical base that has many elements, including physiology, psychology, pathology, pharmacology and sociology. To deliver quality care to patients that is focused, safe and organised it needs to be planned. Documenting the plan of care for a patient and its implementation ensures continuity of care and provides a legal document demonstrating that care has been delivered.

Care can be organised using the nursing process, and nursing models can help focus care to meet the specific needs of patients.

## WHAT IS NURSING THEORY?

Nursing theory is the cognitive knowledge and understanding that is used by practitioners to help them deliver the best possible care based on best evidence. Nursing theory is partly drawn from a range of interconnected subjects from the arts and sciences domains that can be applied to the practice of nursing.[1] This knowledge comes from experiential learning and research and is part of the rich tradition that has been linked to the development of nursing since it first aspired to professional status in the wake of Nightingale. The importance of children's and young people's nurses delivering care that is underpinned by evidence-based theory is perhaps reflected in Nightingale's famous pronouncement articulated in her notes for nursing (1859):[2]

*Children: they are affected by the same things [as adults] but much more quickly and seriously.*[2,p.72]

It is because children are different from adults and become sicker much more quickly that children's nurses need a cognitive toolkit to help them successfully manage the whole care paradigm of sick children. Great Ormond Street's Hospital For Sick Children's most famous matron, Catherine Jane Wood, has left children's nurses a powerful legacy to abide by, for it was she who first indicated that if sick children require special nursing then sick children's nurses would require special training.[3] It is this training in the ability to deliver care based on nursing theory which is the hallmark of the professional nurse.

Despite its history nursing is still a relatively new science and most of the research-based theories of nursing have been produced in the last 30 years, and not all of them necessarily support one another. Much theory has emerged from North America where early female emancipation was responsible for the growth of undergraduate nursing within the university sector. In the contemporary UK setting there have been some criticisms of the way in which North American nursing theory has been imported into our nursing landscape. There may of course have been some slight resentment at this tacit acknowledgement that somehow the UK nursing profession was falling behind its North American counterpart. After all, it was British nurses who through Nightingale and later Mrs Ethel Bedford Fenwick pioneered worldwide nursing as a professional vocation for women. This not withstanding it is North American nurses who have paved the way in developing the underpinning method of delivering care to patients through the use of the nursing process.

The antecedents of the introduction of the nursing process are a reflection that nursing was evolving from the biomedical model in which the nurse primarily provided the care prescribed by the doctor. This medical model is primarily based on pathophysiology and the treatment of disease and does not fully take into account the psychological, social or cultural differences between individual patients. The new age of nursing as pioneered by Florence Nightingale recognised that patients were individuals, and she believed it was the nurse's responsibility to adapt the environment to enable the patient to have the optimum opportunity of recovery.

> **KEY POINTS**
>
> Nursing theory is knowledge that comes from experiential learning and research and is used by the nurse to guide practice

## WHAT IS THE NURSING PROCESS?

The nursing process is a framework for organising individualised nursing care; it involves four stages: assessment, planning, implementation and evaluation. The intention of the nursing process is to enable continuity of care by thorough documentation of information, to provide continuous observations and ensure effective interventions. However, there has been a lot of criticism of the nursing process approach to care as it imposes rigid constraints on practice and is cumbersome and outdated.[4]

Care plans provide an excellent means through which the rights of children and their families can be respected. They enable children and families to be fully informed and share in decision-making about their care.[5,6]

The involvement of children and families in the planning and implementation of care is recognised by professional bodies as vital in the formation of effective partnerships with families and children in the provision of care and healthcare services.[6]

The Nursing and Midwifery Council requires nurses to respect the patient or client as an individual and recognise and respect the role of patients and clients as partners in the contribution they can make to it. This includes identifying their preferences regarding care.[7]

The primary rationale for using the nursing process is the creation of a care plan that is used to determine the nursing care given to an individual patient.

An essential component is that the goals or objectives of the care plan are measurable to enable care to be evaluated and then improved upon.

Before the introduction of the nursing process many nurses delivered patient care in a piecemeal manner, often using task allocation where one nurse might administer all the ward medications and another might perform all the surgical dressings, and so on. In seeing the patient as a series of tasks the holistic nature of nursing was often lost. For many the introduction of the nursing process was liberating and probably heralded the advent of what later became known as primary nursing. Primary nursing facilitated through the use of the nursing process encouraged nurses to provide the total care package to the whole patient, often on a one-to-one basis rather than by functional tasks. Thus the concept of 'my patient and my nurse' became synonymous with nursing practice from the later part of the twentieth century.

It is important to differentiate between the nursing process itself, which is described as a way of thinking about nursing in a logical, problem-solving manner, and the written nursing process documentation or care plan, which must be viewed as a tool of the nursing process.

The nursing process can be perceived as the cognitive vehicle for planning the cooordination of care delivered to a patient. Universally it is the language of nursing, and wherever you work you will use the same basic steps which constitute the nursing process, i.e. care delivered using four steps (APIE or SOAPIE see below). It is important to remember that patient care must be documented and every child should have an individual plan of care which has been determined following a full nursing assessment. In legal terms *if it was not documented it never happened*.

The nursing process (Figure 6.1) can be applied in any nursing healthcare situation and offers nurses a cognitive toolkit to assess, plan, implememnt and evaluate care. The nursing process is easy to use because it is systematic. It's use in practice does however require a number of nursing skills, namely a good understanding of how health problems can impact on an individual child with reference to pathophysiology and social science. Additionally, the use of the nursing process requires nurses to have excellent interpersonal skills of communication with added well-developed listening skills. Finally, the nursing process requires nurses who are technically proficient in delivering care based on best evidence.

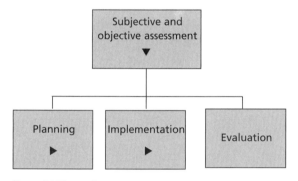

**Figure 6.1** The nursing process.

## What is APIE?

APIE is an acronym for

1 assessment
2 planning
3 implementation
4 evaluation.

However the North Americans prefer to use the same four steps differently (SOAPIE)

## What is SOAPIE?

SOAPIE is an acronym for

1 subjective
2 objective
3 assessment
4 planning
5 implementation
6 evaluation

## USING THE NURSING PROCESS IN YOUR PRACTICE

The whole purpose of using the nursing process is to help you the children's nurse plan and deliver care to child and family which fulfils the whole ethos of nursing as first defined by one of the most influential nursing theorists of the twentieth century, Virginia Henderson. Glasper[8] cites her enduring definition of nursing.

> *The unique function of the nurse is to assist the individual, sick or well, in the performance of those activities contributing to health or its recovery (or to a peaceful death) that he would perform unaided if he had the necessary strength, will or knowledge and to do this in such a way as to help him gain independence as rapidly as possible.*[8,p.91]

Henderson delineated the activities contributing to health as activities of daily living and stressed that professional nurses are responsible for planning, providing and evaluating nursing care in all settings. They do this by assessing how efficiently patients (or families) achieve these activities of daily living.[9]

Children's and young people's nurses in contemplating Henderson's definition of nursing are able to interpret it by seeing the family as a whole in need of the nurse's support to help them in the performance of those activities which are compromised by illness. Clearly, very young children may not be developmentally able to fulfil their own activities of daily living and will rely on the parent to do this for them. The use of the nursing process is thus the hallmark of the professional nurse.

## APIE/SOAPIE in practice

- *Assessing patient's needs or nursing problems subjectively and objectively*: During the assessment stage of the nursing process the nurse must undertake a full and detailed assessment of the child in the context of the family. This will probably be from a parent. This begins with the S element of the SOAPIE nursing process. The S or subjective assessment is sometimes known as 'an across the room assessment' and relies on a nurse's experience and intuition. The ability to observe a child without even interacting with them is a skill that grows with experience, and the subjective cues elicited during this period of observation may be invaluable in helping to identify actual or potential problems. For example, how the child holds him/herself and the child's demeanour and facial expressions can all be subjectively appraised before commencing the O or objective assessment. During this stage the nurses are objectively assessing the child's pulse, respiratory rate, $O_2$ saturations, blood pressure, etc. The whole assessment process can be guided and enhanced by the use of a nursing model.

- *Planning care*: Nursing care has always been planned; however, in recent times the focus of care has changed from the completion of tasks to the provision of holistic care where patients are viewed as individuals with diverse and individual needs.[10]

  Planning care should involve where possible the child and family to uphold the overarching family-centred care philosophy of children's and young person's nursing. Planning care involves reviewing all of the identified needs or patient problems and prioritising them. Glasper[8] discusses how Maslow's hierarchy of human needs can help nurses objectively plan nursing care. Clearly, if a child has compromised respiratory efforts this must be prioritised before planning dietary intake for example. Care plans are frameworks through which nurses apply the nursing process in addressing the needs of their patients. A nursing care plan is a written statement of the patient's nursing problems and the measures that will be used to effect a solution or mediate these problems (Johnson, 1980 cited in Ref. 11).

  Care pathways or critical pathways involve all the multidisciplinary team involved in the treatment and management of a patient and provide a programme of care delivery involving all the professionals: they are thought to provide care that is focused, cost effective and collaborative.[12] For each clinical problem the essential steps involved in the care of the patient are set out and planned with regard to that individual's expected progress. They provide a plan of desired patient outcomes, linked to an estimated time frame and the resources available. They can assist in the application of national evidence-based guidelines into local practice. Care pathways have the advantage of improving teamwork, reducing duplication of documentation and providing continuous records of care for a patient.[13]

  When using care pathways or predetermined core care plans it is important these should still be individualised. Some NHS Trusts have care planning software which allows nurses to produce a care plan for each child. When planning care the nurse must ensure that the goals of care are achievable. Sometimes it is useful to use the acronym SMART when setting objectives of care.

  S  *Specific*. The objectives of care set by the nurse in consultation with the family must accurately specify what it is that will be measured as an indicator of achievement. Hence if the child is dehydrated and needs a certain volume of fluid intake then this can be specified by the hour or day.

  M  *Measurable*. The nurse should be in a position to accurately determine, for example, that the child has drunk the prescribed volume of fluid as specified in the nursing care plan or care pathway.

  A  *Achievable*. For example,. was the specified volume of fluid prescribed for the child achievable in practice? Was the plan successful in achieving the objective set?

  R  *Realistic*. Were the targets set through the nursing plan objectives achievable given the resources available to the nursing staff, etc.?

  T  *Time*. Have you set a time frame for achieving your specific child-focused nursing care plan objectives?

- *Implementing care*: The implementation element of the care plan is crucial as this gives clear directions to the reader of the plan on how the care objectives are to be met. This might include for example specific instructions on the timing of infant feeds or how often a dressing should be changed.

- *Evaluating care*: All objectives of care and the nursing actions to implement them should be evaluated by the primary nurse responsible for the child. Amendments to the nursing care plan are made in light of the evaluations. Once an objective has been achieved for example this can be deleted from the care plan. Conversely, if the recommended action failed to meet the objective then further changes to the care plan will be necessary.

## Writing a care plan

After subjectively and objectively assessing the child, the nurse is then able to list and prioritise the problems that require a nursing intervention. Each nursing problem or unfulfilled need as in the case of a developmentally immature child (or child with complex disabilities) will require an (SMART) objective of care. The actions needed to be undertaken by the nurse or carer to fulfil the objective and thus fulfil the unmet need or problem can be detailed on the care plan. Figure 6.2 is an example of how care plans are usually configured. To fulfil the evaluation stage of the APIE/SOAPIE nursing process formulae, it is necessary to include a review period on the action component of the care plan. This might be an hourly evaluation for a problem such as pyrexia or a daily evaluation for a child with dietary needs.

## WHAT ARE NURSING MODELS?

Nursing models are a combination of theories and concepts that provide a framework for nurses to assess, plan, implement and evaluate the care they give. Unlike two-dimensional models such as maps or three-dimensional models such as model buildings, nursing models cannot be examined in the same way, for they are cognitive. However, like a model car, a nursing model can be used to examine the world of nursing in much the same way as a car designer would examine the model of the car he intends to build before it is built, to assess it for aerodynamics or aesthetics. In this way the use of a nursing model allows nurses to explore the full parameters of their nursing interventions before they have actually delivered them. It is helpful to think of a nursing model as allowing you to build the world of nursing inside your head. Wimpenny[14] has raised doubts about the use of nursing models in contemporary nursing practice and has revealed that there is limited evidence that models are being explicitly used in the clinical domain. This might be explained by the growing trend of using computer-generated care plans or care pathways where the philosophical underpinnings might be hidden or lost. Despite this, it is important to stress that the nursing process is optimised when used in conjunction with a nursing model.

| Identified problem or or need | Objective of care | Action to be implemented |
|---|---|---|
| 1 | | |
| 2 | | |

**Figure 6.2** Sample care plan design.

## Benefits of care plans

- Improved quality of care
- Improved communication
- Evidence-based practice
- Reduced risk of litigation
- Standardised care
- Continuity of care
- Patient and staff satisfaction (Figure 6.3, page 68)

There are many nursing models that have been proposed by nursing theorists[15] but it is beyond the scope of this text to consider them all in detail. There are several models which are commonly used in the nursing of sick children and young people. The commonest are 'activities of daily living models', which include Henderson,[9] Roper *et al.*[16] and Orem (cited in Ref. 17). Additionally, a further model is applied to the care of sick children and can be used in conjunction with other models that were

| Problem/need | Objective of care | Plan of care |
|---|---|---|
| **The infant is vomiting and has loose stools** | | |
| Potential problem of dehydration | Prevent dehydration | Maintain intravenous infusion as prescribed |
| | | Offer oral rehydration solution at a ...mL/hour for 24 hours |
| | Document fluid balance | Record intake and output on a fluid balance chart |
| Return to normal dietary intake | Diet and fluid intake will be re-established prior to discharge | Gradually re-introduce normal diet and fluids. Avoid milk until fully recovered |
| To identify the underlying cause of the diarrhoea and vomiting | | |
| **Danger of pyrexia** | | |
| Potential problem of infection causing raised temperature | Early Identification of changes in body temperature and to respond appropriately | Record body temperature 4 hourly or as required |
| **Risk of skin excoriation** | | |
| | Skin excoriation to be kept to a minimum | Keep nappy area clean and dry. Apply barrier creams as required |
| **Potential danger of cross-infection** | Cross-infection will be prevented | Nurse in isolation, adhere to trust policy for isolation of infections |
| **Prevent distress to child and parents caused by isolation** | Child and family distress due to admission and isolation will be prevented | Provide psychological and physical support for child and parents as required |
| | | Support parents and encourage them to provide basic care |
| | | Explain to the family the need for isolation procedures |

**Figure 6.3** Example of care plan for an infant with diarrhoea and vomiting.

essentially designed for adults. Anne Casey's model for children's nursing[18] is all about partnership and has become standard practice in UK children's units. The central premise of these activities of daily living models is that normally people maintain their own functions in these areas, but in times of illness these may be compromised and require support from healthcare professionals. In the case of children some activities of daily living such as keeping the body clean may be compromised simply by developmental age. This is why children's nurses have adopted Casey's theoretical framework based on the notion of partnership and in turn on the philosophy of children's nursing, which believes in the notion of the indivisible family unit where parents (carers) provide essential care until the child is mature enough to do it themselves. Orem's model is sometimes called the self-care model and is orientated towards restoring an individual to a health status where self-care is possible. It is particularly useful in rehabilitation settings for example after childhood head injury.

## The activities of daily living (Henderson[9])

1 Breathe normally.
2 Eat and drink adequately.
3 Eliminate body waste.
4 Move and maintain desirable postures.
5 Sleep and rest.
6 Select suitable clothes, dress and undress.
7 Maintain body temperature within normal range by adjusting clothing and modifying the environment.
8 Keep the body clean and well groomed and protect the integument.
9 Avoid changes in the environment and avoid injuring others.
10 Communicate with others expressing emotions, needs, fears or opinions.
11 Worship according to one's faith.
12 Work in such a way that there is a sense of accomplishment.
13 Play or participate in various forms of recreation.
14 Learn, discover or satisfy the curiosity that leads to normal development and health and use of the available health facilities.

## The activities of daily living (Roper, Logan and Tierney[16])

1 Maintaining a safe environment
2 Breathing
3 Communicating
4 Mobilising
5 Eating and drinking
6 Eliminating
7 Personal cleansing and dressing
8 Maintaining body temperature
9 Working and playing
10 Sleeping
11 Expressing sexuality
12 Dying

## Orem's universal self-care requisites

1 Air
2 Water
3 Food
4 Elimination
5 Activity and rest
6 Solitude and social interaction
7 Hazard prevention
8 Promotion of normality

For further information, visit the websites below on a range of nursing models.[19]

- Virgina Henderson's definitions of nursing: http://www.stti.iupui.edu/library
- Imogene King's general system's framework: http://www.nurses.info/nursing_theory_person_king_imogene.htm
- Betty Neuman's systems model: http://www.neumansystemsmodel.com/
- Dorothea Orem's self-care framework: http://www.muhealth.org/~nursing/scdnt.html
- Hildegard Peplau's theory of interpersonal relations: http://publish.uwo.ca/%7Ecforchuk/peplau/hpcb.html
- Calista Roy's adaptation model: http://www2.bc.edu/~royca/
- Roper et al. Elements of nursing: a model for nursing based on a model of living: http://www.sandiego.edu/nursing/theory/roper.txt

There has been some disapproval of nursing models, and Mckenna[20] among others has been critical of some models because their structure prevents the nurse from being flexible and intuitive when trying to meet the patient's needs. Although Glasper[8] extols the benefits of pre-written core care plans, possibly the antecedents to care pathways, their very creation may shoehorn patients into care categories that ignore their individual needs or preferences. The original intention of pre-written core care plans was to identify only the essential core elements of care associated with, for example, a child in traction. They were never intended to impose care that was not individualised and failed to take into account the child's age, gender, social, emotional and cultural lifestyle.

Wigfiled and Boon[21] have linked the introduction of critical care pathways with attempts by nurses and others to detail the parameters of care provision for specific types of patients. The resultant care pathways attempt to describe the care required for the duration of the patient stay, sometimes on an hour-by-hour basis. Most professional children's nurses would be able to describe the typical pattern of care for a child in their care, particularly if they have considerable experience of nursing a certain type of child such as a child with a fractured femur. Care pathways attempt to make the sequences of care absolutely explicit so that all elements will be documented. This is important in an increasingly litigious climate of healthcare. Hence, critical pathways or integrated care pathways are multidisciplinary approaches to care that are being developed which provide care that is cost-effective, patient focused, multidisciplinary and collaborative. Importantly they are believed to be cost-effective, but little research has been done to evaluate whether care pathways improve the quality of patient care.[22]

Care pathways and care plans are seen by some as important tools in the provision of the holistic, child and family-centred care on which the fundamental principles of the *National service framework for children, young people and maternity services* are built.[23] They are integral to many Department of Health, NHS quality improvement incentives and they have key functions within the national clinical governance framework in safeguarding children and the provision of evidenced-based practice.[24-26]

> **KEY POINTS**
>
> - Nursing models can be used to assess, plan, implement and evaluate care
> - There are many nursing models designed for patients with different needs: Casey's model was specifically designed for caring for children
> - Care pathways can assist in the provision of multidisciplinary goal-focused care

 Go to the website to find the PowerPoint presentation for this chapter and MCQs to test your knowledge. **www.hodderplus.com/childnursingskills**

## REFERENCES

1  Colley S (2003) Nursing theory: its importance to practice. *Nursing Standard* **17**(46): 33–37.
2  Nightingale F (1859) *Notes on nursing: what it is and what it is not*. London. Duckworth and company (1970 reprint).
3  Wood CJ (1888) The training of nurses for sick children. *The Nursing Record* 6 Dec: 507–510.
4  Walsh M (1997/2002) *Watson's clinical nursing and related sciences*. London: Balliere Tindall.
5  United Nations (1991) *The United Nations Convention*. London: HMSO.
6  Royal College of Nursing (1992) *Paediatric nursing: a philosophy of care*. London: RCN.
7  Nursing and Midwifery Council (2004) *Professional code of conduct*. London: NMC.
8  Glasper A (1990) A planned approach to nursing children. In: Salvage J, Kershaw B (eds) *Models for nursing 2*. London: Scutari Press, Ch 10.
9  Henderson V (1978) The concept of nursing. *Journal of Advanced Nursing* **3**: 113–130.
10  Walsh (2001) *Models and critical pathways in clinical nursing: conceptual frameworks for care planning*. Edinburgh: Bailliere Tindall.
11  Hurst K (1993) *Problem solving in nursing practice*. London: Scutari Press.
12  Herring L (1999) Critical care pathways an efficient way to manage care. *Nursing Standard* **13**(47): 11–17, 36–37.
13  Norris AC, Briggs JS (1999) Care pathways and the information for health strategy. *Health Informatics Journal* **5**: 209–212.
14  Wimpenny P (2002) The meaning of models of nursing to practicing nurses. *Journal of Advanced Nursing* **40**: 346–354.
15  Chalmers H ( 1990) Nursing models and their relationship to the nursing process and nursing theory. In: Salvage J, Kershaw B (eds) *Models for nursing 2*. London: Scutari Press.
16  Roper N, Logan W, Tierney A (1983) A nursing model…why the nursing process is useful, when used in an explicit nursing framework. *Nursing Mirror* **156**(21): 17–19.
17  Aggleton P, Chalmers H (2000) *Nursing models and nursing practice*. Basingstoke: Mcmillan.
18  Casey A (2007) Partnership model of nursing. In: Glasper E, McEwing G, Richardson J (eds) *Oxford handbook of children's and young people's nursing*. Oxford: Oxford University Press.
19  Hambridge K, McEwing G (2009) Care of the adult: surgical. In: Glasper EA, McEwing G, Richardson J (eds) *Foundation studies for caring: using a student-based approach*. London: Palgrave. pp 440–477.
20  Mckenna H (1997) *Nursing theories and models*. London: Routlege.

21  Wigfield A, Boon E (1996) Critical care pathway development: the way forward. *British Journal of Nursing* **5**: 736–753.

22  De-Luc K (2000) *Care pathways: an evaluation of their effectiveness. Journal of Advanced Nursing* **32**: 485–496.

23  Department of Health (2004) *Executive summary, national service framework for children, young people and maternity services: change for children – every child matters.* London: HMSO.

24  Department of Health (1997) *The new NHS: modern, dependable.* DH: Leeds.

25  Department of Health (1998) *A first class service quality in the new NHS.* DH: Leeds.

26  Department of Health (2000) *The NHS plan: a plan for investment: a plan for reform.* London: The Stationary Office.

## CHAPTER 7

# Play provision for children in hospital

Katy Weaver and Joanna Groves

## LEARNING OUTCOMES

*Upon completion of this chapter, the reader should be able to accomplish the following:*

1 Appreciate the importance of play in hospital
2 Discuss the effects of hospitalisation on a child
3 Understand the role of the Hospital Play Specialist
4 Describe the types of therapeutic play techniques
5 Use specific play techniques to help children overcome debilitating fears
6 Identify the advantages of play in hospital
7 Explore play resources available and ways of using them more effectively
8 Make simple tools for therapeutic play techniques
9 Use simple therapeutic play techniques in their practice
10 Explore other therapy techniques available to children

## CHAPTER OVERVIEW

Therapeutic play techniques can be hugely beneficial to all members of the multidisciplinary team; however, the techniques used are not often understood and therefore rarely used unless a hospital play specialist is present to provide or facilitate such techniques. The role of the play specialist is still quite misunderstood, and so it is hoped that this chapter will give paediatric staff an insight into the role of the hospital play specialist, therapeutic play techniques used and how they can use these to their advantage in their own practice. The chapter aims to provide a better understanding of play in hospital and the importance both to the patient and to their families.

## 'NORMAL' PLAY

*Play is at the very centre of a healthy child's life. From the earliest age, playing helps children to learn, to relate to other people and to have fun.*[1]

*The food and drink of mental growth, play, is an essential requirement for a child's well-being and development.*[2]

Play is essentially the language of children; through play they are able to learn about their environment and, of course, themselves. Children are able to play from a very young age and so play becomes a useful tool for communicating before even the skills for verbal communication are acquired. It allows the child to learn, discover and experiment in an enjoyable way.[3]

The five main areas in which children develop are physical and sensory (gross and fine motor/manipulative skills), intellectual, social, emotional and language/cognitive. While playing and having fun, children develop in all areas without really being aware.

Children are unknowingly involved in different types of play depending on their age and stage of development. As they get older their social skills and ability to interact with others develop and adapt to the environment.

The four types of play are:

- *Solitary play*: The child will play alone/independently and pay no attention to others playing around him/her.
- *Parallel play*: Children may be playing the same game or activity and are aware of the presence of peers but they are not talking or interacting with each other and play independently.
- *Associative play*: Children are playing the same game or they are attending the activities of their peers; they are not interacting actively with each other but they are sharing and taking turns.
- *Cooperative play*: Children are working or playing together and interacting with their peers. They are able to organise their play activities and cooperate with each other to reach a common goal.

Some simple but effective messy activity ideas include gloop, jelly play, shaving foam/baked beans play and play dough. Please see the website to see how to make these.

There are lots of other activities that can really help to build a rapport with a child, among many other benefits. Board games, computer games, role play/pretend activities, story books and art and craft activities are all great fun and very adaptable to individual needs.

Be aware of cross-infection and health and safety issues, including allergies. Also, patients should have their own materials to play with, which can be discarded when they are finished or saved for that same patient to continue playing with later unless they can be washed effectively. All toys must be washable.

## EFFECTS OF HOSPITALISATION

Every child responds to hospitalisation in a different way: some will sail through, seemingly unaffected, while others will experience varied levels of anxiety/distress and other long-term effects. These could include:

- loss of concentration;
- relationships with peers and siblings affected;
- temperament changes due to loss of boundaries/control:
- loss of 'normal life' and what it entails, e.g. home, school, friends, etc.;
- loss of confidence and self-esteem;
- possible regression educationally and socially;
- poor coping techniques when faced with strong feelings of fear and anxiety;
- development of phobias.

Taylor *et al.*[4] explains that hospital experiences are stressful for children, the degree of which is varying.

*There are many factors that may affect a child's responses to hospitalisation including the child's previous experiences (of separation/ hospital visits etc), exhibited symptoms or lack of, relationship with parent/carer (we will use the term 'parent' from this point to refer to the child's primary carer) and the parents' own thoughts and feelings about upcoming visits and admissions to hospital. Of course, issues during the hospitalisation may also play a big part in influencing responses, such as the length of the child's stay, whether a parent/carer is present throughout the child's stay and the relationship the carers have with the hospital staff.*

Children, and many adults, are likely to be worried about a hospital admission; not only are they worried about physical pain they may have to endure, but they are also being confronted with a situation they are likely to know little about. Fear of the unknown will play a big part in the child's anxiety levels and illustrates the importance of preparation, sharing information and of any misconceptions being addressed at the earliest opportunity. There is an element also of children not knowing what is expected of them and how they should behave, particularly if it is their first experience of hospital. Discipline and boundaries are important for normal development in children and this remains true when a child is in hospital, although it may be difficult because of the child's individual circumstances. Ultimately maintaining boundaries will help the child to know what is expected of them and maintain a level of normality.

There will of course be times when exceptions need to be made and some lenience is necessary.

It is important to consider the child's individual needs and circumstances and be aware that all children display their emotions differently and so negative feelings may not be easy to detect. The parent/carer is usually able to help in this area as they will, in most cases, know their child better than anyone and will be able to compare behaviours with those displayed at home in a familiar and comfortable environment. The range of emotions experienced by a child during a hospital stay will be varied and sometimes difficult to deal with and express.

Feelings of vulnerability are inevitable when children are faced with an unfamiliar environment (with strange sights, sounds and smells, etc.), a number of people they don't know talking about things they may not always understand and the possibility of unpleasant/invasive procedures being performed with little notice. As well as all of this, they have had to leave behind family and friends, which may introduce separation anxiety/issues for the child and feelings of isolation.

The child's illness will also weigh on the child's mind and heighten feelings of fear, worry and uncertainty. Of course, this may be dependent on the child's concept of illness and the way they interpret it; this could depend on previous personal experiences of 'illness'. For example, a child with a tummy ache may find this more upsetting than being told they need surgery, because of associated feelings and lack of understanding.

Limitations as a result of any illness or disability may restrict the child further and increase their level of dependence on parents and medical staff. The pursuit of independence and psychological autonomy begins from birth,[5] and so the sudden loss of independence, and privacy can be very difficult to adjust to and can seriously affect confidence and self-esteem levels. The child also has to adjust to physical changes and self-image issues (i.e. loss of hair, scarring) and may at some point be reliant on medical equipment. A lack of routine and freedom may lead to boredom and frustration. These issues will affect children in different ways, depending on their age. Teenagers are often more self-conscious of their appearance and might find a change of body image difficult to accept, whereas a younger school age child may feel isolated or 'different' if physically unable to keep up with peers and the activities they participate in.

Children who have to visit the hospital frequently or endure long stays will experience interruptions in their education and as a result of this may fall behind, which can be a big worry at a time when it is so important to 'fit in'. It is unfortunately quite common for children to develop fears and phobias; this is often due to the child's medical requirements that don't always allow us the luxury of time. Children have also been found to suffer other psychological effects, such as withdrawal, depression and aggression.[6] Loss of concentration and regression are also common, and some children may go on to experience post-hospital disturbances.

It's worth remembering also that a well-prepared happy child is likely to be more compliant and recover faster, adding a cost-effective aspect to the play service. Play input helps to reduce the length of hospital stays and the amount of medical staff time that is required, and there is also evidence to suggest that play intervention reduces the need for children to be anaesthetised for medical procedures.[7]

Evidence of this is shown in an audit undertaken on a paediatric oncology unit within a regional radiotherapy centre. Over a 5-year period (1994–9) all patients between the ages of 2 and 5 years were subjected to a play preparation programme before radiotherapy, and data were collected. The data showed that the need for sedation was very low for a procedure which children of this age are often routinely sedated; this was due to an effective play preparation programme. Of the 62 children having radiotherapy during this period only six were sedated for the whole of their treatment, 52 required no sedation at all and no general anaesthetics were given. Also, of 1030 treatment days only 111 of those days required sedation.[8]

## PLAY IN HOSPITAL

*The hospital experience, whether it is as an in- or out-patient, presents the child or young person with a very particular challenge.*[9]

Having a Hospital Play Specialist or another member of staff dedicated to leading and facilitating play in hospital offers many benefits to the child, family and hospital staff. It provides opportunities to:

- *Provide a link to home* by allowing 'normal' play, children are able to act out scenes from home (i.e. role play) and remember things from home that they may not have seen for some time (i.e. photos and sound games). This is particularly important for long-stay patients or babies who have never been at home.
- *Aid normality.*
- *Boost/regain confidence and self-esteem* and allowing children to take some control back into their life; this could include giving the child an active part in their treatment, e.g. choosing to have oral medication in liquid or tablet form.
- *Minimise regression.*
- *Improve concentration skills.*
- *Enable the child to fulfil medical requirements in an enjoyable way.*
- *Act as an outlet for emotions*, giving children the opportunity to express their feelings, frustrations and tension in an appropriate manner. For example, a child in traction might like to play with balloons, Velcro darts or play dough to release tension.

- *Reduce stress and anxiety.*
- *Facilitate communication.*
- *Enable information to be passed on* in an appropriate and enjoyable manner, empowering the child and enabling informed consent.
- *Adapt games/activities for all children*, whatever their needs.
- *Aid all areas of development.*
- *Encourage parents and siblings to be involved.*
- *Provide often much needed boundaries*: without a 'normal' routine and unusual circumstances boundaries are slackened or lost completely leaving children feeling unsure and out of control;
- *Aid compliance with medical procedures.*
- *Help to divert thoughts* and occupy and stimulate minds and provide fun – escapism!

## THE ROLE OF THE HOSPITAL PLAY SPECIALIST

The role of the play specialist varies considerably depending on the area/department in which they are based; however, the main principles remain the same (Figure 7.1).

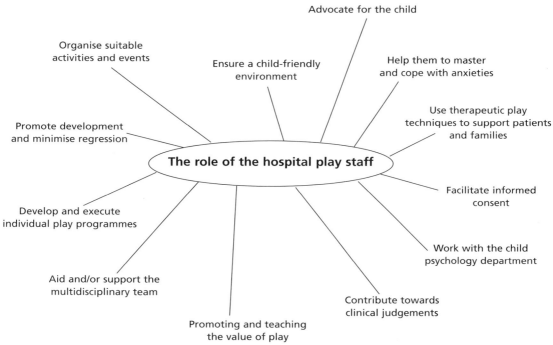

**Figure 7.1** Spider chart.

# THERAPEUTIC PLAY TECHNIQUES

The Department of Health[7] suggest in the Standard for Hospital Services that play techniques should be encouraged among the multidisciplinary team, adopting techniques modelled/taught by the hospital play specialist. Table 7.1 shows some of the more common therapeutic play techniques. These techniques can also be used to complement other traditional methods of pain control, but not replace them.

**Table 7.1** Therapeutic play techniques

| Therapeutic play techniques | |
|---|---|
| Preparation | Playing through an experience in anticipation: talking and sharing information, making plans and discussing options, photographs/books, role play with dolls/teddies and even the child themselves using real equipment wherever possible |
| Distraction/diversionary play | Involving the child in an activity, usually interactive to take the child's focus away from the procedure |
| Post-procedural play | Evaluating the procedure in an appropriate way with the child; reinforce positive behaviour with praise and rewards to promote confidence and self-esteem when faced with medical procedures in the future. It enables children to reflect on and make sense of the hospital experience[9] |
| Relaxation | Progressive muscle relaxation whereby regions of the body are relaxed in sequence to help control pain, nausea and vomiting and for stress management. Can include counting and deep breathing exercises |
| Guided imagery | This is used in conjunction with relaxation (above). Whitaker[10] describes guided imagery as 'a therapeutic technique that allows two people to communicate based on a reality that one of them has chosen to construe through a process of imaging' |
| Desensitisation and needle play | A process in which the child is subjected to controlled exposure of a feared object or situation until the feared object/situation then becomes associated with comfortable emotional state and a situation of which they are in control.[2] Needle play can assist in this but it is well planned and supervised |
| Modelling, role play and expressive arts | Children are encouraged to observe real procedures that show good coping skills; videos and books can be used too. This, in theory, gives them confidence and helps them to cope also. Art can be a fun way to express feelings and can take many forms. For example, syringe painting often helps children who are anxious about needles |

# PREPARATION: HOW TO PREPARE CHILDREN FOR A PROCEDURE

*The idea is simple: there is still much in hospitals that is unfamiliar, worrying and threatening and the more one can be prepared for an event, in order to offset the fear of the unknown, the better one copes.*[2]

The aims of preparation are to help the child to understand his or her illness and treatment, and to provide the opportunity to correct any mis-conceptions the child or family may have.

Preparation gives the child an opportunity to ask questions and express any feelings they may be experiencing through play activities.

Preparation is crucial to enable informed consent. Having a treatment or procedure explained to a child and family in a way that they can understand can ease the consent procedure and allow them to feel more comfortable with the procedure.

*Children are likely to experience changes from their normal routine in what they see, hear, touch and smell and should be prepared in all areas.*[2]

*It is evident that hospitalisation generated a range of fears and concerns for these children. The children's fears about unfamiliar routines, procedures and health professionals indicates the importance of preparatory procedures.*[11]

## THE STAGES OF PREPARATION

### Pre-admission

Preparation for a hospital admission should ideally begin at home. A pre-admission booklet should be sent out containing information about the ward, information about any planned procedure, advice on preparation activities that parents can carry out at home, as well as a list of children's books about hospital and any relevant, recommended websites that can be accessed.

Children and families should be invited to an informal visit to the ward or department they will be visiting. This allows opportunities for the child and family to ask any questions they may have, meet some of the staff and see the area they will be visiting for themselves.

A study of 203 children (7–12 years of age) was carried out between January 2004 and January 2005 in one of the largest acute-care hospitals in Hong Kong to examine the effects of therapeutic play on outcomes of children undergoing day surgery. The results showed that children who had received therapeutic play techniques 1 week before surgery reported significantly lower anxiety scores during both pre- and postoperative periods and showed fewer negative emotions at induction of anaesthesia. The therapeutic play included a tour of the unit, operating room and recovery room, a doll demonstration and the opportunity to touch and explore the real equipment. This is in comparison to a group of children who received routine information preparation involving a briefing session on pre- and postoperative care. The children that received therapeutic play preparation also had lower pain scores postoperatively.[12]

### On admission

The key factors for a child on admission are building a trusting relationship with the staff. Establish what toys, games or hobbies the child may like and allow time for normal play before introducing any hospital play.

This time can also allow the staff to assess the child before they carry out any preparation. The National Association of Hospital Play Staff (NAHPS)[13] states the following should be taken into account:

- age of child
- cognitive development
- emotional maturity
- individual vulnerability
- previous hospital/medical experiences
- cultural background and language
- coping strategies
- parental anxiety.

*Play preparation does not necessarily require elaborate organisation. Hospital dressing up clothes and equipment can be a part of the play provision on the wards so that children can dress up and enact events that are about to happen or have happened.*[4]

## PROCEDURE: General preparation

| Procedural steps | Evidence-based rationale |
| --- | --- |
| 1 Get to know the child first to build rapport and develop a level of trust | To ensure a level of trust is established with the child and to ensure that the correct information is shared |
| 2 When devising a plan with the child for a procedure, you need to be practical – don't make promises you can't keep | To maintain an element of trust and ensure that targets are achievable wherever possible, however small, to boost confidence and self-esteem |
| 3 Consider the environment | An environment full of distractions/interruptions, 'scary' sights, etc. will make preparation difficult and probably less effective for all involved |

| 4 Gain information prior to preparation | To ensure that the information you share with the patient is as accurate as it can be |
|---|---|
| 5 Be honest at all times but ensure the information you give is age appropriate; this applies to both the language/wording you use and the content of the information | To ensure a level of trust is established with the child and to ensure that the correct information is shared |
| 6 *Communication*: be aware of verbal and non-verbal communication (consider your tone of voice, body language and the child's eye level) *Language*: if the child or family has any specific words they use for things such as 'special sleep' or 'zip' for scars, try to use these in the explanations for consistency. If the child has no particular phraseology always use the real names for things to avoid confusion | It is essential to ensure that information is given to the child and family in a way that is understood and interpreted correctly |
| 7 Play sessions must always be supervised | To ensure safety at all times and to make sure that therapeutic play is beneficial and appropriate |
| 8 Document all therapeutic play input following local documentation guidelines/policies | This will aid planning and the monitoring of progression and inform other staff of your input and the patient's needs |
| 9 Assess the patient's individual needs, taking into consideration any contributing factors, and devise an individual play plan | To enable you to select the most appropriate and effective preparation technique and plan how to execute the plan and the aims |
| 10 Execute the chosen preparation techniques following the plan and assessing the patient's responses and behaviour throughout | To allow you to evaluate and adapt the techniques accordingly as session progresses |
| 11 Evaluate every session and document this on the individual play plan | This will allow you to assess any progress and plan for subsequent preparation sessions including any necessary changes |

## Methods of preparation

When you have taken into account all of the above an appropriate method should be selected, depending on the age of the child. An assessment of their stage of development and level of understanding should be taken into consideration, to give the child the information they need to be able to cope with the procedure.

Parents should be involved in the preparation process. The aims and benefits of play preparation should be discussed as well as their own understanding of the procedure. It should also be discussed with the parents about the importance of siblings being involved and also having access to preparation.

*Many parents need to be prepared themselves for their child's forthcoming operation. All parents want to do the best they can for their child but most lack the relevant* detailed information about the pre-operative procedures and are usually very anxious to co-operate with ward preparation schemes.[14]

It is worth bearing in mind that parents and carers usually like to be involved and with some guidance and support is able to help their child through a procedure/treatment/hospital visit. Therefore, parents can also benefit hugely from being involved in play preparation sessions.

Timing of preparation should be carefully considered. A younger child may not be able to retain the information if it is given too far in advance, whereas a teenager may benefit from preparation a few days before the procedure to allow them time to process it and develop any coping strategies.

*Where possible the timing of the preparation should be dictated by the child and parent.[13]*

A child or teenager who is particularly anxious may not be able to absorb all the information at once and a few preparation sessions may be needed.

Be aware that preparing a child can increase any anxiety as they become aware of the implications of the upcoming procedure, but this should be addressed appropriately during the preparation session.

*Stay with the child and parents offering reassurance and further explanation where needed.*[13]

Before starting any preparation you should be familiar with the ward routines and policies relating to the procedure. Try to spend a little time observing and assessing the child, taking into account their age, level of understanding and any previous experiences of illness or hospital, good and bad.

Discuss the procedure with the staff who will be involved and most importantly the person who will be carrying out the procedure; this will help to ensure you all know your roles and have a good idea of the plan. Good communication is essential in preparation to ensure the child and parents receive the correct and relevant information.

Once you have all the information you need you can set aside some time to sit with the child and family, preferably in a quiet room/cubicle away from distractions and interruptions.

You will of course have a good knowledge by this stage of the child and family and so you can tailor your preparation techniques to suit. Explaining the procedure from start to finish can really help some children to understand what will happen and what is required of them. You should also at this stage address any options open to the child to give them as much control over the procedure as possible. They may prefer to lie down for the blood test or chose what DVD they watch during the procedure. Writing these down and putting together a plan might help to reassure the child and give them a greater level of involvement. It will also be beneficial to you when relaying information to other professionals involved.

Reassurance should be given that fears and anxieties are perfectly normal reactions and be aware of any implications the procedure may have on the child.

Coping strategies should be discussed and encouraged at this stage, a child may benefit from the suggestion of deep breathing activities,

relaxation or ideas for distraction techniques. Any past strategies should be discussed and reviewed as to whether they were beneficial.

Role play and small world role play toys can be very beneficial when preparing a child. You can act out the procedure with the child, using real equipment where possible, according to the plan you have devised together. You could take turns in doing the procedure on each other or on a doll/teddy and this will give you the opportunity to reinforce things you may have already discussed (e.g. 'Take a nice deep breath teddy' or 'Isn't teddy clever at staying still'). This is a good opportunity also to practise relaxation and deep-breathing techniques together. Make sure you allow the child opportunities to ask questions, and repetition can help to reinforce the information.

Looking at storybooks and photograph books (showing procedures in stages) together is a good way to prepare and prompt discussion. You could ask questions throughout about how the child might feel copying the child in the photo and address any issues that arise.

Allowing the child to look at and try out some of the medical equipment they may come into contact with, such as blood pressure cuffs, thermometers, saturation probes, etc., can ease some of the anxieties that may surround coming into hospital. You could take them for a visit to the ward area or theatre, which can also be a good way of preparing the child and encouraging them to trust hospital staff.

Preparation is a valuable tool for reducing the long- and short-term effects of a hospital admission as well as helping to speed up recovery.

Kain *et al.*[15] discuss a study they executed involving a preparation programme for children undergoing surgery, which targets the family as a whole. They randomly assigned 408 children and their families to one of four groups, consisting of a control group receiving standard care, a parental presence during anaesthesia induction group, an advance group, which received family-centred behavioural preparation, and an oral midazolam group (sedation administered). The study showed that the children in the advance group displayed significantly less anxiety in the waiting area, required significantly less analgesia in the recovery room and were discharged from the recovery room earlier than those children in the three other groups. This shows that family-centred preparation can have a positive influence on both pre-operative anxiety and postoperative outcomes.

Table 7.2 shows examples of play preparation materials for different age groups. Remember, 'An informed child is a less vulnerable child'.[16]

**Table 7.2** Play preparation materials

| Age (years) | Play materials | Uses | Benefits |
|---|---|---|---|
| 2–10 | Dolls: calico, adapted preparation dolls and puppets | Role play: to show procedure, how to behave | Easy for child to identify |
| 2+ | Playmobil® or an equivalent small world role play toys | Role play, discussion, good for checking current knowledge and giving more | Easy for child to identify |
| 3+ | Simple picture books of hospital experiences Leaflets | Information for child and parents Information for parents and can be more procedure specific | Can use again and again at own pace Beneficial for parents to ensure they are well informed and better able to support their child |
| 4+ | Photo books: a collection of photos put together to show the child what happens during their hospital stay/procedure | Discussion, detailed explanation of procedure | Can also make their own to show family, friends or school and can include siblings |
| 6+ | DVDs/videos that show children modelling what happens during a stay in hospital, a visit or a procedure | Discussion, detailed explanation of procedure | Good for child reluctant to play or participate. Can use again and again at own pace |

## ADAPTING AND USING DOLLS FOR PREPARATION

For younger children a useful way to prepare them for a procedure may be to adapt a doll. Simple dolls can be adapted to meet a purpose using real medical equipment as long as it is safe (i.e. no needles are left in the doll). It may be necessary to choose a doll that best accommodates the adaptations you would like to make, and a little imagination may be necessary to make certain adaptations! Don't use a patient's own doll unless they specifically request it, it could be very upsetting for a child to see their favourite doll/teddy with a bandage or cannula. There are also pre-adapted dolls/teddies available to buy (please see Useful websites, page 88).

Calico dolls are simple stuffed fabric doll shapes made out of calico material (available in different skin tones). These are useful as they are very adaptable and easily personalised by the child with a face and clothes, etc. These dolls can be used as a way of showing the child what will happen to them and what they may see on the outside of their bodies following the procedure.

### How to make calico dolls

Please see the website for instructions and patterns to make these dolls.

You can use dolls to demonstrate procedures such as inserting a cannula, a gastrostomy button and placing a plaster or dressing on the doll in the relevant place. You can even draw or sew stitches onto the doll to show where a scar may be.

It is important that the children are able to take part in this but are supervised by a play specialist or nurse who can answer any questions or anxieties that may arise. You can also take it in turns in being the nurse, allowing the child to be more involved. Don't forget that you can use these role play sessions to introduce coping techniques and discuss how the child would like things to work when it is their turn to have the procedure.

Remember that you need to be aware of health and safety issues at all times, as well as infection control policies. Fabric calico dolls should be given to the child as they are personal; they cannot be washed and so should not be handled by other patients.

## DIVERSIONARY PLAY/DISTRACTION THERAPY: HOW TO DISTRACT DURING PROCEDURES

Distraction is a technique used primarily to divert the child's focus and attention away from a procedure in an attempt to lessen anxiety levels, help the child to stay calm and compliant/cooperative during the procedure.[17] The results of a study carried out by Windich-Biermeier et al.[18] indicated that, in comparison with other participants, those who participated in distraction during their procedure (venous port access or venepuncture for the sake of this study) demonstrated significantly less distress and fear. Distraction has also been shown to reduce the sensation of pain.

Murphy and Carr[19] reviewed 21 studies on the efficacy of paediatric pain management in patients aged 1–19 years of age. Their findings of the evidence reviewed supported the use of psychological interventions (including distraction, relaxation and play therapy) as the evidence showed that these techniques are effective in reducing pain and distress associated with painful medical procedures, and also for children experiencing recurrent abdominal pain and those with persistent tension or migraine headaches.

Medical procedures can trigger all sorts of negative feelings and emotions resulting in emotional turmoil for the child. The range of emotions they experience could include fear, panic, worry, anger, disgust and resentment or sometimes all of them and others. The reason for these may be a result of the child's previous experiences, pre-conceptions or even the attitude of the parents and staff but, whatever the cause of all these emotions, it is hoped that successful distraction can offer a barrier from this and any associated physical pain.

*Nonpharmacologic interventions, such as distraction, have been shown to be powerful adjuncts in reducing pain and anxiety in children with both acute and chronic painful conditions.*[20]

Distraction is a technique that doesn't necessarily require a lot of training, the tools are readily available and it is a skill that can empower medical staff and parents.[21]

Before attempting distraction with any child there are a few aspects to be considered in advance: a useful tip to remember is to be as well prepared yourself as possible, stay calm and be adaptable. Successful distraction involves constant observation of the child to ensure the techniques used are effective and adapted accordingly. Some things to consider when distracting a child are the techniques/tools, positioning of the child (for example, on a parent's lap for comfort and feelings of security), timing (of the distraction and the procedure itself) and who is going to be present. Be aware of the environment and how the child may perceive it; lots of people and noise is not going to promote a calm and relaxed approach and may make the child less perceptive to any distraction techniques used. Involving the child and encouraging them to actively participate and make their own choices regarding distraction can also be hugely beneficial, to both the distracter and the child (Figure 7.2).

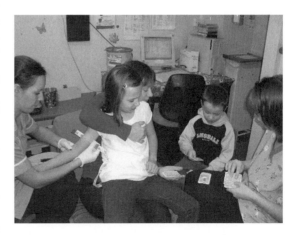

**Figure 7.2** Child being distracted during a blood test.

There are many tools that can be used for distraction which need to be considered when assessing the child's needs, age, stage of development and their likes and dislikes. Some children are more receptive to this than others, but don't be disheartened and remember that any achievement, however small, is a positive step, and positive reinforcement of these is imperative. It's always useful, wherever circumstances allow, to evaluate the procedure/distraction afterwards, as this allows any issues to be addressed instantly and plans for future procedures to be made. This is where documentation is vital, as successful techniques can be recorded and reviewed when needed.

Communication skills are important, as they are with any interaction with a child, and the family may have specific needs (such as interpreters, hearing and visual impairments and other special individual needs). Language used should be age and stage appropriate and consistent with the language used at home, and body language and tone of voice need to be considered as children will respond better when approached in a friendly cheerful manner at eye level. Try to allow children time to respond, don't hurry or interrupt and be aware of and respond to the child's cues. This is all common sense but is vital and will help to maximise the benefits of play intervention.

Russell and Smart[22] explain that the use of distraction techniques could in fact reduce the amount, or frequency of administration, of analgesia.

## PROCEDURE: General distraction

| Procedure steps | Evidence-based rationale |
| --- | --- |
| Follow steps 1–8 for General preparation (page 77), plus | |
| 1 Assess the patient's individual needs and consult any existing individual play plans | To ensure needs are met and input is appropriate |
| 2 Discuss and plan preferred distraction techniques with patient if appropriate | Allows the patient to be involved and have some control |
| 3 Execute agreed/planned distraction method as procedure is performed. Evaluate effectiveness throughout | Enables you to assess the situation and adapt techniques as and when necessary |
| 4 Post-procedural play: evaluate procedure and distraction techniques used | Helps children to interpret the experience, agree on changes for next time and feel more confident/ positive about the procedure, whatever the outcome |
| 5 Document the play input | This information can be used for future reference for other required procedures and informs others of the input given and its outcome |

## DISTRACTION TECHNIQUES

### Guided imagery

This is a technique that involves the use of the child's imagery, guided by an adult, as a coping technique and a form of pain management. Any adult can practise it, although some training in this skill is required. Any child who is able to use their imagination could benefit from this technique, and when used to complement medical methods of pain control can be very useful; however, it is not meant as a substitute for pharmacological pain control.

Guided imagery can be very effective, but as with any form of play intervention it is important to assess the child's individual needs in advance, if possible, to discover if the technique is appropriate. For example, some children with special needs will find this difficult and impractical and it won't be appropriate for all.

This technique works best when the child is in a comfortable and relaxed state and so relaxation techniques are very beneficial; it's a great way to reduce anxiety and enhance the child's feelings of self-control.[23]

Once the child is relaxed (these techniques are explained further below) the imagery, which is chosen by the child in advance, begins. Simple forms of imagery can be facilitated with the use of music or sound tapes, which can help to encourage children to imagine a familiar experience or event that they enjoy. For example, seaside sounds, football commentator recordings or a song that reminds them of an experience.

## Relaxation and deep-breathing exercises

*The more relaxed your child is, the less pain he will feel.*

*Helping children cope with needles –*
*a guide for parents*
*Action for Sick Children*

Relaxation therapy is a technique used to help control pain, manage stress levels and control nausea and vomiting. It is useful to have a little time to begin this before a procedure is started, as it can be very difficult to calm an already anxious and stressed child. It is useful to consider the environment when considering relaxation therapy to reduce the likelihood of interruption/ distractions, and once the child is comfortable and settled you can start the process.

Focusing the child on his/her breathing is a good way to start; there are many ways this can be done that can be adapted to suit the child. One way is to place one hand on the chest area and the other on the tummy and discuss the movements, and then ask him/her to adopt the deep-breathing techniques, concentrating on slow deep breaths in through the nose and exhaling through the mouth. Once this is established you can draw attention to the different movements of the chest and tummy. Another way is to inhale through the nose, imagining all the air travelling all the way down to the toes, and when exhaling through the mouth, imagining that all the tension from that area is being blown away. Repeat the process while moving up the body and focusing on different areas. You can use colours as an image to support this technique, where the child breaths in a colour they find calming and exhale a colour that may symbolise to them anxiety or tension until it has all disappeared.

Once the breathing technique is established, progressive muscle relaxation can begin, working up the child's body (from toes to head and neck) and making a conscious effort to be aware of tensions and release them is a really good way to relax a child and help them to realise that we are sometimes tense but unaware of it. A good way of illustrating this is to ask the child if they feel relaxed and then gently lift the child's hand a little by the wrist over a soft surface. If the child is relaxed the child's hand will fall; if not, it will remain in the air where you left it. There are many visual ways to approach relaxation; you could use colours, where the child imagines a calming/ relaxing/favourite colour working it's way up the body and relaxing all the muscles on its way. Some children may respond well to a feeling of warmth slowly spreading through the body or a heavy sinking sensation as the muscles relax. You can tie imagery in with this also: for example, the child could imagine being on a cloud or floating in the sea. The possibilities are endless and will depend on the child.

When finishing relaxation therapy it is a good idea to bring children out slowly when they are ready; there is no set method for this but counting works well. For example asking the child to count backwards and when they reach 1 they can slowly open their eyes.

This technique is also an adjuvant pain control method, but not a replacement for pharmacological methods.

## Interactive toys and activities

When it comes to distraction using toys and activities the possibilities are endless, as long as you are guided by the child's needs and responses. Some popular examples include books, jokes, bubbles, puppets, I-Spy, sensory toys, counting games, card games, videos/DVDs, singing, making faces, hand-held computers and simply just talking about their favourite chosen topic.

It is useful to have a distraction box handy: this is a box that contains a variety of attention catching and interactive toys and activities. These are simple to put together yourself and can include items that you find work well for you when distracting. It might include finger puppets, wind-up moving animals, find the object books, 'Snap' cards and sensory toys (Figure 7.3, page 84). Please see the website for more ideas and information on Starlight Distraction Boxes.

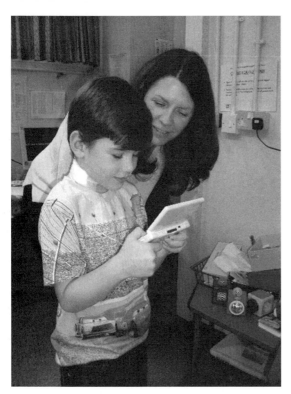

**Figure 7.3** Child engrossed in his hand-held computer, which can be a useful distraction tool.

They are a great resource to have with you when working with children: just reach for your distraction box and look at what's inside with the child and choose something to use as your distraction tool. Together you can choose a toy that might distract the child enough for the whole procedure or you might need to systematically work your way through the entire contents of the box to maintain the child's attention (Figure 7.4)!

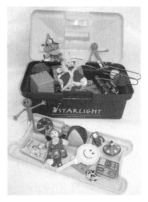

**Figure 7.4** Starlight children's foundation distraction box. (reproduced with permission from Starlight Children's Foundation).

## BEING RESOURCEFUL

Toys and play equipment can be expensive but they are not essential to providing good play opportunities for children of any age or stage of development. With a little imagination you can create fun and exciting activities with little cost implications. After all, how often is it the case that children receive expensive gifts and open them only to spend the next few hours busy playing with the boxes.

Here are some examples of cheaper alternatives:

- Pots/pans with a wooden spoon make a great set of drums.
- Empty drink bottle can be cleaned and filled with different things to create shakers when secured safely (i.e. sand, water, glitter, rice, etc.).
- Make your own dressing up clothes and facemasks using unwanted clothing and paper plates.
- Decorate the windows with suitable paints/tissue paper: placing silver foil to reflect lights and decorating lamps can create a relaxing room for children. These suggestions can be adapted for children with special needs, and provide lots of sensory stimulation.

Please see the website for more ideas.

Remember safety and infection control issues and that all children need supervision. Homemade toys will not meet safety standards and so always assess the risk and take the necessary precautions at all times.

- Positioning: make sure the child doesn't see things they have specifically requested not to also ensure that their position allows them to be comfortable and feel secure
- Be aware of the child's choices and plans
- Be aware of your tone of voice and body language, as children can pick up on feelings of anxiety. A calm and confident approach by staff is far more likely to instil feelings of security and trust in the child
- If the child is not prepared or might benefit from further preparation, it may be necessary to temporarily delay a procedure to accommodate this if it is possible

## POST-PROCEDURAL PLAY: WHY IT IS IMPORTANT

This should always be offered to the child routinely. It can take practically any form and should include praise, certificates and/or stickers. This form of play allows children to evaluate the procedure/experience by looking at, discussing and playing out both the positive and the negative aspects. It helps us to change and improve plans for future hospital experiences and can make a huge difference by ensuring that negative aspects are addressed at the time and the experience ends on a positive note, despite what the experience itself was actually like. All parts of the experience should be looked at, including any of the coping strategies that were used. Allow the child the opportunity to express any feelings following the procedure: how it went, how it felt, etc.

Post-procedural play is useful in helping to reveal aspects that can be improved on for next time; if other interventions might be required, the adults involved should be made aware of this.

## PLAY AND RECOVERY

Play is an important part of recovery, and toys, games and activities are incredibly versatile and can be adapted to meet the individual needs of patients. This may be particularly important for patients who may have undergone medical procedures or surgery. It often takes only minor alterations to enable children to take part in activities that may otherwise be difficult because of medical

restrictions/limitations. Ensuring you have the tools necessary to accommodate play, such as trays or magnetic puzzles for bed-bound patients who may need to lie flat. Don't forgot that patients can be moved into the play room or outside on their beds or in a wheel chair if necessary, or perhaps moving a child near a window to play I-Spy games, among others, may be very much appreciated if a child is unable to go outside. Play activities may be available to all patients, but we do need to ensure we give the patients the support to accommodate play and enable them to participate.

For those patients who may have experienced some loss of function, due to either injury or illness, it is important to devise activities that particularly help to rebuild confidence and self-esteem levels.

## INDIVIDUAL REFERRALS

Fear is a perfectly natural response in both children and adults when faced with a potentially threatening event or procedure.[24] However, sometimes this fear develops into extreme levels that are seemingly disproportionate to the situation itself. This level of fear and anxiety in relation to hospitals and procedures can result in a variety of consequences, some of which may have a negative effect on a child's health/wellbeing.

One of the main aims of therapeutic play interventions is to prevent such fears developing in the first place, but unfortunately some children have negative first experiences of hospital because of the circumstances that they (or a family/friend) have experienced. Other possible causes of such fears/phobias developing are previous experiences, attitudes of parents and perceived misconceptions, whatever there origin.

There are many techniques that can be used to approach fears and phobias but they often take time, and in these cases it is beneficial to work with children on a one-to-one basis where the child/family and play specialist can build a rapport. Through discussion and observation, the play specialist can investigate the roots of the fears and the child's needs can be assessed. This enables the play specialist to devise a personalised individual play plan, which will help the child to address the issues and ultimately develop a plan for procedures and coping techniques that work well for them with the support of the play specialist.

Referral systems vary between trusts, but it is worth familiarising yourself with the guidelines in your hospital so that you are aware of support available from the play team (Figure 7.5).

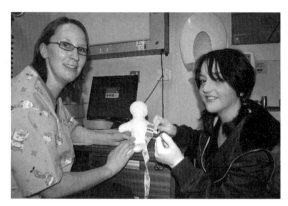

**Figure 7.5** Preparation using a calico doll for role play.

## USING DESENSITISATION

*This form of play should only be undertaken by a qualified Hospital Play Specialist or a member of staff who has attended a 'needle play' workshop and has shown competency in practical assessment.*[25]

Desensitisation is a technique that can be used with children during individual play sessions once a rapport has been built between the child and play specialist and must always be carried out under professional supervision. Each child should of course be assessed first to enable the professional to decide if this technique is appropriate – careful consideration is vital.

It involves controlled slow and increasing exposure of a feared item or situation (i.e. a needle) to the child at a pace of which they are in control. For example, if a needle is the feared object you might begin by introducing the needle to a child while still in its wrapper with a little distance between you and the child. You could then slowly progress, and hopefully the child will gain the confidence to handle the needle and investigate it themselves.

There are of course rules and guidelines that need to be discussed with the child and family and followed when using this technique to ensure safety of all involved at all times: constant supervision is essential. An individual detailed plan should be devised for every child and sessions should be evaluated to ensure progress is monitored constantly.

Desensitisation isn't specific to needles and can be used to desensitise children to uniformed staff, a certain area (i.e. treatment room) or medical equipment such as scanners.

## NEEDLE PLAY

This form of play should be carefully supervised at all times and should be undertaken only by a qualified hospital play specialist or a member of staff that has attended a workshop and demonstrated the necessary competencies in using the technique. However, it can be highly beneficial to children who have developed a fear/phobia of needles or, in fact, any form of medical equipment. Needle play allows us to work through procedures using real equipment in an attempt to familiarise children with the equipment and ultimately allay fears considerably.

The use of specialist dolls, such as specially adapted venesection dolls, are really useful for needle play and give children the opportunity to actively participate in role play situations such as taking blood. Calico dolls (mentioned previously) can also be used in a similar way. This type of play can also form part of a desensitisation plan.

These are the four stages of needle play from the guidelines developed by NAHPS.

- *Stage 1: Assessment* At this stage the role and benefits of needle play should be discussed with both the parent/carer and the child. They are then able to make an informed decision whether they feel this technique might be appropriate and beneficial to the child. It should be explained to the child and carers that needle play is a great way to teach children about procedures and improve their understanding. It also allows the opportunity for feelings to be discussed and underlying issues to be discovered and addressed in an appropriate manner. It is imperative at this stage to ensure that you are well informed regarding the procedure, the child and family, previous experiences and individual needs (including age/stage of development and emotional maturity). The play specialist should allow themselves time to build a rapport with the child initially through non-directed play.

- *Stage 2: Preparation* The child needs to be made aware of the possible dangers of handling needles outside the needle play session and of why it is safe to do this type of play in a controlled environment. The more practical plans should be taken care of too, making sure that the environment time restrictions are considered. It is often useful to discuss some simple rules and boundaries as an extra safety precaution for all involved.

  The procedure should first be demonstrated using appropriate equipment and visual aids by the professional leading the session, which is why it is important that you have all the information you need and that you are well prepared in advance. Allow time for questions during and after the session.

- *Stage 3: Procedure* Support the child and family through the procedure offering distraction therapy, if this is what the child wants. Give the child choices whenever it is possible to do so in an effort to return the element of control; the child will have made most of these decisions during stage 2 but they are not set in stone and can be changed accordingly.

- *Stage 4: Post-procedure* Give feedback to the child and praise their achievements, however minor, even if the procedure wasn't as successful as you

had hoped. A post-procedural play plan should be devised and followed if necessary.

Discuss plans for future hospital visits/procedures and whether further needle play sessions might be beneficial. It is important to recognise your limitations and involve other professionals for advice and support if necessary (perhaps the psychologist).[25]

There are also guidelines for professional practice that must be adhered to; this information is available on the NAHPS website (details below). For more information, see the National Association of Hospital Play Staff guideline on needle play.[25] These techniques are not always appropriate and so the child's needs, age, stage of development and emotional maturity should be assessed and considered in advance. Information on the profession and useful information and support can be found on the NAHPS website: www.nahps.org.uk.

Be sure to document any play interventions used with a child so that others can see what techniques have worked and are aware of any plans in place. It also promotes consistency and enables you to look back and see what worked well with the child and what didn't work well if you see them again.

Please see the website for further information.

---

 Go to the website to find the PowerPoint presentation for this chapter and MCQs to test your knowledge. **www.hodderplus.com/childnursingskills**

---

## REFERENCES

1  National Association for Hospital Play Staff (NAHPS) www.nahps.org.uk/ (accessed 14 April 2008).

2  Lansdown R (1996) *Children in hospital: a guide for families and carers.* New York: Oxford University Press.

3  Chambers M (2007) The importance of play. In: Glasper EA, McEwing G, and Richardson J (eds) *Oxford handbook of children's and young people's nursing.* New York: Oxford University Press.

4  Taylor J, Müller D, Wattley L, Harris P (1999) *Nursing children: psychology research and practice,* 3rd edition. Cheltenham: Stanley Thornes.

5  Dixon SD, Stein MT (2006) *Encounters with children: paediatric behaviour and development,* 4th edition. Philadelphia: Mosby Elsevier.

6  Mathiasen L, Butterworth D (2001) The role of play in the hospitalisation of young children. *Neonatal Paediatric and Child Health Nursing* 4(3): 23–26.

7  Department of Health (2003) *Getting the right start: the national service framework for children, young people and maternity services – standard for hospital services.* London: DH.

8  Scott L, Langton F, O'Donoghue. J (2002) Minimising the use of sedation/anaesthesia in young children receiving radiotherapy through an effective play preparation programme. *European Journal of Oncology Nursing* 6(1): 15–22.

9  Walker J (2006) *Play for health: delivering and auditing quality in hospital play services.* London: NAHPS.

10 Whitaker BH (2006) Distraction therapy and guided imagery. Course at Weston House, Great Ormond Street Hospital for Children 9, 10 and 24 November 2006.

11 Coyne C (2006) Children's experiences of hospitalization. *Journal of Child Health Care* **10**: 326–336.

12 William LI, Lopez V, Lee TLI (2007) Effects of preoperative therapeutic play on outcomes of school-age children undergoing day surgery. *Research in Nursing and Health* **30**: 320–332.

13 National Association of Hospital Play Staff (2002) *Guidelines for professional practice: No. 5. Play preparation*. London: NAHPS.

14 National Association of Hospital Play Staff (1987) *Lets play: No. 7. Preparation for surgery and unpleasant procedures*. London, NAHPS.

15 Kain ZN, Caldwell-Andrews AA, Mayes LC, *et al.* (2007) Family-centered preparation for surgery improves peri-operative outcomes in children: a randomized controlled trial. *Anesthesiology* **106**(1): 65–74.

16 Collier J, Mackinlay D (1993) Play at Work: Play preparation guidelines for the multidisciplinary team. *In Child Health*. London: DH, pp.123–5.

17 Woon R (2004) Hospital play therapy: helping children cope with hospitalisation through therapeutic play. *Singapore Nursing Journal* **31**(1): 16–19.

18 Windich-Biermeier A, Sjoberg I, Conkin Dale J, *et al.* (2007) Effects of distraction on pain, fear, and distress during venous port access and venepuncture in children and adolescents with cancer. *Journal of Paediatric Oncology Nursing* **24**(1) 8–19.

19 Murphy E, Carr A (2000) *What works with children and adolescents? A critical review of psychological interventions with children, adolescents and their families*. London: Routledge.

20 Sinha M, Christopher NC, Fenn R, Reeves. L (2006) Evaluation of nonpharmacologic methods of pain and anxiety management for laceration repair in the pediatric emergency department. *Pediatrics* **117**: 1162–1168.

21 Stubenrauch JM (2007) Striving for distraction. *American Journal of Nursing* **107**(3): 94.

22 Russell C, Smart S (2007) Guided imagery and distraction therapy in paediatric hospice care. *Paediatric Nursing* **19**(2): 24–25.

23 Miles BS (2002) *Imagine a rainbow: a child's guide for soothing pain*. Washington: Magination Press .

24 Weaver K, Battrick C, Glasper EA (2007) Developing a hospital play guideline and protocol for sick children with debilitating fears. *Journal of Children's and Young People's Nursing* **1**(3): 143.

25 National Association of Hospital Play Staff (2002) *Guidelines for Professional practice. No. 7, Needle Play*. London: NAHPS.

## USEFUL WEBSITES

National Association of Hospital Play Staff:
www.nahps.org.uk
Hospital Play Staff Education Trust: www.hpset.org.uk
Southampton General Hospital: www.suht.nhs.uk
Action for Sick Children: www.actionforsickchildren.org
Department of Health: www.dh.gov.uk
McKinnon Medical: www.mckinnon-medical.co.uk
Sparkle Box: www.sparklebox.co.uk
Play England: www.playengland.org.uk
Association for Children's Palliative Care:
www.act.org.uk
Forum for Nursery Staff: www.nurserynurseforum.com
Information for Play Workers: www.playworkers.co.uk
Silkysteps (early learning resources) www.silkysteps.com
Children and Young People Now: www.cypnow.co.uk

## CHAPTER 8

# Manual handling for children's and young people's nursing

Marion Aylott

## LEARNING OUTCOMES

*Upon completion of this chapter, the reader should be able to accomplish the following:*

1 Define moving and handling
2 Demonstrate awareness of the legislation and the employer/employee responsibility to ensure risk assessment is undertaken, reviewed regularly and documented
3 Cite the biomechanical principles of safer handling of people, which must be applied to all handling tasks
4 Discuss the principles of hoist use and the types of hoist available
5 Develop awareness of recommended techniques and equipment that might assist a procedure

## KEY WORDS

Moving and handling    Task load
Individual environment    Risk assessment
Equipment safety    Child handler

## CHAPTER OVERVIEW

Many people don't think about their back until they are in pain, but by then it is too late, as the damage has often been done. Nearly 80 per cent of people have back pain at some stage in their lives, and the statistics are even higher in nurses, irrespective of specialty.[1] Nurses caring for children and young people appear to under-rate the importance of manual handling in the child population. Size and weight of the child are not the only considerations: posture awareness is crucial. Taking care of your back involves more than just safe lifting.

Sick children and young people and those with physical disabilities, particularly those aged between 5 and 12 years, often require special assistance to perform everyday tasks such as getting into bed or taking a bath. Even as a child ages and is able to accomplish more tasks independently, he/she may still depend on parents or a caregiver to transfer into or out of a wheelchair to accomplish these tasks.

Safe lifting is important to everyone. Most people lift, lower, push, pull, carry or move many things throughout the day. However, most injuries are usually the result of repeated strain that has happened over many years.[1] Yet, this risk can be reduced if people understand how to conduct manual handling tasks/activities correctly and look after their back. Don't wait until you have pain to do something about back care!

The aim of this chapter is to provide practical guidelines that facilitate the safer moving of the patient using mechanical assistance, ensuring both the health and safety of staff and the patient.

When using risk assessment terminology within this chapter, the infant or child will sometimes be identified as 'load'. This is not meant to denigrate the child, but to put the practical considerations of care in the context of performing a moving and handling assessment, plan and procedure. Also, when describing the 'person' carrying out the moving and handling task, the term 'handler' will be used, as this is quite often a parent or other caregiver working with or under the instruction and responsibility of a nurse.[2] Nurses should act as positive role models.

---

**Definition**

Moving and handling is any action required as part of a person's job that involves movement of a person or inanimate object by hands or bodily force. This includes activities such as lifting, lowering, pushing, pulling, carrying and supporting a load.[3]

---

## MOVING AND HANDLING: A CHILD-FRIENDLY APPROACH

Children's nurses handle their patient population differently from adult nurses as part of a developmental approach. For example, it is generally considered reasonable for a children's nurse to 'lift' and hold an infant or attend to children on or near the floor. Therefore, moving and handling requires some unique consideration. This is especially important as many children's nurses consider it acceptable to adopt the quickest, simplest 'child-friendly' method to complete a task as opposed to the safer approach.[1]

Application of safe principles of moving and handling practice extends to education and informing the child, parents and others caregivers of the safest handling techniques for the child and themselves to ensure their ability to continue caring without injury to themselves or the child.[7] Every year significant numbers of parents are forced to give up caring for their child because of

illness or injury.[4] The *National strategy for carers*[4] suggests that many of these physical injuries could be avoided if carers were taught how to move their child in a safer way. Possibly the most effective way to teach parents about safer handling is to work with them individually when the handling tasks are carried out.[5] The child and parents have the right to be consulted in respect of their care and informed about the options available in the provision of that care.[6]

## WHAT DOES THE LAW SAY?

A practical understanding of the law is essential for all those involved in the manual handling of adults and children whether in 'hands-on', managing, commissioning or advisory roles. There are three pieces of legislation that relate to the moving and handling of children: the Health and Safety at Work Act (HSWA)[7] the Manual Handling Operations Regulations (MHOR)[3] and person entitlement under human rights legislation.[6]

HSWA[7] remains the basis of health and safety legislation, and sets out the general duties which employers have towards employees and members of the public, and employees have to themselves and to each other. Section 3(1), states that 'employers must ensure, as far as reasonably practicable, the health, safety and welfare of their employees whilst at work and any other persons affected by their business activities.' Therefore, this applies not only to healthcare professionals as employees but also to informal carers, that is parents. Failure to offer parents advice about avoiding identified moving and handling risks could result in a breach of duty to care.

The MHOR regulations add to the duties placed on employers by the HSWA. MHOR requires a risk assessment approach and to avoid lifting wherever *reasonably practicable* when moving and handling objects or people. The purpose of the legislation and regulations are to reduce the risk of injury from manual handling (Table 8.1, page 91).

Many handling operations, e.g. lifting a teacup, will involve a negligible handling risk. Therefore the HSC[3] (Health and Safety Commission) give a general guide to the weight limits at which risk assessment should be triggered but these are not hard and fast rules and there is no simple answer (Figure 8.1, page 91). But they assume that the

**Table 8.1** Employer and employee legal duties[3,7] (data obtained from HSC[3])

| The employer's duties | The employee's duties |
|---|---|
| **Avoid** the need for hazardous manual handling as far as is reasonably practicable | Follow appropriate systems of work laid down for their safety |
| **Assess** the risk of injury from any hazardous manual handling that can't be avoided | Make proper use of equipment provided to minimise the risk of injury |
| **Reduce** the risk of injury from hazardous manual handling, as far as reasonably practicable | Cooperate with the employer on health and safety matters. If a care assistant fails to use a hoist that has been provided, they are putting themselves at risk of injury. The employer is unlikely to be liable |
| | Apply the duties of employers, as appropriate, to their own manual handling activities |
| | Take care to ensure that their activities do not put others at risk |

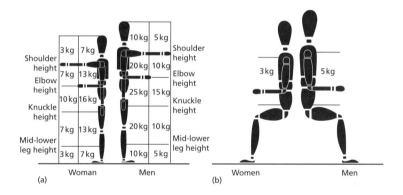

**Figure 8.1** Guideline weight limits for lifting and lowering (redrawn from HSC[3] under the terms of the Click-Use Licence).

**VIGNETTE**

**Question:** When can/can't I manually 'lift' children?

**Answer:** You can, but the Law says that whenever possible manual lifting should be avoided! The only 'acceptable' reasons to 'lift' a child or any person[7] include drowning, fire, collapsing building, bomb.

But avoiding manual lifting of infants and young children in particular can be challenging as many routine 'everyday' tasks involve repetitive and/or awkward movements and posture. Your safety and that of the child is paramount.

handling is taking place in reasonable working conditions with an inanimate load that is easily grasped with both hands, which is not directly applicable to any human, child or otherwise. Arbitrary weight limits are no substitute for a proper risk assessment.

**KEY POINT**

During any person-handling task, if the handler is required to lift more than 16 kg (female) or 25 kg (male) of a child's weight in good standing posture, then consider the child fully dependent, conduct a risk assessment and use assistive handling devices

## WHAT DOES THE NMC SAY?

The NMC[2] states that as a registered nurse or midwife you are personally accountable for your practice. In caring for your patients and in relation to manual handling, you must

- respect the individual (do not treat patients merely as manual handling 'loads' – they are people);
- obtain consent before you give any care (discuss the options with the child and/or family; do not treat people just as loads to be shifted or hoisted);
- cooperate with others in the team (such as physiotherapists, back care advisors, occupational therapists);
- maintain your professional knowledge and competence (manual handling training is compulsory – you need to keep up to date);
- act to identify and minimise risk (risk assessment – use appropriate skills, techniques and equipment).

## DISPELLING COMMON MYTHS

1 Manual handling assessment and techniques are not so important because children are not heavy and can be lifted easily.
   - Manual handling in child health areas involves the broadest variance in weight of load (from a neonate weighing less than 1 kg to an adolescent who could weigh over 50 kg).
   - Children are often awkward, wriggly, bulky and top heavy loads (head is a third to a half of the weight).
   - A child's moving and handling ability is not just dependent on ability to move but on their developmental age, capability and level of compliance.
   - A high proportion of normal care routines can involve poor positioning or posture or repetitive strain.
2 Manual handling assessment and techniques are not so important because few children are immobile or bedridden.
   - Infants and toddlers are totally dependent on others. Manual handling is pivotal to their everyday care.
   - Manual handling of children involves a range of activities, some of which directly involve the child and others which are peripheral, e.g. setting up a high chair.

- Infants, young children and those with special needs may be unable to understand commands and may actively resist any manoeuvre.
- Acute/chronic illness, injury, disablement, surgery pain, fear or procedures permanently or temporarily alter the child's manual-handling needs.
- Normal essential processes of cuddling, feeding and holding infants and young children involves the lifting and holding of a load.

3 Manual handling assessment and techniques are not so important because parents do most of the moving and handling.
   - In hospital children receive care from their parents and caregivers as well as staff. Therefore, nursing staff are responsible for educating parents and carers in safe moving and handling as well as being role models of 'best' practice.

## YOUR BACK

The spinal column is the centre of postural control and the spinal column protects the spinal cord.[8] It is built to provide stability and at the same time allow flexibility. These two seemingly incompatible functions of support (inflexibility) and movement (flexibility) are at opposite ends of a spectrum of movement, and this fact is one reason why the spine is so vulnerable to injury. The spine is constructed of 24 vertebrae, stacked from the pelvis to the skull in a gentle 'S' curve (Figure 8.2, page 92). The two curvatures of the spine contribute to the spring-like capacity of the spine and allow the vertebral column to withstand higher loads than if it were straight.[8] The functions of the spine are

Support: S
Transmit: T
Attachment: A
Movement: M
Protect: P
Shock absorber: S

---

**KEY POINT**

The lumbar spine is the most injured area, followed by the cervical spine. This is because they are the most mobile and, therefore, vulnerable areas

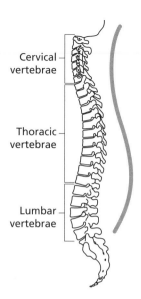

**Figure 8.2** Spine 'S' shape.

Located between the vertebrae are intervertebral discs, which are dense cartilage with a jelly-like centre (Figure 8.3). These act as the shock absorbers for the spine.[8] Although the vertebrae are designed to withstand certain compressive loads, uneven forces from high-risk activities, e.g. bending or twisting can result in uneven wear and movement of inner material. Excess spinal pressure can cause these discs to be compressed until they rupture; this is known as herniation.[8]

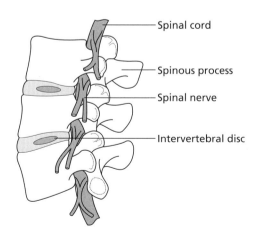

**Figure 8.3** Anatomy of the healthy spine.

| KEY POINT | Overexertion is the most common cause of back injuries and force is the most important risk factor |
|---|---|

## BIOMECHANICAL PRINCIPLES TO PROTECT YOUR BACK

For efficient posture for moving and handling:

- maintain a natural posture and head up whenever possible during manual handling, keeping your 'spine in line';
- always create a good, stable base, by widening your stance within comfortable limits, placing one foot in front of the other, about shoulder width apart, with your knees slightly bent;
- keep any load, or point of force, as close to your vertical centre of gravity as possible;
- use the large leg and buttock muscles to provide the power during manual handling using a lunge technique that is transferring your body weight from front to back leg.

Please see the website for (further) information  on protecting your back.

## BEST PRACTICE STARTS WITH RISK ASSESSMENT

The key to safe nursing work is careful analysis of the factors that that explain the risk involved in providing patient care.[3] ELITE (Table 8.1, page 91) (sometimes called ELIOT) is the suggested format for recording risk assessments in this chapter, which focuses on ergonomic assessments of the characteristics of five key factors: environment, load, individual, task, equipment. Risk assessment is an extremely useful tool, and employed correctly it is the singular most effective way of reducing work place injuries.[9]

| KEY POINT | Basic risk assessment should consider |
|---|---|
| | E  environment |
| | L  load |
| | I  individual capability |
| | T  task |
| | E  equipment |

The only way to eliminate the risk associated with the handling task is to not perform it. This involves facilitating the movement of the child by themselves through

- the provision of an appropriate environment;
- the provision of equipment such as electronic beds, walking aids;
- encouraging and coaching the child to move themselves.

However, in many situations it is just not practical or possible for a child to move themselves without assistance. Therefore, the focus shifts to controlling the risk. You should try to remove or control as many of the risks as possible to reduce the risks as low as reasonably practicable.[9]

Doing a risk assessment is not the end of the process:

- review the assessment regularly;
- review the outcomes with the person being assisted;
- analyse any adverse incidents/near misses;
- carry out internal/external audits.

It is essential that all manual handling incidents/near misses are reported using the Trust's Adverse Incident Reporting System.[10] This allows the Trust to be aware of any issues that may arise with regard to managing the hazards associated with manual handling. Recording near misses can alert managers to an issue, not highlighted before. This allows risk to be managed in a more pro-active way rather than just addressing issues after someone gets hurt.

| | |
|---|---|
| **KEY POINT** | Risk assessments are the most important and effective recent safety legislation |

## A DEVELOPMENTAL APPROACH TO RISK

Many of the challenges to risk assessment with regards to manual handling of children are related to the nature of the child and all that it encompasses. As children (on the whole) come in various sizes, most importantly they are smaller than the average adult and thus pose postural difficulties for the handler immediately. For example, when walking with a child there is a tendency for the handler to stoop or be oversupportive and manually carry part of the child's weight. In this circumstance, walking on knees or wheeling by the side of the child while seated on a therapy stool might be biomechanically preferable but not always practicable. The everyday equipment of a child, e.g. cots, chairs, pushchairs and beds, are designed with the child's safety and 'preference' in mind, not the handlers. The larger, heavier child must be treated as adult from a physical manual handling perspective while continuing to manage the psycho-emotional aspects of the child in a child-friendly and appropriate manner. The greatest risk, however, lies with the infant and toddler, whom it is generally considered 'acceptable' to lift from and to high and low levels, including the floor, and carry over comparatively longer distances than one would carry an older and larger child.[1]

### Infants

- Infants have immature neurology resulting in poor muscle tone and an inability to bear weight or support themselves.[11]
- Carers need to take complete control in regards to selection of the technique and supporting their weight.
- Common caring activities for a baby are repetitive and put the carer at risk of poor positioning/posture, e.g. nappy changing, bathing.
- Moving and handling is further compromised when infants are attached to equipment, e.g. monitors, infusions, oxygen and ventilation delivery devices.

### Toddlers

- Toddlers need help with virtually all activities of daily living.
- From the age of 1 year, toddlers are able to follow simple instructions but also resist and struggle.
- Many moving and handling needs are as for the infant but their weight is greatly increased.
- Toddlers are short so handlers often stoop down to their level or squat.

- Toddlers need help to mobilise or supervision, i.e. holding hands to walk.

## Children

- Young children may not be able to understand or follow more than 'simple' instructions.
- Children may not be compliant.
- Children may have disabilities that impair movement or complicate moving and handling procedures, i.e. seizures, contractures, loss of muscle tone, a tendency for muscle spasm.

## Adolescents

- Most adolescents are able to understand and follow instructions and assist in moving and handling procedures if they want to!
- They have greater weight, including bariatric.
- They may be reluctant to cooperate (hoisting, sliding).
- They fear loss of control/privacy and dignity.
- Those with cognitive deficits, e.g. attention deficit/hyperactivity disorder, may not appreciate the safety implications of manoeuvres.

**VIGNETTE**

**Question:** What is appropriate footwear and clothing?

**Discussion:** Shoes should cover the toes. They should be a full shoe (not clogs) and flat. Clothing should be suitable for the tasks. If you are wearing uniform ensure it is not too tight and allows easy movement. Jewellery (particularly rings and watches) can create a hazard for the handler in that they can catch on fabrics while moving a child or they can injure the child being moved. Be aware that items in pockets can sometimes cause injury in the same way that belts do.

## MANUAL HANDLING QUESTIONS

Brooks[11] presents a simple tool consisting of five manual handling questions, which provide a principles-based approach to assessment and decision-making before performing a moving or handling task. These questions, answered in sequence prompt the handler to think in advance systematically through a moving and handling problem with the aim of leading the handler to use an appropriate intervention.

## PROCEDURE: Manual handling questions[11]

| Procedural steps | Evidence-based rationale |
|---|---|
| 1 What do you consider to be normal movement for the task? | Knowing what the common patterns of normal movement are, helps us in dealing with people who have some movement dysfunction or some psychological factors that are limiting their movement When giving instructions to people it is important to always start with the head as this initiates movement for the rest of the body |
| 2 Can you teach the child to do this unaided? How? Give clear, developmentally appropriate instruction for each movement following the planned approach each time to avoid confusion, aid learning and promote independence If 'no', go to 3 | Work safe. Provide guidance about the direction and timing of the movement and momentary stabilisation of some body parts to enable the child to complete the movement. An important focus in rehabilitation is enabling the child to be an active participant in the acquisition of skills. There is a strong body of evidence supporting the need for opportunities to practise to improve physical abilities Children learn by repetition and therefore need to be guided to move in the same way by all to reinforce learning |

## PROCEDURE: Manual handling questions[11] (continued)

| | |
|---|---|
| **3** If the child not completely unaided, is there equipment available that would mean that the child could do this for themselves? How? For example, bed lever, slide sheet, variable height or profiling bed If 'no', go to 4 | Always ask 'Do I need to handle manually? Can I ask or guide the child to move? Can I use a handling aid to move the child?' The child must take their own body weight. At no point does the handler carry the weight or any part of the weight of the child if over 16 kg (female) 25 kg (male)[3] Mechanical handling aids can reduce the risk of injury when used correctly. Remember that although they will eliminate many of the manual handling risks their use will introduce others[9] |
| **4** If the child is unable to perform the task themselves, what is the minimum of assistance one and then two people can give: (a) without equipment; (b) with equipment? | All repositioning tasks with a dependent/immobile child using mechanical devices should be performed by at least two handlers[9] |
| **5** Are there unsafe ways of doing this that I must avoid? If so, what are they? | Consider here any element of care that may threaten the handler(s) and child's safety, e.g. an infant may be dropped during a manual lift if the caregiver suddenly develops back pain or damage[12] |

## Selecting appropriate moving and handling equipment

Appropriate moving and handling aids are selected based on the level of dependency of the child. An individual child handling plan should be developed for each child whose mobility level is assessed as requiring supervision or limited assistance (see Figure 8.4 for an algorithm to help decision).

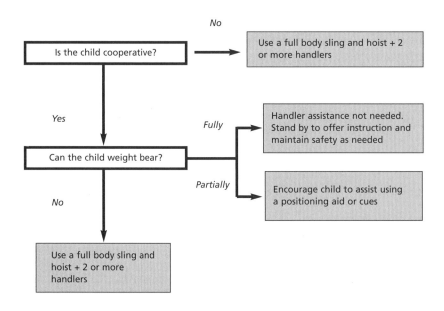

**Figure 8.4** Manual handling algorithm.

# LIFTING AN INFANT

Infants and young children are often positioned in the centre of cots and beds (some with fixed heights), or on the floor. Although it is natural to pick up an infant if crying to give comfort or to give care, it might be more appropriate to get down to their level. However, following consideration of the recommended safe handling loads,[3] and the distance over which the lift is required, there will be circumstances where a 'lift' is considered reasonably practicable and low risk (see Figure 8.1, page 91).

### The procedural goal is to

1 Lift and hold infant safely with minimal risk to caregiver
2 Deliver safe and compassionate handling of infant.

## PROCEDURE: Lifting an infant

| Procedural steps | Evidence-based rationale |
|---|---|
| 1 Prepare the *environment*<br>Where is the child going to be placed? Make sure your route is clear of obstructions and that there is somewhere to put the child down safely. For a long lift, i.e. floor to shoulder height, consider resting the infant mid-way on a bed or nappy bench to change grip | Prevent avoidable accidents: a clutter-free environment allows for free movement of the handler and promotes safety for the child |
| 2 Consider the *load*<br>Weight?<br>Stability?<br>The infant form is an awkward, unpredictable load | Ensure that the infant is light enough to lift and is stable and unlikely to wriggle or spasm. Infants over 13 kg (female) or 20 kg (male) or likely to be awkward should be lifted from the floor using a hoist if possible[3] |
| 3 Consider the *individual*<br>Are you 'fit' for the task?<br>Do you need help with the load? | If the child is cooperative (stable), use two handlers (max 22 kg female; max 34 kg male handlers)[3]<br>This task carries a greater risk for new or expectant mothers[19] |
| 4 Consider *equipment* needs<br>If a close approach to the infant is not possible, try sliding the infant towards you on a slide sheet first | Sliding requires less effort than lifting[12] |
| 5 Plan the *task*<br>• Stand as close to the infant as possible, spread your feet to shoulder width distance apart.<br>• Place the leading leg as far forward as is comfortable<br>• Bend your knees so that the hands when holding the infant are as nearly level with your waist as possible and<br>• Maintain your back in a neutral position[10]<br>• Lean forward a little over the infant if necessary to get a good grip.<br>• Bend your hips and knees instead of bending your waist to allow your leg muscles to take the infant's weight.<br>• *Lift the infant smoothly*; raise your head as the lift begins, keeping control of the load<br>• If you must turn while carrying the load, turn using your feet, not your torso<br>• Keep the infant trunk close to your trunk for as long as possible<br>• If precise positioning of the infant is necessary, place the infant down then adjust or place the infant down on a slide sheet first, then slide into desired position | • A stable base of support, increases stability and minimises the force required[13]. Human capacity is reduced when stooping<br>• A secure grip helps to ensure that there is no danger of slippage and dropping the infant<br>• Larger leg muscles offer more leverage reducing the strain on your back. Tighten abdominal muscles as these support the spine when lifting.[14] If the infant is at waist height if you are in the high kneeling position less stress is placed on the back. In general, the faster the muscle is contracting the less force it can generate and the greater the risk of injury that exists[15]<br>• Twisting amplifies the negative results of forces on the lower back<br>• A trunk-to-trunk position keeps the heaviest part of the load close to your spine exerting less force, and helps balance[9]<br>• This helps to avoid needless repetition of lift which reduces capacity. Sliding requires less effort than lifting |

## DELIVERING CARE AT A LOW WORKING LEVEL

Low-level working postures are recognised as one of the factors that potentially contribute to musculoskeletal disorders (MSDs).[9] For safety, care is often delivered to children at a low working level, usually on a mat on the floor, yet this same consideration may place staff at risk due to adoption of stooping posture.[9] Work in this extreme and static posture is associated with higher levels of MSDs and, therefore, stooping should be avoided if at all possible; the provision of a low stool may enable staff to avoid this posture[15].

### The procedural goal is to

1 Deliver care safely with minimal risk to caregiver
2 Maximise child independence and autonomy.

## PROCEDURE: Working at low level

| Procedural steps | Evidence-based rationale |
|---|---|
| 1 Prepare the *environment*<br>Is it absolutely necessary to work at floor level?<br>Where are you going to be working and for how long?<br>If possible, raise the level of the activity<br>Make sure the area is clear of obstructions and hazards, e.g. liquid spills | Reaching to the floor involves unavoidable excessive spinal flexion, increasing lumbar spinal pressure[15]<br>If low-kneeling, use a small cushion under the hips to help gain a better position and increase reach[15]<br>Prevent avoidable accidents: a clutter-free environment allows for free and safe movement of the handler |
| 2 Consider *equipment* needs<br>Where are you going to be kneeling, sitting?<br>Have you got an appropriate surface to kneel on or appropriate height chair or stool? | When working at low level for a prolonged period of time (over 15 minutes), sit on a low stool in preference to kneeling or squatting.[15] A kneeling stool can reduce knee flexion and improve spinal posture[15] |
| 3 Consider the *load*<br>What is the estimated weight of the load?<br>Avoid working in this position for more than 15 minutes at a time?. | Ensure that the working load does not exceed 7 kg (female) or 10 kg (male) if the load is close to the body[3]<br>Fixed postures put strain on the body because of the increase in the static muscle effort required to maintain the body in balance. In the back this can lead to an increase in intradiscal pressure[7] |
| 4 Consider the *individual*<br>Are you 'fit' for the task?<br>Do you have any pre-existing ankle, knee, hip conditions? | Kneeling involves flexion of the spine, static contraction of the spinal extensor muscles, increased compression loading and hence an increase in intradisc pressure[15]<br>Extreme joint angles in squatting is associated with ankle, knee, hip and back strain[15] |
| 5 Plan the *task*<br>• When working at low level, avoid stooping. Bend your knees (kneel or squat) rather than your back<br>• Sitting on the floor either with crossed legs or legs out straight is preferred<br>• Remember lifting capacity from floor level is much reduced, especially if lifting with one hand[15] The ability to exert force is greater when kneeling on one knee compared to kneeling on two especially when force is applied at waist height and close to the body.[15] It also allows greater mobility and reach | • Stooping causes increased compressive loading on the intervertebral discs and facet joints, tension in the extensor ligaments and static-muscle loading[9]<br>• Sitting on the floor lowers the centre of gravity and therefore increases stability.[15] It also puts less stress on the spine as long as twisting is avoided[16]<br>• In kneeling, the centre of gravity is low and therefore the body is relatively stable |

## LATERAL TRANSFER ASSIST DEVICES

When you consider the injuries that occur to healthcare employees involved in patient handling and movement, transferring is the primary concern reported; in one study the incidence rates for back-related injuries in hospitals were 10.1 per 100 employees, and 25 per cent of those were due to lateral transfers.[17] Lateral transfers require the handlers to use different muscle groups such as the arms and shoulders rather than the legs, and often require the task to be carried out in less than desirable postures. Lateral transfer devices help to reduce strains/sprains in employees performing these tasks. Lateral transfer assist devices, such as slide sheets and transfer boards, reduce the forces and awkward postures required for transferring children between adjacent surfaces because of their friction-reducing properties,. Transfer assist devices do not reduce the weight of a patient and should not be used to lift, carry, or support the whole or a large part of a child's body weight. There are three principle types:

- air assist device
- transfer board, e.g. PAT-Slide
- mechanical transfer aid.

Please see the website for further information on each device.

Though an child might be considered 'light' by nursing staff, usually after the age of 1 year they are always well above the weight limits recommended.[15] Therefore, unless the child is able to do most of the repositioning or lateral transfer by themselves, a lateral transfer aid should always be used to avoid injury to the handler(s) and the child.

### Transferring a child using a transfer board and slide sheet

A transfer board is a non-mechanical device that can reduce the forces or awkward postures associated with lateral transfer activities through its slippery vinyl covering and bridge a gap between two surfaces. When properly used, this device can reduce the risk of musculoskeletal injury (MSI) to handlers.[8] Transfer assist devices used in combination with each other, such as a slide sheet with a transfer board, require less force than using only one device.

#### The procedural goal is to

Use the lateral transfer board, e.g. PAT-Slide, to

- provide a safer means of moving and transferring a child between two flat and even surfaces with minimal short-term discomfort;
- facilitate independence and maintain the dignity of the child being moved or transferred;
- eliminate or minimise risk factors that can lead to injury to the handler or child.

#### Equipment

Slide sheet (so even less force required)
Pillow
Transfer board

## PROCEDURE: Transferring a child

| Procedural steps | Evidence-based rationale |
|---|---|
| **1** Prepare the *equipment*<br>• *Never use a slide board if you have not been trained in its use* | All users require training prior to use[3,7] |
| • Use the slide board in conjunction with a slide sheet, which is placed between the child and the slide board | Less force required of handlers |
| **2** Prepare the *environment*<br>• Place the bed and trolley side-by-side and lock the wheels of bed and trolley | To prevent inadvertent movement of either surface |
| • Raise bed to waist level and slightly above level of trolley | To avoid extended reach and minimise forward flexion[17] |
| • Lower head of bed (slight Trendelenberg position) according to child tolerance | Use gravity to assist the transfer |

## PROCEDURE:  Transferring a child (continued)

| | |
|---|---|
| **3** Prepare the *load* <br>• Assess the child's need for pain medication <br>• Review care plan for any activity restrictions <br>• Explain the purpose and describe details of the transfer to the child and parents as appropriate. <br>• Provide for child privacy. <br>• Educate child regarding ways to assist in transfer as appropriate <br>• If able, ask the child to position themselves at the edge of bed nearest stretcher before slide board is put into place <br>• Or, roll the child onto their side using an appropriate technique, position the slide board with slide sheet on top under the child and roll the child into a supine position on the board <br>• Position child's head on a pillow with majority of pillow on side of move | Maintain comfort <br>To avoid causing unforeseen harm <br>To gain informed consent and cooperation[2] <br><br><br>To promote independence <br><br>To prevent skin injury and promote comfort |
| **4** Consider the *individual* <br>• Handlers must have undergone training in lateral slide use <br>• Two handlers are required to use the slide board safely if the child is fully dependent | Minimum number of handlers considered necessary to maintain safety[9] <br>Skills competence[3,7] |
| **5** During the task <br>• Assume good posture <br>• Handlers position their hands down in handles at the child's hip and shoulder <br>• Keep arms straight <br>• Position legs in lunge position with body weight on front leg <br>• Gently slide the child using good body positioning <br>• One handler coordinates the task 'ready, set, slide' <br>• Keeping arms straight, handlers move their weight from front to back leg | Do not try and pull with arms (keep straight throughout move). The move is done through the stronger leg and buttock muscles by shifting body weight from front to back leg[17] |

## USING A SLIDE SHEET TO REPOSITION A CHILD IN BED

The slide sheet (or the more child friendly 'Slippery Sam') allows easy movement of the body on the supporting surface as it reduces friction by allowing one layer to slide over the other. A slide sheet is made from nylon sailcloth, which slides on itself, thus reducing the friction between the child and the surface. The advantage of the slide sheet over other techniques is that the movement required in its use is a slide, not a lift. This, therefore, reduces the strain on the handler(s). It is used to

• move a child in bed
• reposition a child up or across the bed

• turn a child over in bed
• assist car transfers
• reposition a child in a chair.

### The procedural goal is to

• minimise the risk of injury to the child and to reduce unnecessary handling of the child;
• minimise the risk of injury to handlers who are required to move and handle the child in and around the bed.

### Equipment

Slide sheet
Pillows

## PROCEDURE:  Using a slide sheet

| Procedural steps | Evidence-based rationale |
| --- | --- |
| **1** Prepare the *environment*<br>Remove any obstacles, clutter or spillages from the area | To prevent untoward accidents |
| Adjust the bed height to waist level of the handlers<br>Ensure that the bed brakes are on and working | To reduce reaching and forward flexion of handlers |
| **2** Consider the *individual*<br>*Never use a slide sheet if you have not been trained in its use*<br>Always use at least two handlers who have undergone training in lateral slide use | All users require training prior to use;[3,7] ensure skills competence<br>Minimum number of handlers considered necessary to maintain safety |
| **3** Prepare the *equipment*<br>Select the appropriate sized slide sheet for the child and task<br>If using the slide sheet with the child in a lying position, select a size that allows the slide sheet to reach from above the shoulders to below child's knees | This minimises the degree of spinal loading on the handler[17] |
| Always have two layers of slide sheet (either one folded or two separate sheets)<br>For a child weighing over 90 kg or those with contractures or muscle spasm, it is recommended that a larger slide sheet or two slide sheets (one on top of the other) are used<br>Examine the slide sheet for cleanliness, wear and damage to material and stitching before each use. Do not use if there is any evidence of soiling or wear or damage to the sling<br>Fold with the open end facing the direction of travel (generally) | The safest method for moving a dependent or partially dependent child using a slide sheet[18]<br>To increase the sliding surface and minimise the required forces |
| **4** Prepare the *load*<br>Assess the child's need for pain medication<br>Review care plan for any activity restrictions<br>Explain the purpose and describe details of the transfer to the child and parents as appropriate<br>Provide for child privacy | Maintain comfort<br>To avoid causing unforeseen harm<br>To gain informed consent and cooperation[2] |
| Encourage the child to assist as much as they can; educate child regarding ways to assist in transfer as appropriate<br>If able, ask the child to position themselves at the edge of bed nearest stretcher before slide board is put into place<br>Or, roll the child onto their side using an appropriate technique; place the slide sheet under the child by rolling up one edge and placing it under the child up to and including at least the child's buttocks and shoulders. Roll the child onto their other side and pull rolled up edge through | To promote the child's independence[19] and to reduce the amount of effort required by the handlers |

## PROCEDURE: Using a slide sheet (continued)

| | |
|---|---|
| Or, if the child is not too heavy, there is no necessity to move the child as the slide sheet can be positioned under the child's buttocks by placing your flat palms on the top of the slide sheet. Push down on the mattress as the slide sheet is positioned underneath the child's buttocks  Position child's head on a pillow with majority of pillow on side of move | To prevent skin injury and promote comfort[6] |
| 5 During the task:  Assume good posture  When using a slide sheet it is important to grasp the sheet, holding the top layer only, at the level of the child's shoulder and hip with palms facing upwards and arms kept close to the body at all times  If the child is assisting with pushing, make sure that their foot/feet and/or hand(s) are off the slide sheet  Position your legs in lunge position with body weight on front leg  One handler coordinates the task 'ready, set, slide'  Keeping arms straight, handlers move their weight from front to back leg  *Do not lift* the child being moved – slide  Move slowly!  Be aware of the distance between the child and the side of the bed  Remove slide sheet by pulling on bottom layer of the sheet against the top layer | Remember the principles of manual handling; the handlers' stance and posture is a key factor affecting spinal loading The power of the transfer comes from using your legs and bodyweight[9]  To prevent them from sliding off and to increase  their stability  For safety purposes, the child's buttocks should be no closer than 15 cm from the edge of the bed[18]  To reduce skin friction, the slide sheet is pulled on itself and not against the child's skin[17] |

## USING A HOIST

A hoist is a mechanical device used to transfer the full weight of a person in a lying, semi-reclined or sitting position. It consists of a central mast, boom with a rotating spreader bar and hooks to attach the sling, and an adjustable U-shaped base on castors or wheels. Hoists can be divided into three categories:

- Fixed, floor-mounted hoists are used mainly when bathing.
- Overhead hoists are usually electrically operated. They may be fixed permanently overhead or mounted on mobile frames.
- Mobile hoists are the largest of the three categories, and can be operated hydraulically or electrically.

There are a multitude of different slings available with varying designs and functions. Each patient will have to be assessed for the correct sling according to their needs. The most important considerations are the size, type and fabric of the sling. The choice of hoist sling will depend on

- the amount of support required;
- tasks which need to be undertaken;
- the comfort of the child being lifted;
- the ability of the child being lifted;
- the ability of the handler.

Generally speaking, the more fabric there is in a sling, the more support it will offer and the larger the area over which to spread the weight of the individual. Hence, hammock slings, which have more fabric, distribute pressure over a larger area and are usually the most comfortable. This is particularly important for children who are susceptible to pain. The spread between the points of suspension for the sling will also affect how the child is supported. The greater the spread between the suspension points the more open the sling will be. Although this may make the user feel more comfortable, the child may feel less supported.

### The procedural goal is to

- minimise the risk of injury to the child when you use a mechanical hoist;
- minimise the risk of injury to the handler when using a mechanical hoist.

## PROCEDURE: Using a mobile hoist

| Procedural steps | Evidence-based rationale |
|---|---|
| **1** Consider the *individual* <br><br> *Never use a hoist or sling that you have not been trained to use* | All users require training prior to use[3,7] for skills competence in order to take responsibility for knowing how equipment works |
| Gather the appropriate equipment and other handlers needed. Use a minimum of two handlers when using a mobile hoist. When a ceiling track hoist, a gantry hoist or a stand-aid is used, there may be circumstances where only one handler is needed, unless the child's risk assessment dictates otherwise | This is not a ruling from any specific professional body, nor an instruction from the manufacturers; it is considered to be safe practice.[9] A child is at risk of injury when being hoisted, particularly to head and feet. A single handler may find it difficult to facilitate the move as well as all aspects of the child's safety. When moving a mobile hoist (with child in situ) a second handler may be required to keep the child from swingin |
| Ensure that your team members know their role. Rehearse if necessary | Procedures with two or more caregivers require communication and coordination |
| **2** Prepare the *equipment* <br> Battery is charged (if electrical) <br> Pump works (if hydraulic) <br> Check that there are no parts missing and that all parts of the hoist are operational | So that there is sufficient power for use <br> All electric hoists should have a manual override system in case of loss of power during a move. Handler(s) should be familiar with the override systems of the hoist |
| The weight of the child should not exceed the safe working load (SWL). This will be marked somewhere on the hoist, usually the mast | The SWL is the capacity that the hoist has been designed to work at safely |
| Ensure that the hoist has been serviced every 6 months and there is a visible date/coloured plastic inspection tag attached to the hoist and sling is in-date (identifies them as having passed the inspection and are safe to use) <br> Irrespective of manufacturer, ensure that the hoist/sling interface is compatible, i.e. the type of attachment between the hoist's spreader bar and the sling must be the same. For example, do not use a sling with 'loop' type attachments with a hoist that has 'stud' type attachments on its spreader bar | Hoists and slings are subject to the Lifting Operations and Lifting Equipment Regulations (LOLER),[18] and you must comply with these regulations. If the equipment has not been inspected within the specified time period, i.e. does not have the appropriate coloured plastic inspection tag, do not use it – report it! To use it would be negligent <br> Some slings are incompatible with some hoists. There is also the risk of wrongly attaching the slings. Often manufacturers, because of liability, stipulate only their own slings can be used on their hoists. |

## PROCEDURE: Using a mobile hoist (continued)

| | |
|---|---|
| | However, some companies will give written permission for their slings to be used on compatible hoists manufactured by other companies |
| Examine the sling for cleanliness. Do not use if there is any evidence of soiling or wear or damage to the sling. Do not use disposable single patient use slings for bathing, or get them wet; in accordance with manufacturer's instructions they should be disposed of if they become wet and they should not be washed or cleaned | This is an important infection control issue to consider when slings are shared between patients. Do not use soiled slings. Ideally, slings should be patient allocated and/or laundered between patients. Disposable slings should be considered for use on patients with known infections or who are incontinent |
| Examine the sling for wear and damage to material and stitching, clips, straps before each use, e.g. holes, ladders, loose stitching, frayed material. Do not use a sling that is faulty, worn or soiled; discard and get a replacement | Slings do not last indefinitely. They may become worn and laundering will contribute to general wear and tear compromising safety over time. Damaged slings should be retired from use and replaced immediately[19] |
| Check that the sling is appropriate for the manoeuvre and patient size, shape and weight. Re-assess if patient has changed shape, size or weight, e.g. amputation, weight loss/gain | Follow manufacturer's instruction or coding system. If patient falls between two sizes, always use the smaller size[19] |
| | *Beware*: Although many manufacturers colour code their slings for size, there is no consistency between companies. Colour coding of slings can prove very confusing as corresponding sizes can vary from one company to another, in the way that shoe sizes often vary |
| **3 Prepare the *environment*** | |
| Organise the physical environment: ensure that there is sufficient space; remove any obstacles, e.g. rugs, trailing leads. Mop up spills if necessary Organise the equipment; ensure the wheels of the bed or chair are locked as necessary, the bed/stretcher is adjusted to the correct working height | To avoid adverse events and accidents To ensure safe completion of the task |
| Before beginning the procedure, check that the furniture or equipment, e.g. wheelchair, that you are transferring the patient to is ready and is correctly positioned so that the patient is moved only a minimum distance | Although there is no specific guidance on what distance a hoist may be moved with a patient in situ; hoists are designed to transfer, not transport. Do not move the child on the hoist, move the equipment to the child. Note that moving a bariatric child on a hoist is a high-risk activity Consider also the issues of patient comfort and dignity |
| **4 Prepare the *load*** | |
| Explain to the child and parents (if present) what you are doing and why Check for any vulnerable areas/issues, e.g. delicate skin, wounds, painful joints, catheters, respiratory compromise, paralysis, obesity Check with the child what they do for themselves, e.g. assisting with sling placing, moving own limbs Coach the child; tell them what action you plan and expect from them. Show them what to do, and then help them move through the activity | To gain the child's consent and cooperation[4] To avoid negative medical consequences of wrong sling choice[19] |

## PROCEDURE:  Using a mobile hoist (continued)

**5** During the *task*

As you begin the procedure, remain mindful of your posture; do not stoop over the patient as you put the sling on, e.g. raise the bed, kneel or squat down

To select the correct size sling

- Place the sling against the child and measure it from the top of the head to the base of the spine. (If it is not a full-body sling it should be measured starting at shoulder level)
- Measure the leg piece of the sling against the child from the back of the seat to the knee (or the floor to the knee). The leg piece should extend about 10 inches (25.4 cm) past the knee to fit correctly
- Make sure the sling fits the body width by holding the sling level with the shoulders. There should be a couple of inches extra width on both sides

Inserting a sling in bed

- Raise the bed to a good height
- Roll the child from side to side remembering to use normal patterns of movement
- Fold or roll the sling so that the child's spine will be in the middle of the sling ensuring that the handles and labels are on the outside of the sling
- Place the leg straps under the legs, bending the knees if necessary
- Some slings require the straps to be crossed over to maintain dignity

Inserting a sling in a chair

- Lean the child forward in the chair and slide the sling behind them. It may be necessary to fold the sling in half to do this
- Place the sling behind the child so that the centre of the sling is in line with the child's spine ensuring that the handles and labels are on the outside of the sling
- Slide the sling down behind the child until the bottom of the sling meets the seat
- Gently pull the leg straps round to the front and bring them under the knee
- If the leg needs to be raised to position the leg strap, do not lift it
- Use a sliding sheet to slide the child's foot onto the handler's thigh
- Aim to bring in the boom and spreader bar from one side
- Attach the sling connection to the spreader bar according to manufacturer's instructions
- Attach the shoulder sling connections. The legs should be positioned carefully. Give due consideration to dignity and hip status

*Think back*. Remember, a hoist does not resolve all your manual handling risk. Position yourself throughout the procedure using the principles of body mechanics (as described above)

It is important to have a sling that fits the child correctly.[19] If the sling is too large there is a risk of the child slipping out of the sling. A sling that is too small can result in the spreader bar coming too close to the face. The sling can be tight in the crotch and cause discomfort, and the sling may not provide enough support for the back

Always maintain good posture when inserting a sling. Position yourself throughout the procedure using the principles of body mechanics

Do *not* stand up and bend over to lift one or both of the legs of the child to position the sling underneath[19]

When trying out new slings, remember that it may take a few attempts to find the most comfortable position, and that the first sling that is tried may not be the correct size and/or shape

This can reduce the feeling that the spreader bar will touch the face of the child in the sling

Improper use of pull straps may result in injury to the patient and/or handler or damage the sling

Loops on the slings are for positioning the person

## PROCEDURE:  Using a mobile hoist (continued)

| | |
|---|---|
| • Ensure that leg supports are placed smoothly (not twisted). Bad fit is indicated when clips/loops only just appear between legs or leg supports dig into the backs of knees | correctly in the sling, not for trying to make a sling that is too big or too small fit him/her. It may take several attempts to successfully position the child so that he/she is comfortable. Once this has been achieved, it is worth marking the loops that have been used to avoid wasting time in the future |
| • Check that sling attachment clips are in the correct position before operating the lift | Do not put brakes on while hoist in use as the, pivot arm has to overcompensate for weight being carried and find its own centre of gravity. The hoist will automatically move towards the child when the weight is taken, rather than it moving away |
| • When using a mobile hoist, ensure that the hoist brakes are 'off' except when the hoist is in storage/not in use; when hoisting on an incline; or when adjusting a patient's clothing while they are suspended by the hoist | This will affect the hoist's stability |
| • When using a stand-aid, the brakes should be on while hoisting the patient into a standing position, but should be off when lowering the patient into a seated position | |
| • Do not push/pull the hoist's spreader bar excessively, or let the child hold on to the spreader bar | |
| • If appropriate, ask the child, being lifted to operate the controls | Provides the child with some element of independence and allows the handler both hands free to assist |
| Once the child starts to be raised | During the lift, the child will 'settle' into the lift: |
| • Ensure that the sling adequately supports the head (if using a sling with a head support) and that the child's buttocks are not beginning to slip through the sling opening | • should this happen, stop the lift procedure immediately and re-adjust the sling[19] |
| • Re-check that the sling hoops are securely attached to the spreader bar and 'in-tension' | • should this happen, stop the lift procedure immediately and retry with a smaller sling size[19] |
| • Re-check that the straps are not rucked-up under the legs | |
| • Check that the child feels safe and comfortable | |
| During the remainder of the lift | |
| • Ask the second handler to be vigilant of the position of the child's head in relation to the spreader bar, and especially so if the patient has any medical items in situ, e.g. a nasogastric tube, Hickman catheter, shunt | |
| • Raise and transfer the child smoothly and efficiently. If necessary remind the second handler to prevent the sling from swinging or moving unduly | |
| • Be aware to avoid twisting your trunk if manoeuvring a hoist in a confined space – do not force it, walk it round | When moving a hoist, employ the principles of safe handling; maintain a good posture and push rather than pull, if possible to prevent MSDs |
| • Minimise the amount of time that the child remains suspended in a sling | To promote comfort |
| As the child is lowered | |
| • Be mindful of the child's head as you lower the spreader bar to detach the sling | |
| • Ensure that the child is correctly positioned in the new location | |
| • Remove the sling carefully to avoid damage to the child's skin | To prevent further manual handling once the sling is removed[19] |

## THE BARIATRIC CHILD

The number of obese children has tripled in 20 years. Ten per cent of 6-year-olds are obese, rising to 17 per cent of 15-year-olds. Defining the term 'bariatric' poses a challenge, as there are many classification systems. Internationally, bariatric is defined as a body mass index (BMI) greater than 30.[20] The term 'bariatric' relates to those patients who weigh more than 25 stone (100 kg).[9] There are a few limitations of using weight and BMI categories. The above ranges can be used for people 20 years and over. For children and teenagers it doesn't work this way. Their body proportions are still developing and the formula has to be adjusted. There are implications both for health and for the moving and handling of the bariatric child. Risk assessment, adequate and suitable equipment provision, and training are essential in bariatric handling. The increased strain on the child's joints, cardiovascular system, range of movement and posture all make it more difficult for them to move and be moved.

There is a common misconception that bariatric patients can be accommodated by simply asking for equipment designed for a 'large size'. Most of the attention focuses on a bed and lift to accommodate the bariatric child. In fact, there are many aspects related to equipment that need to be considered. Knowing the weight capacity of existing equipment is critical for safety. Bariatric equipment may be indicated by using a label indicating 'EC' (expanded capacity) and weight limits. In addition to patient handling/movement equipment, the weight capacity of bedside recliner chairs or toilets must be considered.

Three tasks which prove very challenging and place handlers at a high risk for injury include

- insertion of slings
- repositioning
- turning.

Currently, manufacturers are working on designing slings that can be left under bariatric patients who have to be moved frequently. The advantages to this would be less strain on the handlers to turn the child to the side or log roll them to insert the sling, less time taken to perform the task of repositioning because the sling would already be there and, most important, less risk and exposure to injury. Although there is no evidence or literature on leaving slings under patients and patient outcomes, this decision should be carefully weighed. Questions for consideration:

1 Is the child's skin compromised?
2 How breathable is the sling?
3 Does the sling present rough uneven edges which can cause pressure points if left underneath?
4 Can the sling be left under the sheet and tucked into mattress when not in use?

Leaving a sling under a child can be advantageous to handler safety but may be detrimental to the child and clinical judgment should be used to determine the safest course of action. More research needs to be done in this area.

## CONCLUSION

Caring for your back, whether at home or at work, is your responsibility. It is important that you take every opportunity to learn and update yourself at least annually in safe moving and handling so that you can try to prevent back pain and injury. There is no completely safe and proper method for lifting and handling people, but there are general principles for lowering the risks of injury. It is important to use good lifting methods, have correct posture and take part in regular exercise. Prevention is always better than cure, especially in the case of back injuries.

Clearly it would not be possible to publish in any book every alternative moving and handling method and technique. Therefore, the aim of this chapter is to develop the reader's problem-solving abilities, enabling them to solve everyday moving and handling challenges.

This chapter provides a broad introduction to the topic of safe lifting and back care, fundamental information on the basic principles of manual handling and has given pointers on how to conduct a manual handling risk assessment. Beyond the specific strategies outlined, foremost is the need for a mind-set of 'safety first.' Yet we all know that vigilance, although necessary, is not sufficient to make the care we deliver safer. Beyond individual vigilance, employees have a legal duty to take reasonable care of their own health and safety and that of others who may be affected by what they do or not do, and organisational adherence to legislation must be established.

Go to the website to find the PowerPoint presentation for this chapter and MCQs to test your knowledge. **www.hodderplus.com/childnursingskills**

# REFERENCES

1 Jolley S (2007) Manual handling: lifting, lowering, pushing, pulling, carrying, supporting. *Paediatric Nursing* 18(7): 18.

2 Nursing and Midwifery Council (2008) *The code: standards of conduct performance and ethics for nurses and midwives*. London, NMC (http://www.nmc-uk.org/aFrameDisplay.aspx?DocumentID=3954).

3 Health and Safety Commission (HSC) (2004) *Manual handling operations regulations 1992* (as amended). Sudbury: HSE Books (http://www.opsi.gov.uk/si/si1999/19993242.htm).

4 Commission for Social Care Inspection (2008) *National strategy for Carers*. London: CSCI.

5 Andrews S, Bennett M (2007) Shouldering the burden of care. *The Column*, 19(3), 10–13.

6 The Children Act 2004 c31 s6.

7 Health and Safety Executive (HSE) (1974) Health and Safety at Work Act, etc. Act, 1974. London, HMSO (http://wwwhse.gov.uk/legislation/hswa.pdf).

8 McCance KL, Huether SE (2006) *Pathophysiology: the biologic basis for disease in adults and children*. 5th edition. St Louis: Elsevier.

9 Smith J (ed.) (2005) *The guide to the handling of people*. 5th edition. Teddington: ARJO, RCN & National Back Exchange.

10 Health and Safety Executive HSE (1995) *Reporting of injuries, diseases, and dangerous occurrences regulations 1995* (RIDDOR). London: HMSO.

11 Brooks AS (2008) Manual handling questions. *The Column* 20(1): 11–13.

12 Alexander P (2008) The changing face of manual handling in the community. *British Journal of Community Nursing* 13(7): 316–322.

13 Pellino TA, Owen B, Knapp L, Noack J (2006) The evaluation of mechanical devices for lateral transfers on perceived exertion and patient comfort. *Orthopaedic Nursing* 25(1): 4–10.

14 Sanders MJ, Morse T (2005) The ergonomics of caring for children: an exploratory study. *American Journal of Occupational Therapy* 59(3): 285–295.

15 Croshaw C (2007) To kneel or not to kneel: that is the question. The Column: *Journal of the National Back Exchange* 19(3), 14–21.

16 Baptiste A, Sruthi V, Boda MS (2006) Friction-reducing devices for lateral patient transfers: a clinical evaluation. *AAOHN Journal*, 54(4): 10–14.

17 Nelson A, Collins J, Siddharthen K (2008) Links between safe patient handling and patient outcomes in long-term care. *Rehabilitation Nursing* 33(1): 32–43.

18 Health and Safety Commission (2000) *Lifting operations and lifting equipment regulations (LOLER) 1998, approved code of practice and guidance*. London: HSC (http://www.hse.gov.uk/lau/lacs/90–4.htm).

19 Bakewell J (2007) Which sling and why? A product guide. *International Journal of Therapy and Rehabilitation*, 14(9): 424–429.

20 World Health Organization (2009) *Obesity: preventing and managing the global epidemic*. Geneva: WHO.

## CHAPTER 9

# Assessment and vital signs: a comprehensive review

Elizabeth Gormley-Fleming

## LEARNING OUTCOMES

*Upon completion of this chapter, the reader should be able to accomplish the following:*

1 Define the assessment phase of the nursing process
2 Discuss the purpose of assessment in nursing practice
3 Identify and apply the skills required for undertaking a systematic nursing assessment
4 Differentiate between objective and subjective data collection
5 Describe the various methods that may be employed to obtain objective data collection during physical assessment
6 Describe the procedures used to assess vital signs, temperature, pulse, respirations, blood pressure, capillary refill time and oxygen saturation level
7 Recognise normal vital sign values for infants and children of all ages
8 Identify rationale for using different routes when assessing temperature, pulse and capillary refill time
9 Describe and explain the role of electrocardiograph monitoring in infants and children
10 Describe the procedure for assessing neurological status in infants and children and be able to recognise abnormalities
11 Describe the procedures used to assess growth in the infant and child

## CHAPTER OVERVIEW

Central to the delivery of safe and effective nursing care is the nurse's ability to assess accurately the infant and child. It is the keystone of effective and safe practice and is a fundamental skill. Each child has unique healthcare needs, and the first question a nurse should ask is 'What information do I require if I am to nurse them effectively and safely?' Assessment leads to the identification of health problems and then to the development of care plans. This chapter is concerned primarily with the collection of physical data but will also consider the role of systematic assessment.

## AIM OF ASSESSMENT

The aim of assessment is to obtain information about the child that will form a baseline on which to plan care and initiate treatment. The seriously ill child must be identified and managed immediately before a complete assessment is undertaken.

The child's personal details, social history, developmental status, and psychological and physiological needs should be addressed. This will require multiple nursing skills and will necessitate classification and the analysis of data from a variety of sources.

There are many frameworks available to aid the process of assessment and these should identify the health needs of the child who requires the

| **Definition** | |
| --- | --- |
| **Assessment** may be defined as the gathering of information and formulation of judgements in partnership with the child and family. It is a continuous process. It will include physiological, physical, psychological, social and the spiritual aspect of the child and the effect that their health problem is having on their development and family life. | Assessment is the gathering of subjective and objective data. Subjective data will be ascertained from talking to the child and parent/carer and objective from the findings of auscultation, vital sign recordings, inspection, percussion and palpation. Assessment should be holistic but in the emergency situation an expedient and focused assessment may initially be undertaken when the seriously ill or injured child presents. |

intervention of the healthcare team. There are also many tools available, some of which are validated, that will assist in the assessment of specific areas, such as skin integrity, level of consciousness and mouth care. In child health a partnership approach to assessment is advocated.[1]

# SYSTEMATIC ASSESSMENT

Systematic assessment is a rigorous approach to the collection of subjective and objective data. It entails examination and review of the systems of the body.

## Approaching the child

The approach to the child and family by the nurse is of particular importance at the assessment phase, as anxiety and fear may be present in both the child and parents. A sympathetic approach is required and the child's cooperation and trust need to be gained before the objective assessment is undertaken, except in the case of a life-threatening event. Mock examinations of the child's teddy for example may help to allay fears as will allowing them to handle equipment that may be used.

Prior to any communication, it is essential to evaluate the child visually as you approach them. This will provide you with immediate information regarding the state of their current health, nutritional state, level of hygiene and care, interaction with environment and carers, and general demeanour. Developmental milestones can be noticed at this stage also.

Commence the assessment with the most non-threatening aspect, first having given detailed explanations to the child and family. Any holding that is required should be gentle.[2] Remember your own behaviour: a smiling, talking nurse will appear less threatening to the child and family. Warm, clean hands are also essential.

## The child's age

The assessment should be adapted to reflect the age of the child. This may require the nurse to be resourceful and employ distraction techniques and games in order to achieve a complete assessment. It should never be performed under duress. Parents can facilitate the assessment process if informed of what is required of them. Cultural sensitivities should be considered. The following points should be considered for the various groups of children that require assessment:

- Babies may either be assessed in the parent's arms or on the examination couch/cot with parents close by.
- Toddlers are best assessed on the parent's lap or over the parent's shoulder. Parents are reassuring for the child at this age.
- Young children can be initially assessed when playing, and then will require a quiet private area for a more detailed physical assessment. They may have some understanding of their body parts and may like to examine the equipment being used.
- School-aged children will be aware of various body parts, will generally be cooperative and value their parents' presence.
- Young people will be concerned about their privacy and this must be maintained. Be sensitive to their needs and wishes. They may or may not want their parents present.

## Privacy and dignity

A warm, comfortable area is essential when undertaking assessment of the child. When undressing the child, it is best done in stages only exposing the areas that need to be. The child and parents should be involved. Sensitivity when questioning is important to avoid embarrassment to the child and family.

## Subjective data

This is the information obtained from the child and parents and it will assist with creating a profile of current health status. This should include the presenting complaint, past health history, the mother's antenatal history, birth history and neonatal history (infants and young children only), any known allergies, immunisation status, current medication, developmental history, psychosocial history, family and social history, along with a detailed account of their normal personal habits: eating, drinking, elimination, activity, sleeping, play/work and sexual activity as appropriate. This is a vital part of the assessment process and will be determined by the severity of the child's illness, which may focus the assessment initially but will require completion at a later stage.

## Objective data

This is the information obtained by the nurse and is collated by inspection, palpation, percussion and auscultation along with a range of medical devices. This is best done by a system-based approach. The most frequently performed skills are discussed in the remainder of this chapter.

## PHYSICAL ASSESSMENT

### Temperature

Fever is a common symptom in infants and children and usually occurs as a result of infection, inflammation or as an immune response. Body temperature is a precisely controlled homeostatic mechanism that regulates heat gained and heat lost from the body. Accurate temperature assessment is of crucial importance as it will determine the decisions made about the clinical management of the infant or child.

A normal core body temperature for a newborn infant will be between 36.5°C and 37.6°C.[3] As the child grows, the normal body temperature reflects a decreasing basic metabolic rate, and for an older child a range of 36°C to 37.5°C may be considered to be within normal parameters, but this will vary depending on the site measured.

Infants and young children are at risk of hypothermia due to larger body surface area to body weight ratio and larger head to body ratio.[4] Infants less than 6 months of age cannot shiver to generate heat and will maintain body heat through non-shivering thermogenesis. This occurs with the secretion of noradrenaline (norepinephrine), resulting in the breakdown of brown fat and the creation of heat. This is an energy-requiring process and increases the infant's oxygen consumption.

Clinical *hypothermia* is a core body temperature of less than 35°C. Hypothermia can be classified as mild, moderate, deep and profound.[5] Hypothermia is mulitfactorial in origin and may be a result of environmental exposure, drugs that affect thermoregulation or metabolic conditions.

*Hyperthermia* is a significant rise in body temperature and may be non-infectious in origin: drug allergy, status epilepticus, malignancy, heat stroke and malignant hyperthermia are some of the possible causes.

Temperature in infants and children may be easily measured at several body sites and the routine sites are indicated in Table 9.1. There are

**Table 9.1** Routes for temperature measurement

| Child's age | Route | Device |
|---|---|---|
| Infant under 4 weeks of age | Axilla | Electronic thermometer6 |
| 4 weeks to 5 years | Axilla Tympanic | Electronic thermometer Chemical dot thermometer Infrared tympanic thermometer[6] |
| 5 years and older | Oral Axilla Tympanic | Electronic thermometer Chemical dot thermometer |
| Should be used only in the critically ill child or in Intensive Care Units and if no other route is available | Rectal | Electronic probe |

advantages and disadvantages for all sites. The ideal technique for measuring temperature should be that it is rapid, painless and it reproduces measurements that accurately reflect core temperature.

## Thermometers

The most frequently used temperature measurement devices in children are:

- electronic intermittent thermometers, which can be used orally or in the axilla;
- infrared thermometers, which measure the temperature by collecting emitted thermal radiation from a specific site, usually the ear canal;
- single-use chemical dot thermometers, which may be used orally or in the axilla, have thermosensitive chemical dots which change colour to indicate the temperature measurement;
- electronic continuous thermometers, which are used during general anaesthesia, treatment of hypothermia or hyperthermia and other situations where continuous monitoring may be required.

Selection will depend on the age of the child, clinical condition of the child, availability of equipment, and preference of the child, if they can articulate this.

As temperature is frequently measured, reliability and consistency of recording is important and is achieved by using the same type of thermometer and site each time measurement is required.

Mercury thermometers must not be used as they are hazardous if broken; vapours can be inhaled causing significant toxicity.[3]

### Indications for measuring temperature are

- on admission to determine a baseline for assessment and future measurement;
- to monitor any changes in temperature; this can occur suddenly in children;
- at parental request.

### The procedural goal is to

- accurately assess and measure core body temperature.

### Equipment

Thermometer
Clean disposable probe cover
Watch with second hand

## PROCEDURE: Tympanic temperature measurement

| Procedural steps | Evidence-based rationale |
|---|---|
| **1** Wash hands | To minimise the risk of cross-infection |
| **2** Explain procedure to child and parents | To gain cooperation |
| **3** Place the infant either in the supine position or sitting on parent's knee, if old enough to sit; stabilise their head and turn it 90° to gain access. For children older than 1 year, position on parent's lap with head secure | To gain access to ear canal |
| **4** Remove probe from thermometer base and observe lens, which should be clean and free from cracks | Clean and maintain as per manufacturer's instructions Alcohol-based wipes should not be used as they may cause a false high measurement |
| **5** **Children <1 year of age** For children under 1 year of age, if you are measuring the right ear, hold thermometer in right hand, and vice versa if using left ear | Allows greater control over sudden movements |
| **6** Pull pinna of the ear straight back and downwards. Approach the ear from behind to direct the tip | The tip must be aimed at tympanic membrane if accurate measurement is to be obtained |

## PROCEDURE: Tympanic temperature measurement (continued)

| | |
|---|---|
| of the probe anteriorly to make sure the thermometer tip will be aimed at the tympanic membrane | |
| 7  Place probe in the ear as far as possible to seal the canal | Provision of accurate measurement of temperature by preventing air from entering ear canal causing a false low measurement |
| 8  Turn on scanner and leave in ear canal until audible alarm confirming temperature measurement has sounded | Early removal will provide inaccurate measurement |
| 9  Remove probe and read temperature | |
| 10  Document measurement on observation chart, noting which ear was used | Evidence of procedure<br>The same ear should be used when recording the temperature frequently and the child needs to be in the same ambient temperature for 20 minutes to provide greater accuracy[7] |
| 11  Dispose of disposable cover and wash hands | To minimise the risk of cross-infection |
| 12  **Children >1 year of age**<br>Pull the pinna up and backwards in children older than 1 year of age | The tip must be aimed at tympanic membrane if accurate measurement is to be obtained |
| 13  Follow steps 6–10 as described above | |

## PROCEDURE: Axillary route: Electronic and chemical dot thermometers

| Procedural steps | Evidence-based rationale |
|---|---|
| 1  Wash hands | To minimise the risk of cross-infection |
| 2  Remove probe from protective holder and ensure it is intact and clean | Clean as per manufacturer's instructions if required |
| 3  Place protective sheath on probe and place under infants or child's axilla, ensuring it is placed in the centre of the axilla with the arm firmly against the side of the chest | To achieve accurate measurement |
| 4  Turn on scanner and wait until audible tone can be heard indicating that measurement has been recorded | To achieve accurate measurement |
| 5  Remove probe, note reading and document in observation chart. Document which axilla has been used as it is important that the same arm is used for repeated measurements | There may be a variation on temperature between right and left |
| 6  Dispose of probe sheath, replace probe in holder and wash hands | To minimise the risk of cross-infection and to provide evidence of care<br>Probe covers are single-use only |
| 7  If you are using chemical dot thermometer, ensure chemically active strip is placed facing torso and leave in situ as per manufacturer's instructions which maybe up to 3 minutes | False low reading will occur if positioned incorrectly |

## PROCEDURE: Oral route

| Procedural steps | Evidence-based rationale |
| --- | --- |
| 1 Wash hands | To minimise the risk of cross-infection |
| 2 Check that child has had nothing to eat or drink within last 20 minutes | Mastication and drinking hot or cold liquids can cause a significant change in oral temperature measurement Smoking can also cause significant changes in oral temperature measurement as can mouth breathing |
| 3 Assess the cooperation of the child and their ability to hold the thermometer in their mouth before commencing procedure | Child needs to be able to cooperate to obtain accurate measurement |
| 4 Place the oral probe covered with a disposable sheath or disposable thermometer under the child's tongue in the posterior sublinguinal pocket | Must be in posterior sublingual pocket to maintain accurate measurement. Changes in core temperature are most accurately reflected here[8] |
| 5 Turn on scanner and wait for audible tone to sound. Remove from child's mouth and note reading. If you are using chemical dot thermometer, leave in situ for 60 seconds prior to removal and then note reading | Needs to be in situ as per manufacturer's instructions to obtain accurate measurement |
| 6 Dispose of probe cover/chemical dot thermometer and wash hands | To minimise the risk of cross-infection |
| 7 Document measurement in observation chart | To provide evidence of care and to enable care to be planned |

There are many factors to consider when measuring temperature: temperature measurement devices, sites used, patient preference which all have an impact on the management of fever or hypothermia. A holistic approach must be adopted and temperature measurement must also include general observation of the child.

- Is child shivering, moving or lying still?
- Position of child: curled up or extended?
- Skin colour: pale or flushed?
- Are they sweating?
- Body hair: piloerection?
- Respiratory rate.
- Heart rate.
- Level of consciousness.
- Urine output and faecal loss.

## CARDIOVASCULAR ASSESSMENT

Cardiovascular assessment entails inspection, palpation of pulse, auscultation of heart sounds and taking blood pressure. These are basic skills that are essential in determining the improvement or deterioration of the child.

## Pulse

A pulse is a pressure wave transmitted through the arterial tree with each cardiac cycle as the arteries expand and recoil.[8] Palpation of the pulse is an important aspect of cardiovascular assessment in infants and children. Normal ranges of pulse rate must be known (Table 9.2, page 115).

A pulse can be palpated in an artery that lies close to the surface of the body; thus, the radial, femoral, brachial and carotid pulses may be easily palpated. Rate, rhythm and volume must be noted and documented. Other locations of palpable pulses are the temporal artery, facial artery, popliteal artery, posterior tibial artery and dorsalis pedis artery as outlined in Figure 9.1, page 115.

Cardiac output is the product of heart rate and ventricular stroke volume. Cardiac output relative to body weight is highest in infancy. High cardiac output in infants and children is achieved by high heart rates. Thus, bradycardia is a serious sign in the infant and child and must be acted upon vigorously, as inadequate circulation will lead to inadequate tissue perfusion.[9] The stroke volume increases with age and the heart rate decreases. The heart rate will

**Table 9.2** Normal heart rates for children of different ages[9]

| Age | Approximate range: awake (bpm*) | Average (bpm*) |
|---|---|---|
| Newborn to 3 months | 95–205 | 140 |
| 3 months to 2 years | 100–180 | 130 |
| 2–10 years | 60–140 | 80 |
| >10 years | 60–100 | 75 |

*bpm, beats per minute.

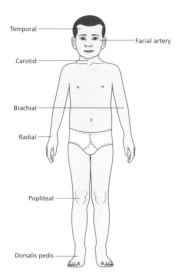

**Figure 9.1** Location of pulse points.

also increase with exercise, excitement, anxiety and fever. The presence of 1°C of fever may increase the heart rate by 10 beats per minute. All of these stressors will increase the child's metabolic rate, thus creating an increased need for more oxygen. The child responds to this by increasing the heart rate: sinus tachycardia. Children do not have the ability to increase their stroke volume to increase tissue perfusion like adults do.

### Indications for taking a pulse

- as a baseline assessment on admission so comparisons can be made;
- following surgery to assess for cardiovascular stability;
- when a child is receiving intravenous fluids, medication and blood or blood products;
- when caring for a child with a head injury or any suspected alteration in levels of consciousness;
- following any procedure where sedation has been administered;
- before the administration of cardioglycosides;
- when treating a child with hypertension – the pulse rate should be determined along with rhythm and volume and this must be compared with baseline;
- in the presence of infection;
- as part of pain assessment;
- as part of routine monitoring.

## Auscultation

Auscultation of the apex of the heart is the gold standard for assessing heart rate in infants and children less than two years of age. It may be necessary to prioritise the order of the physical assessment and auscultation of the heart is best

---

## Definitions

**Bradycardia:** a heart rate of < 80 beats per minute in a child under 1 year of age and < 60 beats per minute in a child > 1 year of age, commonly as a result of hypoxia, acidosis, respiratory or circulatory failure.[9]

**Tachycardia:** a heart rate of > 180 beats per minute in a child < 1 year of age and a heart rate of > 160 beats per minute in a child > 1 year of age.[9] This is frequently a physiological response due to pain, fear, fever. However, it may occasionally be due to cardiac arrhythmias.

**Sinus rhythm:** normal regular rhythm on of the heart

performed when the infant or child is asleep or quiet. The first (mitral and tricuspid valve closure) and second (aortic and pulmonary valve closure) heart sounds 'lub-dub' should be heard. Any other sounds heard should be discussed with medical staff.

### The procedural goal is to

• measure heart rate to determine cardiovascular function and make comparisons.

### Equipment

Stethoscope
Alcohol-based swab
Watch with second hand

### Apical heart beat

Children under 2 years of age should have an apical heart beat recorded as they have a rapid heart rate and locating a pulse in small area of an extremity for palpation can lead to inaccurate measurement being recorded. However, comparisons between distal and proximal pulses may need to be made for strength of pulse so the practitioner needs to be able to accurately locate all pulse sites in the infant. In an emergency situation when no stethoscope is available, the brachial pulse should be utilised for assessing pulse data.

## PROCEDURE: Measuring heart rate

| Procedural steps | Evidence-based rationale |
|---|---|
| 1 Wash hands and clean diaphragm of stethoscope | To minimise risk of transmission of infection |
| 2 Remove clothing from chest | To gain access to fourth intercostal space |
| 3 Distract infant if not sleeping | A quiet infant will provide a resting pulse rate |
| 4 Place stethoscope over fourth intercostal space in the midclavicular line. Place stethoscope over fifth intercostal space in the midclavicular line if recording apex beat in an older child | Location of cardiac apex in infants. In infants and young children, palpation of a pulse in an extremity is difficult to achieve for the required amount of time to count the rate<br>Auscultation of apex is the most accurate method of counting heart rate in infants[10] |
| 5 Count heart rate for 60 seconds | Sufficient time required to detect irregularities and to note volume |
| 6 Note rate, rhythm and volume | Each 'lub-dub' sound is one beat |
| 7 Document apical rate on observation chart, clean stethoscope and wash hands | Evidence of care given and enables comparisons to be made<br>To minimise risk of transmission of infection |

## PROCEDURE: Palpation of peripheral pulse

| Procedural steps | Evidence-based rationale |
|---|---|
| 1 Wash hands | To minimise risk of transmission of infection |
| 2 If possible measure the pulse under the same conditions. If not possible, document changes: crying, distressed, combative | Ensures consistency and continuity of measurements |
| 3 Place second and third finger gently above the artery from which pulse is being recorded | Thumb and forefinger have their own pulses so may be mistaken for patients own pulse. Too much pressure will occlude pulse and cause patient discomfort |
| 4 Count for 1 full minute | Sufficient time required to detect irregularities and to note volume |
| 5 Note rate, rhythm and volume. If any concerns cross-check with apex beat | Enables comparisons to be made<br>Peripheral pulses should be consistent with apex beat |
| 6 Document and wash hands | Evidence of care given and enables comparisons to be made<br>To minimise risk of transmission of infection |

## Palpation of peripheral pulse

The radial pulse is generally the site of choice when measuring the pulse rate in children over 2 years of age as it is the most accessible site. Occasionally this site may not be available so another site may have to be used.

### Pulse volume

The volume of the central pulses (femoral, axillary and carotid) should be graded according to the criteria in Table 9.3. Pulse volume gives a subjective indication of stroke volume. As stroke volume decreases so will the pulse volume, with the peripheral pulses (radial) decreasing in volume earlier in the presence of circulatory shock. Simultaneous palpation of central and peripheral pulses may be useful in determining the degree of compensation.[9] Caution must be maintained when assessing pulse volume in the child with fever, vasoconstriction, and when the room temperature is cold.

**Table 9.3** Grading of pulses[11]

| Grade | Description |
| --- | --- |
| 0 | Not palpable |
| +1 | Difficult to palpate. Thready and weak. Easily obliterated |
| +2 | Difficult to palpate and may be obliterated easily with pressure |
| +3 | Easy to palpate. Not easily obliterated with pressure. Normal pulse volume |
| +4 | Strong, bounding and not obliterated with pressure |

**VIGNETTE**

**Problem:** When palpating a child's radial pulse you notice that it increases and then decreases. The child is not exhibiting any other signs or symptoms.

**Discussion:** Sinus arrhythmia is normal and common in children; on inspiration the heart rate increases and on expiration it decreases.

## Blood pressure

Non-invasive blood pressure (BP) measurement is an essential part of the physical assessment and should be left until last to avoid upsetting the child. Blood pressure may be defined as the force exerted against the walls of the vessels in which it is contained.[8] It is cardiac output systemic vascular resistance. Blood pressure is read as systolic over diastolic. Blood ejected from the left ventricle into the arterial vessels provides the peak pressure of blood and this is referred to as the systolic blood pressure. Diastolic pressure is the minimum pressure of the blood against the walls of the arteries following closure of the aortic valve. Systemic vascular resistance increases with age and this is reflected in the range of normal blood pressure measurements (Table 9.4). These normal values are only reliable if the same methods of measurement, limb and cuff size are used in clinical practice. A normal BP is defined as a systolic and diastolic BP less than the 90th percentile for age and sex.[11] Children have the ability to compensate effectively when their cardiac output is decreased; thus hypotension is a late and pre-terminal sign which requires immediate resuscitation.

**Table 9.4** Blood pressure ranges by age of child[9]

| Age | Normal systolic blood pressure (mmHg) | Lower limit |
| --- | --- | --- |
| 0–1 month | >60 | 50–60 |
| 1–12 months | 80 | 70 |
| 1–10 years | 90+ (2 × age in years) | 70 + (2 × age in years) |
| >10 years | 120 | 90 |

### Measurement of blood pressure

Blood pressure is usually measured by auscultation with a manual aneroid sphygmomanometer or by oscillometry using electronic devices such as a Dinamap™. Doppler technique can also be used. Oscillometry provides a digital read-out for the systolic and diastolic and mean arterial pressures and is probably the most common method used in practice. It works on the principle that blood flowing through the artery between systolic and diastolic pressure causes vibrations in the arterial wall, which are detected and transduced into electrical signals.[12] Blood pressure measured by this method is generally higher and correlates with direct radial arterial pressure values.[13] Users of electronic devices need to be aware of their limitations and follow the manufacturers instructions. They are sensitive to movement and will adversely affect the measurement. Other errors in measurement such as pulse volume and rhythm will not be detected by the electronic device, thus indicating the need for manual recordings.[14] Conversely, oscillometry eliminates some other problems associated with auscultation, such as the inability to hear the soft sounds and the exact numbers at which Korotkoff sounds are audible (Table 9.5). Korotkoff sounds are not reliably heard in all children under the age of 1 year and in some of those under 5 years of age, thus indicating the need for oscillometry and Doppler.[4]

There are many factors that affect blood pressure. Human error such as faulty technique,[15] inadequate education[16] and incorrect cuff size are contributing factors. Sucking, crying, movement and eating may also effect the accuracy of blood pressure readings.[17]

**Table 9.5** Korotkoff's sounds

| Korotkoff's sound | Description |
| --- | --- |
| Phase 1 | A clear tapping sound |
| Phase 2 | A blowing or swishing sound |
| Phase 3 | A softer tapping sound than phase 1 |
| Phase 4 | Sound becomes faint or muffled |
| Phase 5 | Disappearance of all sound |

### Sites from which blood pressure may be measured

The sites from which blood pressure may be measured in infants and children are:

- upper arm: brachial artery, the site of choice due to accessibility;
- lower arm: radial artery;
- thigh: popliteal artery;
- calf or ankle: posterior tibial artery.

Whichever site is chosen should be documented in care records.

Blood pressure measurement may differ when other sites are used. Systolic pressure in the lower limbs is greater than the upper limbs generally. Systolic pressure in the calf is greater than that of the thigh. This may be 10–15 mmHg (1.33–2.00 kPa).

### Cuff size

One of the most important components in recording an infant's or child's BP is choosing the correct cuff size, whether their blood pressure is being recorded manually or electronically. The cuff size should not be determined by the manufacturer's sizing on the cuff but on the child's arm dimensions. 'Undercuffing' – too narrow or too short a bladder – can lead to overestimation of BP and 'overcuffing' – too wide or too long – may lead to underestimation.[18] The cuff should be two-thirds of the distance from the elbow to the shoulder or the upper thigh, and the bladder of the cuff should cover 100 per cent of the circumference of the arm.[3,17] The cuff used should be documented so continuity of care can be provided.

### Indications for measuring blood pressure

- It provides a baseline of the child's condition on admission.
- It aids in assessing the infant's and child's cardiovascular system.
- It may be used to monitor the effect of medication, e.g. antihypertension medication, cytotoxics.
- It may assist in the diagnosis of disease, e.g. cardiac disease, renal disease.

- It monitors variations in a child's condition.
- Following surgery the child's blood pressure should be measured so a base line of comparisons may be made.
- When receiving blood or blood products or intravenous fluids.
- It may identify an additional health need that is not immediate obvious, e.g. undiagnosed real disease or a neurological defect.

### The procedural goal is to

- accurately measure a child's blood pressure.

### Equipment (manual blood pressure measurement)

Sphygmomanometer (manual)
Various size cuffs
Paediatric stethoscope

## PROCEDURE: Measuring blood pressure

| Procedural steps | Evidence-based rationale |
|---|---|
| 1 Explain procedure to the child and family, telling them how it will feel | To ensure their understanding and gaining their consent. |
| 2 Wash hands | To minimise risk of transmission of infection |
| 3 Ensure the infant/child is resting/sitting quietly for as long possible. Ideally, this should be between 1 and 3 minutes. The child might wish to sit on parent's lap. BP should be recorded before any other anxiety-inducing procedures. Use diversion techniques | To obtain an accurate reading. Normal blood pressure is measured with the patient sitting and calm[11] |
| 4 Remove restrictive clothing from arm/leg | Tight or restrictive clothing will affect accuracy of reading[19] |
| 5 Select correct size cuff | To obtain accurate reading |
| 6 Ensure arm is supported and positioned at heart level. Right arm is preferable[10] | Muscle contraction in an unsupported arm can raise diastolic measurement and an arm positioned above heart level can lead to an underestimation of BP.[18] Right arm is consistently used for development of blood pressure standard |
| 7 Apply cuff snugly around arm ensuring that the centre of the bladder covers the brachial artery | To obtain accurate reading |
| 8 Place sphygmomanometer at eye level | To obtain accurate reading |
| 9 Palpate for brachial pulse | |
| 10 Close air escape valve and inflate cuff until radial pulse can no longer be palpated. Continue to | To avoid a low systolic pressure not being accurately measured |

## PROCEDURE: Measuring blood pressure (continued)

| | |
|---|---|
| inflate cuff to another 20 mmHg (2.67 kPa) higher than estimated systolic pressure | Pressure exerted by the inflated cuff prevents blood flow through the artery |
| 11 Place diaphragm of stethoscope gently over pulse point of brachial artery, ensuring it is not tucked under edge of cuff | Too much pressure will distort sounds |
| 12 Release air valve slowly to deflate the cuff 2–3 mmHg per second (0.27–0.40 kPa) | Slower deflation rates may cause arm pain from venous congestion leading to false low readings, and fast deflation rates can lead to an imprecise reading[20] |
| 13 Note first Korotkoff sound, a clear tapping sound, and record as systolic value. Record diastolic pressure at the fourth Korotkoff sound, a low-pitched muffled sound for children up to 12 years of age. Record fifth Korotkoff sound, disappearance of all sound for children aged 13–18 years | To ensure an accurate reading is recorded |
| 14 Remove cuff and replace child's clothing | Promote patient comfort and dignity |
| 15 Document readings on observation chart and in care records, noting limb, position, cuff size and method of measurement | For comparisons to be made, facilitate care planning and continuity of care[21,22] |
| 16 Wash hands and clean equipment and store correctly | To minimise risk of transmission of infection |

### Automated measurement of blood pressure

This should be done in accordance with the manufacturer's instructions and steps 1–7 and 14–16 outlined above followed.

When you are using an automated device, the first reading should be discarded.[23] Movement will affect measurement and often leads to machine alarming, which can be distressing for the child. A sequence of abnormal readings obtained by automated measurements should be checked with a manual sphygmomanometer.

Automated devices need to be calibrated on a regular basis to ensure accuracy of measurement.

### Capillary refill time

Capillary refill time (CRT) is the rate at which blood returns to the capillary bed after digital compression. CRT should always be measured when you are assessing the sick infant and child.

It is a very useful, non-invasive and quick method of determining the efficacy of respiratory function and degree of dehydration and is an early indicator of shock. It should never be measured in isolation and should always be considered along with other clinical signs.[24]

**VIGNETTE**

**Problem:** You cannot locate the correct size BP cuff to record a child's BP.

**Discussion:** When the correct size cuff is not available an oversized cuff is preferable than an undersized one. Alternatively, use a different site. Ensure correct documentation by recording cuff used and site used for measurement.

### Procedural goal

• assessment of degree of shock and hydration.

### Sites used for assessing CRT

• Fingers
• Sternum-at heart level
• Toes
• Forehead

**VIGNETTE**

**Problem:** You notice that room temperature is very cool

**Discussion:** CRT is affected by body exposure to cold environments and ambient temperature should always be considered when interpreting the results, as should consideration be given to room lighting.

## PROCEDURE: Measuring CRT

| Procedural steps | Evidence-based rationale |
|---|---|
| 1 Assess the need for measuring CRT | Tissues require oxygen and blood flow through the capillary bed for survival |
| 2 Wash hands | To minimise the risk of cross-infection |
| 3 If using digits or toes, raise the limb to heart level if possible | Reduces the effect of gravity on the result |
| 4 Apply moderate pressure with your forefinger to the chosen site for 5 seconds | CRT is the return rate of blood to the capillary bed after compression |
| 5 Remove pressure source and while counting in seconds note when reperfusion occurs, i.e. when skin returns to normal colour | Normal value is accepted as <2 seconds in infants and children, <3 seconds in neonates |
| 6 Return limb to resting position | Patient comfort |
| 7 If CRT is >2 seconds, report to medical staff at once | Delayed CRT may be indicative of poor peripheral perfusion and an early indicator of shock. A refill time of >3 seconds in a child is associated with >10% dehydration[25] |
| 8 Document procedure noting site used, findings and action taken | Provide evidence of care and facilitate planning of care[21,22] |

The skin of the sternum and forehead are best for estimating CRT as peripheral circulation can be delayed even in good health.

### Electrocardiograph

An electrocardiograph (ECG) measures the electrical activity of the cardiac muscle, which is displayed on an oscilloscope and may be printed out on calibrated graph paper. This may then be analysed and evaluated. It is a non-invasive diagnostic tool and may be used in conjunction with other tests such as echocardiogram or cardiac catheterisation. ECG is now frequently used to complement cardiovascular assessment and to continuously monitor the haemodynamic status of the child. The ECG may be performed intermittently or continuously. Interpretation of the ECG is essential if arrhythmias are to be recognised and treated. The information an ECG supplies to the clinician includes:

- heart rate and rhythm
- abnormalities of conduction
- effects of electrolyte imbalance
- presence of ischaemia
- effect of drug therapy
- hypertrophy of cardiac muscle
- pericardial disease.[26]

The electrical activity of the heart is presented diagrammatically in Figure 9.2.

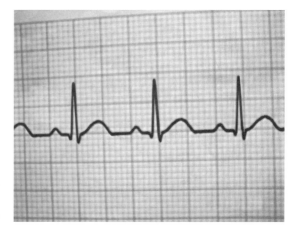

Figure 9.2 Normal sinus trace.

The *P wave* represents the contraction and depolarisation of the atria.

The *PR interval* is a measurement of the time taken for the electrical impulses from the sinoatrial node to travel through the atrial muscle, atrioventricular node, bundle of His and to reach the ventricular muscle mass.

The *QRS complex* represents the spread of ventricular depolarisation.

The *T wave* is produced by ventricular repolarisation: resting electrical state.

The age of the child is significant when undertaking ECG monitoring you are as the contribution of each chamber of the heart changes with growth. At birth in the term infant, right ventricular dominance is present, changing to left ventricular dominance by 1 month of age and to an adult pattern by 6 months of age.[27] The T wave will be positive/upright during the first 4 days of life, changing to a negative position until adolescence is reached, when it will adopt a positive position again.

An ECG may be recorded with either 3, 6 or 12 leads, with 12 leads being used to provide the optimal recording. Three-lead ECG monitoring is commonly used for bedside monitoring. The leads detect electrical current approaching them and going away from them, giving a positive and negative deflection on the monitor.[28]

### The procedural goal is to

- to provide safe and effective monitoring while being able to recognise abnormalities.

### Equipment required

ECG machine with chest and limb leads
Electrodes, appropriate sizes for age of child
Alcohol swabs

## PROCEDURE: Taking an ECG

| Procedural steps | Evidence-based rationale |
|---|---|
| 1 Explain the procedure to the child and parents and discuss the need for the child to remain as still as possible | To ensure that the child and parents understand need for procedure and gives their consent |
| 2 Wash hands | To reduce the risk of cross-infection |
| 3 Ensure the child is in a comfortable position | Will help in obtaining optimal recording |
| 4 Clean the skin as required. Skin needs to be dry, free from dry skin and greasy lotions/ointments. Body hair may need to be removed | To obtain good contact between skin and electrodes which will reduce electrical artefact |
| 5 Position electrodes as in Tables 9.6 and 9.7 (page 123) | Correct placement of electrodes is important to ensure that electrical impulses are accurately recorded in both the vertical and horizontal plane |
| 6 Attach leads from ECG machine to correct electrodes ensuring leads are not pulling on electrodes or lying over each other | To ensure correct polarity in ECG recording and to reduce electrical artefact |
| 7 Ask child to lie as still as they can | To reduce artefact from muscle movement |
| 8 Turn on ECG machine/monitor | To obtain recording |
| 9 Note tracing and for presence of artefact: check electrodes and connections to leads. | To obtain optimal recording |
| 10 If you are performing a 12-lead ECG, detach printout, label with child's name, hospital number, date and time | To ensure ECG is labelled with correct patient details |
| 11 Remove electrodes gently. If electrodes are to remain in situ for continuous 3-lead bedside monitoring, change as per manufacturer's instructions, usually daily | Prevents dermal abrasions from occurring |
| 12 Clean child's skin by removing any excess gel from electrodes and replace clothing | Promotes comfort and dignity |
| 13 Clean leads as per manufacturer's instructions | To reduce the risk of cross-infection |
| 14 Wash hands and dispose of waste | To reduce the risk of cross-infection |
| 15 Place ECG recording in child's medical notes, document that procedure has been performed and inform nursing and medical colleagues that procedure has been completed | To provide a record of care and to enable data to be used in treatment and care planning[21,22] |

**Table 9.6** Placement of electrocardiogram electrodes for 12-lead ECG

| | |
|---|---|
| Chest electrodes | V1: fourth intercostal space to right of sternum |
| | V2: fourth intercostal space to left of sternum |
| | V3: midway between V2 and V4 |
| | V4: fifth intercostal space at midclavicular line |
| | V5: fifth left intercostal space at anterior axillary line, midway between V4 and V6 |
| | V6: 5 fifth left intercostal space at midaxillary line |
| Limb electrodes | One on each of the upper limbs at the level of the wrists |
| | One on each of the lower limbs just above the ankles. |

**Table 9.7** Placement of electrocardiogram electrodes for 3-lead ECG

| |
|---|
| Two electrodes are placed above the level of the heart: one on the right side of the chest (RA) at the shoulder and one on the left side of the chest (LA) |
| Two electrodes are placed below the level of the heart. One on the centre of the left leg (LL) and one on the right leg (RL) |
| The neutral lead (N) may be placed anywhere but is best to be away from the other leads to avoid interference |

Cardiovascular assessment provides essential information on the circulatory status of the child and the effects of treatment. It entails palpation, inspection and auscultation. Accuracy of assessment and measurement is essential.

## RESPIRATORY ASSESSMENT

The respiratory system supplies oxygen to the body and removes carbon dioxide. This is its prime function and is achieved by diffusion of gases between the air in the alveoli and the blood in the alveolar capillaries.[8] In the newborn term infant a transition occurs from irregular episodic ineffective breathing to regular, rhythmic and effectual breathing within the first 7 days of life.[4] Maturity of the respiratory system is generally completed by the eighth year of life.

The most frequent infection of infancy and childhood is respiratory tract infections; thus it is also the most common reason for infants and young children to attend a GP's surgery. While the majority will be mild and self-limiting, some can be potentially life-threatening. Accurate respiratory assessment is vital in determining the severity of illness in the infant and child. Breathing is usually the first vital sign to alter in the deteriorating infant and child. Respiratory failure can occur due to either acute or chronic pathology and can also be of non-respiratory origin.[8] Failure to recognise respiratory failure will lead to cardiorespiratory arrest, of which outcomes tend to be poor.

The purpose of respiratory assessment is to identify the infant's or child's respiratory status, which will also provide information on cardiovascular function and neurological status.

### Indications for monitoring respiratory rate

- All infants and children should have baseline respiratory assessment undertaken on admission to hospital.
- Evaluation of effect of medication on respiratory system, e.g. bronchodilators, opiates.
- To compare and identify changes: improvements or deterioration in the child's condition following surgery or investigative procedures.
- To assess and monitor the child's condition as part of their ongoing care.
- Monitoring effectiveness of oxygen therapy.
- When the child is receiving intravenous fluids, blood or blood products.

---

### Definitions

**Dyspnoea:** difficulty in breathing accompanied by an awareness of discomfort with breathing.

**Orthopnoea:** shortness of breath when lying down, relieved by sitting upright.

**Tachypnoea:** increase in respiratory rate.

**Bradypnoea:** decrease in respiratory rate but rate remains regular.

**Hyperventilation:** increase in both rate and depth of respirations.

**Hypoventilation:** slow, shallow breathing.

**Hypoxaemia:** low oxygen levels in the blood.

**Cyanosis:** bluish discolouration of the skin or mucous membranes due to lack of oxygen in the blood.

---

Respiratory assessment includes

- inspection
- palpation
- percussion
- auscultation.

These all indicate the efficacy, work of breathing and adequacy of ventilation. A calm gentle approach should be adopted when you are assessing the infant or child with respiratory difficulties (Table 9.8).

**Table 9.8** Normal respiratory rates[9]

| Age in years | Respiratory rate (breaths per minute) |
| --- | --- |
| <1 | 30–40 |
| 1–2 years | 26–34 |
| 2–5 years | 24–30 |
| 6–12 years | 20–24 |
| >12 years | 12–20 |

Respiratory rate may be increased by anxiety, agitation and frustration along with the presence of fever. Respiratory rate must not be considered in isolation but correlated along with the other physiological parameters that will indicate the level of respiratory distress. A respiratory rate of greater than 50 breaths per minute in an infant and child under than 3 years of age and greater than 30 breaths per minute in the older child have been identified as indicators of respiratory dysfunction.[29,30] An increase in body temperature will also cause an increase in respiratory rate.

Infants are obligatory nasal breathers until approximately 6 months of age, so any degree of nasal obstruction will impact on the work of breathing and nutrition.

### Inspection

Visual observation of the infant and child will facilitate accurate assessment of the work of breathing and the following should be observed:

- respiratory rate and rhythm
- work of breathing
- respiratory noises
- colour
- facial expressions
- posture
- altered behaviour
- chest wall shape
- clubbing of the fingers and toes
- cough.

### Equipment needed

Watch with a second hand
Stethoscope
Alcohol swab for cleaning earpieces and diaphragm of stethoscope
Observation chart

# PROCEDURE:  Respiratory assessment

| Procedural steps | Evidence-based rationale |
|---|---|
| **Respiratory rate** | |
| 1 Note the rise and fall of the abdomen in infants and children under the age of 6–7 years<br>A stethoscope should be used when the infant's respiratory rate is counted | In infants and children respiration is primarily diaphragmatic<br>Smaller breaths may be missed if observation alone is used to count respiratory rate[31] |
| 2 Count for 1 full minute for accuracy | Respiration is irregular in infants and young children |
| 3 Chest expansion should be equal and symmetrical | Unequal symmetry may be associated with:<br>• Chest trauma<br>• Pneumonia<br>• Foreign-body inhalation<br>• Pneumothorax |
| 4 Note inspiration–expiration ratio. Normally this is 1:2 | Increased inspiration time may indicate upper-airway obstruction<br>Increased expiration time may indicate lower-airway obstruction |
| **Work of breathing** | |
| 5 Observe the child for any signs of respiratory distress:<br>• Nasal flaring: may be subtle<br>• Expiratory grunting<br>• Use of accessory muscles, especially sternoidmastoid (head bobbing) and abdominal rectus muscle in infants<br>• Recession: subcostal, intercostals, suprasternal<br>• Inability to speak (child) or feed (infant)<br>• See-saw (paradoxical) breathing<br>• Pursed lips | The presence of any of these signs indicates respiratory distress<br>Grunting is an attempt to create a positive end expiratory pressure (PEEP) to prevent airway collapse at the end of expiration<br>The degree of recession is an indicator of respiratory distress<br>Recession occurs when the minute volume is high<br>Recession indicates an increase in respiratory effort and respiratory distress. It can be described as mild, moderate or severe depending on the depth, and this relies on clinical experience and judgement[32]<br>Recession may not be visible in the obese child[33]<br>Children who cannot speak and infants who cannot feed may indicate tiredness, altered consciousness level and/or respiratory distress<br>See-saw breathing is indicative of severe respiratory distress<br>Pursed lips prolong expiration and is a natural method of maintaining a PEEP |
| **Noise** | |
| 6 Listen for noises associated with breathing, noting where they occur in the breathing cycle. Respiratory noise can include:<br>• Wheeze<br>• Stridor<br>• Grunting<br>• Gurgling<br>• Snoring | Normal breathing is quiet  Volume of noise is not an indicator of severity of respiratory distress[9]<br>Noise is an important factor in determining cause of respiratory distress and degree of obstruction<br>Wheeze is indicative of lower-airway narrowing<br>Stridor is indicative of upper-airway disease<br>Grunting is indicative of alveolar collapse<br>Gurgling may indicate presence of vomit or blood in main airway<br>Snoring may suggest partial occlusion of nasopharynx |

## PROCEDURE: Respiratory assessment (continued)

| Posture | |
|---|---|
| 7 Position of infant/child should be noted and maintained undisturbed. This may be the tripod or sniffing position. The child with epiglottitis will be sitting upright, slightly forward and drooling | Infants and children often adopt a position of comfort that promotes maximum oxygenation |
| **Skin colour** | |
| 8 Observe the child's colour. Skin colour needs to be considered in context with the child's ethnicity Skin colour and temperature need to be consistent over trunk and extremities. The newborn baby may have normal peripheral cyanosis | Central cyanosis is best observed on the tongue[34] Nail beds are best observed for peripheral colour, indicating cardiovascular pathology Cyanosis is a pre-terminal sign Peripheral cyanosis is normal in the newborn while they adapt to extrauterine life |
| **Facial expression** | |
| 9 Facial expression should be noted | The infant and child who is in respiratory distress can appear tired, tense or frightened looking[35] |
| **Behaviour** | |
| 10 Observe the infant's and child's behaviour Do they respond appropriately to parent/carer? Are they agitated or drowsy? | Children may present with altered level of consciousness or be agitated due to hypoxaemia Hypercapnoea is indicated in the drowsy and obtunded child[9] |
| **Chest wall shape** | |
| 11 The infant's chest should be round. By the age of 5 years the chest shape should resemble that of an adult. Other deformities such as scoliosis, kyphosis, pectus carinatum, pectus excavatum and hyperinflation (barrel shape) should be noted and documented | The ribs of the infant lie horizontally, which limits expansion |
| **Clubbing of the fingers and toes** | |
| 12 Observe fingers and toes for clubbing. The finger and toe ends become round with a spongy nail fold | A proliferation of nail bed tissue that elevates the nail base towards the skin causes clubbing to occur The severity of clubbing is measured by the degree that the nail bed is elevated[36] |
| **Cough** | |
| 13 The role of the nurse is determining the presence, frequency, depth and sound of the cough and any associated trigger factors. It should be noted if it is productive or non-productive and if the onset was sudden or gradual | Young children are unlikely to produce a sputum sample as they generally swallow their secretions Coughing must be considered in terms of its characteristics and with other symptoms |
| 14 Document all findings in care records and verbally report all abnormalities promptly to senior nursing staff/medical staff | To plan treatment, monitor progress and provide care record[21,22] |

## Auscultation

The chest is auscultated with a stethoscope to assess the quality and characteristics of breath sounds, detect abnormal breath sounds and to evaluate vocal resonance. Abnormal sounds and hoarseness can be detected without the use of a stethoscope and the presence of these indicates the need for more detailed examination. A paediatric stethoscope should be used. The stethoscope diaphragm transmits breath sounds more effectively than the bell. It is difficult to interpret findings from auscultation, so they must be considered in the context of a full physical examination. Skill is required in auscultation of the infant's and child's chest.

## PROCEDURE: Auscultation

| Procedural steps | Evidence-based rationale |
|---|---|
| 1 Explain procedure to child and gain their informed consent | Increase compliance and informed child should enable greater cooperation and completion of procedure |
| 2 Wash hands | To minimise the risk of cross-infection |
| 3 Warm stethoscope in hands and expose child's chest, ensuring privacy and that environment is not cold | Child more likely to cooperate with warm stethoscope |
| 4 Evaluate quality of breath sounds over entire chest:<br>• Main bronchus for bronchial sounds<br>• Anterior and posterior chest (Figure 9.3)<br>• The apices and midaxillary areas should be used with the infant and young child | Assessment of all lobes of the lungs will be performed Listen to a complete respiratory cycle before moving on to the next site as important findings may not be heard if the stethoscope is removed too soon Breath sounds should have normal intensity, pitch and rhythm bilaterally.<br>Infants and young children have thin chest walls so the sounds from one lung can be heard over the entire chest area<br>Absent or diminished breath sounds are likely to identified here as the distance between the lungs is greatest at these points[37] |
| 5 Try to auscultate the infant's/child's chest when they are quiet and not crying. With the older child, encourage them to take deep breaths | If the infant/child continues to cry, they will take a breath at the end of every cry which can be used to assess breath sounds<br>Easier to hear when the child takes deeper breaths |
| 6 Ask the child to repeat a series of words and use stethoscope to listen over entire chest and sides to identify quality of sound | Voice sounds are normally muffled and indistinct through chest<br>Absent or more muffled than usual indicates airway obstruction |
| 7 Document findings and report all abnormalities to senior nursing/medical staff | |
| 8 Wash hands | To minimise the risk of cross-infection |

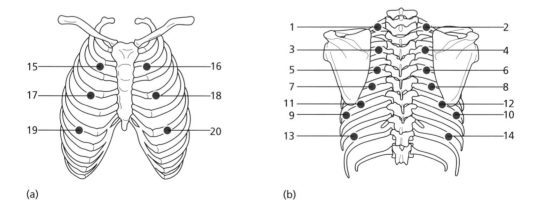

(a)  (b)

**Figure 9.3** Anterior (a) and posterior (b) chest wall. Possible sequence of auscultation of the chest.

---

**Definitions**

*Breath sounds*
**Bronchovesicular:** medium pitched, hollow, blowing sound heard equally on inspiration and expiration in all age groups related to child's developmental stage.

**Vesicular breath sounds:** lower pitched, swishing, soft short expiratory sounds heard in older children but not infants.

**Bronchial/tracheal:** hollow, higher pitched sounds than vesicular breath sounds.

---

## Referred breath sounds

In the infant, because of their small thorax, noise from upper-airway secretions may be heard all over their chest and this is called referred breath sound. Transmitted breath sounds is the other term that may be used.

## Abnormal/added breath sounds

Added breath sounds generally indicate disease. These include wheezing, crackles/crepitations, ronchi and friction rub (Table 9.9). The locations of these sounds are important and their location within the respiratory cycle must be noted. It must also be noted if these sounds change or disappear as the child moves or coughs.

**VIGNETTE**

**Problem:** You are trying to auscultate an infant's chest and they continue to cry despite your best efforts to pacify them.

**Discussion:** Auscultation of breath sounds in a crying child is difficult but at the end of every cry the child will take a deep breath, which can be used to assess their breath sound.

Toddlers should be encouraged to breath deeply by asking them to blow out pretend birthday candles/bubbles or a windmill.

**Table 9.9** Abnormal/added breath sounds

---

**Wheeze:** Due to narrowed or obstructed airways
Continuous and more pronounced on expiration
Associated with asthma

**Crackles/crepitations:** Fine crackles are high pitched, non-continuous and heard at the end of inspiration
Coarse crackles are loud, bubbling and low pitched

**Ronchi:** Heard during inspiration and expiration
Sounds like a snore
May clear with coughing

**Friction rub:** Heard on inspiration; a harsh grating sound
May be due to plural rub

---

# PERCUSSION

There is less reliance on percussion of the chest today, as radiological examination is utilised more frequently. It is sometimes used to assess the resonance of the lungs and underlying organs, such as the liver and heart. Percussion will determine whether the lung is filled with air, fluid or solid matter.[37] When you are percussing the chest the anterior and posterior should be examined using the same sequence as one would use for auscultation. The whole chest should be percussed as this will allow for bilateral comparisons. The chest is percussed for resonance, dullness, flatness and tympany.

## Palpation

Palpitation is used to determine chest movement, respiratory effort, tactile fremitus and deformities of the chest wall. This is a difficult skill to perform in the infant and young child so findings must be considered in context with a complete examination.

## PROCEDURE:  Percussion

| Procedural steps | Evidence-based rationale |
| --- | --- |
| **1** Wash hands | To minimise risk of cross-infection |
| **2** Place middle finger only of non-dominant hand on the child's chest at an intercostal space<br>Apply fingertip of dominant hand to tap the finger in direct contact with the chest using a spring-like action. Compare like with like | To elicit the quality of resonance of lungs and underlying organs<br>Normal resonance is a loud, low-pitched, hollow sound and should be heard over the lung<br>Tympany is loud and high pitched, usually heard over stomach<br>Flatness is a soft dull sound and is heard over dense bone and muscle<br>Dullness is a moderately loud thud. It is heard over liver, heart and base of lungs<br>Hyper-resonance is a loud, very low-pitched booming sound. It may be heard over super-inflated lungs[37] |
| **3** Percussion of an infant's chest is achieved by tapping the intercostal space with a fingertip only | |
| **4** Document findings and report abnormalities | To facilitate care planning and treatment[21,22] |

**Problem:** The observation of respiratory distress is a more significance that auscultatory findings in children.

**Discussion:** The child who has tachypnoea and intercostal recession is more likely to have respiratory disease than those who are presenting with abnormal respiratory sounds.

## PROCEDURE:  Palpation

| Procedural steps | Evidence-based rationale |
| --- | --- |
| **1** Wash hands and ensure they are warm | To minimise risk of cross-infection, and warm hands will encourage child to cooperate |
| **2** Place thumbs just touching at sternum and outspread fingers on each side of child's chest over their ribs<br><br>Use fingers to palpate for any abnormalities: growths, areas of tenderness, fractures | Confirms bilateral symmetry of chest movement. When the child takes a deep breath, the distance your thumbs move apart is the degree of chest expansion – normally 1 cm or more[38]<br>None should be found.<br>Crepitus: a crinkly sensation is due to air escaping into the subcutaneous tissues |
| **3** To identify mediastinal deviation the position of the trachea is identified by using one finger for an infant and two for an older child to locate the trachea in the midline.<br>To locate the apex beat, place hand over chest with fingertips in anterior axillary line. The apex beat is located with one finger. Confirm its position by counting down the ribs: the midclavicular line and the fifth intercostal space for children >5 years of age and fourth intercostals space <5 years of age | The trachea can be palpated at the suprasternal notch Children generally dislike this so it needs to be done selectively[34]<br>Displacement of the apex to the left is suggestive of mediastinal shift[38] |
| **4** Wash hands if examination is completed at this point | To minimise risk of cross-infection |

**VIGNETTE**

> **Problem:** When assess a child you note that they are both tachypnoeic and tachycardic.
>
> **Discussion:** Inadequate respirations will have an adverse effect on heart rate as hypoxia leads to tachycardia. Consideration of the child's temperature, medication received and levels of distress may all contribute to a rise in their heart rate so this must be given due consideration when assessing the child's respiratory status, thus indicating the need for frequent if not continuous assessment.

## Pulse oximetry

Pulse oximety is a simple, non-invasive monitoring modality. It is used to measure the percentage of oxygen saturation ($SaO_2$) of haemoglobin in peripheral capillary blood. Pulse oximetry is used in the clinical setting in the hospital and community and the home. It can be used for spot readings or for continual monitoring. Pulse oximetry is based on two physical principles: first, the presence of a pulsatile signal generated by arterial blood, which is reasonably independent of non-pulsatile arterial blood; second, oxygenated and deoxygenated blood have different absorption spectra. Two light-emitting diodes emit red and infrared wavelengths through the tissues to a photodetector, and these work together. The detector measures the colour difference between the oxygenated and deoxygenated haemoglobin during each cardiac cycle so the probe requires a constant supply of arterial blood. This information is then analysed in the calibration algorithm of the microprocessor of the pulse oximeter and the estimated arterial saturation level is displayed. This is displayed as a percentage and a waveform. A normal signal shows a sharp waveform with a clear dicrotic notch.[39] Movement artefact and decreased perfusion will distort the waveform.

### Normal value

In room air 95–99 per cent denotes that the haemoglobin is adequately saturated with oxygen.

### Related physiology

While it is not the remit of this chapter to provide an in-depth understanding of the physiology of breathing, a basic outline is provided.

On inspiration oxygen from inspired air enters the lungs, and by diffusion from the alveoli oxygen enters the blood stream, thus being circulated around the body by the pumping action of the heart.

Normally 98–99% oxygen is transported around the body and tissues by the protein haemoglobin (Hb) contained in the erythrocytes. This is referred to as the arterial haemoglobin saturation $SaO_2$. The remaining 1–2% is dissolved in the plasma and this is referred to as the partial pressure of oxygen ($PaO_2$).[40] Haemoglobin that is saturated with oxygen is referred to as oxyhaemoglobin and haemoglobin that is not saturated is referred to as deoxyhaemoglobin. Normally, when there is a satisfactory amount of oxygen in plasma there will be an increased amount of oxygen bound to the haemoglobin and when there is less oxygen in the plasma, there will be less bound to the haemoglobin. Thus the $PaO_2$ and $SaO_2$ can both indicate the level of oxygen in the blood. Oxygen affinity is also higher or lower in the presence of haemoglobin variants. Fetal haemoglobin has a high affinity whereas sickle cell haemoglobin has a low affinity.

Infants have a higher metabolic rate and therefore greater demand for oxygen, which is the main reason for their increased respiratory rates. Thus, oxygen levels are more significant in infants and children and they decompensate quickly if oxygen levels are not stabilised. As children age, the mechanisms of breathing change.

The concentration of haemoglobin in the blood varies with age and gender, with newborns having a Hb of 15–24 g/dL compared with a 12-year-old whose Hb is in the range of 11–15 g/dL.[41] Males tend to have a higher Hb than females by the time they reach adolescence.

However, pulse oximetry cannot detect anaemia, so the nurse needs to be aware of the patient's haemoglobin level otherwise a false high reading will occur. Oximetry measures the percentage of haemoglobin that is saturated by oxygen, so if there is less haemoglobin available then the saturated blood will have reduced oxygen-carrying capacity, which is not reflected in the oximetry readings, making the child at an increased risk of hypoxia.

### Indications for use/clinical application

Pulse oximetry should be used to monitor infants and children and as a screening tool when the following conditions are present:

- the potential for respiratory failure;[9]
- respiratory illness;
- haemodynamic instability;
- the need for sedation or anaesthesia;
- the need for oxygen therapy;
- when complex surgical procedures of > 6 hours have been undergone;[17]
- when the child is under 1 year of age and post surgery;
- when administration of continuous respiratory depressant medication, e.g. patient controlled analgesia, is being given
- during intradepartmental or intra-hospital transportation of infants and children who are at risk of respiratory compromise or who are already receiving oxygen therapy.

### Limitations

Pulse oximetry has a number of limitations that the user needs to be aware of as these may lead to inaccurate readings.

- When the child has low cardiac output, hypothermia or vasoconstriction, peripheral perfusion may be impaired and as oximetry relies on detecting a pulse, it may be difficult for the sensor to detect a true signal.[42]
- When the $SaO_2$ is <70% pulse oximetry is unreliable due to the presence of carboxyhaemoglobin, which the two wavelengths of light cannot distinguish.
- Elevated methaemoglobin, caused by either structural changes of iron in the haemoglobin or drug induced as with local anaesthesia, may lead to tissue hypoxia as oxygen binding to haemoglobin is inhibited.[43,44]
- Smoke inhalation and carbon monoxide poisoning. The oximeter cannot distinguish between haemoglobin saturated with oxygen and that saturated with carbon monoxide.
- Motion artefact accounts for a significant number of errors and false alarms; thus shivering can cause problems with detecting saturation level and give a false high pulse.
- The use of intravenous dyes such as methylene blue can give false low readings, so nurses need to know which dye has been used and what the half-life of this is.
- The presence of oedema will lead to inaccurate measurement of saturation level.
- Inaccurate reading will also occur in the presence of nail varnish and acrylic nails.[45,46] Dried blood and dirt will also affect the accuracy of readings and need to be removed.
- Inaccurate readings have been reported in people with dark skin and in pigmented patients.[47] This has not been reported in jaundiced patients.
- Bright overhead lighting and external light may cause overestimation of saturation level.[48]
- Various studies[49-51] on the use of pulse oximetry as a monitoring tool for patients with sickle cell anaemia having acute vaso-occlusive disease have reached different conclusions about the accuracy of the readings with up to 8 per cent bias. Therefore, the nurse should state the child's diagnosis when reporting saturation levels.

### Equipment

Pulse oximeter
Probe: appropriate size

### The procedural goal is to

- identify the effectiveness of oxygen transportation in the tissues and cells of the infant/child.

## PROCEDURE: Pulse oximetry

| Procedural steps | Evidence-based rationale |
| --- | --- |
| **1** Wash hands | To minimise the risk of cross-infection |
| **2** Explain to the child and parents that an oxygen saturation reading is required and obtain consent | To provide understanding of why procedure is necessary and therefore obtain informed consent |
| **3** Make sure equipment is clean and working | To minimise the risk of cross-infection and that equipment is suitable for use |
| **4** Select correct probe | Some probes are weight specific and incorrect size may lead to inaccurate readings |

## PROCEDURE: Pulse oximetry (continued)

| | |
|---|---|
| **5** Perform baseline assessment prior to attaching the probe, this should include respiratory rate and heart rate/pulse. Skin colour and respiratory effort should be noted | Correlation between monitor's data and patient's data can be identified |
| **6** Place the probe on the appropriate site:<br>*Infant/young child:* on the foot either the outer aspect at the base of the little toe or on the big toe. The Achilles area may also be used<br>The probe may also be placed across the palm of the hand with the probe at the base of the little finger<br>*Older child:* the probe may be placed on the fingertip, on the toe or on the ear lobe<br>Probe site used should be documented in care records | The ear lobe is used when the child has poor perfusion as this is considered a central location because of the large percentage of blood flow to the head and brain<br>Accurate readings will only be possible if the probe is placed correctly |
| **7** Secure probe to infant/child following manufacturer's instructions. Check it is not too tight | To avoid burning of child's skin and to avoid pressure ulceration/necrosis |
| **8** Connect lead to monitor and turn it on and watch for saturation level, waveform and pulse rate. Check pulse rate corresponds to patient's | To identify if probe is functioning correctly |
| **9** Note oxygen saturation level and document. Note if child is also receiving oxygen<br>If saturation levels < 95% in room air, notify medical staff | Provides documentary evidence of procedure and enables planning of care |
| **10** Identify parameters for setting of alarms. This will include both high and low limits of oxygen saturation level and pulse rate. Document these in care records. This may be done in discussion with medical staff | Neonates are at risk of retinopathy of prematurity when receiving a high concentration of oxygen, and a target oxygen saturation of 85–95% has been suggested[52]<br>For the child with a chronic respiratory disease, a lower normal level may need to be agreed with medical staff as they are unlikely to achieve a reading in the normal range[53] |
| **11** If infant/child is being continuously monitored then remove probe every 2 hours, check skin condition and reposition on a different location. Document in care record | To prevent burns and pressure ulcers occurring[11,54]<br>To provide a record of care and to ensure communication of potential problems |
| **12** If the reading is to be intermittent, then remove probe from child and turn off monitor<br>If using a hand-held monitor, clean as per manufacturers instructions. If probe<br>Is disposable, then dispose in clinical waste | To ensure comfort for child and freedom of movement<br>Comply with infection control precautions |
| **13** For continual monitoring, document readings as indicated by patient's condition and local policy | To provide a record of care and to ensure communication of potential problems[21,22] |
| **14** On completion of monitoring, turn off monitor, remove probe, clean equipment and maintain in storage as per manufacturer's instructions | To minimise the risk of cross-infection<br>Correct storage and maintenance will ensure equipment is ready for use when next required |
| **15** Wash hands | To minimise the risk of cross-infection |

Respiratory assessment is complex and detailed with data being obtained by subjective and objective means. The efficacy and work of breathing needs careful assessment and consideration of the child's developmental stage is paramount.

## AUXOLOGY

### Growth

All infants and children who attend any healthcare setting should have their growth measured.

Accurate measurement of height, length, weight, and head and chest circumference is a vital part in the overall assessment of the infant and child in order to assure health, identify nutritional status and to identify the impact of disease on the child. Growth can be accurately assessed only by taking at least two measurements of the various

parameters.[38] This information must then be transposed onto the relevant growth charts for the child's age and sex before it can be interpreted. Current standard for this in the UK is the chart based on the WHO Child Growth Standard advocated by the Royal College of Paediatrics and Child Health (2009).[55]

### Length

In children under 2 years of age, length should be measured even after they have developed the ability to stand independently.

#### The procedural goal is to

- accurately assess the infant's and child's length

#### Equipment

Measuring board or other length measuring device
Percentile chart and/or personal health record

## PROCEDURE: Length measurement

| Procedural steps | Evidence-based rationale |
|---|---|
| 1 Have parent remove any hats, hair decorations and shoes | Will give false measurement |
| 2 Wash hands | To minimise the risk of cross-infection |
| 3 Use parent or assistant to hold infant's head in the midline and to gently push down on the knees until straight | With the normally flexed posture of the infant their body must be extended to obtain an accurate measurement |
| 4 Position the heels of the feet on the footboard and record the length to the nearest millimetre[56] | To ensure accuracy |
| 5 Repeat for accuracy | If a discrepancy is identified between measurements, take an average reading for documentation purposes |
| 6 Plot the measurement on the age and gender appropriate percentile chart and in the care records making sure they are dated and signed | To assist with the planning of treatment and care Evidence that the procedure was performed[21,22] |
| 7 Wash hands | To minimise the risk of cross-infection |

### Height

From the age of 2 years and if standing independently, children may have their height recorded upright with a stadiometer.

#### The procedural goal is to

- record accurately measurement the child's height.

## PROCEDURE: Height measurement

| Procedural steps | Evidence-based rationale |
|---|---|
| **1** Remove shoes, hat and hair decorations | Greater accuracy of reading |
| **2** Wash hands | To minimise the risk of cross-infection. |
| **3** Stand child straight with back to the wall and their head should be erect in the midline position | |
| **4** The child's shoulders, buttocks and heels should touch the wall, and the outer cantus of the eye should be on the same horizontal plane as the external auditory canal<br>Ensure feet are flat on the floor | Positioning of the head ensures consistency in placement of the head piece on the crown of the head |
| **5** Move head piece down to touch crown | |
| **6** Note the height reading to nearest millimetre[56] | Ensure accuracy |
| **7** Document height reading on percentile chart and care records | To assist with the planning of treatment and care[21,22]<br>Evidence that the procedure was performed |
| **8** Wash hands | To minimise the risk of cross-infection |

### Weight

Weight is measured with an age appropriate scale: an electronic digital platform scale for an infant which will measure weight to the nearest 10 g and either a standing or sitting scale for a child, depending on their condition, that will measure to the nearest 100 g.

The scale must be calibrated in accordance with hospital policy and the manufacturer's instructions.

### The procedural goal is to

- Measure accurately the infant's and child's weight.

### Equipment

Scales – calibrated accurately
Percentile chart

## PROCEDURE: Weight measurement

| Procedural steps | Evidence-based rationale |
|---|---|
| **1** Ask the parent to assist in the removal of the infant's/child's clothing. Infants should be weighed naked, toddlers in their under garments and children in their outdoor clothing, with heavy items and shoes removed.<br>If child is wearing a prosthetic device or other medical device that cannot be removed, document this when recording weight | By minimising the amount of clothing, comparisons can be made with previous weight<br>Respect the privacy and dignity of the child |
| **2** Ensure room is warm and private | To prevent infant and child from becoming cold.<br>Promotion of dignity |
| **3** Wash hands | To minimise the risk of cross-infection |
| **Procedure for infant** | |
| **4** Place infant on scale and remain close at hand. Place your hand lightly above their body | Infants move quickly and safety is paramount |

## PROCEDURE:  Weight measurement (continued)

| | |
|---|---|
| 5 Distract infant and note reading when the infant stops moving | It takes a few seconds of inactivity for the scale to reach the infant's actual weight |
| 6 Record the weight to the nearest 10 g | |
| 7 If repeated measurements are required it is important to weigh at the same time every day | |
| 8 Document the weight on percentile chart and in care records | Provide evidence of care and planning of care[21,22] |
| 9 Clean scale in accordance with hospital policy and manufacturer's instructions<br>Replace paper sheet | Reduce transmission of cross-infection and promotion of asepsis |
| **Procedure for child** | |
| 4 Ask child to stand still on weighing scale. It may be necessary to provide distraction technique | Any movement will give a false reading |
| 5 Note weight to nearest 100 g | |
| 6 Document the weight on percentile chart and in care records | Provide evidence of care and planning of care[21,22] |
| 7 Wash hands | To minimise the risk of cross-infection. |

### Head circumference (occipitofrontal [OFC])

Rapid growth of the head occurs during the first 6 months of an infant's life, and the size of the skull is closely related to the size of the brain. Routinely infants and children have their head circumference measured at birth and again at 6–8 weeks.[57] Children up to the age of 3 years or those with questionable head size should have head circumference recorded at regular intervals.

### The procedural goal is to

- Measure accurately infant's/child's head circumference

### Equipment

Disposable flexible non-stretch measuring-tape with centimetre and millimetre markings
Percentile chart

## PROCEDURE:  Head circumference measurement

| Procedural steps | Evidence-based rationale |
|---|---|
| 1 Wash hands | To minimise the risk of cross-infection. |
| 2 Remove any hat or head gear that child is wearing | |
| 3 Wrap tape around the head at the supraorbital prominence, above the ears and around the occipital prominence taking care to prevent a paper cut | This is the usual point of largest head circumference |
| 4 Record the circumference to the nearest 0.5 cm | |
| 5 Repeat measurement three times at slightly different points | The largest measurement should be recorded as the actual OFC[38] |
| 6 Dispose of tape and wash hands | To minimise the risk of cross-infection |
| 7 Plot on percentile chart and in care records | Provide evidence of care and planning of care[21,22] |

### Chest circumference

Chest circumference may be measured until 1 year of age. It is a useful measurement to compare with head circumference when there may be concern about growth of either the head or the chest.

### The procedural goal is to

• Measure accurately the chest circumference

### Equipment

Disposable non-stretch measuring-tape with centimetre and millimetre markings

## PROCEDURE: Chest circumference measurement

| Procedural steps | Evidence-based rationale |
|---|---|
| 1 Wash hands | To minimise the risk of cross-infection |
| 2 Remove all upper-body clothing | To gain access to chest |
| 3 Wrap the tape measure around the chest just under the axilla and at the nipple line | Correct positioning is essential for accuracy |
| 4 Note the circumference measurement to the nearest 0.5 cm | |
| 5 Compare with head circumference measurement | The head and chest circumference will approximately be equal until the age of 1 year when the chest circumference begins to surpass the head circumference |
| 6 Dispose of tape measure and wash hands | To minimise the risk of cross-infection |
| 7 Document in care records | Provide evidence of care and planning of care[21,22] |

### Body mass index

Body mass index (BMI) is considered one of the best methods of quantifying obesity[34] and is used in assessment of growth in contemporary practice as the prevalence of obesity in childhood increases. BMI is categorised as normal, overweight, obese or morbidly obese (Table 9.10).

Body mass index is determined by the calculation of the weight in kilograms/height in metres squared.

**Table 9.10** Body mass index (BMI) categories

| Category | BMI |
|---|---|
| Normal | 19–27 |
| Overweight | 28–30 |
| Obese | 30–40 |
| Morbidly obese | >40 |

BMI = weight (kg)/height (m$^2$)
For example: a child is 16.5 kg and 91 cm in height. The height needs to be in metres squared, so when converted it is 0.8281 m$^2$
BMI = 16.5/0.8281
BMI = 19.9, in the normal category.

## BLOOD GLUCOSE

Glucose is an essential source for all body tissues, including the brain and the myocardium, thus low levels of serum glucose (hypoglycaemia) can have potential serious consequences, such as seizures and reduced cardiac output. Neonates are prone to hypoglycaemia and require frequent testing of their blood glucose levels. High blood sugar (hyperglycaemia) may also have adverse neurological outcomes. The normal blood glucose level is between 3–6 mmol/L for infants and children. The accepted norm for the neonates is 2.6 mmol/L.[38]

The blood glucose level is frequently monitored at the bedside and in the community for many clinically indicated reasons, with the management of type 1 diabetes being the most common. This is performed using glucose-sensitive strips and a blood glucose meter. Point-of-care testing with hand-held blood glucose devices requires strict quality controls and formal training.[58,59] Blood glucose meters should be used in accordance with standard operating procedures.

Blood may be taken from capillary, venous or arterial routes. This will be determined by the access available to blood sampling and the clinical condition of the child. Capillary sampling is frequently used. Infants and children have high energy requirements and low glucose stores and may become hypoglycaemic quickly, thus necessitating the need for rapid and frequent bedside testing. Parameters need to be identified on an individual basis of what action to take when blood glucose levels are outside the accepted range. Depending on the result and the condition of the child, the true blood glucose level may be required by laboratory analysis.

## Signs of hypoglycaemia include

- pallor
- irritability
- jitters
- headache
- sweating
- seizures
- loss of consciousness.

## Indications for testing blood glucose level

- following a prolonged seizure;
- sudden change in level of consciousness;
- sudden deterioration in condition;
- when a child becomes septic;
- management of diabetes type 1 and diabetic ketoacidosis;
- prolonged fasting prior to surgery.

### The procedural goal is to

- measure capillary glucose level.

### Equipment

Glucose-sensitive strip (compatible to glucose meter)
Hand-held glucose meter
Finger-pricking device with appropriate lancet
Cotton wool/gauze
Disposable gloves
Sharps box

## PROCEDURE: Blood glucose measurement

| Procedural steps | Evidence-based rationale |
| --- | --- |
| 1 Perform quality control checks on glucose meter before bringing it to child's bedside: (a) monitor and test strips have been calibrated together; (b) test strips have not been exposed to air; (c) strips are in date; (d) check high and low internal quality controls have been carried out with results logged and signed; (e) equipment is clean<br>Assemble required equipment before approaching bedside: attach disposable lancet to finger-pricking device | To ensure accurate result and to promote patient safety |
| 2 Explain procedure to child and family and obtain consent | Facilitates cooperation and reduces anxiety |
| 3 Ask child to wash hands in warm soapy water and rinse well or in the case of an infant parent may wish to wash heel | Ensures a non-contaminated result as any glucose on hands will be removed during washing<br>Warm water will promote blood flow to finger<br>Alcohol-based swabs or rubs should be avoided as they will react with the reagent in the strips giving a false reading |
| 4 Keep heel or fingers warm | Encourages a good blood flow[60] |
| 5 Wash own hands and wear gloves | To minimise risk of cross-infection and to maintain universal precautions |
| 6 Turn on glucose testing meter | |
| 7 Place test strip into meter as per manufacturer's instructions | Ensures accuracy of results |

## PROCEDURE: Blood glucose measurement (continued)

| | |
|---|---|
| **8** Hold the child's finger or heel securely and prick the side of the child's finger or their heel with the finger-pricking device. In the infant, the heel will be used | The side of the finger is less painful and easier from which to obtain a hanging droplet of blood<br>Finger-pricking device reduces pain to finger or heel due to measured depth of lancet<br>The site should be rotated to reduce pain, risk of infection and toughening<br>Young children use pincer action to pick up objects and repeated pricking will be painful[61] |
| **9** Milk the finger or heel until there is a reasonable sized drop of blood hanging from it | A drop of blood is required to ensure full coverage of test strip and accuracy of results |
| **10** Bring the test strip towards the drop of blood and drop the blood onto the strip. Some test strips are hydrophilic and will soak the blood up from the side or bottom of the strip | Insufficient blood coverage of test strip will give an inaccurate result<br>The window on the test strip will allow visual verification of correctly applied blood |
| **11** When the test strip has soaked up sufficient blood the monitor will commence testing. This procedure will depend on the monitor | Ensures accuracy of result |
| **12** Meter will sound audible tone when test is complete. Note result and document immediately in care records. Report any abnormal readings to medical staff as appropriate. All 'HI' and 'LO' readings must be reported | Ensure accuracy of result and provide evidence of procedure, which will facilitate care planning |
| **13** Dispose of all waste appropriately: lancet in sharps bin, gloves, test strip and cotton wool/gauze in clinical waste | To reduce risk of cross-infection and prevent needlestick injury |
| **14** Check the child's heel/finger for bleeding and make them comfortable | To ensure the child is comfortable |
| **15** Wash hands and store equipment safely | To minimise risk of cross-infection and to maintain equipment in working order |
| **16** Document results in care record | Provide evidence of care and planning of care[21,22] |

Blood glucose monitoring can provide vital information on the physiological status of the acutely ill child, thus competence in this skill is essential.

## NEUROLOGICAL OBSERVATIONS

Neurological observations are essential when evaluating the integrity of the nervous system. As a baseline assessment the neurological status of a child must be recorded when an alteration in brain function is suspected or spinal injury has been sustained. Deterioration in the level of consciousness may occur rapidly and may have fatal consequences. Early identification of deteriorating brain function may be life saving and may prevent further brain insult. The most commonly used tool to assist practitioners with this is the Glasgow Coma Scale (GCS),[62] as recommended by the National Institute for Health and Clinical Excellence.[63]

The Adelaide scale[64] and the modified version of the GCS have been designed for use with younger children.

Neurological function is assessed by observation and measurement of five essential areas:

- level of consciousness
- papillary action
- motor function
- sensory function
- vital signs: temperature, pulse rate, blood pressure and respiratory rate.

### Glasgow Coma Scale

The GCS is designed to assess the integrity of normal brain function and is the best tool for consistent assessment (Table 9.11). The scores

**Table 9.11** Glasgow Coma Scale

| Feature | Response | Score |
| --- | --- | --- |
| Eye opening | Spontaneous | 4 |
| | Open to speech | 3 |
| | Open to pain | 2 |
| | No eye opening | 1 |
| Best verbal response | Orientated | 5 |
| | Confused | 4 |
| | Inappropriate words | 3 |
| | Incomprehensible sounds | 2 |
| | No verbal response | 1 |
| Best motor response | Obeys commands | 6 |
| | Localises to pain | 5 |
| | Withdrawal from pain | 4 |
| | Flexion to pain | 3 |
| | Extension to pain | 2 |
| | No motor response | 1 |

derived from the GCS provide a baseline for comparison with future scores determining improvement, deterioration or no change in the child's condition.

The GCS is a three-part assessment which consists of eye opening, verbal response and motor response. These three categories of behaviour reflect the activity in the higher centres of the brain. Numeric values are assigned to the level of response for each category. It is the sum of these values that provides the objective measurement of the child's level of consciousness. A score of 15 indicates an unaltered level of consciousness. A score of 12 requires very close monitoring, whereas a score of 8 or below signifies coma, indicating the need for intubation and ventilation, and a score of 3 indicates deep coma.[63]

Neurological assessment of the child who is sedated is difficult, so additional methods of assessment of brain function may be required such as electroencephalograms (EEGs). When you are caring for the child who has developmental delay, it is essential that parents/carers are actively involved in identification of normal behaviours, and it is imperative that these are documented accurately.

In order to improve accuracy of assessment and interobserver reliability, a complete set of neurological observations should be recorded at the commencement of the shift by the oncoming nurse and the nurse who has been caring for the child.

The level of stimulus should be increased on an incremental basis to determine the level of consciousness and to provide an accurate response.

The assessment should be made on the child's developmental level before their illness.

## Consciousness

Consciousness has been defined as a general awareness of one's self and the surrounding environment; it is a dynamic state and is subject to change.[65] It comprises awareness and arousability. Consciousness may range on a continuum from alert wakefulness to deep coma.

### Arousability

Arousability or wakefulness is a function of the reticular activating system (RAS).

### Awareness

Awareness and cognition are functions of the cerebral cortex, which are activated via the thalamic portion of the reticular activating system.

## Assessment of level of consciousness

### Eye opening to assess the arousal mechanism

Spontaneous eye opening on approaching a child indicates an intact RAS and will score 4 on the GCS. In the visually impaired child, the arousal system should still be intact. Ocular movement should also be assessed, as abnormal movement may indicate underlying pathology.[66]

Eye opening to verbal commands scores 3. This observation should be made without touching the child. Speak to the child in a normal tone of voice initially. The tone of voice should be gradually increased. Ask parents/carers to speak to the child as they may respond better to a familiar voice.

Eye opening to pain scores 2. Touch or shake the child's shoulder gently, initially to avoid undue distress. If there is no response to this then a deeper stimulus is required, and a peripheral stimulus needs to be applied. Explain why this needs to be done to the parents and child before applying any stimulus.

### Stimuli

#### Peripheral stimulation

The third or fourth finger should be used as a peripheral stimulus, as they are more sensitive.[67] Apply pressure to the lateral outer aspect of the third or fourth finger with a pen, rotating the point of stimulus on each assessment. Pain should only be felt momentarily.

Sternal rub and nail bed pressure must not be used for continuous assessment as both may lead to bruising and long-term discomfort.[68]

#### Central stimuli

*Supraorbital pressure*: just below the inner aspect of the eyebrow a notch may be felt by running a finger along the supraorbital margin. A branch of the facial nerve runs through this. Apply pressure to this notch by resting a hand on the child's head; the flat of the thumb or knuckle is placed on the supraorbital ridge under the eyebrow. Apply gradual pressure and increase for a maximum of 30 seconds. If there is no facial trauma or fractures suspected then supraorbital pressure may be applied.

*Trapezius muscle pinch*: using the thumb and two fingers, gently pinch the trapezius muscles where the neck meets the shoulders and twist slightly for 30 seconds. This may be used for children over 5 years old.

*Jaw margin pressure*: rest the flat of the thumb against the corner of the maxillary and mandibular junction and apply increasing pressure for a maximum of 30 seconds.

It is important that competency in these skills are achieved before independent practice.

Peripheral stimulus must be used as this stage of the assessment, as painful central stimulus tends to make patients close their eyes, inducing a grimace, which is not the desired response.[62] It is important to document which stimulus was used and this stimulus must be consistently used.

No eye opening-score 1. A score of 1 is recorded when there is no response to a painful stimulus. Sufficient stimulus must be applied before agreeing on a score of 1.

If a child has facial fractures or their eyes are closed as a result of swelling, it will be difficult to perform an accurate assessment of their level of arousal. This will need to be documented as 'C' on their neurological chart, with subsequent written documentation in their healthcare record.

The child who is in a long-term coma may have their eyes open but will not be able to demonstrate awareness.

#### Verbal response

This response provides information about the level of cognition and awareness, indicating function of the higher cognitive centres of the brain.

Best response scores 5: ask the child their name, where they are, what school they go to or the name of their sibling. Are they listening to what they are being asked? Do they seem to be aware of their surroundings? If the child is a toddler, are the words they are saying normal for them; confirm this with their parents. Is the infant babbling or cooing? Note the child's/infant's cry. Is it appropriate, can they be consoled or distracted, are there any other associated factors: fear, pain, hunger or thirst? If the cry is high pitched then medical help must be summoned immediately. If these questions are answered correctly, then they may be classed as orientated.

Confused scores 4: if the child provides confusing or inappropriate answers to the above questions, then it must be documented that they are confused.

Inappropriate words score 3: absence of, limited or inappropriate speech may be present. Words rather than sentences may be offered.

Incomprehensible sounds scores 2: this may include babbling, moaning or groaning in response to speech or painful stimulus. If there is damage to the speech centre of the brain, the child will be unable to talk but may be alert and aware; a score of 2 still needs to be recorded unless alternative communication devices are in place.

No verbal response scores 1: there is no vocalisation to painful stimuli.

### Grimace

If the child has a tracheostomy or endotracheal

**Table 9.12** Grimace score to assess best verbal response[71]

| Verbal response | Grimace |
| --- | --- |
| Score 5 | Facial or mouthing activity is seen with developmentally appropriate voice stimulation. This may include sucking and coughing |
| Score 4 | No response to verbal stimuli but there may be a response to light touch |
| Score 3 | Vigorous response to painful stimuli |
| Score 2 | Mild response to painful stimuli |
| Score 1 | No response to painful stimuli |

tube in situ they will be unable to respond verbally, as will a child less than 8 months of age. Also, the neurological status of a child who does not speak or understand English may be assessed by a grimace score as outlined in Table 9.12.

If the child has no comprehension of the English language, adequate assessment of this component of the GCS cannot be undertaken.

### Motor response

This determines if the child is aware of their environment and can obey simple commands. The best motor response should be tested on both arms. Lower-limb responses reflect spinal function.[69]

Obeys commands scores 6: ask the child to undertake an activity such as lift their arm, squeeze your hand/finger and let go (to discount primitive grasp reflex) or to show you their teeth. Observe for normal infant movements. Both limbs should be assessed noting the power in the child's hands to grip and their ability to release the grip. A normal response scores 6.

Localising to pain scores 5: this is the response to a central painful stimulus. It involves the higher centres of the brain recognising the stimulus and trying to remove it. To classify as localisation the child must move their hand to the point of the stimulation. Observation of the child and their reaction to the presence of an oxygen mask, nasogastric tubes or intravenous cannula, which they may be attempting to remove, or pushing you away when you are situating these devices, will provide you with information about their response to stimulus without constant need for the administration of a painful stimulus.[70] Infants will withdraw upon touch.

Withdrawal from pain scores 4: the child will move away from the pain or will flex their arm towards the source of pain but not in an attempt to push it away as they fail to locate the source of the painful stimulus.

Flexion to pain scores 3: decorticate posture will be adopted when a painful stimulus is applied. This is a slow response and can be recognised by the child flexing the upper arms and rotating their wrist. The thumb may come through the fingers. This demonstrates a malfunction in the motor pathway between the cerebral cortex and brain stem. This score has the potential for a poor outcome.

Extension to pain scores 2: decerebrate posturing. This indicates damage to the brain stem or blockage in the motor pathway. The elbow is straightened with internal rotation of the shoulder and wrist. The legs will also extend with the toes pointing downwards when a painful central stimulus is applied. This score has the potential for a poor outcome

No motor response scores 1. If there is no response to painful stimulus this indicates that the brain is incapable of processing any sensory input or motor activity.

## Additional assessment of neurological function

In addition to the GCS, careful assessment of pupils, motor function, sensory function and vital signs must be conducted.

### Pupils

The reaction of the pupils to light is an important part of the neurological assessment. Pupil constriction and dilatation is controlled by the oculomotor nerve (cranial nerve III) and alterations in this function may be indicative of pressure on this nerve or brain stem damage (Table 9.13, page 142). The inability of the pupils to accommodate may be due to midbrain injury.

**Table 9.13** Pupil size examination[72]

| Pupil | Indication |
|---|---|
| Pupils equal and pin point | Opiates or pontine lesion |
| Pupils equal, small and reactive | Metabolic encephalopathy |
| Pupils mixed size, fixed | Midbrain lesion |
| Pupils mixed size and reactive | Metabolic lesion |
| Pupils unequal, dilated, unreactive | Third cranial nerve palsy |
| Pupils unequal, small and reactive | Horner's syndrome |

To assess the pupil the size, shape, equality, reaction to light and position should be noted. Deviation of eyes should be noted as should eye movement: do they move together or not move together.

It is best to assess pupils in a slightly darkened room. Normal pupils are round.[70] A normal reaction is when the pupils are equal and reacting to light (PEARL).

Ask the child to open their eyes, noting the size, shape and equality of the pupils. Compare the size of the pupils with the neurological observation chart. Document the size of the pupils. This is measured in millimetres

Cover one of the child's eyes and shine the light from a pen torch into the other pupil. The pupil should constrict immediately and dilate upon removal of the light. Repeat this with the other eye and document findings on the neurological observation chart as brisk (+), sluggish (S) or no reaction (−).

While observing one pupil, shine light into the other pupil and the observed pupil should also constrict. Repeat this with the other eye. This is a result of the cross-over of the optic nerve at the optic chiasma and is referred to as the consensual response.[72]

If the child is asleep, they try to rouse them first; this may be difficult in the child who is in a deep sleep or who has been sedated. The pupils may be a little sluggish to begin with. It may be necessary to hold the eyelids open; both eyelids should be open simultaneously.

The reaction of the pupils may be affected by pharmacological preparations and this must be considered when you are assessing pupillary reaction.

It is essential to gain the cooperation of the child when pupil activity is assessed: the frightened child may not be a willing participant. Any congenital eye defects such as squints or deviations should be noted on the initial assessment and documented.

### Motor function

The ability to move may be affected by damage to any part of the motor nervous system. This will involve assessing all four limbs.

Muscle strength is assessed by asking the child to push and pull their arms and legs towards you and away from you while you act as resistance. The developmental age of the child will have to be considered. For a young child, observe how they are holding an object such as a favourite toy/bottle and note their reaction to you removing it to assess the upper limbs. To assess the lower-limb strength see how they stand (if not contraindicated) and hold their body weight.

### The procedural goal is to

- to evaluate neurological function.

### Equipment

Pen torch
Thermometer
Blood pressure monitor
Stethoscope
Pencil
Neurological observation chart

## PROCEDURE:  Neurological assessment

| Procedural steps | Evidence-based rationale |
|---|---|
| **1** Explain the procedure to the child and parents even if the child is unconscious | Consent will be obtained and the procedure will be understood[22]<br>Hearing may not be impaired in the unconscious child |
| **2** Wash hands | To reduce the risk of cross-infection |
| **3** Observe the child prior to commencing the neurological assessment, noting their movements, interaction with their environment, speech and behaviour | Will provide information about neurological status |
| **4** Identify whether the child is receiving any medication or has any pre-existing health condition that may influence their neurological assessment | To enable an accurate assessment of neurological status to be performed |
| **5** Assess and record any observation that does not require physical intervention such as respiratory rate. Note the characteristics of respiration and the pattern | Reduces distress on the child<br>Respiratory insufficiency may be a sign of brain stem compression[73]<br>Abnormal respirations may contribute to pain, hypovolaemia, sepsis or fever |
| **6** Record the child's temperature at specified intervals | Damage to the hypothalamus may reflect in severely abnormal temperatures. Hyperpyrexia may be a result of pressure on the hypothalamus. Hypothermia can affect conscious levels due to decreased cerebral blood flow |
| **7** Measure the child's heart rate/pulse at specified intervals | Tachycardia may be present initially in response to hypoxia from raised intracranial pressure (ICP). This will then become a bradycardia if the ICP is not treated because of excessive pressure on the medulla oblongata. This is a late sign[9]<br>Tachycardia may also be present because of pain, fever, hypovolaemia or sepsis |
| **8** Measure the child's blood pressure at specified intervals | Hypertension is a late sign of raised ICP. In the presence of bradycardia and respiratory depression (Cushing's triad), this is a very late and serious sign and one that carries a high mortality rate[9]<br>Other causes should be considered for hypertension, such as pain and fear |
| **9** Observe the child, noting their interaction with their parents and the environment. Talk to them noting the degree of alertness: whether they are restless, lethargic or drowsy. Ask them their name, do they know where they are, what day it is (older child) and details of their family, school or friends. If assessing a toddler, are the words and noises they make normal for them. Confirm answers with parents. If the child is sedated, intubated or non-verbal, assess using grimace score | To establish level of consciousness. If the child is disorientated, changes will occur in these answers[70]<br>When a verbal response is not possible a grimace score can be used[74] |

## PROCEDURE:  Neurological assessment (continued)

| | |
|---|---|
| 10 Evaluate motor response by asking child to squeeze your fingers and to release them. Ask them to stick out their tongue. When assessing an infant see if they move towards a noisy toy and move their lower limbs if tickled | To assess motor response ensuring responses are equal and purposeful. A young baby will have a reflexive grasp |
| 11 Apply a sufficient painful stimulus as discussed earlier if the child does not respond | A deteriorating neurological status may be elicited by the child's inability to localise to pain and respond to it purposefully[70] Infants cannot localise but should withdraw their limb from the stimulus |
| 12 Ask the child to open their eyes and assist if the child cannot do so, noting the size, shape and equality of the pupils | Normal pupils are round[71] abnormality may be an indication of brain damage |
| 13 Assess the pupils' reaction to light as described above noting their ability to constrict which should be brisk; consensual light reflex any abnormal eye movements should be noted | Pupils should be equal in size and react to light briskly indicating an intact brain stem in the area that regulates pupil constriction. The presence of consensual light reflex indicates intact connections in the area of the brain stem. Abnormal eye movements may indicate damage to the cranial nerve |
| 14 Assess limb strength and spontaneity of movement on both sides of the child's body as described above | To indicate muscle tone. If hypertonia or hypotonia is present, note which limb is affected or if all limbs are equally affected, which would indicate brain damage. |
| 15 Document all findings on neurological observation chart, precisely recording the child's/infant's best response, total score for GCS component and report all abnormalities at once. If a stimulus was used note which one, where it was applied, how much pressure was required to elicit a response and how the child/infant responded | Accurate records provide continuity of care and promote patient safety[21,22] |

Rapid assessment of neurological status is determined by the AVPU score.

    A – alert

    V – voice

    P – pain

    U – unresponsive to painful stimuli.

An alert response equates to 15 on the GCS. A child who is unresponsive to painful stimuli equates to 8 or less on the GCS.[9] The AVPU score should be used only for rapid assessment, with the full GCS assessment being undertaken as soon as possible.

**VIGNETTE**

**Problem:** When performing neurological observations on a child you notice that there is a watery discharge from their nose (rhinorrhea).

**Discussion:** A watery discharge from the nose or ears may indicate a possible base of skull fracture and this should be tested for glucose with a Detrostix, as it may be cerebrospinal fluid.

Neurological assessment of the infant and child requires meticulous attention to detail as their neurological status can deteriorate rapidly. Initial assessment and family involvement is essential when trying to establish what behaviours are normal or abnormal for the child. Neurological observations should never be omitted.

Assessment of the child is complex and detailed. The general appearance of the child is a subjective impression of their heath status, behaviour, social skills, interaction with parents and environment, and should be the initial assessment. Measurement of temperature, cardiovascular and respiratory assessment constitutes the physiological approach to assessment. Neurological assessment addresses the motor, sensory and cerebellar function along with cranial nerve function. Assessment of growth is measured against standard growth charts and should be undertaken as part of the physical assessment.

Go to the website to find the PowerPoint presentation for this chapter and MCQs to test your knowledge. **www.hodderplus.com/childnursingskills**

# REFERENCES

1 Casey A (2006) Assessing and planning care in partnership. Chapter 7. In: Galsper EA, Richardson J (eds) *A textbook of children's and young peoples nursing*. Edinburgh: Churchill Livingstone.

2 Royal College of Nursing. (2003) *Guidelines for practice. Restraining, holding still and containing children*. London: RCN.

3 Hockenberry M, Wilson. D, Winkelstein M (2005). *Wong's nursing care of infants and children*, 7th edition. St Louis: Elsevier Mosby.

4 MacGregor J (2008) *Introduction to the anatomy, physiology of children*, 2nd edition. London: Routledge.

5 Fergusson D (2008) *Clinical assessment and monitoring in children*. Oxford: Blackwell Publishing.

6 National Institute for Clinical Excellence (2007) *Feverish illness in children. Assessment, management in children younger than 5 years*. Guideline 47. London: NICE.

7 Childs C, Harrison R, Hodkinson C (1999) Tympanic membrane temperature as a measure of core temperature. *Archives of Disease in Childhood* 80(3): 262–266.

8 Marieb E (2005) *Essentials of human anatomy: physiology*. San Francisco: Benjamin Cummings Publishing Company.

9 Resuscitation Council UK (2008) *Paediatric immediate life support*, 1st edition. London: RCUK.

10 Sarti, A. Savron F Casotto V, Cuttini M (2005) Heartbeat assessment in infants: a comparison of four clinical methods. *Pediatric Critical Care Medicine* 6(2) 212–215.

11 Whaley L, Wong D (1999) *Nursing care of infants and children*, 6th edition. St Louis: Mosby.

12 Berger A (2001) Oscillatory blood pressure monitoring devices. *British Medical Journal* **323**(20): 919.

13 Gillman MW, Cook NR (1995) Blood pressure measurement in childhood epidemiological studies. *Circulation* **92**: 1049–1057.

14 Beevers G, Lip G, O'Brien E (2001) Blood pressure measurement. Part 1. Sphygmomanometry: factors common to all techniques. *British Medical Journal* **322**(7292): 981–985.

15 Gillepsie A, Curizo J (1998) Blood pressure measurement: assessing staff knowledge. *Nursing Standard* **12**(23) 35–37.

16 Beevers M, Beevers G (1996) Blood Pressure measurement in the next century: a plea for stability. *Blood Pressure Monitor* **1**(2): 117–120.

17 Royal College of Nursing (2007) *Standards for assessing, measuring and monitoring vital signs in infants, children and young people*. London: RCN.

18 Medicines and Health Care Products Regulatory Agency (2006) *Measuring blood pressure top ten tips*. London: DH.

19 Petrie J, O' Brian E, Litler W, deSwiet M (1997) *Recommendations on blood pressure measurement*, 2nd edition. London: British Hypertension Society.

20 Jowett N (1997) *Cardiovascular monitoring*. London: Whurr.

21 Nursing, Midwifery Council (2007) *Record keeping*. London: NMC.

22 Nursing, Midwifery Council (2008) *The Code. Standards for conduct, performance and ethics for nurses and midwives*. London: NMC.

23 Schnell K (2006) Evidence-based practice: non

invasive blood pressure measurement in children. *Pediatric Nursing* **32**(3) 263–267.

24 Cruse L (2004) Physiological measures in Intensive care. *Paediatric Nursing* **16**(9) 14–17.

25 Mccance K, Huether S (2006) *Pathophysiology: the biological basis for disease in adults and children*, 5th edition. St Louis: Mosby.

26 Curley M A, Moloney-Harmon PA (2001) *Critical care nursing of infants and children*, 2nd edition. Philadelphia: WB Saunders.

27 Williams C, Asquith J (2000) *Paediatric intensive care nursing*. Edinburgh: Churchill Livingstone.

28 Jacobson S (2000) Electrocadiography. In: Woods SL, Froelicher ES, Motzer S (eds) *Cardiac nursing*. Philadelphia: Lippincott.

29 Candy D (2001) Clinical paediatrics and child health. WB Saunders: Edinburgh.

30 Bloomfield T (2002) Tachypnea. *Pediatrics in Review* **23**(8): 294–295.

31 Hewson P, Humphries SM, Roberton DM, *et al.* (1990) Markers of serious illness in infants under 6 months old presenting to a children's hospital. *Archives of Disease of Childhood* **65**(7) 750–756.

32 Gormley-Fleming E (2006) Assessing children. In: Peate I, Whiting. L (eds) *Caring for children and their families*. Chichester: Wiley, Chapter 9.

33 Davis F (2004) *Spotting the sick child*. London: DH (DVD).

34 Lissauer T, Clayden G (2007) *Illustrated textbook of paediatrics*, 3rd edition. Mosby: Edinburgh.

35 Gill D, O'Brien N (2002) *Paediatric clinical examination made easy*, 4th edition. Edinburgh: Churchill Livingstone.

36 Bickley L (2003) *Bates guide to physical examination and history taking*, 8th edition. Philadelphia: Lippincott, Williams, Wilkins.

37 London M, Ladewig D, Ball J, *et al.* (2007) *Maternal and child health nursing*, 2nd edition. Upper Saddle River.

38 Rudolf M, Levene M (2006) *Paediatrics and child health*, 2nd edition. Oxford: Blackwell Publishing.

39 Jurban A (1999) Pulse oximetry. *Critical Care* **3**: 11–17.

40 Tortora G, Derrickson. B (2006) *Principles of anatomy and physiology*, 11th edition. Danvers: Wiley.

41 Neill S, Knowles H (2004) *The biology of child health. A reader in development and assessment*. Basingstoke: Palgrave Macmillan.

42 Villanueva R, Bell C, Kain Z, Colongo K (1999) Effects of peripheral perfusion on accuracy of pulse oximetry in children. *Journal of Clinical Anaesthesia* **11**: 317–322.

43 Coleman MD, Coleman NA (1996) Drug induced methaemoglobinaemia. Treatment issues. *Drug Safety* **14**(6) 394–405

44 Woodrow P (1999) Pulse oximetry. *Emergency Nurse* **7**(5) 33–38.

45 Hinkelbein J, Genzwuerker H, Sogl R, Fielder F (2007) Effects of nail polish on oxygen saturation determined by pulse oximetry in critically ill patients. *Resuscitation* **72**: 82–91.

46 Hinkelbein J, Koehler H, Genzwuerker, H, Fielder F (2007). Artificial acrylic fingernails may alter pulse oximetry measurement. *Resuscitation* **74**: 75–82.

47 Jurban A (1998) Pulse oximetry. In: Tobin M (ed.) *Principles and practices in intensive care monitoring*. New York: McGraw Hill.

48 Stoneham M, Saville G. Wilson I (1994) Knowledge about pulse oximetry among medical and nursing staff. *Lancet* **344**: 1339–1342.

49 Homi J, Levee L, Higgs D, *et al.* (1997) Pulse oximetry in a cohort study of sickle cell disease. *Clinical and Laboratory Haematology* **19**: 17–22.

50 Kress J, Pohlamn A, Hall J (1999) Determination of haemoglobin saturation in patients with acute sickle chest syndrome. A comparison of arterial blood gases and pulse oximetry. *Chest* **115**: 1316–1320

51 Comber J, Lopez B (1996) Evaluation of pulse oximetry in sickle cell anaemia patients presenting to the emergency department in acute vaso-occlusive crisis. *American Journal of Emergency Medicine* **14**: 16–18.

52 Levene M, Tudehope D, Sinha S (2008) *Neonatal medicine*, 4th edition. Oxford: Blackwell Publishing.

53 Ashurst S (1995) Clinical oxygen therapy. *British Journal of Nursing* **4**(9): 504–514.

54 Chandler T (2000) Oxygen saturation monitoring. *Paediatric Nursing* **12**(8): 37–42.

55 Royal College of Paediatrics and Child Health (2009) *Growth reference charts for use in the UK*. London: RCPCH http://www.rcpch.ac.uk/Research/UK-WHO-Growth-Charts (accessed 20 August 2009).

56 Patel L, Dixon M, David TJ (2003) Growth and growth charts in cystic fibrosis. *Journal of Royal Society of Medicine* **96**(43): 35–41.

57 Hall DMB, Elliman D (2003) *Health for all children*, 4th edition. Oxford: Oxford University Press.

58 Department of Health (1996) Extra-laboratory use of blood glucose meters and test strips: contraindications, training and advices to users. Medical Device Agency Adverse Incident Safety centre Safety Notice. 9616. June.

59 Medical Device Agency (2002) *Management and use of IVD point of care test devices*. London: MDA.

60 Cowan T (1997) Blood glucose monitoring devices. *Professional Nurse* **12**(8): 593–597.

61 Page N, Mackowiak L, Bratt K (1999) Identifying

and caring for the child with new onset Type 1 diabetes. *Journal of the Society of Pediatric Nurses* **4**(3): 128–130.

62  Jennett B, Teasdale G (1974) Assessment of coma and impaired consciousness. *Lancet* **2**(7872): 81–84.

63  National Institute for Clinical Excellence (2003) *Triage, assessment, investigation and early management of head injuries in infants and children and adults.* Clinical guideline 4. London: NICE.

64  Simpson D, Reilly P (1982) Paediatric coma scale. *Lancet* **2**(8295): 450.

65  Hickey J (2002) *The clinical practice of neurological and neurosurgical nursing,* 5th edition. Philadelphia: Lippincott.

66  Downey D, Leigh R (1998) Eye movements: pathophysiology, examination and clinical importance. *Journal of Neuroscience Nursing* **30**(1): 15–23.

67  Frawley P (1990) Neurological observations. *Nursing Times* **86**(35): 29–34.

68  Fairley D, Cosgrove S (1999) Glasgow Coma Scale: Improving nursing practice through clinical effectiveness. *Nursing in Critical Care* **4**(6): 276–279.

69  Aucken S, Crawford B (1998) Neurological assessment. In: Guerrero D (ed.) *Neuro-oncology for nurses.* London: Whurr Publishers.

70  Shah S (1999) Neurological assessment. *Nursing Standard* **13**(22): 49–56.

71  Tatman A, Warren A, Williams A, *et al.* (1997) Development of paediatric coma scale in intensive care clinical practice. *Archives of Disease in Childhood* **77**(6): 519–521.

72  Fuller G (1993) *Neurological examinations made easy.* Edinburgh: Churchill Livingstone.

73  Hazinski MF (1999) *Manual of pediatric critical care.* Mosby: St Louis.

74  Warren A (2000) Paediatric coma scoring researched and benchmarked. *Paediatric Nursing* **12**(3): 14–18.

# Medicines administration

Carol Hall

## LEARNING OUTCOMES

*Upon completion of this chapter, the reader should be able to accomplish the following:*

1 Define 'medicine administration' within a wider context of 'medicines management' for children
2 Identify legal requirements and responsibilities of nurses in the administration of medicines to children and young people, including administration of controlled drugs
3 Discuss the importance of communication and decision-making in ensuring safe and effective medicines use by children
4 Identify steps in preparing to give a medicine, including identification of routes for administration
5 Describe critical points relating to giving and recording medicines safely
6 Describe some processes for safe calculation of medicines
7 Identify organizational and management elements of medicine administration including administration and management of controlled medicines and consideration of administering medicines under patient group directions

## KEY WORDS

Medicines management    Medicines administration
Calculation    Patient safety

## CHAPTER OVERVIEW

Administering medicines to children is a part of everyday nursing practice that is complex and multifaceted. It is a part of clinical practice with some clear theoretical components and thus needs to be considered both practically and theoretically to deliver care which is both safe and effective. This chapter is pragmatic and practical, leading the reader through specific elements of the role of the nurse in the practice of administering medicines to children and the knowledge required. The chapter defines medicines administration, and the associated legal definitions and responsibilities which impact on nursing. Processes for calculation of medicines and procedural practices for administering medicines are also explained. Specific consideration of nursing skills and communication is essential for medicines administration with children and young people, and this is achieved using decision-making exercises to illustrate problem-solving skills needed. While problem-solving and decision-making are critical for delivery of effective nursing care by children's nurses who are regularly giving medicines to children, it can be secondary in consideration to more technical and legal considerations. This is unfortunate, because the capacity to make effective decisions can mean the difference between quality care and the occurence of errors and unsafe practice. In this chapter, problem-solving and decision-making are emphasised.

A key consideration in administering medicines to children is ensuring their safety, and medication error is a concern in nursing generally.

It is important to recognise that medication error can occur at any point in the medicine management process; it is intended not to include a separate section on this element but to draw attention to key considerations throughout the chapter.

To participate in medicines administration most effectively, the children's nurse needs to combine a range of skills, including technical capacity and knowledge, understanding of legal and ethical issues, and communication and decision-making abilities.

## MEDICINE ADMINISTRATION

The first consideration for nurses proposing to administer a medicine should be to think about what their activity actually is, in the context of all care given to a child or young person. This may sound strange, because, if you are asked to administer a medicine, the first apparent activity is to get the child's prescription chart (properly known as the medicine administration record, MAR) and identify what should be given. However, this is one point in a series of events undertaken by a multiprofessional team, and for safety and legal reasons it is important that nurses are aware of how this focal point of preparing to give a medicine is situated within a wider context.

In professional and legal terms 'medicine administration' is therefore properly defined within the context of 'medicines management'. This is a wider term, which includes the medicine manufacturers, licencers (in the UK this is the Medications and Healthcare Products Regulatory Agency, MRHA), distributors, purchasers, pharmacists, prescribers (including doctors, nurses and other professionals allied to medicine) and finally the nurse or carer who gives the medicine to the child.

For children's nurses, this means that all medicine must be administered safely, cost-effectively and in a way that ensures that the child is fully able to benefit from their treatment. It is important for nursing to continually evaluate against this standard in order to enable best practice.

## LEGAL REQUIREMENTS AND RESPONSIBILITIES FOR PRACTITIONERS WORKING WITH CHILDREN

Before a medicine can be prescribed to be administered to an individual child, there are many steps through which one needs to proceed both legally and in development as part of medicines management.

---

### Definitions

**Medicine:** (a) Any substance or combination of substances presented as having properties for treating or preventing disease in human beings or (b) any substance or combination of substances which may be used in or administered to human beings either with a view to restoring, correcting or modifying physiological functions by exerting a pharmacological, immunological or metabolic action, or to making a medical diagnosis.[1]

**Medicine administration:** The administration of any medicinal product for a medicinal purpose, including therapeutic treatment or prevention of disease, diagnosis of disease, contraception, induction of anaesthesia, or otherwise preventing or interfering with the normal operation of a physiological function.[2]

**Medicines management:** The clinical, cost-effective and safe use of medicines to ensure patients get the maximum benefit from the medicines they need, while at the same time minimising potential harm.[3]

Children's nurses need to be aware of these as they affect both storage and administration practices relating to medicinal treatment. This section will address manufacture and labelling, and prescribing while a later section will look specifically at legal requirements relating to the use of controlled medicines.

Medications manufactured must be tested to stringent standards and the product should be appropriately licensed for use with children. This is, however, sometimes difficult. There is a dearth of testing of medication with children and thus limitations relating to the marketing authorisations (previously called licences) issued, even for sometimes commonly used treatments. A fuller discussion about the complexities of prescribing and administering 'off-licence' and 'off-label' drugs to children is addressed within the British National Formulary for children.[4] If the child is an NHS patient, the medicine must be available and recognised for use in accordance with the National Institute for Health and Clinical Excellence (NICE) guidance for prescribing in the NHS, according to the disorder and then appropriately prescribed in the correct dose by a qualified and authorised practitioner. The medication must also be dispensed by a pharmacist in an appropriate carrier (e.g. syrup, tablet, etc.) to give the child concerned, and in accordance with regulations defined by the legal classification of the medicine.

## MEDICINE NAMES AND LABELLING

In the UK, medicines are labelled in two ways. The brand name and the generic product name. So, for example, Calpol is a brand name for one children's formulation of the drug with the generic UK name paracetamol. This year, a further requirement has been added in light of increasing international health care activity. The European Directive 92/27/EEC[21] specifies the requirements for the labelling of medicines, and outlines the format and content of patient information leaflets to be supplied with every medicine; the directive also requires the use of Recommended International Non-proprietary Names for drugs (RiNN),[4] which are now recognised through common international names. This has meant that, for some medication, changes in the names have occurred. For paracetamol this requires the inclusion of the RiNN acetaminaphen within formulary as found within the BNFc.[4]

> **KEY POINTS**
> - Nurses must be aware of brand (proprietary) and national and international generic (non-proprietary) drug names
> - Confusion of drug names can cause errors in medicine administration

> **VIGNETTE**
>
> **Problem:** George is 15 days old and born 6 weeks prematurely. He has been prescribed caffeine citrate as a respiratory stimulant. In checking the prescription, the nurse identifies that this medicine is not licenced for use with neonates like George.
>
> **Discussion:** This is correct and it is a difficult situation. However, the use of caffeine is well documented in the literature and guidance for its use is given in the BNFc.[4] Further The BNFc identifies that there is no caffiene product licensed for use with neonates. In George's case, the absence of a respiratory stimulant may mean an increased risk of respiratory arrest or a prolonged period of artificial ventilation. The prescription and decision to give is one which needs to be made by the medical and nursing staff, but the benefits in George's care may be seen to outweigh the legal concerns.

> **VIGNETTE**
>
> **Look at the Wayne Jowett Inquiry.**[5] Reading through the main conclusions of this Inquiry, try to identify how many different professionals influenced Wayne's care. What errors were made and why? What could have been done differently?
>
> **Discussion:** Investigators found errors had occurred throughout a system of medicines management, by a range of professionals, which had culminated in a final fatal error. This has long been recognised both by researchers in the field[6,7] and by the National Patient Safety Agency (NPSA),[8] who provide monitoring and guidance in respect of medication error in the UK.

KEY POINTS

- Children's nurses often administer medicines at the end of a series of multiprofessional events and are responsible for ensuring that the medication given is appropriate for the child who receives it
- Nurses must be vigilant for unusual prescriptions, doses or routes. For children's nurses this is especially challenging because children are less able to determine which medicines they might usually take or by which route when compared with adult patients

## PROFESSIONAL REQUIREMENTS AND RESPONSIBILITIES IN ADMINISTERING MEDICINE

In order to administer a medicine to a child, nurses must be working within legal parameters, but they must also work within the guidance of their professional body and within local policies issued by the institution in which they work. All medicines should be administered by a registered nurse; student nurses can participate in the administration of patient-specified prescriptions under the direct supervision of a registered nurse.[9] Student nurses must additionally work within the guidance of their universities. This can lead to dissonance when one set of guidance may be broader than another.

KEY POINTS

- All nurses must be mindful of professional and legal guidance
- Nurses who move around healthcare settings during their practice should check local policy and procedures surrounding medicine administration as a priority prior to participation
- It is not acceptable to administer medicine if the local policy does not allow this, even if the nurse has been used to doing this elsewhere

VIGNETTE

**Problem:** Charlotte is a student nurse. As part of her second-year allocation to nursing clinical practice, she is on placement in a Hospital Trust where she has not worked before. During her induction, she discovers that she will not be permitted to second-check medicines for children during her placement, even though in her last Health Trust she was allowed to do this. Charlotte is frustrated and cross – she feels as though her skills are not being used. What should she do?

**Discussion:** Second-checking of medicines for children is recognised as good practice by the NMC[9] in children's nursing, but it is not an absolute requirement, except when giving 'controlled medicines'. Also, while the first checker must be a registered practitioner, there is no professional stipulation about who can second-check a medicine. Local policy defines when second-checking is required, and identifies who those checking the medicines must be. Local policy also offers the main means for vicarious liability (insurance) if an adverse event arises, and it is the measure by which the employer judges professional responsibility.

## COMMUNICATION, ASSESSMENT AND DECISION-MAKING IN GIVING MEDICINES TO CHILDREN

Up to now this chapter has focused upon the general principles, and the legal and professional considerations in the administration of medicines. This serves as context for considering the practical nursing role. The next step is to consider the delivery of nursing practice, including the child or young person and their carers. This section will consider the importance of communication and the initial assessment in medicine administration, which is identified as a priority within the NICE guidelines[10] relating to medicines adherence.

Nursing practice plays a part as the first point of contact with the child and their family, and can also be the final point of contact on or after discharge. Effective communication and assessment in relation to medicine administration can determine the difference between an excellent experience of medicinal treatment and a sub-optimum one.[10]

Consider the following situation.

VIGNETTE

**Problem:** James aged 6 years has cystic fibrosis, which was diagnosed at birth. He is usually managed effectively at home by his family and his school using a range of medications to treat his condition. He has been admitted to hospital this afternoon with a severe chest infection, which requires hospital management and intravenous antibiotic therapy. Now he is admitted the nurse needs to find out the best way to continue James's treatment. What should be done?

**Discussion:** In this scenario, communication is needed to establish effective continuation of James treatment from home and to determine the best way for him to receive appropriate new medicines in hospital. The nurse or doctor will need to assess his medicine management as part of the admission procedure and communicate requirements to the pharmacist. Communication will be essential at all levels, with James, his family and with the multiprofessional team, to ensure medicine administration is established which will be effective.

KEY POINTS

- Communication, assessment and effective decision-making are critical in administering medicines to children
- Nurses need to communicate with a range of professional and lay people
- Children's developmental ability should also be considered

The following procedural guideline relates to admitting a patient to a care setting. It identifies the nurses need to include communication and also to use skill in decision-making in order to create and document an effective care assessment.

## GAINING CONSENT FOR MEDICINE ADMINISTRATION

Gaining consent can be complex and requires sensitive use of communication skills. It is important to check in the initial assessment documentation and to ask the family who will

## PROCEDURE: Admission of a child requiring medicinal treatment to a care setting

| Procedural steps | Evidence-based rationale |
| --- | --- |
| 1 Identify what medications a child has received prior to admission to the care environment (in other care settings) | To ensure that medication effects can be monitored, medication is not repeated inappropriately and consideration is taken in respect of medicines interactions if new treatments are prescribed |
| 2 Retrieve and safely store any personal medicines brought to the care environment medicine) | To ensure that medicine can continue to be used where appropriate and that it is stored safely away from other children and in accordance with legal requirements for the institution[2,11] Also to ensure storage within the requirements of the medication (some medicines should be refrigerated[4]) |
| 3 Decide whether the child needs to receive medication on admission | To ensure treatment can commence promptly and most efficiently |
| 4 Ensure the child is wearing a name band including their name, hospital number, consultant name and care location | It is essential to be able to correctly identify patients when medicines are to be given[9] |
| 5 Arrange for required medicines to be prescribed by a qualified practitioner | To ensure continuity of treatment and rapid commencement of new intervention |
| 6 Arrange for the pharmacy to assess need and provide any required medicines | Rapid arrangement of any dispensing from the pharmacy will enable new treatment to be commenced and continuation of existing treatment most effectively[12] |
| 7 Assess whether the child has any allergies to medicines | To prevent reaction to medicine occurring |

## PROCEDURE: Admission of a child requiring medicinal treatment to a care setting

| | |
|---|---|
| **8** Determine child's developmental stage, and past experience and that of the family | Nurses must take into account a patient's physical needs and learning ability in order to communicate effectively about medicines and ensure appropriate information is given[10] |
| **9** Assess how a medicine has been taken at home in relation to the prescription (concordance) | To ensure that the medication given is being used in an optimum way which is safe and effective[12] |
| **10** Discuss with child and carers who will give medicines while in hospital | Consultation with the patient and carer is essential to ensure continuity and acceptable participation as well as appropriate preparation and education where needed[10] |
| **11** Identify what utensils are required to administer the child's medicine | Giving a medicine to a child using similar means will help with tolerance and familiarity |
| **12** Identify what form of medication is preferred by the child | Giving a similar form of medicine will aid familiarity and assist in tolerance |
| **13** Document admission assessment within care plan or pathway documents | The care plan or pathway is a legal record of patient care[9] |

be giving the medicine. If the parent or the child themselves is administering (self-administration), then the nurse's role will be different from when the medicine is to be given by the nurse. In the former case, the institution will have procedures for self-administration of medicines by children or their families. The nurse's role in this situation will be one of education about new medications and preparation and assessment for self-administration roles in practice. If the patient or their family is self-administering medicines, it is the responsibility of the registered nurse to ensure that the medication is being administered as it has been prescribed.[9]

If the nurse is administering the medicine, the age and developmental stage of the child needs to be assessed with care to determine their capacity to offer reasonable consent. Where the child is unable to do this, the person with parental responsibility should expect to be asked prior to the prescribed treatment.[5] In community settings where medicines are bought over the counter and not prescribed, written permission must be attained by the person with parental responsibility for all children under 16 years of age.[13]

As well as consent, it is also important to gain the permission of the child. Sometimes this is difficult, because it may not be possible to offer many choices to children about their medicines. If a

course of treatment has been prescribed, then it is important that this must be followed and younger children may not have a full appreciation of this. While there is much debate about the refusal of young children to take medicines and the relative benefits or disadvantages of them acting in this way, very careful consideration is required prior to the prescription regarding the need for the medication and the formulation of the substance and the route to be given. This will affect their concordance and ultimately on the effect of the treatment if every dose is accompanied by distress. Families are less likely to continue with a treatment that is very difficult for them, and indeed children's nurses interviewed by Hall[14] identified that attempting to make children take medicine when they do not want to could be a challenging part of their work.

In practice, nurses need to exercise thought in the way that they communicate with young children over the taking of a medicine. They should not imply choice when actually there may not be one but should try to allow the child to become empowered through making other decisions which may be possible. Consider the following vignette.

Depending upon the age of the child, it is also important to consider when you are going to advise them that their medicine is ready to be given. For a very young child it is not reasonable to ask for consent and then go away to prepare the medicine

**Problem:** Katie is 3 years old and has been in hospital following a meningococcal meningitis infection. She has been receiving antibiotics intravenously but is now well enough to go home provided she continues to take her medicines orally. These taste unpleasant to Katie, but it is essential she finishes the course of treatment. The nurses are giving Katie her medicines in hospital.

The following dialogue takes place.

Nurse: Katie, it is time for your medicine now – would you like a drink afterwards?

Katie: Don't like medsin...

Nurse: I know, but it is not too much, just one little bit and then you can have your drink...what would you like?

[Katie prefers to take her medicine from a single use oral syringe and likes to push the plunger to take the medicine herself]

Katie: No medsin...Blackcurrant

Nurse: Look, it is in the syringe – do you want to push or shall Mummy help you?

Katie: Me...

**Discussion:** The nurse assessed the situation with regards Katie's age and developmental ability. She gave Katie choices where she could reasonably have them in relation to taking a drink after her medicine and in relation to the way the medicine was to be administered. She was not able to offer the choice about taking the medicine so this was not offered at all. This is not always going to work, however, and it is recognised that on some occasions reconsidering the route or method of administration as a result of refusal may be necessary. This should also be resolved before the child returns to a home setting as it is likely that concordance with taking medicines may be compromised if this is not achieved.

as they will not understand this arrangement. Consent may be attained from the parents, but permission from the children needs to be negotiated just before administration takes place. However, with older children it is acceptable to gain permission by saying 'I am just going to get your medicine ready – is this alright?' This will allow the medicine to be prepared without interruption and will also allow the young person time to prepare themselves for their medications.

## PREPARING AND GIVING MEDICINES TO CHILDREN

In the preparation stage, the medicine will be retrieved from its appropriate storage and prepared for administration according to the prescription record. The person who requires treatment will have an MAR chart; although there are some differences, this is similar in the community setting or in hospital, but in schools medicine administration may be recorded within a medicine administration record book held by the school in accordance with local policy, as there is currently no legal requirement for them to keep individual records.[13] Although sometimes identified as a prescription chart, this is technically incorrect as the prescription is the element where the medicine is prescribed and not the component that includes the ordering and recording of medicines given.[9]

Using the MAR it is possible to identify which medicines are required by the child and when they should be given. The record needs to be checked scrupulously on each occasion that it is used in order to determine that all information is completed and is considered at the date and time of review. At this time a first and, if needed, a second checker should be working together in accordance with local policy and with the NMC 2008 Guidance for the Administration of Medicines.

### Helpful hints

1 To review a medicine administration chart, work from the top left-hand side of the chart to the bottom right hand side of the chart on every page examining each component. This helps to ensure all the information is read.
2 Read out the information aloud. This enables a second checker to hear what is being said and the reader to hear themselves, thus allowing a further form of checking.

If all checks of the medicine administration prescription and record are correct, the preparatory process towards the administration of the medicine may continue. Once the medicine to be given is identified then it can be reconsidered. The key points to be considered here include the route of administration and whether any calculation has to be made.

## PROCEDURE: Checking the medicine administration record

| Procedural steps | Evidence-based rationale |
|---|---|
| **1** Full name | The child must be positively identified prior to administering any medication.[9] |
| **2** Date of birth | To further determine identity |
| **3** Address or patient number | To finally establish unique identity |
| **4** Weight of the child | To determine the size of the child. Medications should be prescribed in accordance with the child's weight and children's nurses should know the ranges and dose per weight in kilograms of the medicine to be given[4] |
| **5** Height and body mass index (BMI) of child, if included | Height and BMI can enable a more accurate account of child size for treatment with specific medicines[4] |
| **6** Identify known allergies | Allergic reaction to medication can cause medical injury or fatality[4] |
| **7** Check whether any 'once only' or 'as needed drugs' are to be given or have been given | To determine need for administration and to avoid overdose if medicine has been previously given |
| **8** Check which regular medicines need to be administered at the correct time on the date required | To determine need for administration and to avoid overdose if medicine has been previously given |
| **9** Check that the prescription has been correctly written and signed by an authorised prescriber | Nurses must ensure that the prescription is completed properly before administering medicines, to ensure safe administration practice[9] |
| **10** Check that the prescription is concordant with the child's age, size and can be administered within the marketing authorisation | To prevent administration where calculation or licensing errors may have occurred within the prescription[4] |
| **11** Ensure that the prescription has been checked by a pharmacist (where necessary) and the medication has been dispensed | To ensure the medication is appropriate and available for the child |
| **12** Ensure that the route of the medicine identified for administration is appropriate for the medication prescribed | Medicine administered by an inappropriate route for the prescription can cause medical injury or fatality[5] |
| **13** Check that that the medicine to be given is within the start and stop dates identified by the prescriber. | To ensure the prescription is administered appropriately as part of the regular treatment |
| **14** Check that the medicine has not already been given | To prevent overdose |
| **15** Ensure that following receipt of the medicine by the patient the record is signed at the correct date and time. | The nurse must make a clear, accurate and immediate record of all medicine administered, intentionally withheld or refused by the patient, ensuring the signature is clear and legible[9] |

## ROUTE OF ADMINISTRATION

There are different routes by which medicine may be administered. Table 10.1 provides a useful summary.

There are key principles in the administration of medicines through any route and this chapter will offer procedural guidance for preparation and administration in a general sense. It is not possible to consider procedural guidelines for all of the routes identified; however, reference to Healy's chapter in this book indicates specific procedural guidance for the use of inhalers and nebulisers; other specific procedures for administering medicines to children using different routes can are addressed by Trigg and Mohammed.[15] Issues relating specifically to the administration of cytotoxic medicines can be found in detail within the *Royal Marsden Manual of Clinical Procedures*.[20]

**Table 10.1** Routes for administration of medicine*

| Route | Notes |
| --- | --- |
| Oral | Including anything swallowed to the stomach or via nasogastric or nasojejunal tubes or via percutaneous endoscopic gastrostomy tube (PEG tube) |
| Sublingual/buccal | Allowed to dissolve under the tongue or in the cheek |
| Topical/local | Including application into eyes, ears, or insertion into vagina, rectum |
| Transdermal | Through slow-release patches adhered to the skin |
| Inhalation | Including via masks, nebulisers, breathing tubes and pressurised metered dose inhalers (pMDI) and spacer systems |
| Intravenously/Intra-arterially | Administered into a vein or artery by a doctor or nurse with appropriate advanced qualifications. (Venously: this could be via a peripheral cannula or directly to one of the large veins close to the heart via a central line or peripherally inserted central catheter (PiCC) system or an implanted system such as portacath) |
| Subcutaneously/subdermally | By injection under the cutaneous or subdermal skin layers |
| Intramuscularly | By injection into muscle layers |
| Intrathecally | Administered by appropriately qualified practitioner into the thecal cavity via a lumbar puncture procedure |
| Intra-osseously | Administered by appropriately qualified practitioner into bone cavity (used for urgent access) |
| Other | It is possible for appropriately qualified practitioners to use other routes (e.g. into body cavities such as the pleural space or peritoneal cavity) in specific circumstances. |

*Adapted from Hall[19] (with permission).

# ADMINISTRATION

Any administration of medicine must be considered in relation to the individual child's capacity to actually take the treatment, and in respect of the impact that the treatment may have on them. Considerable care has been taken within children's healthcare to minimise unnecessary use of routes such as intramuscular injection and the use of intravenous peripheral cannulae for long-term treatments. This is because the use of needles with young children can be distressing and uncomfortable and can create painful associations with nursing and medical care that may remain as unpleasant memories. Where intensive treatment is needed long term, for example in the case of treatment for cancer, the insertion of central venous lines may be preferable. A clear and concise consideration of the types of intravenous routes used in children's nursing can be found at the cancerbackup website in the section on children's cancers (www.cancerbackup.org.uk).

Other children needing long-term medication include those with special needs, for whom long-term treatment with anticonvulsants may be necessary. Many children with such needs have percutaneous endogastric feeding tubes formed for feeding purposes and these can be used for the administration of medicines, thus bypassing the need for administering the medications by mouth. Feeding via nasogastric and percutaneous routes have specific procedural guidelines, which are usually issued locally and these should be followed.

## PROCEDURE: Administering a medicine to a child or young person

| Procedural steps | Evidence-based rationale |
|---|---|
| 1 Identify when the medicine needs to be given and check the medicines administration record (see previous guideline) | Medicines must be given in timely manner in order to ensure optimum benefits from treatments |
| 2 Explain planned process to child or young person and their carer using appropriate language and terminology | Healthcare professionals should adapt their consultation style to the needs of individual patients so that all patients have the opportunity to be involved in decisions about their medicines at the level they wish[10] |
| 3 Check child's care pathway or plan for specific requirements | You must be aware of the patient's plan of care (care plan/pathway).[9] Maintaining consistency and adherence,[10] e.g. ensuring the child has the usual drink or cup, will facilitate their participation in the process |
| 4 Decide to check alone or with a second checker according to the substance to be given and to local policy | |
| 5 Identify an appropriate place to check medicine away from interruptions and distractions | |
| 6 Prioritise if a number of medicines need to be given at once | If two types of medication are required via different routes (e.g. intravenous and oral) at the same time this will need to be managed to enable optimum treatment. Some medicines require a specific timing or conditions for best effect[4] |
| 7 Decide if there is any reason not to administer the medicine at this time and record accordingly | You must administer or withhold in the context of the patient's condition[9] |
| 8 Collect equipment required to give the medicine | Thinking ahead to ensure what is needed is readily available for use will enable the best delivery of the medication |

## PROCEDURE:  Administering a medicine to a child or young person (continued)

| | |
|---|---|
| **9** Wash hands and put on any protective clothing required | To meet local policy requirements and to prevent contamination and cross-infection. If medicine is to be given via a peripherally inserted central catheter (PiCC) or central line, an aseptic no-touch technique will be required. If a topical cream is to be applied, then gloves will be worn by the administering practitioner to protect from absorption of the medication through their own skin |
| **10** Retrieve the medicine from appropriate place of storage | |
| **11** Ensure that the medicine selected is<br>(a)  in date | You must check the expiry date (where it exists) of the medicine to be administered.[9] Out of date medicines may have deteriorated |
| (b)  the correct formulation for the route to be given and appropriate for the child's preferences | To prevent error and optimise the best possible outcome in terms of concordance and medicines management |
| (c)  the best dose strength for the prescription | To ensure economical and safe practice in medicines management. Medicines are dispensed in different strengths |
| (d)  the correct medicine according to the prescription | You must check that the prescription or the label on medicine dispensed is clearly written and unambiguous.[9] Getting the wrong medication from storage is dangerous. Checking the medicine label with the prescription simultaneously reduces risk of error. Most medicines are prescribed for individual patients but sometimes stock medicines or injectables may be used. The nurse must determine the most appropriate stock solution with thought given to the best use of the medicines in terms of child preference and the costs involved |
| **12** Check if the prescribed dose is correct for the weight or BMI of the child | You must have considered the dosage, weight where appropriate, method of administration, route and timing[9]<br>All children's medicines are calculated on the basis of milligrams per kilogram per day.[4] Nurses must check the medicine and the dose for weight required. Use of BMI and surface area in children is restricted mostly to specialised areas and a calculator can be found for this in the BNFc online at www.bnfc.org.uk |
| **13** Calculate the volume of the medicine to be given | Calculation of the correct amount of medication must be made |
| **14** Ensure the medication is placed into an appropriate receptacle for administration | Medicine must be measured as accurately as possible using the available equipment, and the nurse must decide on the best use of this, e.g. putting 5 mL into a 50 mL medicine pot makes accuracy difficult.<br>In neonatal care accuracy of even a few millilitres may be clinically significant and small 1 mL syringes may be most accurate |

## PROCEDURE:  Administering a medicine to a child or young person (continued)

| | |
|---|---|
| **15** Medication which is not needed is returned to place of secure storage or disposed of in accordance with local policy and legal requirement. | |
| **16** Complete identity checks for child and reiterate final permissions using appropriate means of communication and play to aid explanation. Check finally for allergies | You must be certain of the identity of the patient to whom the medicine is to be administered.[9] Establish the most effective way of communicating with each patient and, if necessary, consider ways of making information accessible and understandable (e.g. using pictures, symbols, large print, different languages, an interpreter or a patient advocate).[10] You must check that the patient is not allergic to the medicine before administering[9] |
| **17** Ensure medicine is given in an appropriate place, ensuring privacy and maintaining 'safe' play space | Children must have safe spaces to play where medical and nursing intervention does not take place |
| **18** Ensure the child is prepared: has protective clothing (e.g. bib) or tissues if needed, a drink, etc., and is sitting comfortably. An infant may need to be held | |
| **19** Ensure medication is given in accordance with the prescription, local policy and the child's and family preferences | NMC[9]: In the case of children, when arrangements have been made for parents/carers or patients to administer their own medicinal products prior to discharge or rehabilitation, the registrant should ascertain that the medicinal product has been taken as prescribed |
| **20** Record when the medicine has been administered on the MAR, to ensure a legal record of the medicine administered | You must make a clear, accurate and immediate record of all medicine administered, intentionally withheld or refused by the patient, ensuring the signature is clear and legible; it is also your responsibility to ensure that a record is made when delegating the task of administering medicine[9] |
| **21** Safely dispose of receptacles for administration and any waste, remove protective clothing and wash hands | A registrant must dispose of medicinal products in accordance with legislation[9] |
| **22** Offer support for the child and family and education about the medicine given | Parents need to be aware of the main features of their child's treatments and how to manage them effectively and concordantly. At home they need to know what to do if the prescribed medicine is taken inappropriately and implications if medicine is not taken. Parents and older children may need education in the best way to administer medicine and support following discharge from the care setting. Nurses have a role in offering advice and information |
| **23** Monitor for effectiveness of the treatment with pre- and post-considerations (i.e. temperature or pain assessment or peak flow readings | You must know the therapeutic uses of the medicine to be administered, its normal dosage, side-effects, precautions and contraindications[9] The children's nurse must determine and report the effectiveness of the prescribed treatment appropriately and consider alternatives with the multiprofessional team to enhance effectiveness if |

## PROCEDURE: Administering a medicine to a child or young person (continued)

| | |
|---|---|
| | necessary. Different evaluative measurement tools are available depending upon the condition and the treatment required |
| **24** Monitor for reactions to the medication and report and treat accordingly. | You must contact the prescriber or another authorised prescriber without delay when the patient develops a reaction to the medicine or when assessment of the patient indicates that the medicine is no longer suitable[9] <br> Side-effects of medicines for children are identified in the BNFc[4] and must be part of the nurses knowledge in administering medicine to a child <br> The children's nurse should also review the child if they vomit and the medicine is not absorbed. A decision may need to be taken with regards re-administration if the child vomits immediately |

**KEY POINTS**

- Administering medicines to children is a role in practice which requires the application of considerable knowledge and practical skill
- Practice must concord with legal and professional guidance
- The student nurse must work closely with the registrant to learn these skills effectively and become competent for registered practice
- Student nurses must not administer medicines unsupervised at any time

## CALCULATION OF MEDICINE DOSES WITHIN CHILDREN'S NURSING

Calculating medicines for children has greater complexity than for adults. This is because adult patients are larger in size, they are not growing, have wider tolerance between doses than children and have a slower metabolic rate. This means an optimum dose of medication can be more easily obtained by using a standardised dose for which the medication is manufactured and stocked in bulk.

For example, the administration of the analgesic paracetamol for an adult is likely to be tablets or capsules, each of 250 mg, for which the person can take two, up to three times a day. For younger children, paracetamol is administered in syrup formulation and although this is calculated for home use for infants over 3 months, this is a guide from the manufacturer in accordance with the marketing authorisation, which works on the basis

**VIGNETTE**

**Identify the following:** a can of cola; a child's box drink; a small bottle of contact lens solution; a tube of superglue.

What are the volumes included on the packaging? Look at the size of the packaging and pour the drinks out to see how much is included. Think about what you would do if you calculated a medicine from a prescription and the answer was 330 mL.

**Discussion:** Looking at the volumes on the side of the packets: the can of cola usually contains around 330 mL of fluid, the child's box drink around 150 mL of fluid, the contact lens solution around 30 mL and the tube of superglue around 10 mL.

Of course, none of these substances should be given to small children: it is the volumes which are of interest. This illustrates that if, when calculating an oral medicine, the answer suggests that the child should be receiving 330 mL, then this is the volume the size of a can of coke! This would indicate that there is probably a problem in the calculation, in the prescription or the stock medicine selected. Administering 5 or 10 mL would be usual whereas 330 mL would be exceptionally unusual.

of a safe dose for the age group rather than focusing on the weight of the individual child to achieve an optimum dose. In young children, variations in weight are proportionately large and can influence optimum dose management.

| KEY POINTS |
|---|
| • Magnitude errors in calculation are the most common in prescribing and administering and nurses should be vigilant[8] |
| • Making a realistic estimate of the medication to be given may reduce errors |
| • Calculating medicines needs practice and checking is essential |

Within the UK, the system of measures used is the Système Internationale or SI units. Medication doses for children are calculated by weight in milligrams per kilogram of body weight per dose (divided into doses over a 24-hour period). 'Dose for weight' requirements are identified within the BNFc and are used by prescribers, pharmacists and nurses to ensure that the optimum amount of medicine is given for an individual child.

To calculate the dose for weight for a medicine to be given to a child, the following formula can be used: dose for weight at mg per kg per dose weight of the child in kg. This should be checked against the maximum daily dose, which is divided into the required number of doses.

### Calculating an initial prescription of paracetamol

For a simple calculation of dose for weight for a child aged 4 months of age weighing 4.5 kg with severe symptoms. The calculation would be as follows: 20 mg of paracetamol $\times$ 4.5 kg (infants weight) = $20 \times 4.5$ = 90 mg maximum per dose.[4]

Once the dose is established, the volume of medicine to be given can be determined. It is important to understand the volumes and measures concerned in calculating medicines for children and creating some reasoned estimates that can be visualised before finally calculating an answer.

## PROCEDURE: Calculating the volume of medicines to be given to a child

| Procedural steps | Evidence-based rationale |
|---|---|
| **1** In order to achieve this some information is needed | The MAR prescription states that a baby needs 90 mg of paracetamol suspension orally. All other checks have been performed and you are ready to calculate |
| **2** Look at the evidence and determine your realistic estimate | The medicine bottle including dose per mL volume of syrup to include paracetamol syrup 120 mg in 5 mL |
| **3** Now consider how much less… | There are 120 mg in every 5 mL of paracetamol in the medicine bottle. The baby needs 90 mg of suspension<br>Fact 1: 90 mg is less than 120 mg so the amount to be given will be less than 5mL<br>Fact 2: 90 mg is more than 60 mg (which is half of 120 mg contained in 5 mL)<br>Fact 3: The dose will be between 2.5 mL (60 mg) and 5 mL (120 mg). It definitely will not be more or less than this volume |
| **4** Now calculate whether you need to or continue to refine your estimate | A calculation can be made on the basis of these estimated parameters using a formula like the one offered below, or, in this case, it is possible to continue to refine the estimate until the answer is achieved<br>It is important to note that there are many ways of calculating medicine dosages and different methods suit different people and different situations |
|    (a) Achieving an answer through refining the estimate | This can again be illustrated using the same prescription requirement, but may be more difficult to achieve with small numbers and other methods may need to be used<br>Given Fact 3 above 90 mg is halfway between 60 mg and 120 mg – so the answer will be halfway between 2.5 mL and 5 mL = 3.75 mL or if every 60 mg is equal to 2.5 mL then every 30 mg is equal to 1.25 mL so 2.5 + 1.25 = 3.75 mL |

## PROCEDURE: Calculating the volume of medicines to be given to a child

| (b)  Achieving an answer through following a formula | This formula an be used to achieve most children's medicines calculations<br>MAR The prescribed dose in mg the unit of volume dispensed in mL<br>The dispensed unit dose in mg prescription = 90 mg ´<br>Dispensed unit volume of syrup = 5mL<br>Dispensed unit dose = 120 mg<br>90/120 $\times$ 5<br>90/120 can be divided by 10 and then by 3 to reduce the numbers to the lowest common denominator<br>9/12 $\times$ 5 and then 3/4 $\times$ 5 = 15/4 = 3.75 mL |
|---|---|

Although the calculation has been identified, it is not the end of the process. Skill is needed to ensure that the volume in millilitres is correctly measured into the receptacle before giving to the patient and this requires judgement of measurement and skill in ensuring the child takes all of the medicine. If the medicine tastes unpleasant, there may be a temptation to mix it with other substances to make it more palatable. This is not usually recommended. If the child has their medicine hidden in their drink, it raises issues about the disguised use of medicines. Even if the child is aware of the medication, it is diluted in a larger volume making it difficult to determine how much of the medicine has been taken by the child if the drink is not finished. Discussion with the pharmacist and with the child and their family about making medicines more palatable is an important consideration.

Finally, it is important to consider nursing management issues in the administration of medicines to children. Elements for consideration include legal aspects of administering medicines, the provision for administration of medicine under a patient group direction, nurse prescribing within children's nursing and the discharge of patients to other care settings with medicines.

## LEGAL CLASSIFICATION OF MEDICINES AND CONTROLLED DRUGS

All medicines are classified in accordance with the Medicines Act.[2] This Act determines in UK law whether a medicine is available by prescription only or may be sold by a pharmacist or may be freely available to purchase. Some Medicines are further subject to more specific control through the Misuse of Drugs Act (1971) and through subsequent regulations. The current regulations appertain to the Misuse of Drugs act (1971) and control of dangerous drugs (2001) regulations. These identify control of medicines within schedules numbered 1 to 5, with each having different criteria for management and storage by professionals. For nursing, management of controlled substances applies mainly to drugs within schedules 2 and 3. These classifications determine how medicines are handled by nurses, collected from pharmacy and stored in practice settings as well as given to children who need them. A final set of regulations is Dangerous Drugs, England, Scotland: The Controlled Drugs Supervision and Use Regulations (2006), which identifies that in an organisation there must be a nominated person with a legal responsibility for ensuring patient safety in relation to medicinal treatment. In hospitals, this person is usually the chief pharmacist. It is important for nurses to know who the designated person is within their institution.

## PROCEDURE: Extra considerations in the administration of controlled medicine in the hospital setting

| Procedural steps | Evidence-based rationale |
|---|---|
| 1 Check MAR, prepare child and family; clean hands and apply protective clothing as per previous procedural guidance | A controlled medicine requires the same preparation of the family as any other. Families may need extra support in understanding why these medicines are needed and that their child will not become addicted[16] |
| 2 Retrieve the Ward Controlled Medicine Record Book from place of storage | All clinical areas must have a contemporaneous record of controlled drugs stored and used |
| 3 Registered practitioner and checker to retrieve keys to controlled drug cupboards. Registrant and second checker unlock cupboards and identify medication to be administered | Keys for controlled medicines cupboards must be held and the location of them known at all times by the person in charge of the clinical area |
| 4 Check the number of tablets or ampoules in the cupboards against the stock register. If these are the same, then remove the number required for the prescription | Stocks of controlled medicines should be checked every 24 hours by two people, one of whom must be a registered nurse, in accordance with legislation and local policy |
| 5 Complete the controlled medicines record to identify the existent amount of tablets or ampoules or fluid volume and the amount removed for this patient's prescription | You must make a clear, accurate and immediate record of all medicine administered, intentionally withheld or refused by the patient, ensuring the signature is clear and legible; it is also your responsibility to ensure that a record is made when delegating the task of administering medicine[9] |
| 6 If not all of the medicine is required and it is not possible to return it (e.g. half ampoules) then waste must be disposed of appropriately and the written record should state this | A registrant must dispose of medicinal products in accordance with legislation[9] |
| 7 Return remaining medicine to the cupboard and lock away | Controlled medicines should be stored in accordance with the requirements of the law (1971, 2001, 2006) |
| 8 Take the medicine to the patient and complete as per medicine administration procedural guideline, including monitoring, evaluation and clearing away | A controlled medicine requires the same preparation of the family as any other |
| 9 Once the medicine has been administered, registrant and second checker to sign MAR and sign Controlled Drug Record Book. | You must make a clear, accurate and immediate record of all medicine administered, intentionally withheld or refused by the patient, ensuring the signature is clear and legible; it is also your responsibility to ensure that a record is made when delegating the task of administering medicine[9] |

## DISCHARGING CHILDREN AND YOUNG PEOPLE WITH CONTINUING MEDICATION NEEDS

The role of the nurse in relation to medicines administration is critical when considering discharging the child or young person from an area. Without effective planning information and education, future treatment to be continued in the home could be poorly adhered to or misunderstood or given inappropriately, leading to injury or even fatality.

Planning for discharge should begin early. If the child or the parent will be expected to administer medicines at home, the process must be explained, they should have the chance to practise in the care setting and must be assessed as being able to achieve an effective practice.[9] The correct equipment is supplied and the parents must know how it should be used. Patient information needs to be supplied and this may take the form of verbal discussion but also supportive education through leaflets or websites. Contact information should also be given for further advice. Any medicine to be taken home should be ordered in advance of the proposed discharge time to minimise waiting times for patents.

After the child has gone home, parents might telephone for advice about the management of medicines. Nurses therefore need to know how to respond appropriately on the telephone, how to make a full assessment of the situation and what advice should be given.

## MANAGEMENT OF ADVERSE EVENTS

> *As a registrant, if you make an error you must take any action to prevent any potential harm to the patient and report as soon as possible the prescriber, your line manager or employer (according to local policy) and document your actions.[9]*

In nursing and health care it is recognised that the reporting of incidents and near misses can help professionals to learn about how to make the patient experience safer. The NPSA has a Medication Zone on its website, which offers details on this view, and the NMC Standards for the Administration of Medicines clearly identifies the benefits of taking such an approach. However, the perceived impact of making a mistake is sometimes challenging to manage and you may find if you are in this position it is difficult to make decisions and to feel confident. This is not unusual, and getting support from colleagues or from your professional union may be helpful to you. It is also sensible to identify the untoward incident form in use in the locality, and think about the information that may have to be included before any event happens.

## PATIENT GROUP DIRECTIONS AND NURSE PRESCRIBING

While these considerations are included for reference within the chapter, these represent roles which are expected only of qualified nurses. According to current professional guidance from the NMC,[9] students must always be supervised in the administration of medicines and should not participate in the administration of medicines arranged under Patient Group Directions (PGDs). Indeed, it is recommended that the majority of medicines administered within the clinical setting should be on a patient-specific basis.[17] All nurses, however, must understand what patient group directions are, and how they may be used. Commonly used PGDs in children's nursing include topical application of local anaesthetic creams prior to intravenous injections or blood-taking procedures in the hospital or clinic, and also vaccinations in the community setting.

## NURSE PRESCRIBING

Nurse prescribing is an extended role for registrants in medicines management and takes two forms.

- Independent prescribing, where the nurse is qualified to prescribe any licensed medication for any medication within their competence.
- Supplementary prescribing, where the nurse is qualified to prescribe certain medicines within a clinical management plan.[18]

The benefits of such prescribing to children and their families is to allow a more efficient and flexible service that can meet needs rapidly and reduce the number of practitioners involved with a child's care.

# CONCLUSION

This chapter has addressed some key issues in the administration of drugs to children and young people. This is a complex area with many facets for which justice cannot be done within a chapter this size. However, where possible, further reference material has been included for development.

---

### Definition

**Patient Group Directions (PGDs)**, in existence since August 2000, constitute a legal framework which allows certain health care professionals to supply and administer medicines to groups of patients that fit the criteria laid out in the PGD. So, a healthcare professional could supply (for example, provide an inhaler or tablets) and/or administer a medicine (for example, give an injection or a suppository) directly to a patient without the need for a prescription or an instruction from a prescriber. PGDs allow the supply and administration of specified medicines to patients who fall into a group defined in the PGD; using a PGD is not a form of prescribing.[17,p.6]

Guidance on the use of PGDs is contained within Health Service Circular (HSC) 2000/026.

---

 Go to the website to find the PowerPoint presentation for this chapter and MCQs to test your knowledge. **www.hodderplus.com/childnursingskills**

---

# REFERENCES

1  European Parliament and Council (2001) *Directive 2001/83/EC on the Community code relating to medicinal products for human use*. 6 November Brussels
2  Medicines Act (1968) Co 67. London: HMSO.
3  Medicines and Health Care Regulatory Agency (2008) *Marketing authorisation*. www.mhra.gov.uk/accessed (accessed 3 May 2008).
4  Paediatric Formularies Committee (2007) *BNF for children*. London: British Medical Association, the Royal Pharmaceutical Society of Great Britain, the Royal College of Paediatrics and Child Health, and the Neonatal and Paediatric Pharmacists Group.
5  Department of Health (2001) *Medicines management*. London: HMSO
6  Leape L (2002) Reporting of adverse events. *New England Journal of Medicine* **347**: 1633–1638.
7  Cohen MR (2000) Why error reporting systems should be voluntary (Editorial). *British Medical Journal* **320**: 728–729.
8  National Patient Safety Agency (2007) *Safety in doses: improving the use of Medicines in the NHS*. London; NPSA.
9  Nursing and Midwifery Council (NMC) (2008/2009) *Standards for medicines management*. London: NMC www.nmc-uk.org/

aArticle.aspx?ArticleID=2995 (Accessed 26 February 2009).
10  National Institute for Health and Clinical Excellence (NICE) (2009) Medicines adherence. Clinical guideline CG76 www.nice.org.uk/Guidance/CG76.
11  Misuse of Drugs Act (1971) London: HMSO.
12  National Institute for Health and Clinical Excellence (NICE) (2007) *Patient safety guidance*. PSG001 technical patient safety solutions for medicines reconciliation on admission of adults to hospital: Guidance. www.nice.org.uk/guidance/index.jsp?action= download&o=38560 (accessed 25 February 2009).
13  Department for Education and Science (2005) *Managing medicines in schools and early years settings*. DFES-1448- London: DfES.
14  Hall C (2002) *An evaluation of nurse preparation and practice in administering medicine to children*. PhD thesis. The University of Nottingham School of Education, Nottingham.
15  Trigg E, Mohammed T (2006) *Practices in children's nursing: guidelines for hospital and community*. Edinburgh: Churchill Livingstone.
16  Hall C, Jones C (2007) Controlled drug administration. In: Glasper A, McEwing G,

Richardson J (2007) *Oxford handbook of children's and young peoples nursing.* Oxford: Oxford University Press.

17  National Prescribing Centre (2004) *Patient group directions: a practical guide and framework of competencies for all professionals using patient group directions: Incorporating an overview of existing mechanisms for the supply and prescribing of medicines.* London: NPC. www.npc.co.uk/pdf/pgd.pdf (accessed 26 February 2009).

18  Department of Health (2008) *The non-medical prescribing programme: Whats new?* London: DH www.dh.gov.uk/en/Healthcare/ Medicinespharmacyandindustry/Prescriptions/ TheNon-MedicalPrescribingProgramme/ Supplementaryprescribing/index (accessed 25 February 2009).

20  Hall C (2009) Medicines. In: Mallik M, Hall C, Howard D (2009) *Nursing knowledge and practice: foundations for decision making,* 3rd edition. Edinburgh: Elsevier, Chapter 10.

21  Dougherty L, Lister S (2007) *The Royal Marsden manual of clinical nursing procedures,* 7th edition. Oxford: Blackwell Publishing.

22  European Economic Community (1992) Council Directive 92/27/EEC of 31 March 1992 on the labelling of medicinal products for human use and on package leaflets. *Official Journal* L 113, 30/04/1992 pp. 0008–0012.

## FURTHER READING

Health Act (2006) *Part 3 drugs, medicines and pharmacies: supervision of management and use of controlled drugs.* London: The Stationery Office, Chapter 1, www.opsi.gov.uk (accessed 26 February 2009).

Medicines and Health Care Regulatory Agency (2004) cited by Nursing and Midwifery Council (2008b) *Standards for Medicines Management* (revised edition 09/01/09) London: NMC.

## USEFUL WEBSITES

www.cancerbackup.org.uk
www.bnfc.org.uk

# Undertaking emergency life support

Jan Heath

## LEARNING OUTCOMES

*Upon completion of this chapter, the reader should be able to accomplish the following:*

1 Have an understanding of the principles of resuscitation
2 Recognise the need for basic and advanced life support
3 Be familiar with the ABCD approach to resuscitation
4 Understand the use of a defibrillator
5 Be able to identify between shockable and non-shockable rhythms
6 Consider where to gain access to practical resuscitation training and practice on mannequins under the guidance of an experienced trainer

## BASIC PRINCIPLES

Major organs, the brain, heart, liver and kidney, require a good blood supply to deliver oxygen. When this is interrupted the risk of major organ failure is high.

As directed by the Resuscitation Council use the following format for basic life support (BLS), which is fundamentally the same for all victims with slight variations according to age.

Infant: birth to 1 year
Child: 1 year to puberty
Adult: young adult to senior citizen.

In order to reduce this risk BLS must be performed when cardiopulmonary arrest occurs.

## Definition

**Cardiac arrest** is an emergency situation that with prompt and effective treatment may reverse the situation where breathing and circulation has stopped.

A cardiac arrest occurs where there is no cardiac output and breathing has stopped.

A **respiratory arrest** occurs where the heart is still beating but breathing has stopped.

## WHY DO CHILDREN COLLAPSE?

Children collapse for a number of reasons including the following:

- trauma
- drowning
- congenital abnormalities
- respiratory disease
- anaphylaxis
- infections.

Primary cardiac events are rare in children but a major cause of collapse for adults.

## PREVENTION OF COLLAPSE

Adults are more likely to have a cardiac arrest from coronary artery disease, which is referred to as a primary cardiac arrest.

Children and infants rarely have a cardiac arrest as a primary event but rather as a catastrophe following other events, such as respiratory distress or trauma, or as respiratory and/or circulatory failure with the progression of an illness such as meningitis.

Early intervention is the key to preventing cardiac arrest occurring and reduce major organ failure, which can also lead to a cardiac arrest.

The outcome from cardiopulmonary arrest in paediatrics is poor. Early recognition and treatment of very poorly children is essential to avoid cardiac arrest.[1]

## EXAMPLES OF APPLICATIONS TO REDUCE THE RISK OF CARDIAC ARREST

- Prevention of accidents
  - Road safety schemes
  - Playground safety
  - Fire safety
  - Safe storage of harmful substances
- Reduce the effects of accidents
  - Promotion of cycle helmets
  - Guidance to use fireworks with care
- Education in the management of injury
  - First aid training for babysitters/child carers
  - Paediatric life support courses (EPLS/APLS)

Different age groups are at different risks hence need appropriate intervention.

## PRINCIPLES OF RESUSCITATION

Dealing with seriously ill children is difficult and can be very frightening. Using a systematic approach provides key points to remember. Throughout this chapter the ABCD approach will be applied:

A = airway
B = breathing
C = circulation
D = disability.

Early intervention in a child who appears very unwell is vital.

The Resuscitation Council Guidelines[2] aim to be as simple as possible. Many people who have no experience in resuscitating children worry about causing harm, but doing nothing to a collapsed child is very harmful.

The guidelines released in 2005 therefore address the potential of applying the same guidelines to children as to adults.

Doing something certainly improves the chance of survival; therefore, for the lay person the ratio for compressions in paediatrics is the same as that for adults, i.e. a ratio of 30 compressions to two ventilations.[3]

For those rescuers with a duty to respond, including healthcare staff,[3] the ratio should be 15 compressions to two ventilations.

The management of a collapsed child should include basic life support when a cardiac arrest has occurred until more help has arrived, whereby advanced life support should be provided. This requires recognition of the cause of the collapse where known, and identification of the cardiac arrhythmia to enable the treatment algorithm to be applied. The cardiac arrest rhythms must be recognised: these may be:

- shockable: ventricular fibrillation (VF)/pulseless ventricular tachycardia (VT);
- non-shockable: pulseless electrical activity (PEA)/asystole.

The management of these will be covered later.

## BASIC LIFE SUPPORT (BLS)

This is not difficult; it consists of a few key facts, which must be followed in a systematic way.

Resuscitation Council Guidelines are set by a recognised respected organisation, supporting evidence from practice.[3]

These guidelines should be practised and rehearsed using appropriate training manikins under the supervision of an experienced life support trainer to help you feel comfortable in delivering these psychomotor skills:

- danger
- response: assessment
- help
- airway
- breathing
- CPR.

## Check for danger

- Ensure you are safe before approaching the casualty.
- Make sure you are safe from hazards from, for example, fire, water, and electricity.
- In hospital, consider any hazards such as needlestick injury; are there any sharps on the bed?
- Will you hurt your back trying to move a collapsed child on your own?
- Treat all body fluids as potential dangers and put on gloves to minimise risk of infection.
- When approaching look for any clues that may suggest why this child has collapsed as they may dictate the way the emergency is managed, e.g. empty bottles of hazardous substances? Is there any suspicion of trauma?

## Assessment

Consider the following.

- Is it safe for you to go near the victim?
- What is the problem?
- Is the victim conscious?
- Is the victim able to maintain his or her own airway and breathing?
- Is the victim unconscious?
- Is the victim unable to maintain his or her own airway?
- Is the victim breathing?
- Do you have any help?

Addressing these questions in a logical manner will dictate the management of the event.

If you are alone with a paediatric collapse provide 1 minute of BLS before going for help.

## How to summon help

Out of hospital use the emergency services number 999 or 112.

In hospital use the universal 2222 number, stating where the emergency is and that a paediatric cardiac arrest team is required.[4]

If you are alone call for someone to help you. Do not leave the child to go for help or to use a phone. If not alone ask someone to phone for the emergency medical services (EMS): tell them to give the following information:

- precise location;
- type of emergency e.g. baby unable to be roused in cot, road traffic accident;
- how many victims and estimated age;
- severity of the incident, e.g. bleeding.

## PROCEDURE: Basic life support: initial steps

| Procedural steps | Evidence-based rationale |
| --- | --- |
| **1** *Danger*<br>Is it safe to approach?<br>Look for any signs of what may have led to the emergency | Do not put yourself or other rescuers in danger. For example, if the child is highly infectious apply gloves, gown and mask<br>Are there any signs of trauma or blood loss for example? |
| **2** *Response*<br>Assess by talking and touching the child<br>Assess by putting a hand on the child's forehead and squeeze their arm gently while calling their name; ask 'Are you alright' | The child may look unconscious but may be roused by disturbing him<br>Never shake a child to stimulate as this may cause injury |

| PROCEDURE:  Basic life support: initial steps (continued) |
|---|

| | |
|---|---|
| **3** Note time of collapse<br>Call for help<br>If more than one person present, send someone<br>to get help, ask them to come back to you once<br>they have called for help<br>In hospital call 2222<br>Out of hospital call 999/112<br>State location of the emergency and in hospital<br>that a paediatric team is required in the community<br>Gve a summary of the emergency | Early interventions will improve outcome<br><br>A specialist cardiac arrest team will be required<br>to help<br>Additional assistance is required and transfer to a<br>hospital is essential even if the child responds to BLS<br>Essential that the responding team know where to go<br>and what they will be attending |

## Airway

Open the airway.

The aim is to move the tongue away from the posterior pharyngeal wall.

### In the infant

Place the head in the neutral position with your fingertips on the bony part of the infant's jaw and lift the chin upwards, the other hand on the infant's forehead.

### In the child

You should only put a finger into the child's mouth if you can see or suspect there is something in their mouth, which you are confident you can remove with a single finger sweep.

To achieve the same manoeuvre the head and neck need to be tilted more (Figure 11.1).

If there is still difficulty in opening the airway, attempt the jaw thrust manoeuvre: place two fingers behind each side of the child's jaw bone and push the jaw forward (Figure 11.2).

Push your lower jaw forwards so that your bottom teeth are in front of your upper teeth is a good indicator of the position you are trying to replicate in the victim. This is of course more difficult in smaller children who do not as yet have full dentition (Figure 11.2)

Only when this step is complete should you proceed to Breathing.

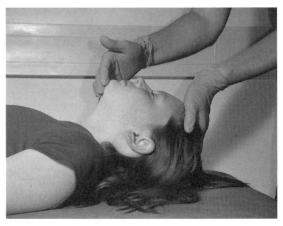

**Figure 11.1** Chin lift and head tilt.

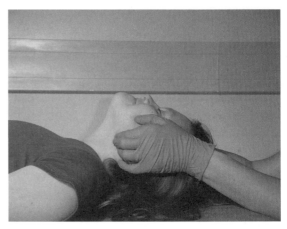

Figure **11.2** Jaw thrust.

## PROCEDURE: Basic life support steps

| Procedural steps | Evidence-based rationale |
| --- | --- |
| **1** Parents may be present; if so quickly explain simply what has occurred and why help is required | Without delaying progress it is important the parents are given information and support |
| **2** Airway: assess<br>Look in the mouth for any debris or foreign body.<br><br>Never perform a blind finger sweep, only remove what you can see or, if safe to do so, turn the head to the side to allow fluid to drain out | This may be done with the child in the position you found them in.<br>This may push the object back in to the airway. If there is a foreign body back blows or chest thrusts may be required |
| **3** Airway: opening<br>If there is no obstruction perform the head tilt/chin lift<br>Position: an infant's head should be in the neutral position<br>A child's head should be in the 'sniffing the morning air' position | To facilitate ventilation<br>This will lift the tongue from the posterior pharyngeal wall<br>This accommodates the larger occiput in the infant and avoids putting pressure on the trachea<br>Care must be taken to avoid pressure on the soft tissue under the chin to avoid occluding the airway |
| **4** Breathing: assess<br>Look at the chest<br>Listen for breath sounds<br><br><br>Feel for breath on your cheek or the back of your hand | Watch for chest movement reflecting air being taken in or indeed attempts made to breath out<br>No noise indicates no efforts to breathe but there may be noisy respirations, wheeze, grunting or stridor for example.<br>This may be helpful if it is dark or noisy and difficult to confirm respirations by looking or listening |

## Breathing

Is the victim breathing?

- Look: is the chest moving?
- Listen: can you hear any breath sounds from the child's mouth or nose?
- Feel: can you feel expired air from the victim on your cheek?

Do this assessment for no more than 10 seconds. If there is no breathing or only occasional ineffective gasps, deliver rescue breaths.
This may prevent respiratory arrest proceeding to cardiopulmonary arrest.

### Rescue breaths

Five initial breaths should be attempted; during these slow breaths any gag or cough response to your actions will contribute to your assessment of the victim.

If there is no equipment available, expired air respiration can be performed by applying your mouth to the victims mouth or mouth, and nose as appropriate. However, there are ranges of simple devices on the market that may be used if you know how to use them.

*Infants*
To deliver rescue breaths in infants, cover the mouth and nose where possible to create a seal to deliver expired air rescue breaths. The head should be in the neutral position; apply chin lift.

*Children*
To deliver rescue breaths in children, occlude the nose by pinching the nostrils and perform mouth-to-mouth, blow steadily into the victims mouth for 1–1.5 seconds, watching for chest movement.

If no chest movement is seen you must reposition the victim's head and repeat.

Give five initial rescue breaths before moving to circulation.

### Airway equipment

In hospitals there should be equipment for managing the airway:

- self-inflating bags
- pocket masks
- Guedal airways.

## PROCEDURE: Rescue breaths

| Procedural steps | Evidence-based rationale |
| --- | --- |
| **1** If there is breathing, turn the victim into the recovery position | The recovery position helps maintain a clear airway for an unconscious victim |
| **2** Breathing: if no spontaneous respiration<br>Deliver five rescue breaths<br>In the absence of any equipment, mouth-to-mouth is required<br>A pocket mask may be used | To provide oxygenation<br>Apply your mouth over the infant's mouth and nose<br>Apply your mouth over the child's mouth and pinch the nose<br>Deliver enough breath to make the chest wall move |
| A bag–valve–mask device may be used, preferably attached to oxygen | This will deliver a greater concentration of oxygen and should always be available in hospital. Added oxygen will improve oxygenation to the tissues. Room air only contains 21 per cent oxygen<br>Training is required before attempting to use such a device |

### Self-inflating bags

Most commonly used are self-inflating bags (Figure 11.3). The principle of using these is basic. While pressure is applied to the bag by the rescuer's hand, air moves past the one-way valve to the mask and into the victim's patent airway. When this pressure is relieved, the elasticity of the bag allows it to be automatically refilled as air enters through another entry from the reservoir. As this occurs the first valve closes to prevent rebreathing. These bags have an additional oxygen port to enrich the air supply and a reservoir that will facilitate a higher oxygen concentration.

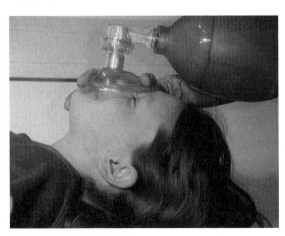

**Figure 11.3** Self-inflating bag.

The bags used for children should have a pressure-limiting valve to prevent over inflation of the lungs.

Training should be obtained before using these devices in practice.

When a child has been unable to breath for whatever reason, it is important to be able to deliver as much oxygen as possible.

Consider the following:

- room air contains 21 per cent oxygen;
- expired air contains approximately 16 per cent oxygen.

Hence using a bag mask device with no added oxygen, only 21 per cent oxygen will be delivered as room air.

Once there is access to a source of oxygen it should be used. Small oxygen cylinders may have a flow of only 4 L of oxygen per minute available, and as such will deliver a lower percentage oxygen to the victim than piped oxygen from the wall flow meters, where up to 10–15 L can be delivered; this can deliver over 85 per cent oxygen to the patient, depending on which device is used.

Wherever possible a bag–mask–valve system should be used with an oxygen reservoir bag and high-flow oxygen supply.

The efficiency of the system is assessed by witnessing chest wall movement.

If despite repositioning you are still unable to move the chest the potential for there to be a foreign body airway obstruction must be considered and dealt with. See foreign body airway obstruction, page 181 (FBAO).

Remember, the equipment is only as good as the individual using it. If you do not use these devices on a regular basis you must attend training sessions to reinforce your skills.

*Guedal airways*

These devices may be used to help maintain a clear airway.

The size varies for different-sized children. A useful way to measure a Guedal airway is to place the flange at the middle of the lips; across the side of the child's face the end of the airway should lie adjacent to the angle of the jaw (Figure 11.4a). The airway is inserted by opening the child's mouth and sliding the airway over the tongue in the position it is required to lie (Figure 11.4b).

## Circulation

Assess for signs of life. Take no more than 10 seconds to assess for any movement, swallowing, coughing or normal breathing, not gasps.

Assess for a pulse if you are trained to do so, remember even experienced individuals find this is can be very difficult.

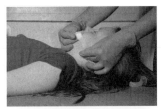
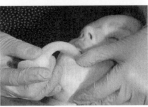

Figure **11.4 (a, b)** Sizing and inserting a Guedal airway.

*Infants:* Feel for a brachial pulse inside the inner aspect of the upper arm.

*Children:* Feel for the carotid pulse in the neck.

If there is no pulse, proceed to manage circulation with chest compressions.

If there is a pulse continue with rescue breaths only, one every 3 seconds.

If the victim is breathing but unconscious, put into the recovery position.

If there is no circulation as suggested by colour, a lifeless appearance, no pulse or a slow pulse with poor perfusion or you are really unsure, start chest compressions with rescue breathing.

## PROCEDURE: Chest compressions

| Procedural steps | Evidence-based rationale |
|---|---|
| 1 *Circulation* <br> Assess for colour, signs of life. If there are signs of life, e.g. swallowing or gasping, support respirations only at a rate of 1 breath every 3 seconds <br> If there are no signs of life, start chest compressions | To maintain oxygenation <br><br><br><br> *Infants:* compress the sternum by approximately one third of the depth using the tips of two fingers on the lower third of the sternum <br> *Children:* locate the landmarks by positioning yourself above the child's chest; compress the chest by one-third of the depth using the heel of one hand in smaller children and possibly two hands in larger children |

## Infants

Compress the sternum by approximately one-third of the depth using the tips of two fingers on the lower third of the sternum. This is good for the single rescuer. For a two-person rescue the chest compression technique may be better using the encircling technique, whereby the person doing chest compressions places both thumbs flat, side by side on the lower third of the sternum with the thumb tips pointing towards the infants head, spread the rest of both hands, fingers together to encircle the lower part of the infants rib cage, press down with the thumbs depressing the chest, again one-third of the depth of the infant's chest.

## Children

Locate the landmarks by positioning yourself above the child's chest, compress the chest by one-third of the depth using the heel of one hand in smaller children and possibly two hands in larger children (Figure 11.5)

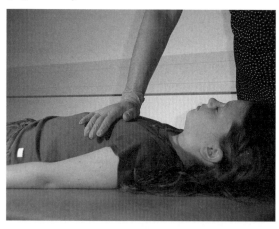

Figure **11.5** External chest compression on a child.

The aim is to deliver 100 compressions over 1 minute, but this is interrupted by ventilations every 15 compressions.

Remember the ratio 15 compressions to two breaths (Figure 11.6).

## Recovery position

For the unconscious child breathing unaided, the recovery position is used to reduce the risk of aspiration of vomit or secretions. This also prevents the tongue falling back to a position that could obstruct the airway, as shown in Figures 11.7a–c, page 175.

**Paediatric Basic Life Support (Healthcare professionals with a duty to respond)**

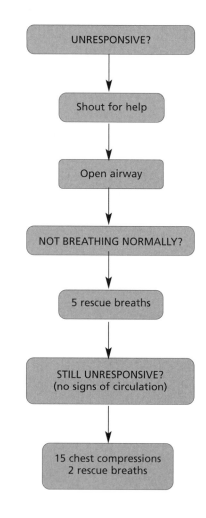

After 1 minute call resuscitation team then continue CPR

Figure **11.6** Basic life support algorithm (reproduced with permission from Resuscitation Council UK).

If there is a risk of cervical spine trauma then the recovery position should not be used.

## ADVANCED LIFE SUPPORT

Please see the website for information on cardiac monitoring.

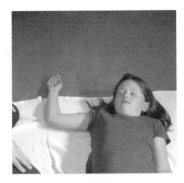

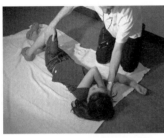

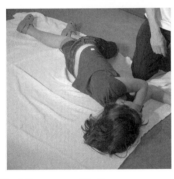

Figure **11.7 (a–c)** Recovery positions.

## Cardiac arrest rhythms

Children are most likely to collapse because they become hypoxic from respiratory problems, circulatory failure or metabolic disturbances. The heart becomes short of oxygen and slows down: bradycardia. If the rate becomes too slow to maintain adequate tissue oxygenation cardiac arrest is possible. Hence by treating the hypoxia early, cardiac arrest may be prevented.

In the event of cardiac arrest, the rhythms to treat are:

- shockable: VF/pulseless (VT);
- non-shockable: PEA/asystole.

### *Ventricular fibrillation (VF)*

This is abnormal chaotic waveform, where the ventricle is unable to contract properly and does not eject blood from the ventricle through the carotid arteries. Pulses will not be palpable.

The incidence in children is small, less than 20 per cent.[5]

### *Pulseless ventricular tachycardia (VT)*

This is uncommon in children. It is a wide QRS complex with a rate in excess of 120 with no palpable pulse. It should be treated the same as VF.

## Causes of cardiopulmonary arrest

There are many complex medical conditions that may cause children to collapse.

A helpful aide-memoire is to consider the four Hs and four Ts for eliminating the potential cause of collapse:

- hypoxia
- hypovolaemia
- hypothermia
- hypo/hyperkalaemia
- tension pneumothorax
- thromboembolism
- toxicity
- tamponade.

Many cardiac arrests may seemingly be due to a number of these causes in which case all should be addressed and treatment delivered as necessary.

### *Hypoxia*

This is lack of oxygen preventing healthy cell metabolism.

Every patient who has a cardiac arrest will be hypoxic. Consider if difficulty in breathing prior to the event has contributed to the event, e.g. pneumonia, cystic fibrosis or neuromuscular disorders, making respiration inadequate.

Treat by managing the airway and delivering as high a concentration of oxygen as possible.

### *Hypovolaemia*

This is lack of circulating fluid. There may be obvious blood loss from trauma or surgery. Fluid loss may also be due to burns, severe diarrhoea and vomiting or by redistribution of shock because of sepsis.

Treat by inserting large-bore intravenous cannulae or intraosseous cannulae and infusing replacement fluid. It may be necessary for surgical intervention as a matter of urgency.

### Hypothermia

Temperatures measured centrally which are less than 30°C will have a significant effect on cell metabolism and alter the pH of the blood, which will cause severe cell death. Such severe temperature drops may occur in extreme weather conditions, and in cases of near drowning, even in seemingly warm water conditions.

Treat by active warming procedures such as covering the victim's head, infusing warm intravenous fluids, instillation of warm fluid into body cavities, such as the bladder and abdomen.

### Hypo/hyperkalaemia

Potassium is vital in nerve and muscle excitation, which is essential for the electrical conduction of impulses in the cardiac cycle and muscle contraction of the heart's chambers.

A severe rise or fall of potassium levels can cause major problems.

Normal potassium levels are 3.5–5.5 mmol/L. Problems with potassium levels may occur during severe fluid loss, as may occur with gastrointestinal problems, and in patients who cannot excrete potassium correctly, as is possible with renal failure.

### Tension pneumothorax

The sudden collapse of a lung usually under pressure will change the pressure within the thoracic cavity and can compromise cardiac output as the heart struggles to pump against the pressure. This may occur as a result of acute lung injury and during mechanical ventilation of the newborn. Patients with underlying lung pathology are more vulnerable to such events.

Treatment is by assessing which side of the chest is affected: there is diminished chest movement on the side of the tension pneumothorax. A cannula is then inserted by an experienced practitioner into the second intracostal space in the midclavicular line. Air will be heard to hiss out through the cannula and the lung should reinflate. A definitive drain should be inserted into the affected side as soon as possible.

### Thromboembolism

Blood clots in coronary arteries are the most common cause of cardiac arrest in adults. This is very rare in children but the presence of pulmonary embolism can result in cardiac arrest. Within this category is also the obstruction of the airway by an inhaled foreign body.

Treatment of embolism is complex, but an embolism should be suspected after prolonged bed rest or long-bone fractures.

Management of inhaled foreign bodies is covered in this chapter (page 181).

### Toxicity

To result in cardiac arrest the heart or central nervous system will have been affected by a substance, which produces devastating effects. The causative substance must be identified and if possible the antidote given. For example, giving narloxone can reverse opiates. However, supportive measures such as giving artificial respiration must be provided to treat the patient while antidotes are given.

Anaphylaxis is a cause of collapse within this category, specific management of which is covered elsewhere in this chapter (page 183).

### Tamponade

A collection of blood or fluid in the pericardial sac can reduce the ability of the heart to eject blood from the ventricles. The most common cause for this is blunt chest trauma after a fall, but it can also occur after cardiac surgery.

Treatment is by aspirating the excess fluid blood from the pericardial space.

## Management of a cardiac arrest

The Resuscitation Council produces clear, concise guidelines and it is this guidance that is followed here.[3]

The treatment algorithms are designed to be easy to follow; each step should be followed assuming the preceding steps have been completed (Figure 11.8, page 178).

### Treatment of non-shockable rhythms

CPR and adrenaline (epinephrine) are key treatments in cardiac arrests where electrical complexes are present without a palpable pulse or if there is no electrical activity and no pulse.

- Perform CPR 15 compressions to two breaths.
- Give adrenalin (epinephrine) 1:10 000 solution

## PROCEDURE: Assessing cardiac arrest

| Procedural steps | Evidence-based rationale |
|---|---|
| **1** Four Hs<br>Hypoxia<br><br>Hypovolaemia<br><br>Hypothermia<br>Hypo/hyperkalaemia | <br>Maximise oxygenation and ventilation Treat respiratory dysfunction<br>Assess what fluid loss is the cause of collapse. Replace fluid and treat cause<br>Measure temperature and actively warm.<br>Get access to recent blood results and correct the metabolic disturbance |
| **2** Four Ts<br>Toxicity<br>Tamponade<br><br><br>Tension pneumothorax<br><br>Thromboembolic | <br>Know the toxic event and treat<br>Assess the chest for signs of and assist a clinician who is competent to drain the collection of fluid in the pericardial space<br>Assess the chest for air entry, assist a clinical to decompress the chest if necessary<br>Rare: consider specific treatment for the embolic episode. |
| **3** Cannulation<br>Insertion of a cannula using an aseptic technique During advanced life support adrenaline (epinephrine) is required for which an intravenous cannula is required<br><br>If a cannula cannot be inserted within 90 seconds an intraosseous cannula should be inserted | This is an invasive procedure and local and systemic infections should be avoided<br>adrenaline (epinephrine) supports circulation by vasoconstriction ofperipheral vessels and vasodilation of central vessels<br>Intraosseous cannulation is usually performed in the anteromedial surface of the tibia in children under 6 years<br>Over 6 years the medial aspect of the tibia |

10 µg/kg as soon as intravenous access is established.

- After 2 minutes of CPR check the monitor; if unchanged continue with CPR.
- Give adrenaline (epinephrine) every 3–5 minutes.
- Consider the four Hs and four Ts as potentially reversible causes.
- In addition, check the patient's glucose and electrolytes, and correct if abnormal.

### Treatment of shockable rhythms

Defibrillation is the key factor in giving the victim any chance of survival.

- Deliver a shock at 4 J/kg as soon as a defibrillator is present with a trained operator.
- Immediately after delivering the shock, recommence CPR without checking for a pulse.
- After 2 minutes check the rhythm; if still a

shockable rhythm, deliver another shock at 4 J/kg followed by a further 2 minutes of CPR.

- After 2 minutes check the monitor; if there is no change give adrenaline (epinephrine) at 10 µg/kg IV/IO (intravenous/intraosseous) and deliver the third shock at 4 J/kg. The CPR delivered after this shock will circulate the drug.
- Continue CPR for a further 2 minutes.
- If VF/VT persists administer amiodarone 5 mg/kg as a bolus intravenously before the fourth shock.
- Continuation of this treatment is required if the child does not respond to treatment with shocks at 4 J/kg followed by 2 minutes of CPR and adrenaline (epinephrine) administered at alternate cycles.
- Pulse checks are not recommended unless signs of life occur, which may suggest a return of a spontaneous circulation.

## Paediatric Advanced Life Support

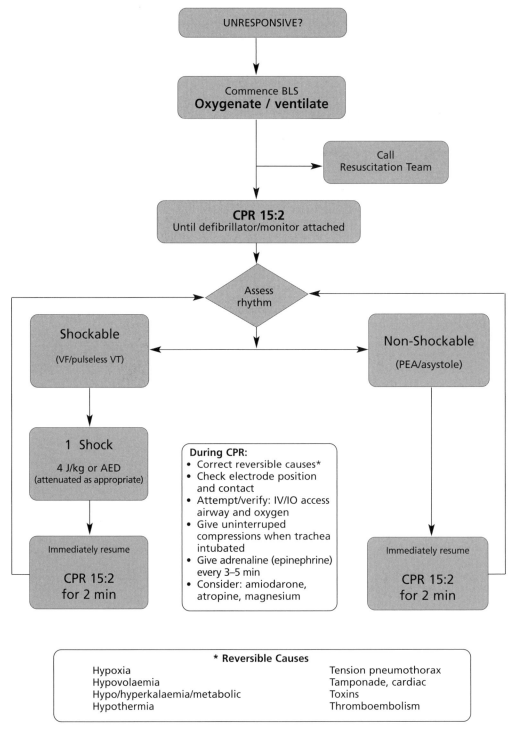

Figure **11.8** Advanced life support (ALS) treatment algorithm (reproduced with permission from Resuscitation Council UK).

### Defibrillation

Defibrillation is a skill, which must be acquired, and competence assessed before using in practice. This skill should be refreshed regularly as it is rarely required in children since the incidence of shockable cardiac arrest rhythms is small.

Defibrillation if the key treatment for patients in VF.

Defibrillation causes a simultaneous depolarisation of the myocardium that basically stops the electrical activity of the heart and aims to allow the normal conduction system to start again. This is done by applying pads or paddles on to the chest and discharging an electrical current across the chest.

## PROCEDURE: Cardiac arrest managements

| Procedural steps | Evidence-based rationale |
|---|---|
| **1** Cardiac arrest management<br>Rhythm recognition<br>Attach an ECG monitor to the patient | Required to define treatment progression |
| **2** Shockable rhythm: VF or pulseless VT<br>Treat with defibrillation as soon as possible, continue with BLS until defibrillation is possible<br>Deliver BLS between shocks<br>Safe use of defibrillator | VF or pulseless VT are only terminated by delivery of an electric shock using a defibrillator<br>Potential hazards to the victim or staff if not used by individuals trained in the use of a defibrillator |
| **3** Non-shockable rhythm: pulseless electrical activity (PEA) | Ensure BLS is in progress<br>Cause of collapse is required to assist with appropriate treatment |

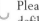

Please see the website for information on defibrillators

### Position of pads/paddles

When applying pads or paddles on the chest, one should be just below the right clavicle and the other in the left anterior axillary line.

Paddles are held in the hands of the operator and require defibrillation gel pads placed on to the chest first to provide a better conduction of electricity into the chest and a reduction in the damage to the skin.

Small gel pads are not produced, so adult-sized gel pads need to be cut to size.

Self-adhesive pads may be used that stick to the patient's chest. These pads are connected to the defibrillator and are operated from the machine; these are known as hands-free pads.

### Pad/paddle size

There are appropriate pads for children, which should be 8–12 cm in size, and 4.5 cm for infants.

The chest should be dry, free from dressings and pacing wires.

It is important that the gel pads together with the paddles placed on top or the self-adhesive pads do not touch when on the chest as this will cause arching of the energy when discharged from the defibrillator.

### Automated external defibrillation

These units analyse the patient's rhythm and direct treatment using spoken prompts.[6]

There are insufficient data regarding the use of automated external defibrillation (AED) units in infants, thus manual defibrillators should be accessible for infants less than 12 months old.

### Energy levels

For manual defibrillators each shock should be calculated as 4 J/kg.

AED units, which are designed to recognise paediatric shockable rhythms and should be used for children aged 1–8 years, deliver a paediatric attenuated energy level which is approximately 50–75 J.

For AED units for a child over 8 years use the adult shock energy.

*Safety*

Everyone attending a cardiac arrest must be aware of the potential hazards of defibrillation.

This is particularly important in paediatrics where such an intervention is not a common practice and more people will be less familiar with the procedure.

The following aspects must be considered.

- *Dry surfaces:* the victim' chest skin must be dry.
- *Metal:* the defibrillator pads should not be placed over metal, such as pacing wires, transdermal medication or jewellery.
- *People:* when delivering the shock no one should be touching the bed, the patient, intravenous fluids or breathing circuits.
- *Oxygen:* remove all free-flowing oxygen devices, such as a mask or ventilation bags using a mask, and place at least 1 metre away from the patient. Ventilators and ventilation bags may be left connected if it is a closed circuit.

*To perform defibrillation using an AED*

1 Confirm cardiac arrest.
2 Begin CPR.
3 Turn on defibrillator and apply appropriate sized pads to patient's bare chest.
4 Press the analyse button and stop CPR.
5 If a shock is advised look all around to ensure that no one is touching the patient or bed.
6 Press the charge button.
7 Tell everyone to stand clear.
8 Press the shock button and deliver the shock.
9 Recommence CPR for 2 minutes.
10 Continue as directed by the ALS shockable rhythm algorithm.
10 If no shock is advised by the AED recommence CPR and continue as directed by the AED.

*To perform defibrillation using a manual defibrillator*

1 Confirm cardiac arrest.
2 Begin CPR.
3 Turn on the defibrillator and attach self-adhesive pads, or apply paddles or attach 3-lead ECG electrodes; pause CPR and assess the rhythm.

4 If a shockable rhythm VF or pulseless VT, select appropriate energy level (4 J/kg).
5 Another person should continue to carry out CPR.
6 When the energy has been selected tell, everyone to stand clear if using paddles and apply to the chest, placing the paddles on top of the gel pads.
7 Press the charge button on the paddles.
8 When the machine has charged to the required energy, press the buttons on both paddles to release the energy.
9 If using self-adhesive pads, ensure everyone is clear of the bed and press the charge button on the machine.
10 When charged to the correct energy, press both discharge buttons to deliver the shock.
11 Recommence CPR for 2 minutes.

## DRUG DELIVERY

Airway and breathing must be addressed initially during a paediatric cardiac arrest. Circulation should be managed with chest compressions in the absence of palpable pulses. Circulatory access may then be established. This is not easy with small children and infants with compromised circulation.

Peripheral venous access is necessary.

If you are unable to acquire peripheral veins to cannulate the intraosseous route may be an option. It is easier and quicker to establish than the central venous route, with all the positive attributes but less complications.[7]

Intraosseous cannulation is usually performed in the anteromedial surface of the tibia in children under 6 years; place the cannula about 3 cm below the tibial tuberosity to avoid the growth plate.

In children over 6 years, the medial aspect of the tibia is 3 cm above the medial malleolus.[8]

These are invasive procedures and should be performed using universal infection control and safety precautions, i.e. gloves, aseptic techniques and care of sharps. If all else fails and if an endotracheal tube is in situ some drugs may be given via the endotracheal tube. When this is used the dose should be 10 times that of the intravenous dose. However, if possible this route should be avoided as it can have a paradoxical effect.

## Drugs used in cardiac arrests

### Adrenaline (epinephrine)

This is the major drug used in cardiac arrests, although there have been no clinical trials in humans.

Adrenaline (epinephrine) causes vaso-constriction and increases the blood supply to the coronary arteries that helps cardiac performance. The dose for children in cardiac arrest in 10 µg/kg using 1:10 000 adrenaline (epinephrine) (1 mg/10 mL)

This should be given intravenously or via an intraosseous cannula.

Other drugs found on cardiac arrest trolleys have a less significant part to play. Please see the website for information on other drugs.

## FOREIGN BODY AIRWAY OBSTRUCTION

Choking in children is a frightening yet common occurrence. Children often put things in their mouths, such as sweets, pieces of toys, beads and pieces of food, while playing. Remember the anatomy of the upper airway; items that are in the nostril can be inhaled into the upper airway, which is shaped like a cone, and thus inhaled objects can become lodged in the larynx and cause the child to asphyxiate. Small children may put items into their nostrils, which can be a problem in itself but the situation may become worse if the item is then inhaled.

Simple yet effective methods can be used for such problems.

When dealing with an airway obstruction, the aim is to force air out of the lungs by sudden inward and upward movement, which in turn should push the obstruction out of the airway. This is the same principle as a powerful cough; however, the choking victim is unable to cough for him or herself.

If the child is coughing then encourage them to do so.

## Signs and symptoms of a foreign body airway obstruction

- Child otherwise well.
- Child witnessed eating or playing with objects likely to obstruct airways.
- Child suddenly silent or unable to breathe (Figure 11.9).

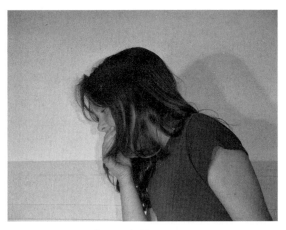

Figure **11.9** Child in distress choking.

### Infants

To provide intervention for a choking infant, their size is advantageous. The best position is to turn the infant face down supporting their chin with the fingers of your left hand; the body of your hand can then support their chest, with the baby's face down lower than their chest. Apply up to five firm back slaps between the shoulder blades. It may be easier to support the infant on your knee. If this does not solve the problem, turn the baby on to their back on a firm surface, which again may be your thigh; make sure the baby's head is lower than their chest and apply chest thrusts.

### Children

In small children, when giving backslaps (Figure 11.10, page 182) you may need to place them across your lap, then kneel behind them to give abdominal thrusts (Figure 11.11, page 182).

Do not attempt blind finger sweeps; this may push the object further down and cause injury.

In an infant, it is dangerous to give abdominal thrusts, use chests thrusts instead. These are performed in the same position as compressions but each thrust is sharper and more vigorous, as it aims to relieve the obstruction.

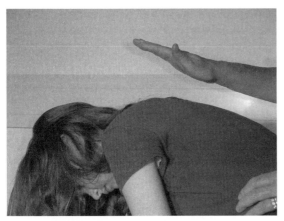

Figure **11.10** Back blows to a child.

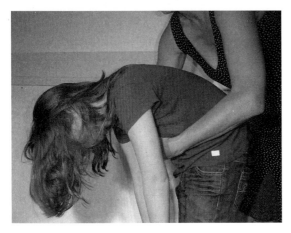

Figure **11.11** Abdominal thrusts to a child.

# EQUIPMENT USED WHEN ATTENDING SERIOUSLY ILL CHILDREN

Children vary enormously in size and as such there needs to be a range of sizes for some of the equipment used.

Age is not a great indicator to select which kit to use; weight is a better determinant. Alternatively, the useful formula to calculate weight as referred to earlier may be used.

Equipment should be the same on all trolleys and have a familiar layout. Staff should know how to use all equipment within the area they work. Equipment should be checked as per local policy but at least daily; when this check is made, any missing or faulty equipment should be dealt with at that time.

Suction and oxygen points should be fitted with the correct connections; if wall-mounted suction and oxygen is not accessible, then appropriate portable units should be provided.

Children rarely need to be defibrillated; however, a defibrillator should be available to attend all paediatric emergencies, particularly for the monitoring capacity of the units. Staff on a paediatric cardiac arrest team should be capable of using a defibrillator. Defibrillators used for paediatric emergencies should have the smaller paddles, which may be accessed under the adult paddles or may be added over the larger units. Find someone to show you how to do this; never change the paddles when the machine is turned on.

The ideal contents of a cardiac arrest trolley are listed in *Cardiopulmonary resuscitation: Standards for clinical practice and training* (see Further Reading, page 187):

## Case study

You are on duty in the emergency department when a call is received alerting the department that a 6-year-old has had a severe asthmatic attack at school.

The activity in preparing for the child arrival should include the following using the ABCD approach.

**Airway and breathing**
Prepare oxygen delivery kit, mask with rebreathe bag attached to oxygen with a flow meter capable of delivering high flow oxygen.

Bag mask device with oxygen attached and reservoir bag.

Intubation equipment with a straight blade laryngoscope, clean with light working, size 5, 5.5 and 6

Size of endotracheal tube is calculated by using the following formulae, age/4 + 4, i.e. 6/4 + 4 = 5.5

A tube size above and below should be prepared.

**Suction equipment**
Bougie
Tape to secure the tube and appropriate connections
**Circulation**
Cannulae to establish an IV line

Drugs as requested with a working knowledge of the potential weight of the child
$(6 \times 2) + 8 = 20$ kg
Or $(6 + 4) \times 2 = 20$ kg

Fluids may be prepared by calculating the required volume as 20 mL/kg
i.e. $20 \times 20$ mL = 400 mL

It is helpful to take a moment to think of a number of potential scenarios and practice doing the calculations for weight and endotracheal tube size; do not make life difficult and use years only rather than a child aged 4 years and 3 months!

Many parents do not know their child's weight, and certainly not in kilograms!

Remember the estimations of weight for those infants aged 1 year and less.

**Example of an application**
A 6-month-old is being brought in with a 3-day history of vomiting and diarrhoea
Consider the weight of the baby
Make a list of the equipment you might prepare and the drugs and fluid you may get ready
**Equipment**
Oxygen
Self-inflating bag
Cannulae and intraosseous needles
Intravenous infusion equipment
Blood specimen bottles
**Drugs**
Glucose
Adrenaline (epinephrine)
Crystalloid fluids
normal saline

# CARE OF THE CARER

Resuscitation of a child is emotive for families and staff caring for that child both in and out of hospital. It is important that after paediatric resuscitation, particularly any unsuccessful attempt, a debriefing session should be held.

## When not to resuscitate

Resuscitation is not always appropriate and for some children with life-limiting conditions it may be agreed that any attempt to resuscitate the child would not be beneficial.

This is never an easy subject and every case must be considered with great care. It should wherever possible involve the most senior clinicians available.

In hospital this decision activates a 'Do not attempt resuscitation' order (DNAR). This must involve the following considerations.

- Recognition that a cardiac arrest is a possible course of events; the DNAR order must be made before the event, with agreement between the medical staff looking after the patient, all other

members of the team looking after the patient and the family.
- Quality of the patient's life and expected prognosis.

The DNAR order must be communicated to all members of staff caring for the patient. It must be written in the patient's medical notes and must be dated and signed.

A DNAR order must be regularly reviewed and may be changed at any time that the patient's condition warrants such a decision.

## Parents

When a child is being resuscitated, provision should be made to consider the presence of relatives. Parents may wish to be there to see what efforts have been put into the resuscitation.[9]

An experienced member of staff must stay with them and keep them informed of progress and interventions. This person can also prevent the relatives disturbing the staff during this difficult time.

It has been shown that when parents have been present at resuscitation, they have fewer difficulties after the event. The person delegated to look after the relatives should not be the most inexperienced member of the team; they must be supportive and be able to ensure their presence does not affect the delivery of treatment required.[10]

It is the team leader who makes the decision to end the resuscitation not the parents. Clearly, this is a difficult role and must be done in a sensitive and empathic manner.

# ANAPHYLAXIS

Anaphylaxis is a rare but life-threatening reaction to an allergen.[11] There is not a conclusive definition for anaphylaxis but it should be considered when more than two systems are affected: skin, respiratory, circulatory and neurological or gastroenterological systems.

Other features are usually present:

- erythema
- generalised pruritis
- wheeze
- rhinitis
- conjunctivitis
- itching of palate/external auditory meatus
- nausea, vomiting, abdominal pain

- palpitations
- urticaria
- angio-oedema
- sense of impending doom.

## What happens during anaphylaxis?

An anaphylactic reaction occurs following exposure to an allergen to which a person has been sensitised. People who have asthma and allergies are at high risk of anaphylaxis.[11]

Repeated exposure results in specific immunoglobulin (Ig)E antibodies recognising the allergen and creating a reaction to it. This encourages mast cells to release inflammatory mediators that cause an anaphylactic reaction. It is the rapid release of large quantities of mediators that causes leakage of capillaries and mucosal oedema, causing cardiovascular and respiratory shock.

It may be due to a whole host of things, most commonly

- food, e.g. sea food, egg, peanuts, bananas
- drugs, e.g. antibiotics
- latex,
- stinging insects, e.g. wasps.

When dealing with patients presenting with difficulty breathing, severe rashes or circulatory problems following exposure to elements which may cause anaphylaxis, urgent action is required.

## How to treat

Act immediately. If out of hospital ask someone to dial 999.

Remove the item causing the event if possible, i.e. stop the antibiotics: it is too late if it is something that has been eaten. If it is due to an insect sting, immediately scrape away any insect parts at the site of the sting. Avoid squeezing.[12]

Put the victim in a position where they are able to breathe more easily if possible; the victim may feel very faint or look very pale. If so, lie the victim down.

Give 100 per cent oxygen if possible. An experienced anaesthetist is mandatory if the child is in hospital (Figure 11.12, page 185).

### Medication for anaphylaxis in children

Give adrenaline (epinephrine) to all children with signs of circulatory failure, airway swelling or difficulty with respirations associated with an anaphylactic reaction. Repeat adrenaline (epinephrine) after 5 minutes if there is no improvement.

For the dose of adrenaline (epinephrine) refer to Table 11.1. This must be given intramuscularly, unless you are experienced with titrating doses of IV adrenaline, and should be used only by experienced specialists.[13]

After the adrenaline (epinephrine), it may be appropriate to give an antihistamine (chlorphenamine).

If the patient does not respond to the adrenaline (epinephrine) it is advisable to give intravenous fluids. The fluid of choice is 20 mL/kg of crystalloid. Examples of crystalloids are Hartman's solution and normal saline (0.9 per cent).

For severe reactions or patients with asthma hydrocortisone may follow.

Antihistamine, fluids and hydrocortisone should be given only after adrenaline (epinephrine), which is a life-saving drug in anaphylaxis.

Adrenaline (epinephrine) is carried by a large number of the population, who should be capable of administering the drug themselves if in a situation where they find themselves unwittingly exposed to the toxin to which they are allergic to. There are a number of very helpful websites to support the use of patient-administered adrenaline (epinephrine).

## THE RESUSCITATION TEAM

Each organisation will have its own action plan to attend individuals who collapse.

There should be a team that responds to victims of cardiac arrest. The composition of the team will vary within different organisations but should have a minimum of two doctors trained to deal with such emergencies. The team should collectively have the skills to deal with:

- airway interventions
- routes for drug administration
- monitoring and defibrillation
- knowledge of drugs and fluids
- post-resuscitation management.

Ideally there should be a separate paediatric team with appropriately trained individuals.

Anaphylactic reaction?

Airway, Breathing, Circulation, Disability, Exposure

**Diagnosis** – look for:
- Acute onset of illness
- Life-threatening Airway and/or Breathing and/or Circulation problems[1]
- And usually skin changes

- **Call for help**
- Lie patient flat
- Raise patient's legs

Adrenaline (ephinephrine)[2]

**When skills and equipment available:**
- Establish airway
- High flow oxygen
- IV fluid challenge[3]        **Monitor:**
- Chlorphenamine[4]          - Pulse oximetry
- Hydrocortisone[5]          - ECG
                             - Blood pressure

[1]Life-threatening problems:
**Airway:**        swelling, hoarseness, stridor
**Breathing:**     rapid breathing, wheeze fatigue, cyanosis $SpO_2$ < 92%, confusion
**Circulation:**   pale, clammy, low blood pressure, faintness, drowsy/coma

[2]Adrenaline (*give IM unless experienced with IV adrenaline*)
IM doses of 1:1000 adrenaline (repeat after 5 min if no better)

- Adult:                      500 micrograms IM (0.5 mL)
- Child more than 12 years:   500 micrograms IM (0.5 mL)
- Child 6–12 years:           300 micrograms IM (0.3 mL)
- Child less than 6 years:    150 micrograms IM (0.15 mL)

Adrenaline IV to be given **only by experienced specialists**
Titrate: Adults 50 micrograms; Children 1 microgram/kg

[3]**IV fluid challenge:**

Adult – 500–1000 mL
Child – crystalloid 20 mL/kg

Stop IV colloid
if this might be the cause
of anaphylaxis

| | [4]Chlorphenamine (IM or slow IV) | [5]Hydrocortisone (IM or slow IV) |
|---|---|---|
| Adult or child more than 12 years | 10 mg | 200 mg |
| Child 6–12 years | 5 mg | 100 mg |
| Child 6 months to 6 years | 2.5 mg | 50 mg |
| Child less than 6 months | 250 micrograms/kg | 25 mg |

**Figure 11.12** Treatment for anaphylactic reactions (reproduced with permission from Resuscitation Council UK).

**Table 11.1** Dose for adrenaline (epinephrine)*

| Age (years) | Dose of IM adrenaline (1:1000) |
| --- | --- |
| <6 | 150 µg (0.15 mL) |
| 6–12 | 300 µg (0.3 mL) |
| >12 | 500 µg (0.5 mL) |

*Working Group of the Resuscitation Council (UK) January (2008) Emergency treatment of anaphylactic reactions.

## TRAINING IN PAEDIATRIC RESUSCITATION

Members of paediatric cardiac arrest teams should be encouraged to attend one of the national paediatric resuscitation courses; for example, the European Paediatric Life Support Course, Advanced Paediatric Life Support Course or the Newborn Life Support Course. Details of all of these are available from www.resus.org.uk or wwwalsg.org

## HAEMORRHAGE

In cases of severe bleeding
1. Manage of the wound.
2. Reassure.
3. Put on sterile gloves.
4. Assess the situation and call for help.
5. Reassure the conscious child.
6. Where is the blood coming from?
7. If the bleeding is from a limb raise and support the limb with caution – there might be a broken bone.
8. Apply with pressure a clean dressing pad to the wound and bandage the pad firmly to control the blood loss.
9. If the blood oozes through the first dressing do not remove, as this will disturb any coagulation but cover with a second dressing. However, if this second dressing becomes soaked with blood remove both dressings and start again with a new dressing.
10. Reassess the child throughout where possible.
11. Keep the child lying down and treat for shock.

 Go to the website to find the PowerPoint presentation for this chapter and MCQs to test your knowledge. **www.hodderplus.com/childnursingskills**

## REFERENCES

1 O'Rourke PP (1986) Outcome of children who are apneic and pulseless in the emergency room. *Critical Care Medicine* **14**: 466–47.
2 European Resuscitation Council (2005) *European Resuscitation Council guidelines for resuscitation 2005*. Resuscitation 67: (Suppl 1): S1–S190.
3 http://www.resus.org.uk/pages/teachPLS.htm.
4 National Patient Safety Agency Alert 2004.
5 Reis AG, Nadkarni V, Perondi MB, et al. (2002) A prospective investigation into the epidemiology of in hospital pediatric cardiopulmonary resuscitation using the international Utstein reporting style. *Pediatrics* **9**: 200–209.
6 Samson R, Berg R, Bingham R, et al. (2003) Use of automated external defibrillators for children: an update. An advisory statement from the Pediatric Advanced Life Support Task Force, International Liaison Committee on Resuscitation. *Resuscitation* **57**: 237–437.
7 Chiang VW, Baskin MN (2000) Uses and complications of central venous catheters inserted in a pediatric emergency department. *Pediatric Emergency Care* **16**: 230–232.
8 Boon JM, Gorry DLA, Miering JH (2003) Finding an ideal site for intraosseous infusion. Tibia: an anatomical study. *Clinical Anatomy* **16**: 15–18.
9 Beckman AW, Sloan BK, Moore GP, et al. (2002) Should parents be present during emergency department procedures on children, and who should make that decision? A survey of emergency

physicians and nurse attitudes. *Academic Emergency Medicine* 9: 154–158.

10 Meyers TA, Eichhorn DJ, Guzzetta CE, *et al.* (2001) Family presence during invasive procedures and resuscitation. *American Journal of Nursing* 100: 32–42.
11 Johannsen SG, Visscher SG, Bieber T, *et al.* (2004) Revised nomenclature for allergy for global use. Report of the Nomenclature Review Committee of the World Allergy Organization, October 2003. *Journal of Allergy and Clinical Immunology* 113: 832–836.
12 Visscher PK, Vetter RS, Camazine S (1996) Removing bee stings. *Lancet* 348: 301–302.
13 McLean-Tooke AP, Bethune CA, Fay AC, Spickett GP (2003) Adrenaline in the treatment of anaphylaxis: what is the evidence? *British Medical Journal* 327: 1332–1335.

## FURTHER READING

Working Group of the Resuscitation Council (UK) (2008) *Emergency treatment of anaphylactic reactions: guidelines for healthcare providers.* London: RCUK.
Royal College of Anaesthetists, Royal College of Physicians of London, Intensive Care Society, The Resuscitation Council. Joint Statement (October 2004, updated June 2008). Cardiopulmonary resuscitation. Standards for clinical practice and training. London: RCUK.
Resuscitation Council (UK) (2006) *European paediatric life support,* 2nd edition. London: RCUK.

## USEFUL WEBSITES

www.epipen.co.uk
www.bsaci.org
www.aagbi.org
www.allergyinschools.org.uk
www.npsa.nhs.uk

## GLOSSARY

ABCD: airway, breathing circulation, disability

AED: automated external defibrillation

Airway: the passage from the mouth and nose to the lungs

ALS: advanced life support

Anaphylaxis: the process, which leads to an anaphylactic reaction

Anaphylactic reaction: the condition that is the result of anaphylaxis

BLS: basic life support: delivery of expired air respiration and chest compressions with minimal equipment

CPR: cardiopulmonary resuscitation

Defibrillation: the delivery of an electric shock into the heart to stop the electrical dysfunction and allow the normal conduction system to recommence

ECG: electrocardiogram

FBAO: foreign body airway obstruction

IM: intramuscular

IO: intraosseous

IV: intravenous

Rescue breath: forcing air into a victims lungs enough to make the chest rise

Respiration: breathing

Ventricular fibrillation (VF): chaotic quivering movement of the muscle in the ventricle of the heart making the heart unable to pump blood out

Ventricular tachycardia (VT): a broad QRS complex regular rhythm greater than 120 beats per minute with and no obvious P waves. If the patient has no pulse with this rhythm it is called pulseless VT and treated as VF.

## CHAPTER 12

# Caring for personal hygiene needs

Joanna Himsworth

## LEARNING OUTCOMES

*Upon completion of this chapter, the reader should be able to accomplish the following:*

1 Understand when and how to 'top and tail' a neonate
2 Provide umbilical cord care
3 Change a nappy and incontinence pad
4 Know how to give a bed bath to a child and bathe an infant
5 Understand the principles and procedures for eye care
6 Understand oral hygiene and be able to assist with tooth brushing
7 Care for nails
8 Understand the fundamentals of skin assessment
9 Recognise the importance of maintaining appropriate records and documentation of personal hygiene procedures
10 Understand the importance of patient safety and know how to prevent cross-infection
11 Recognise the need to promote patient comfort at all times and self-care where possible

## Definitions

**Personal hygiene:** a physical act of cleaning the body to maintain the skin, nails and hair to be kept in optimum condition.[5]

## CHAPTER OVERVIEW

Infants, children and young people all have some similar basic personal hygiene requirements, but dependent on their age they each have their own extra needs. These needs are often the same at home as in hospital, but while in hospital personal hygiene needs often have an added importance.[1] The patient's and parents' ability to meet spersonal hygiene needs may change because of medical treatment and acute or chronic illness. Assisting patients to meet their own personal hygiene needs is a fundamental aspect of nursing care.[2] With current focus on infection prevention we must consider the importance of maintaining personal hygiene to help prevent hospital-acquired infections.[2]

There are many aspects of personal hygiene, such as washing, oral hygiene, hair washing, nail, nappy, eye and umbilical cord care and skin assessment. After *The NHS plan*[3] was launched, focusing on improving the patient experience, *The essence of care*[4] (these are not specific to paediatrics but adult focused, which we have adapted) was brought in to help practitioners enhance nursing practices, become patient focused and take a structured approach by identifying best practice and developing clear action plans to achieve these. Benchmarks were made identifying best care in certain areas, including continence, bladder and bowel control, personal and oral hygiene, privacy, dignity and principles of self-care.[5] These benchmarks are what should be achieved when providing personal care aiming to meet the hygiene needs of patients adequately.[5]

## SKIN HYGIENE

Infants under 28 days old (neonates) do not need a bath every day.[6] It is more than acceptable to 'top and tail', especially neonates who still have their umbilical cord attached[6] (see Cord Care, page 195). When you are bathing or top and tailing a neonate, it is always necessary to consider the environment surrounding the bathing area, as neonates are particularly susceptible to hypothermia.[7] It is important to shut windows and doors and make sure you have everything you will need to hand. The water should be between 32°C and 35°C, which, when you test it using the back of your hand or your elbow, should feel neither hot nor cold.[8] The DH recommend that only plain water is used on infants under 28 days old and that soap or bubble-bath is avoided.[6]

Standard precautions should be used when there is a risk of contact with bodily fluids. Personal protective equipment (PPE) such as disposable gloves and aprons should be worn and disposed of appropriately.

## Top and tailing

### Equipment

Gloves
Apron
Changing mat
Cotton wool or sponge
Water to fill the bowl (32–35°C)
Baby soap (to be used only on infants older that 28 days)
Bowl
Face cloth or gauze swabs (not sterile)
Two warm towels
Clean clothes
Nappy

## PROCEDURE: Top and tailing

| Procedural steps | Evidence-based rationale |
| --- | --- |
| **1** Wash hands before patient contact. Lay the infant on a changing mat and undress them, leaving the nappy on | Prepares the infant and gives opportunity to observe how the infant handles and looks |
| **2** Wrap the infant in a warm towel | Prevents the infant from becoming cold or uncomfortable |
| **3** Use a damp face cloth or gauze swabs to clean the infant's face, neck and head[9] | To maintain hygiene |
| **4** Use the spare warm towel to dry off the infants face, neck and head | Prevents the infant from becoming cold or uncomfortable |
| **5** Remove the towel and nappy. Using wet cotton-wool (under 28 days old) or wet-wipes (over 28 days) clean the nappy area | Opportunity to observe the nappy area for redness, specifically nappy rash and check the nappy to see if it is wet or if the infant has had their bowels open |
| **6** Put on a new nappy and dress the infant in appropriate clothes for the environment | Keeps the infant comfortable |
| **7** Place the infant somewhere safe, such as their cot | Maintains infant's safety. Never leave an infant on a changing mat on their own |
| **8** Discard the nappy and cotton-wool or wet wipe into a clinical waste bin[3] | Prevents cross-infection |
| **9** Discard the water and place the towels in the correct linen bin | Prevents cross-infection |
| **10** If it is disposable, discard the wash bowl. If not, wash out the wash bowl with hot water and detergent. Dry it and put it away | Prevents cross-infection |
| **11** Wash your hands[3] | Prevents cross-infection |
| **12** Maintain appropriate records[10] | Follows NMC guidelines[10] |

# BATHING

When not in hospital most people wash every day and unless their condition contradicts this there should be no reason why patients should not have either a wash, bath or shower daily. The DH[4] states that patients should all receive the level of assistance that is required to help them meet their individual hygiene needs.

The decision of whether a patient requires a wash ('top and tail'), shower or bath should be made with the patient, or if relevant the parents. Downey and Lloyd[2] suggest that the patient's age, mobility and ability to help should always be considered. The patient's level of independence can also afect which mode of washing is most suitable.[11] As well as the practical side you will need to consider the patient's culture and acknowledge the importance of maintaining their dignity and privacy, gaining consent and remembering the importance of verbal and non-verbal communication.[2]

If patients are likely to experience discomfort during the bed bath then it is important to recognise this, undertake a pain assessment and record findings, give analgesia as prescribed if necessary before you start and record the effectiveness. You should ask patients for their preferences of soaps, shampoo and other toiletries, and should always use their own if available.[4] It is important to have all the equipment needed ready before you start so that you do not need to leave your patient either alone and at risk or exposed unnecessary.[2] You can also use this time to assess the patient's skin integrity.

## Indications for a bed bath[12]

- Patient confined to bed for mobility reasons
- Patient too unwell/weak to attend to their own needs

## Indications for a bath or shower

- Patient mobile and physically able
- Patient/parent requests a bath/shower with assistance and it is safe to do so

## Equipment

Two members of staff or nurse and carer
Glide sheet and/or hoist (as needed)
Wash cloth or disposable wipes
Two wash bowls
Two towels
Shower tray for hair washing
Disposable jug
Toiletries (soap, tooth brush and toothpaste, shower gel, shampoo, conditioner and deodorant)
Brush/comb
Hair-dryer
Clean clothes
Clean linen
Laundry bin
PPE: disposable gloves and apron

## PROCEDURE: Bathing a patient

| Procedural steps | Evidence-based rationale |
| --- | --- |
| 1 Discuss patient's needs and preferences with them and negotiate what involvement they or their parents (if present) are going to have | Planning care allows you to gain their verbal consent[10] and to help promote their dignity |
| 2 Prepare the area by shutting the curtains and doors. Put notice on curtain (i.e. use peg) not to disturb unless urgent. Alert other members of staff of what you are doing so as to avoid unnecessary interruption | Promotes patient's dignity and privacy. Maintains a safe environment |
| 3 Consider and risk assess which manual handling techniques and equipment will be needed | To reduce risk to patient and staff |
| 4 Fill bowl with water and check temperature with patient. Wash hands before patient contact | To maintain patient's comfort |

## PROCEDURE: Bathing a patient (continued)

| | |
|---|---|
| 5 Wash and rinse face, neck and ears. Discuss if they use soap on their face. Dry using towel | To maintain patient's comfort and hygiene |
| 6 Undress the top half of patient and cover with dry towel, only exposing one part at a time. Using appropriate soap and wipes wash arms, axillary areas and torso. If the patient is unable to bathe, put on gloves and assist them. Rinse and dry, paying special attention to axillary areas to avoid becoming sore. Assist patient in applying deodorant as required | To maintain patient's dignity and comfort. To promote cleanliness |
| 7 Keep patient covered with sheet or dry towel. Change bowl and water | To maintain patient's dignity and comfort. To prevent cross-contamination |
| 8 Confirm with the patient that the area around their genitals is going to be washed and encourage them to do so. If they are unable, ensure you are wearing gloves, wash and dry the genital area. When washing females remember to wash from front to back. When washing uncircumcised young people remember to draw back the foreskin gently. Do not force the foreskin back or ever pull the foreskin back on infants and children.[6] Cover patient with dry towel or sheet | To maintain patients dignity. To gain consent.[10] To promote cleanliness |
| 9 Remove and discard gloves in clinical waste bin and wash hands. Change the water and bowl | To prevent cross-contamination |
| 10 The legs and feet should be washed and dried | To promote cleanliness |
| 11 Ask the patient to roll onto their side (if appropriate). If they are unable, use a glide sheet to assist them. Wash and dry the patient's back and use the slide sheet to roll them back again | To maintain patient's dignity and comfort. To maintain safe and correct manual handling |
| 12 If the patient wants their hair washed, ask them to move up the bed with their head at the top. To assist them you can tilt the bed down at the head by around 20–30°. If the patient is unable to move up the bed independently, make a risk assessment. If it is safe staff should roll the patient over and slide the glide sheet under and pull it though from the other side. Using the glide sheet, gently pull the patient up the bed. It may be useful to ask a third person to assist by standing at the top of the bed and support the patient's head | To maintain safe and correct manual handling |
| 13 Once the patient is at the top of the bed tilt the bed flat again. Place the patient's head on the hair tray. Fill thejug with warm water and check the temperature with the patient. Place a large bowl on the floor at the bottom of the tray. Covering their face with a towel (if required) slowly pour the water over the hair onto the tray. Wash hair withshampoo and rinse. You may need to empty the bowl on the floor into the sink. Condition hair and rinse again. Towel dry hair | To maintain patient comfort and hygiene |

## PROCEDURE:  Bathing a patient (continued)

| | |
|---|---|
| **14** While covering patient as much as possible, assist patient to dress themselves | To promote patient dignity and comfort |
| **15** Ask patient if they would like their hair blow dried or left to dry naturally. Brush hair and dry as requested | To promote patient comfort |
| **16** To change patient's sheets, gather up new bottom sheet in preparation. Ask patient (if possible) to roll to one side and push bed sheet up to patient. Align new sheet against the old and straighten. Then ask patient to roll over to the other side, warning them that there will be a lump in the middle of the bed. Remove the old sheet and pull the new sheet tight. Check the patient is comfortable | Sheets should be changed daily for patient's hygiene and comfort. If a patient is unable to help roll themselves, use a glide sheet and as many staff as needed |
| **17** Encourage patient to undertake own oral hygiene (see 'Oral hygiene', page 196) | To promote oral hygiene |
| **18** Discard the water and place the towels in the correct linen bin | To prevent cross-infection |
| **19** If disposable, discard the wash bowls. If not, wash out the wash bowl with hot water and detergent. Dry it and put it away | To prevent cross-infection |
| **20** Wash your hands[13] | To prevent cross-infection |
| **21** Maintain appropriate nursing records[10] | To follow NMC guidelines[10] |

## BATHING AN INFANT

Infants do not always need or want to be bathed daily. This should be negotiated with parents, and any medical conditions affecting how often an infant should be bathed should be taken into account and discussed. Parents may be happy to bath their infant but if the child has intravenous (IV) access or a nasogastric tube, the parents may feel intimidated and need support from staff. Some infants enjoy baths more than others and often find it relaxing. It is a good time to fully observe how an infant handles and moves, and for staff to look at their skin condition.

As for 'top and tailing' it is important to prepare first, ensuring you have everything ready and checking that the windows and doors are shut. You should pre-fill the bath with a few centimetres of cold water first and then top the bath up with hot water. This should prevent scalding. To check the temperature you should use the back of your hand or elbow, and the water should feel neither hot nor

cold.[8] The depth of the water will depend on the size of the infant but Lee and Thompson[14] recommend that the water should be between 5 and 8 cm deep to prevent accidental drowning. However, it is important that you never leave an infant in the bath alone at any time. PPE such as disposable gloves and apron should be worn as required.[13]

### Equipment

Clean clothes
Two warm towels
Clean nappy
Dry wipes or wash cloth
Jug
Cotton-wool
Baby bath
Changing mat
Baby soap and shampoo (if over 28 days)
Disposable gloves and apron
Linen bin

# PROCEDURE:  Bathing an infant

| Procedural steps | Evidence-based rationale |
|---|---|
| **1** Wash your hands before patient contact. Place the infant on the changing mat and undress them and remove their nappy | To promote hygiene |
| **2** Wrap the infant in a warm towel, leaving their face exposed | To maintain infant's comfort |
| **3** Using a disposable cloth or face cloth first wipe their face and neck using plain water[15] | Soap should not be used on infant's sensitive face. Maintain infant hygiene |
| **4** To wash their hair, continue to swaddle them in a warm towel and then gently lay them along your non-dominant forearm, supporting their head in your hand. Slowly tip their head towards the baby bath and using your dominant hand splash water onto their head. Apply a small amount of baby shampoo to their head. Using your dominant hand wash their hair. Use either the jug of your cupped hand rinse the infant's hair using the water from the bath. Once their hair is rinsed lay them back on the changing mat and using the spare towel dry their head thoroughly, to prevent heat loss | To maintain infant's comfort and hygiene. To maintain infant's temperature/thermal regulation |
| **5** Leave the infant swaddled on the changing mat and place one hand securely on them. Using your other hand add a small amount of bubble-bath to the bath, remembering that too much can dry out their sensitive skin[15] | Protect infants safety to prevent them rolling or falling |
| **6** Remove the towel and gently move your hand and arm around their back and shoulders, holding on to the distant arm. The infant's neck and head should naturally rest against your forearm providing support. Use your other hand and place it between their legs on their buttocks | To maintain safe and correct manual handling and comfort of infant |
| **7** Slowly and gently lift and lower the infant into the bath. Slide your hand out from under their bottom, while holding their shoulders and arm gently, but firmly. The infant will be half submerged in the bath water now | To maintain safe and correct manual handling and comfort of infant |
| **8** Use your free hand to cup water and wash the infant. The infant's skin is very sensitive and susceptible so special care should be taken[1] especially to the creases around the neck, under the arms, tops of the thighs and genital area[16] | To maintain infant's comfort and hygiene |
| **9** Young infants can become cold very quickly so they should not be in the bath too long.[6] Using the same hold as before, lift the infant out of the bath and back on to the dry towel. Take extra care, as the infant will be wet and slippery[14] | To maintain infant's comfort and temperature regulation. To maintain safe and correct manual handling |
| **10** Wrap the infant back up in the towel. Aim to keep the infant as covered as possible and using the spare towel dry the infant off. Start with the infant's torso, arms, legs and then genital area | To maintain infants comfort and hygiene |

## PROCEDURE: Bathing an infant (continued)

| | |
|---|---|
| **11** Once the infant is completely dry move off the damp towels. Put on a clean nappy and dress the infant appropriately for the environment | To maintain infant's comfort and hygiene |
| **12** Place the infant somewhere safe, like their cot | To maintain the infant's comfort and safety to prevent then rolling or falling |
| **13** Put the used nappy into the clinical waste bin and put the dirty linen in the linen bin | To prevent cross-contamination |
| **14** Wash the bath out with hot water and detergent and then dry completely | To prevent cross-contamination |
| **15** Remove and discard of your gloves and apron as appropriate[13] | To prevent cross-contamination |
| **16** Wash your hands.[13] Check infant is warm, comfortable and safe | To prevent cross-contamination. To maintain the infant's comfort and safety |
| **17** Maintain appropriate records[11] | To follow NMC guidelines[11] |

## EYE CARE

Children and young people will be unlikely to need specific eye care. Eye care will normally be covered when they wash their face with either water or soap and water. However, in young infants and neonates eye care should only be performed when it is clinically indicated by 'sticky eyes'. Lissauer and Fanaroff[17] state that in the first few weeks of life neonates are unable to excrete tears, which serves as a barrier against infection. Neonates are often born with sticky eyes, but it can be a sign of infection so should always be pointed out to the medical team if it has not already been noticed. Eye care may need to be performed up to four times a day until the eyes clear. With good hand washing it is possible to carry out eye care at the same time as changing the infants nappy.

### Equipment

Cooled boiled or sterile water
Sterile container
Sterile gauze (not cotton-wool)
Disposable gloves and apron

## PROCEDURE: Eye care

| Procedural steps | Evidence-based rationale |
|---|---|
| **1** Pour the water into the sterile pot and open the gauze | To prepare equipment first |
| **2** Wash hands before patient contact. Lay the infant supine on a flat surface and swaddle them in a sheet or blanket | To maintain comfort for the infant and keep them as still as possible |
| **3** Leave one hand on the infant and then dip the gauze into the water, squeezing out any excess | To maintain the infant's safety and keep them feeling secure |
| **4** Gently wipe the gauze from the inner edge of the eyes outwards in one single motion. Discard the gauze and repeat as necessary on both eyes | To maintain eye hygiene |
| **5** Remove the sheet or blanket and place the infant somewhere safe, checking that they are safe and comfortable | To maintain infants comfort and safety |
| **6** Discard the water, sterile pot, gauze, apron and gloves in the clinical waste[13] | To prevent cross-contamination |
| **7** Wash your hands[13] | To prevent cross-contamination |
| **8** Maintain appropriate records[10] | To maintain NMC guidelines[10] |

# UMBILICAL CORD CARE

The umbilical cord is routinely clamped at birth.[18] One of the most important aspects of caring for an umbilical cord stump is to keep it clean and dry,[18] as it is a direct portal for infection.[19] It is advised that the cord only be cleaned when clinically indicated, such as if substances have leaked from the nappy.[18,20,21] The umbilical stump will usually dry out and turn black before separating from the skin.[18] There is no set time for the cord to fall off but between days 5 to 15 is considered normal[18,21] It is normal for the stump to have a small amount of oozing and blood but if the area is looking red and inflamed, as well as there being a lot of blood and oozing, then this should be reported as it could be a sign of infection and a swab should be taken.[18] The infant will need to be undressed for access to the umbilical cord stump, so shut the windows and doors to prevent them getting cold. Gather together all the equipment so that you do not need to leave the infant alone at any point. Wash your hands before you start.

## Equipment

Cooled boiled or sterile water
Sterile container
Sterile gauze
Disposable gloves and apron

## PROCEDURE: Umbilical cord care

| Procedural steps | Evidence-based rationale |
| --- | --- |
| 1 Wash hands before patient contact. Lay the infant supine on a flat surface and undress them to get access to the cord stump. You do not need to remove the nappy to do this. If the nappy does need to be changed, do this first. Then place the infant somewhere safe, wash your hands and start again | To maintain infant's comfort |
| 2 Roll the top of nappy down so that it is not sitting on the cord. Examine the stump. If it is clean and dry you do not need to do anything | Allows you to look for signs of infection (blood, smell, oozing), check that the stump is drying out and that no hernias are forming |
| 3 If the cord is wet from urine or faeces, or oozing, then dip the gauze into the water and wipe around the stump once[21] | Maintain cleanliness and help prevent infection The use of antiseptics and baby skin products is not advised as it may hinder the natural healing process[18] |
| 4 Discard the gauze and repeat if necessary | Clean as required, but do so minimally |
| 5 Using a dry piece of gauze wipe once and discard the gauze. Repeat as necessary until the area is dry | Be careful not rub the area. The cord will naturally fall off and should do so naturally.[18] Drying the area helps prevent infection |
| 6 Put the nappy back on the infant and roll the top of the nappy down | The cord is best left exposed as much as possible to dry out,[18] so by rolling the top of the nappy down it airs it and stops it rubbing |
| 7 Dress the infant and place them somewhere safe | To maintain infant's comfort and safety |
| 8 Discard the gauze, water, container, gloves and apron in a clinical waste bin[13] | To help prevent cross-infection |
| 9 Wash you hands[13] and check the infant is comfortable and safe | To help prevent cross-infection |
| 10 Maintain appropriate records[10] | To follow NMC guidelines[10] and allow documentation |

# ORAL HYGIENE

## Definitions

**Oral hygiene:** maintained through effective removal of debris and plaque to ensure that the structure and tissues of the mouth are kept in a healthy condition.[5]

Oral hygiene is central to good health and healthy living[22] and is learned in childhood.[22,23] Therefore, it is important to re-emphasise these practices while in hospital. Good oral hygiene practices involve brushing teeth in a circular motion, twice a day, with an appropriate toothbrush and toothpaste containing fluoride.[24] The main causes of poor oral hygiene in children are poor diet and nutrition, poor dental hygiene and not using toothpaste containing fluoride.[22] In hospital certain patients will be more at risk of poor oral hygiene, such as patients undergoing chemotherapy, patients with a cardiac condition or who have had recent cardiothoracic surgery, patients who are intubated and patients who do not have a swallow.

It is advised that children begin brushing their teeth as soon as they begin teething at around 6 months of age[24] and within the first year of their life.[23] Before this age children do not need to use a toothbrush or toothpaste, but parents should be encouraged to use a cloth to gently sweep the mouth so that children get used to parents performing this task.[23] Infant feeding has a direct impact on oral hygiene, and breastfeeding should be encouraged; parents should follow correct weaning advice.[23] The National Institute for Health and Clinical Excellence[24] suggests that children visit the dentist as early as possible and that they follow the dentist's advice about how often to have check ups, which may vary from once every 3–12 months. Children up to the age of 5 years will need adult assistance in brushing their teeth, but from 3 years and upwards they should be encouraged to try first.[24] Children under the age of 5 years will not have the dexterity or ability to effectively brush their teeth on their own.

Intubated patients or those who do not have a swallow should still have regular oral care performed for their own comfort and health. However, Berry et al.[25] and Cutler and Davis[26] both agree that there is need for standard guidelines on performing oral care in ventilated patients. There are currently a variety of different techniques used to perform oral hygiene and the frequency of how often this occurs varies, for example using suction toothbrushes, mouth sponges, mouthwash, mouth moisturisers, toothpaste or suction every 2–12 hours.[25] When you perform oral hygiene on ventilated or unconscious patients or those without a swallow reflex, it is best to follow local policy as there are currently no standardised guidelines.

### Equipment

Toothbrush
Toothpaste (containing fluoride)
Bowl
Cup of water
Water
Towel
Disposable apron and gloves

## PROCEDURE: Oral hygiene

| Procedural steps | Evidence-based rationale |
|---|---|
| 1 Depending on the age and level of self-sufficiency of the patient you will need to confirm how much help they would like and who will assist them (staff or parent). It is best if the patient can sit upright in a chair or bed or stand. If you are to brush their teeth agree on how they will let you know if they need you stop or pause. Close the doors and curtains and wash your hands before proceeding | To maintain patient's comfort and promoting self-sufficiency. To maintain patient's privacy and dignity |

## PROCEDURE:  Oral hygiene (continued)

| | |
|---|---|
| **2** Put a small amount of toothpaste on the toothbrush and ask the patient to open their mouth | To maintain oral hygiene. Toothpaste with fluoride should be used[22–24] |
| **3** Gently insert the toothbrush into their mouth and begin cleaning their teeth using a circular motion, making sure you clean all the teeth; brush the gums and tongue gently for 2 minutes | NICE guidelines[24] recommend teeth are brushed in a circular action for at least 2 minutes, twice a day. To maintain oral hygiene |
| **4** If the patient becomes uncomfortable, needs to spit or pause then stop immediately | To maintain patient's comfort |
| **5** Once you have finished brushing allow the patient to spit and rinse their mouth with water. If the patient needs their mouth wiping do so with the towel. Check the patient is comfortable | To maintain patient's oral hygiene, comfort and dignity |
| **6** Rinse the toothbrush and leave to dry. Tidy away the patient's toothpaste. Dispose the towel into the linen bin and put the bowl, water, gloves and apron into a clinical waste bin. Wash your hands.[13] Open the curtains and doors (if appropriate) | To prevent cross-infection |
| **7** Maintain appropriate documentation[10] | To maintain accurate documentation and follow NMC guidelines[10] |

## NAPPY CARE

Neonates and infants normally wear nappies, but sometimes children who have previously been toilet trained may need to wear incontinent pads due to medical treatment, acute and chronic conditions. Most children are fully toilet trained around the age of 3 years.[27] It is of high importance that these children and young people are treated with dignity and privacy, as it could be very embarrassing for them. If old enough this procedure should be discussed with the child and who they want in the room. Some may either want their parents there, actively involved or simply there to support them. Other children may want only those absolutely necessary in the room. It is also important to discuss with parents how involved they want to be, as many may feel that this is a nursing role and prefer not to be involved. When you provide this care for neonates and infants it is important to remember that, if the patient has intravenous access, nasogastric tubes or other medical devices attached to them, then parents who normally provide this care may feel intimidated and need your support.

## Changing an infant's nappy

Infants' nappies can need changing up to 10 times a day, as some have their bowels open and pass urine with every feed. Neonates' and infants' skin is very delicate; if it is in constant contact with moisture, bacteria and ammonia (urine and stool),[28] then the skin is at risk of breaking down.[29] It is well documented that nappy rash is one of the most common complications of treatment that affects children in hospital, but through correct hygiene routine this can be prevented.[30] (For guidance on the management of nappy rash please see 'Skin assessment', page 200). The choice of products used is the decision of the infant's parents, but advice is to use only warm water and cotton-wool in infants under 28 days old. It is important to have all your equipment ready, as you must not leave an infant unattended while they are being changed on a changing mat, in case they should roll or fall and hurt themselves.[31]

### Equipment

Clean nappy (paper or towel)
Changing mat
Cotton-wool and warm water or baby wipes (as appropriate)
Disposable gloves and apron

## PROCEDURE: Nappy care

| Procedural steps | Evidence-based rationale |
|---|---|
| **1** Wash hands before patient contact. Lift the infant onto the changing mat, laying them supine. Make sure the infant is comfortable. You may need to turn their head gently to one side. Undress the infant from the waist down | To maintain infant's comfort and safety |
| **2** Remove the infant's nappy by undoing the adhesive tapes and refastening them to the nappy | By refastening the tapes you prevent them from sticking to the infant's delicate skin |
| **3** Securely hold the infant's ankles with your non-dominant hand and gently raise them upwards. Use your dominant hand to gently slide the front of the nappy underneath their bottom. Be aware that infants often urinate on removal of their nappy. As you remove the front of the nappy you may notice the infant has opened their bowels. If they have, use the inside of the front of the nappy to wipe the mess towards the back. Assess skin integrity | To maintain infant's safety, comfort and hygiene |
| **4** Fold the inside of the nappy fully over and gently lay the infant back down. The infant should now be lying on the clean outside of their nappy | To maintain infant's comfort |
| **5** Use warm water and cotton-wool to gently cleanse the infant's skin | |
| **6** When cleansing a male infant you should never pull the foreskin back | Unnecessary and damaging practice[6] |
| **7** When cleansing female infants always clean from the front to the back in one swipe and then discard the cotton-wool. Repeat as needed | This should prevent vaginal and urethral contamination[32] |
| **8** Carefully dry the infant using the cotton-wool on a blotting action, paying special attention to any creases[29] | To prevent to infant getting sore, from not being dried correctly. To maintain infant's comfort and hygiene |
| **9** As before, lift the infant's legs and then slide the open clean nappy underneath their bottom. Lower the infant down, making sure in boys that their penis is tucked in facing downwards. Securely fasten the nappy, but not so tightly that it pinches the skin[29] | To make sure urine flows downwards and not out of the top of the nappy[33] |
| **10** Dress the infant and place them somewhere safe | To maintain infant's comfort and safety |
| **11** Discard the dirty nappy and cotton-wool into a clinical waste bin.[13] Throw the water away and if the bowl is not disposable wash it out with hot water and detergent. Dry the bowl out and allow it to air | To prevent any cross-infection and follow DH guidelines regarding waste disposal |
| **12** Remove gloves and apron and dispose them in the clinical waste bin[13] | To prevent any cross-infection and follow the DH guidelines regarding waste disposal |
| **13** Wash your hands[13] | To prevent cross-infection |
| **14** Maintain appropriate records[10] | To maintain accurate documentation and follow NMC guidelines[10] |

# Changing an incontinence pad in an older child

*Equipment*

Sheet/towel to cover patient
Clean incontinence pad

Wet wipes or water, wipes, bowl and soap
Towel to dry patient
Disposable gloves and apron

| Procedural steps | Evidence-based rationale |
|---|---|
| 1 First, discuss with child and family who will be in the room and doing what. Close all the curtains and windows | To gain verbal consent[10] and maintain child's dignity and privacy |
| 2 Wash hands before any patient contact. Where possible encourage the child to help as much as possible. Assuming the child is already lying on the bed, assist them to remove their clothes below the waist. Cover the child with the sheet or towel | To promote self-care[4]<br>To maintain child's dignity and privacy |
| 3 Remove the sheet or towel at the last minute. Ask or assist the child in removing the incontinence pad. The pad maybe very wet and dirty so be careful not to flick the pad. As before, roll the front of the pad underneath the child's bottom | To maintain patient's privacy and dignity<br>To prevent cross-infection |
| 4 Using the wet-wipes or water and soap ask the child to clean their genital area. Once clean, pass the child the towel and encourage them to fully dry themselves | To promote patient self-care and hygiene |
| 5 If the child has opened their bowels then ask the patient to roll to one side. Carefully remove the dirty pad, wiping their bottom with a clean area | To promote hygiene |
| 6 Using the wet-wipes or wipes, water and soap cleanse the child fully. Use the towel to fully dry them. Assess skin integrity | To promote hygiene |
| 7 Lay a clean incontinence pad out and ask the child to roll back onto it | To promote patient hygiene |
| 8 Pull the front through and fasten. Again, remembering if it is a boy to ensure their penis is facing downwards | To prevent the incontinence pad leaking, resulting in discomfort for the patient |
| 9 Ask or assist the child in getting dressed and into a comfortable position | To promote self-care and patient comfort |
| 10 Discard the used incontinence pad and wipes into a clinical waster bin.[13] Throw the water away and if the bowl is not disposable wash it out with hot water and detergent. Dry the bowl and allow it to air. Place the used towel/sheets into the correct linen bin | To prevent any cross-infection and follow DH guidelines regarding waste disposal |
| 11 Remove gloves and apron and dispose of them in the clinical waste bin[13] | To prevent any cross-infection and follow the DH guidelines regarding waste disposal |
| 12 Wash your hands | To prevent cross-infection |
| 13 Open the curtains and doors as appropriate | To promote patient comfort |
| 14 Maintain appropriate records[10] | To maintain accurate documentation and follow NMC guidelines[10] |

## NAIL CARE

Neonates, infants and children's fingernails and toenails need to be cut so that they don't scratch themselves and their nails can be kept clean. While you are cutting their nails, both neonates and infants may wriggle a lot, so it is often easier for two people to cut nails. It is easier to cut nails after a bath as the nails will be softer. There are a variety of products available to cut children's nails, and this should be the decision of the child's parents.

### Equipment

Children's nail clippers/blunt-nosed scissors
Inco-sheet
Disposable gloves and apron

## PROCEDURE: Nail care

| Procedural steps | Evidence-based rationale |
|---|---|
| 1 Wash hands before patient contact. Lay the neonate or infant on a flat surface, or ask a child to sit comfortably. Place the inco-sheet under the area you will be cutting | To maintain child comfort<br>To prevent cross-infection by containing the nail clippings |
| 2 If the child is unable to comply (assuming parents have given consent) then ask another adult (parent or colleague) to hold the arm or leg | To maintain safety for child and gain consent[10] from either the child or parent |
| 3 Take a gentle but firm grip of the hand and finger, or toe and foot, with your non-dominant hand | To maintain safety of child |
| 4 Hold the clippers or scissors in your dominant hand and cut each nail, following the nail bed. To avoid cutting a jagged edge aim to cut each nail in one clip straight across | To maintain safety and comfort of child |
| 5 If the child is still wriggling it may be easier to push the finger/toe tip down so that the nail is more exposed | This will stop you accidentally nicking the skin around the nail |
| 6 Once finished place the neonate/infant somewhere safe or check the child is comfortable | To maintain safety of child |
| 7 Wash the clippers/scissors in hot water and detergent and leave to dry. Dispose of the inco-sheet with the nail cuttings, gloves and apron | To prevent cross-infection |
| 8 Wash your hands[13] | To prevent cross-infection |
| 9 Maintain appropriate documentation[10] | To follow NMC guidelines[10] |

## SKIN ASSESSMENT

It is widely documented that neonates and children are at risk of developing pressure sores[34] and that adult assessment tools are not suitable to use on neonates and children.[34,35] The skin is the largest organ[1,35] and is made up of three layers: the epidermis, dermis and subcutaneous layer. There are numerous factors that affect children's skin integrity that need consideration: prematurity, birth weight, oedema, congenital abnormalities, physical or mechanical injuries, hypothermia, pressure, ischaemia, necrosis, dehydration, sepsis, mobility, poor perfusion and children who have had recent surgery.[35] Poor skin integrity can affect children's, especially neonates' ability to control their temperature[35] and increases their risk of infection.[1] O'Brien[30] states that nappy rash is often the most frequent complication that affects children in hospital, but this is not the only aspect of skin assessment in children that needs to be performed. There are numerous opportunities to perform a skin assessment: during a nappy or incontinence pad change, while assisting a child in maintaining personal hygiene. An initial skin assessment should always occur and be documented on admission. As simple as it sounds, skin assessments

should be carried out visually.[35]

### Equipment

Disposable gloves and apron

## PROCEDURE: Skin assessment

| Procedural steps | Evidence-based rationale |
| --- | --- |
| 1 Look at the whole body: head (front and back), trunk and extremities. Pay special attention to eyes, ears, umbilicus, nappy area, sites of medical equipment (IV access site, drainage tubes, endotracheal tubes, blood sugar pricks) | To undertake a full skin assessment |
| 2 Observe for areas of dryness, redness, tears, irritation, pressure, infection or breakdown | To undertake a full skin assessment |
| 3 With permission photograph area of skin damage. Any concerns should be reported to nurse in charge immediately | To gain verbal/written consent[10] |
| 4 Wash hands and dispose of apron in clinical waste bin[13] | To prevent cross-infection |
| 5 Document findings in full and report/update nurse in charge and inform medical staff if treatment is required | To maintain appropriate documentation[10] |

 Go to the website to find the PowerPoint presentation for this chapter and MCQs to test your knowledge. **www.hodderplus.com/childnursingskills**

## REFERENCES

1  Mainstone A (2005) Maintaining infant skin health hygiene. *British Journal of Midwifery* **13**(1): 44–47.
2  Downey L, Lloyd H (2008) Bed bathing patients in hospital. *Nursing Standard* **22**(34): 35–40.
3  Department of Health (2000) *The NHS plan: a plan for investment a plan for reform.* London: The Stationery Office.
4  Department of Health (2001) *Essence of care: patient-focused benchmarking for healthcare practitioners.* London: The Stationery Office.
5  Department of Health (2003) *Essences of care: patient-focused benchmarks for clinical governance.* London: The Stationery Office.
6  Department of Health (2006) *Birth to five.* London: The Stationery Office.
7  Rudolf M, Levene M (2006) *Paediatrics and child health*, 2nd edition. Oxford: Blackwell Publishing.

8  Young AE (2004) The management of server burns in children. *Current Paediatrics* **14**: 202–207.
9  White R, Denyer J (2006) *Paediatric skin and wound care.* Aberdeen: Wounds UK.
10  Nursing and Midwifery Council (2004) *Code of professional conduct.* London: NMC.
11  Pegram A, Bloomfield J, Jones A (2007) Clinical skills: bed bathing and personal hygiene needs of patients. *British Journal of Nursing* **16**: 356–358.
12  Baillie L (2005) *Developing practical nursing skills.* London: Hodder Arnold.
13  Department of Health (2003) *Winning ways: working together to reduce healthcare associated infection in England.* London: The Stationery Office.
14  Lee LK, Thompson KM (2007) Parental survey of belief and practices about bathing and water safety and their children: guidance for drowning

prevention. *Accident Analysis Prevention*, **39**: 58–62.

15 Cowan ME, Frost MR (2006) A comparison between detergent baby bath additive and bay soap on skin flora of neonates. *Journal of Hospital Infection* 7: 91–95.

16 Samaniego IA (2003) A sore spot on pediatrics: risk factor in pressure ulcers. *Pediatric Nursing* **29**(4): 278–282.

17 Lissauer T, Fanaroff A (2006) *Neonatology at a glance.* Oxford: Blackwell Publishing.

18 Selkirk L, Blumberg R, Penrice J (2008) A clinical guide to umbilical cord clamping. *British Journal of Midwifery* **16**: 714–716.

19 Boxwell G (2001) *Neonatal intensive care nursing.* London: Routledge.

20 World Health Organization (1998) *Global strategy for infant and young child feeding.* Geneva: World Health Organization.

21 Zupan J, Garner P, Omar AAA (2004) Topical umbilical cord care at birth. *Cochrane Database Systematic Review* **3**: CD001057.

22 Watt R (1999) *Oral health promotion: a guide to effective working in pre-school settings.* London: Health Education Authority.

23 Department of Health (Dental and Ophthalmic Service Division) (2003) *Choosing better oral health: an oral health plan for England.* London: The Stationery Office.

24 National Institute for Clinical Excellence (2004) *Clinical guidelines 19. Dental recall: interval between routine dental examinations.* London: NICE.

25 Berry AM, Davidson PM, Masters J, Rolls K (2007) Review of oral hygiene practices for intensive care patients receiving mechanical ventilation. *American Journal of Critical Care* **16**: 552–563.

26 Cutler CJ, Davis N (2005) Improving oral care in patients receiving mechanical ventilation. *American Journal of Critical Care*, **14**: 389–394.

27 Royal College of Nursing (2006) *Paediatric assessment of toilet training readiness and issuing of products.* London: RCN.

28 Darmstadt GL, Dinulos JG (2000) Neonatal skin care. *Pediatric Clinics of North America* **47**: 375–382.

29 McManus J (2001) Skin breakdown: risk factors, prevention and treatment. *Newborn Infant Nursing Review* **1**(1): 35–42.

30 O'Brien M (2007) Assessing and treating nappy rash in the hospitalised child. *Continence UK* **1**(1): 30–37.

31 Harold SK, Tamura T, Colton K (2003) Reported level of supervision of young children while in the bathtub. *Ambulatory Pediatric* **3**(2): 106–108.

32 Chon DH, Frank CL, Shortliffe LM (2001) Pediatric urinary tract infections. *Pediatric Clinics of North America* **48**: 1441–1459.

33 Lund C (1999) Prevention and management of infant skin breakdown. *Nursing Clinics of North America* **34**: 907–920.

34 Waterlow J (1997) Pressure sores: risk assessment in children. *Paediatric Nursing* **9**(6): 21–24.

35 McGurk V, Holloway, Crutchley A, Izzard H (2004) Skin integrity assessment in neonates and children. *Paediatric Nursing* **16**(3): 15–18.

## CHAPTER 13

# Providing optimum nutrition and hydration

Rachel Howe, Donna Forbes and Colleen Baker

## LEARNING OUTCOMES

*Upon completion of this chapter the reader should be able to accomplish the following:*

1 Assess a child's nutritional status upon admission to hospital
2 Understand normal feeding patterns of an infant and child
3 Recognise a child who is dehydrated
4 List the different methods of enteral or artificial feeding and describe the advantages and disadvantages of each
5 Understand the principles in the safe administration of enteral and parenteral feeds to children
6 Understand the principles of infection control when preparing and administering feeds to children
7 Recognise any potential problems that could develop when a child receives enteral or parenteral feeds
8 Support the child requiring a pH study

## CHAPTER OVERVIEW

Good nutrition is very important in order for infants and children to grow and develop. Childhood disease can often be complicated by poor nutrition.[1] Therefore it is necessary for children's nurses to learn about elements of infant and child feeding. There is little research available on the specific nursing management of nutrition in sick children.[2] Therefore a collaborative assessment, management and treatment plan collectively devised by the child, parents/guardians, children's nurses, doctors and hospital dieticians is best advised. Further reading and practice of certain feeding techniques will be required.

## ASSESSMENT OF FEEDING

An infant or child's feeding pattern is assessed as part of the nursing process during the admission stage. It is important that the child's normal eating and drinking pattern is ascertained. Any likes or dislikes should be noted. The method of infant feeding should be documented, i.e. breastfeeding, partial breastfeeding or formula feeding. The children's nurse may detect actual/potential feeding problems following the assessment. A nursing care plan should be drawn up and communicated with the parent/guardian and healthcare team. The physical assessment of the child provides important indicators about the child's nutritional wellbeing. Each observation will be discussed regarding best practice in monitoring and relevance to clinical practice.

### Weight

Body weight is an important observation to be carried out upon admission of a child to hospital.

Drug dosage is prescribed according to the child's weight, so it is usual to record this observation as soon as possible.[3] A child's true weight is recorded without any clothing and is best practice. However, some children may not comply with removing all clothing so their weight in their night clothes without foot wear is acceptable. An infant's weight should be recorded without any clothing or nappy. It is important to ensure that the room is warm and private when weighing an infant as he/she can become cold quickly. Place a sheet or hand towel on the scales before placing the baby on the scales to be weighed so that he/she does not come into contact with a cold surface. Check that the scales are at zero before placing the infant on the scales to be weighed. The weight should be documented clearly in the clinical notes. Dress the infant as soon as possible after weighing. It is a good idea to record what scales the infant was weighed on if there is more than one scale on the ward.

If daily weights are required it is important to try and weigh the baby at the same time each day, usually in the morning, and on the same scales. Breastfed babies shouldn't need to be weighed every day unless specifically requested. Breastfeeding mothers can have greater anxiety if their baby is weighed too frequently especially if the baby does not appear to be gaining weight. A breastfeeding mother may doubt her ability to adequately feed her baby if she is told her baby is not gaining weight, which in turn could have a negative effect on her milk supply. Therefore it is important to consider why each observation should be carried out rather than just routinely carrying out observations. The weight should be documented clearly in the clinical notes. Consider weighing the child again if he/she is hospitalised for more than a week so that drug dosages can be as accurate as possible. An accurate weight is also essential in the accurate calculation of intravenous fluids.[4]

In an emergency there may not be sufficient time to obtain a child's weight so it can be estimated using the following formula:[5]

age in years + 4) × 2 = approximate weight in kilograms
Example: a 2-year-old's approximate weight would be calculated as follows
2 + 4 = 6 × 2 = 12 kg

Remember for accuracy you should check the child's weight on a scale as soon as it is safe to do so.

## Length

Length or height should be recorded during the admission stage. An accurate length or height is essential for monitoring any endocrine or growth disorders. A supine length (lying down) is recommended for the 0–3 year group. However, for compliance reasons a standing height can be recorded from age 2 years onwards.

A supine length is recorded by placing the child on a flat surface while the child lies on their back. One observer holds the head in contact with a board at the top of the table and another straightens the legs, turns the feet upwards and brings a sliding board towards the child's heels to measure length.

For standing height measurements, the child stands without shoes, with heels and back in contact with an upright wall. Head should be held in position so that the child's eyes look straight forward. A right-angled block, usually weighted, is then slid down the wall until it touches the child's head where the scale is read and the measurement taken.[6]

## Head circumference

Head circumference is usually required only for 0–2-year-olds. The measurement of a child's head circumference helps to detect any developmental problems. Measure the skull circumference using a tape measure around the forehead above the eyebrows and around the occiput. The measurement should be taken twice to ensure accuracy.[6]

## Growth charts

An infant's weight, length and head circumference can be plotted on a centile chart. A centile chart allows for adjustment in the recording of a baby's weight according to its date of birth and gestational age. The centile is a relative position, allowing the baby's measurements to be judged in relation to what would be expected for their age, size and gender.[3] The doctor or dietician measures and plots children on centile charts. Children's nurses can assist with measuring techniques and should know whether or not the infant or child in their care is meeting the expected measurement gains.

The body mass index (BMI) (Table 13.1) is used to determine whether or not an individual's weight is within the range considered to be healthy.[3] The BMI is often referred to if a child is noted to be under- or overweight (i.e. anorexia nervosa or obesity). The BMI is calculated with this formula:

$$\text{weight (kg)}/\text{height}^2(\text{m}) = \text{BMI}$$

**Table 13.1** Body mass index and health status

| Body mass index | Health status |
| --- | --- |
| Below 20 | Underweight |
| 20–24.9 | Ideal |
| 25–29.9 | Overweight |
| 30–39.9 | Obese |
| Over 40 | Extremely obese |

# INFANT FEEDING

An infant or baby is defined as 0–1 year of age. It is important for children's nurses to understand the normal feeding patterns of infants before he/she can assess, manage, treat and educate children and their families about nutrition.[7] The following information should help inform children's nurses about the normal feeding regime.

## Breastfeeding

Breast milk is the best food for newborn babies and beyond to approximately 2 years.[8] From 6 months babies need to be introduced to solid foods so that they receive sufficient iron to grow and develop at a normal rate. Most mothers decide whether or not they will breastfeed their baby in advance of the birth.[7] Children's nurses have a role in promoting breastfeeding whether inside or outside of work. Ireland and the UK have relatively low breastfeeding rates (30–40% uptake) and therefore it is important that we do our best to promote and support breastfeeding. Breastfeeding offers many health benefits and advantages for the baby and mother (Table 13.2).

**Table 13.2** Some of the benefits of breastfeeding for the baby and the mother*

| Benefits of breastfeeding for the baby | Benefits of breastfeeding for the mother |
| --- | --- |
| The nutritional content of breastmilk changes as the baby's requirements change – thus it is the perfect milk for babies<br>Breast milk contains properties to protect immunity and enhance growth and development of the baby<br>Breast feeding reduces incidence of:<br>• gastroenteritis<br>• respiratory illness<br>• ear infections<br>• allergy<br>• diabetes<br>• obesity<br>Breast feeding enhances growth and cognitive development and can even raise IQ<br>When feeding, a breastfed infant gains comfort, warmth and security close to the mother | Economic<br>Saves time, no preparation or sterilisation<br>Breast feeding can reduce incidence of:<br>• breast cancer<br>• ovarian cancer<br>• osteoporosis<br>Breastfeeding facilitates bonding between mother and baby<br>Breastfeeding helps women to regain their pre-pregnancy figure |

*Adapted with permission from HSE.[9]

Children's nurses have an important role in supporting mothers to continue breastfeeding their baby. The Baby Friendly Initiative promoted in the UK and Ireland encourages healthcare professionals to promote and support breastfeeding (Table 13.3).

Therefore most hospitals or community areas offer training and education about breastfeeding for their staff to help keep them up to date about current practices. Find out where you can attend such lectures near your place of work.

Table 13.3 Baby friendly initiative best practice standards for establishing and maintaining lactation and breastfeeding in neonatal units (UNICEF UK)

| Steps | Description |
| --- | --- |
| 1 | Have a written breastfeeding policy which is routinely communicated to all staff |
| 2 | Educate all healthcare staff in the skills necessary to implement the policy |
| 3 | Inform all parents of the benefits of breastmilk and breastfeeding for babies in the neonatal unit |
| 4 | Facilitate skin-to-skin contact (kangaroo care) between mother and baby |
| 5 | Support mothers to initiate and maintain lactation through expression of breastmilk |
| 6 | Support mothers to establish and maintain breastfeeding |
| 7 | Encourage exclusive breastmilk feeding |
| 8 | Avoid the use of teats or dummies for breastfed babies unless clinically indicated |
| 9 | Promote breastfeeding support through local and national networks |

 You can see the careplan on the website which is an example of how staff within The National Children's Hospital (AMNCH) in Tallaght, Dublin, supports the breastfeeding relationship between a mother and her baby admitted to the children's ward.[10]

While breastmilk is the best milk to offer a baby, it is not an option for every mother and baby. Children's nurses need to accept and respect a mother's decision regarding feeding choice. Supporting the mother to feed her baby whatever way she chooses is very important.

## Bottle feeding

Babies who are bottle fed can grow and develop normally. While children's nurses shouldn't promote a particular brand of formula milk it is important that the content and preparation of formula feeds is understood.

### First and second milks

Cow's milk-based infant formula is the alternative to breastmilk.[11] These milks are based on cow's milk protein. First milks are whey (60%) dominant while second milks are casein (80%) dominant. Second milks are thought to give the baby a fuller feeling for longer and are therefore targeted at hungrier babies. First and second milks can be offered to babies aged 0–6 months. Note that a baby can remain on the first milk until 6 months of age, i.e. he/she may not need the second milk.

### Follow-on milks

These milks contain higher levels of iron to meet the growing needs of a baby aged 6–12 months. Therefore follow-on milks are not suitable for babies under 6 months.

New formula milks are marketed all the time. Milk with partially digested protein is available for babies with colic, reflux and/or constipation. Soya infant formula is available for babies who are found to have cow's milk allergy or galactosaemia. Babies found to have cow's milk allergy are also likely to be allergic to goat's milk. The protein in both milks is very similar. Therefore goat's milk is not recommended and is difficult to obtain because of EU regulations preventing its availability.[11] Cow's milk is not suitable for infants under 12 months.

### Preparation of bottle feeds

Infants up to 12 months old require their feeding equipment to be washed well in warm soapy water and sterilised. This is to ensure that any harmful bacteria are removed to prevent ill health.[11] Refer to your hospital's policies and procedures regarding preparation of infant formula feeds in the hospital.

The UNICEF[12,13] guidelines may help to inform your practice regarding sterilisation and preparation of infant formula feeds (see website).

## POSITIONING FOR FEEDING

Breastfed babies can be positioned to allow for comfort of both the mother and child. Figure 13.1 shows various breastfeeding positions. The baby should be offered both breasts at each feeding. Alternating positions of the baby at each feed to promote milking of all the milk ducts is also a good idea and may even help to avoid complications such as mastitis. Good positioning at the breast is important to avoid nipple soreness from poor attachment.

Bottle-fed babies should be well supported in a semi-upright position allowing for good eye contact between the parent and child to help promote bonding. Breaks at the middle and end of feeding to allow wind to escape are a good idea. Position the baby upright on the lap or over one shoulder. Support their head gently by cupping a hand under their chin and use the other hand to gently rub their back. Spoon feeding is best provided for babies and children who are seated in a high chair. Positioning for continuous nasogastric or gastrostomy feeding can be important, i.e. raising the head end of the bed by approximately 30° helps to improve gastric emptying, prevent vomiting and reflux.[7,14] Positioning a child on their right side for an hour after feeding can help aid digestion, but be sure to return the infant to their back to sleep, in line with sudden infant death guidelines.[7]

## FEEDING INFANTS IN SPECIAL CIRCUMSTANCES

Feeding infants found to have abnormalities such as a tongue-tie, cleft lip, cleft palate, cleft lip and cleft palate or a syndrome such as Pierre Robin can be a challenge. However, difficulties feeding infants can be overcome once the parents and healthcare workers discuss options and it can be managed if the parents are supported with feeding.

Breastfeeding is a challenge for a mother with a baby found to have an abnormality. However, it is

**Figure 13.1** Positioning for effective feeding (a) Front hold or cradle position; (b) underarm position; (c) lying-down position. Position for effective bottle feeding (d) semi-upright. (e) sPositiong for effective poon feeding.

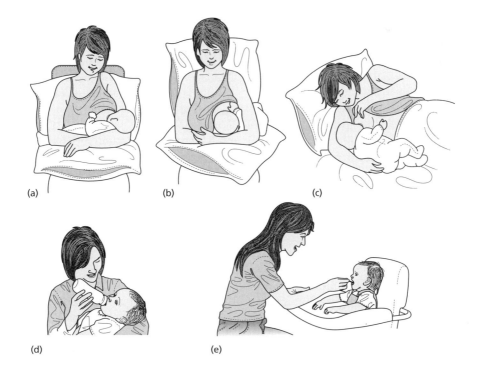

(a)  (b)  (c)

(d)  (e)

very important that breastfeeding is still advocated as being the optimum feeding method for a baby. If a mother wishes to continue breastfeeding her baby then she should be supported by trained staff able to help her. If breastfeeding is not successful following normal attempts to position the baby or if the baby can't maintain their airway or a vacuum because of a cleft palate, then the mother will need to consider expressing her milk. Expressed breast milk can then be offered to her baby using a special device such as a mini-cup or a haberman feeder (Figure 13.2)

Figure 13.2 (a) Mini-cup; (b) Haberman teath and feeder.

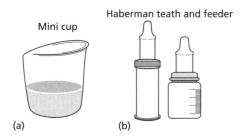

Mini cup

Haberman teath and feeder

(a)                    (b)

### Tongue-tie (ankyloglossia)

Tongue-tie can interfere with breastfeeding if the septum (frenulum) beneath the baby's tongue is restricting movement. Alternative positioning of the baby at the breast may help the baby to feed. Surgery can be performed to release the tongue-tie during the newborn period and feeding usually resumes normally quite quickly post operatively.

### Cleft lip and palate

Babies born with a cleft lip without any palate involvement can usually breast- or bottle feed successfully. When the baby has a cleft palate he/she is unable to maintain adequate vacuum between the tongue and palate, which causes feeding difficulties, particularly when breastfeeding as the baby is unable to suck or obtain enough milk to maintain adequate nutrition. Different leaning or lying positions of the mother and baby at the breast can help. However, it should be acknowledged that feeding, especially breastfeeding a newborn with a cleft lip and palate, can be difficult and teaching a parent to successfully feed their child may be especially challenging for the children's nurse. It is usually necessary for a mother to express her milk and offer expressed breast milk or formula to her

baby using a special device such as a mini-cup, haberman feeder or a nasogastric (NG) tube (discussed later, page 212). The baby should be continually assessed to determine if normal feeding can resume, especially following corrective surgery. If the baby is able to breastfeed even for a few minutes this should be encouraged and then the baby can be supplemented after breastfeeds. Even if the baby can't actually feed from the breast it is important to encourage plenty of mother and baby bonding by placing the baby next to the mother's breasts. Encouraging mother and baby time can help in the long term, especially if breastfeeding is to resume in the future. Further reading and experience regarding cup feeding and the use of a haberman teath will be required.

## INTRODUCING SPOON FEEDS

The WHO[8] and Health Services Executive (HSE)[15] recommend that breastfed babies should not start solids before 24 weeks of age. Breastmilk provides adequate nourishment for babies up to 6 months of age. Introducing solid feeds (also known as the weaning diet) too early can increase the risk of infection and allergies.[16]

When a decision has been made to start spoon feeds the following tips maybe useful. If the baby is in hospital ensure that the parents/guardians are involved with the decision to commence solids.

### Starting solid feeds

- Choose a time when baby is calm and alert. Often lunch or afternoon is a good time.
- Ensure parent/guardian or carer is relatively relaxed.
- Try not to offer spoon feeds when baby is very hungry as it will be too frustrating. Instead try a few spoons either halfway through the milk feed or at the end of a milk feed.
- It is normal for the food to come straight back out of his/her mouth!
- Offer just a few teaspoons at first, gradually building up to food being offered two or three times a day.
- How much, how often and the consistency, texture and range of foods offered need to change as the baby grows and learns.
- First foods to try are often a puréed vegetable, a puréed fruit, baby rice, pureed meat/chicken or a dairy product.

- Foods best avoided include wheat, gluten, eggs, fish, shell fish, liver, soft cheeses, salt, sugar or low-fat foods.
- No honey for under 1-year-olds because of the risk of botulism and no nuts until age 5 because of the risk of choking[11].

Introduce one food at a time building up to a more varied diet by the age of 1 year. Do introduce new foods so that the baby gets used to different tastes and to help widen the range of foods eaten.[16] Altering the consistency and texture of foods is also important as it allows the baby to chew, even without teeth, which helps speech muscles to develop.[11,16] Finger foods can be offered at around 9 months. Cup feeding can be introduced from 6 months and is advocated from 12 months rather than feeding from a bottle.[17] Drinking from a lidless cup rather than a bottle teat may reduce the development of dental carries.[16,17]

## NORMAL DIET FOR OLDER CHILDREN

Children grow and develop fast, so they need a high-quality varied diet with a good balance of energy, protein, vitamins and fibre. The healthy food pyramid (Figure 13.3) is a useful tool to use when discussing a child's diet with children and their parents/guardians.

**Figure 13.3** The Healthy Food Pyramid (adapted with permission) from Health Service Executive (2007) *Healthy Eating for Children.*

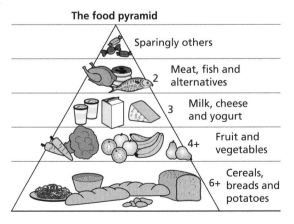

**The food pyramid**

Sparingly others

Meat, fish and alternatives — 2

Milk, cheese and yogurt — 3

Fruit and vegetables — 4+

Cereals, breads and potatoes — 6+

The food pyramid is divided into five shelves, each representing a different food group. A variety of foods from each shelf ensures that the child has a balanced and healthy diet. Most foods should be selected from the bottom two shelves of the pyramid, i.e. fruit, vegetables, cereals, bread or potatoes. Smaller amounts can be given then from the next two shelves, while foods at the top should be taken only sparingly.

Two or three suitable snacks may also be offered to children especially toddlers, who have small appetites but yet need frequent small snacks to help maintain their energy levels. However, snacks should also be healthy and chosen from the following food groups: dairy, fruit, cereals or bread. Food from the top shelf of the pyramid should be reserved for special treats only.

Water should be the drink of choice followed by milk. Low-fat milk is not suitable for children under 2 years of age. Skimmed milk is not suitable for children under 5 years of age.

## NORMAL FLUID AND ENERGY REQUIREMENTS

Newborns, especially breastfed babies, feed 2–3 hourly. By 2 months of age babies may feed every 4 hours, with a longer period between feeds overnight. Breastfed babies feed on demand and dictate the flow and duration to suit their needs. A typical feed intake of formula-fed infants is as follows: 0–6 months 150–200 mL/kg per day and for 6–12 months 120 mL/kg per day.[3] To calculate infant fluid requirements use the following formula:

> Example: a baby weighing 3 kg will have their fluid intake calculated as follows:
> 3 × 200 mL = 600 mL of fluid per day.

The dietician should be consulted regarding calculation of a sick baby's energy requirements per kilogram of body weight in 24 hours. A guide to estimating energy requirements for a healthy baby is 540 kilojoules per kilogram (540 kJ/kg).[3]

> Example: a baby weighing 3 kg will have their energy requirements calculated as follows:
> 3 × 540 kJ = 1620 kJ per day

Each baby's daily fluid and energy requirements need to be divided into equal amounts and offered at each feeding time. The quantity of feeds varies for each baby. To calculate the amount of fluid to be offered at each feed, divide the total requirement by the number of feeds offered in 24 hours:

> Example: a 3-kg baby requiring 600 mL of fluid per day and fed at 4-hourly intervals (six feeds in 24 hours):
> 600 ÷ 6 = 100 mL at each feed

It is advisable to offer an extra 30 mL at each feed to prevent wind/colic and to account for a baby's growing needs or sudden spurts in growth. Therefore, using the above example a 3-kg baby should be offered 130 mL at each feed. Each baby's feeding schedule should be discussed with the parent/carer. It is usual for a formula-fed baby to have a longer interval between feeds at night-time; therefore, 150 mL offered at 4-hourly intervals during the day may be the normal for a 3-kg baby.

**Practice tip:** It is usefull to mark the feeding chart/fluid balance sheet with an asterisk so that you can plan when each baby is due a feed. For example, if a baby wakes at 06.00 h for their first feed you can predict that the next feeds could be due at approximately 10.00 h, 14.00 h, 18.00 h and 22.00 h. Good time management skills are required if a children's nurse has three or four babies to care for during their shift. It will be necessary to coordinate feeding times and therefore assistance will be required from colleagues or the parent/guardian willing to feed their own child.

## Levels of dehydration

A large percentage (60–80%) of an infant's and child's body is made up of water.[2,18] Therefore dehydration can occur very quickly, especially if the infant or child is not drinking and if vomiting/diarrhoea occurs. The levels of dehydration are classified as mild, moderate or severe (Table 13.4).[2,18]

Rapid disturbance in the fluid and electrolyte balance in young children, along with a high metabolic rate, means that there is a lot of waste to excrete. Even small changes in fluid loss can have a large impact on children. The kidneys are immature, particularly in infancy, and are therefore less effective at concentrating urine.[2] Normal urine output is as follows: children, >1 mL/kg/hour; infants 1–2 mL/kg/hour; neonates, 2 mL/kg/hour.

A blood test for urea and electrolytes (U&E) and blood glucose will aid diagnosis of the level of dehydration. Other blood tests such as a full blood count (FBC) will also be taken to help determine the source of infection as well as a urine sample and perhaps swabs for culture and sensitivity. Blood serum electrolytes should be checked before commencing intravenous (IV) fluids. Repeat blood tests should be carried out following 6 hours of therapy in ill patients or 24 hourly if fluid therapy is being continued.[4]

## Treatment of dehydration

*Oral re-hydration therapy* should rehydrate children presenting with mild to moderate dehydration due to vomiting and diarrhoea. Oral rehydration therapy, such as Rapolyte sachets, have been recommended for infants and children in small but frequent quantities.[18] Following 1–2 hours of nil by mouth, offer the child 5–10 mL of solution every 15–20 minutes. Continual reassessment of the child's condition is important to ensure that he/she is responding to the oral rehydration therapy. Further dehydration or fluid overload would be a complication to avoid.

*Intravenous fluid* bolus and maintenance fluids are usually required to manage children presenting with moderate to severe dehydration in order to restore their circulatory volume.[18] The use of

**Table 13.4** The clinical manifestations of dehydration

| Mild dehydration | Moderate dehydration | Severe dehydration |
|---|---|---|
| 5% loss of body weight | 5–9% loss of body weight | >10% loss of body weight |
| Slightly dry mucous membranes | Increased heart rate | Low blood pressure |
| Slightly decreased urine output | Poor tear production | Anuria (absent urine output) |
| Increased thirst | Decreased skin turgor | Lethargic to comatose |
| Irritable | Sunken eyes | |
| | Sunken fontanel | |
| | Oliguria (decreased urine output) | |
| | Restless to lethargic | |

**Table 13.5** Calculation of intravenous fluids.

| Body weight (kg) | Formula |
|---|---|
| <10 | 100 mL/kg/day |
| 11–20 | 1000 mL + 50 mL/kg per kg over 10 kg |
| >20 | 1500 mL + 20 mL/kg per kg over 20 kg |

0.45% saline (half normal saline) or 0.9% saline (normal saline) with dextrose 5% are suitable maintenance fluids for most children.[4] The prescription of IV fluids is calculated per kilogram of body weight by using the formulae in Table 13.5.

> Example: Annabel weighs 13 kg and is dehydrated. Calculate her replacement fluids.
> 1000 mL + 50 mL +50 mL + 50 mL = 1150 ml: intravenous fluids required.

To calculate the hourly rate of intravenous infusion, divide the daily requirement by 24.

> Example: 1150 mL is Annabel's fluid replacement requirement for 24 hours. The hourly rate will be 47.9 mL per hour or when rounded up 48 mL/hour. 1150/24 = 47.9 or rounded up to 48.

### Measuring fluid balance

All intake and output should be measured if an accurate fluid balance is to be monitored (Table 13.6)[2]. can be taught how to assist nurses with maintaining accurate records if they are shown how to measure all drinks offered to children. This allows them to participate in their child's care.

### Reintroduction of food

Intravenous fluids are prescribed to correct dehydration and to help replace the circulatory volume to normal limits. Dehydration is usually corrected within 24–48 hours of commencing IV fluids. Once administration of IV fluids has been completed and the child is tolerating oral fluids well, food can be re-introduced.[18] Breastfed infants should resume breastfeeding with shorter but more frequent feeds. Full-strength feeds can be offered to bottle-fed infants. Babies require all nutrients to maintain adequate hydration and to grow and develop. Therefore it is important to recommence milk feeding as soon as possible to aid adequate nutrition and growth.[11]

## ENTERAL FEEDING

Oral feeding is advocated as much as possible and any decision regarding delivery of food via enteral methods should always be well planned and discussed with all concerned.[19] Parents/guardians may find it difficult to accept that their child requires enteral feeding.[19] Good communication between the child, parents and healthcare workers about the advantages and disadvantages of the type of feeding method proposed should help to relieve

**Table 13.6** Examples of fluid balance

| Oral Intake | Measure and record all intakes of fluids and liquid food stuffs |
|---|---|
| Intravenous Fluids | Record all inputs of intravenous fluids administered including fluid amounts of antibiotics and normal saline flushes |
| Urine | Should be measured either from a urinary catheter, urinal, bedpan, collection bag or nappy. Nappies can be weighed before and after use and the amount of urine passed is estimated by the difference in nappy weight. The volume of fluid in millilitres is equal to the weight in milligrams |
| Vomit | Should be measured and recorded, noting the colour, e.g. green bile, or if there is undigested food present |
| Other outputs | Include sweating (insensible losses), blood samples taken and any diarrhoea. These losses can only be estimated but never the less should be considered |

anxiety and provide information.

Enteral feeding is indicated for children who are unable to take an adequate amount of nutrition orally.[18] If these children are left without supplemental feeds they will become malnourished and will not thrive physically or developmentally. Malnutrition can be acute or chronic.[2,20] Acute malnutrition usually occurs as a result of illness, e.g. pneumonia. Chronic malnutrition occurs in children with chronic diseases or underlying problems, e.g. cystic fibrosis, congenital heart disease, malignancies and chronic kidney disease.

## Nasogastric feeding

Nasogastric (NG) feeding is probably the most common method of enteral feeding seen in clinical practice and the community.[19] Nasogastric feeding is usually commenced until a decision has been made regarding a more long term-feeding method such as gastrostomy tube feeding. An NG tube can be used to administer medications as well as nutrition. Insertion of an NG tube is a clinical procedure and the nurse who is inserting the NG tube should work within his/her scope of practice. There are two main types of NG tubes: polyvinylchloride (PVC) for short-term use and polyurethane (silk tubes) for more long-term use.[21] There are different sized NG tubes, i.e. French gauge 6, 8 and 10 for children. Some tubes have a guide wire to help pass the NG tube, which is removed once the tube is correctly in place. Check which type and tube size is required for the child with reference to local guidelines and procedures. Children's nurses should refer to their hospital clinical guidelines regarding the insertion of an NG tube.

### Guidelines on the insertion of a nasogastric tube[22]

1 The insertion of an NG tube in a child is an invasive procedure and a traumatic experience, both for the child and parents/guardians. For this reason the assistance of another healthcare worker is necessary to help relax and distract the child. It is unreasonable to expect the parent/guardian to do this. However, this does not mean that the parent/guardian cannot be present for the procedure.[21] Whenever possible explain the procedure to the child and family to reduce any distress.

2 Wash hands dry and put on plastic apron to prevent cross-infection.

3 Clean work surface/trolley/tray according to the Infection Control Policy and wipe down with alcohol wipes. Always allow the surface to dry as it cleanses as it dries.

4 Prepare trolley/tray and place equipment on the clean trolley/tray.

5 Get tape ready.

**Figure 13.4** Measuring tube for (a) children (b) baby. (Reproduced with permission from Bradford and Airedale Teaching Primary Care Trust NHS (2007) Community Children's Team Nasogastric Feeding Policy and Procedure.)

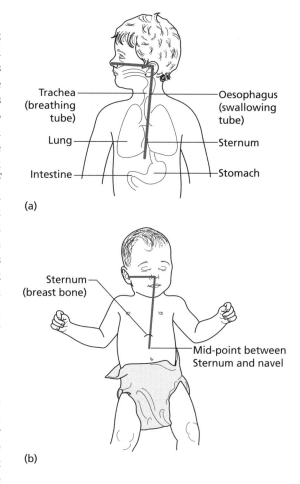

(a)

(b)

6 Have pH indicator strip ready.

7 Take an appropriate sized NG tube out of the sterile packaging. Ensure the tube is not damaged while doing so.

8 Measure the length of tube to be inserted by

placing the tip of the tube at the end of the child's nose. Extend the tube to bottom of the child's earlobe, and then downwards to the end of the xiphoid process.[23] Alternatively measure from the end of the nose to the earlobe and then to a point midway between the xiphoid process and the navel.[21] The black measure mark on the tube will act as a guide as to how much of the tube is to be inserted (Figure 13.4).

9 Position the child so as to access the nostril. Encourage the older child to sit upright in the semi-recumbent position. Sucrose on a soother used with infants along with wrapping the infant in a blanket may provide some comfort.[24]

10 Wash hands thoroughly, dry and put on disposable non-sterile gloves to prevent bacterial contamination of the tube and leakage of body fluids on the hands.

11 Maintain your hold on the end of the tube that remains on the exterior and at the mark at the pre-measured length.

12 Lubricate the end that is passed into the stomach through the nostril with either KY gel or water.

13 Gently pass the tube into the child's nostril. Angle the tube slightly upwards and gently guide it over the back of the nose into the nasopharynx.

14 Continue to pass the tube downwards. As the tube gets to the back of the child's throat, the child will gag. At this stage encourage a baby to suck on a soother or try to persuade the older child to have a sip of water or swallow. Be aware of the child's fasting status. Advance the tube as the child swallows. This will help ease any discomfort and reduce the risk of the tube passing into the trachea.

15 When the pre-measured mark on the tube reaches the child's nostril, the end of the tube should be in the stomach.

16 Securely attach the tube to the child's cheek with adhesive tape/tegaderm.

17 Check the correct position of the NG tube. Recent research shows the use of auscultation using air (via a syringe) and a stethoscope is no longer acceptable to confirm the position of the NG tube.[25]

18 Connect a 5-mL syringe to the tube and withdraw on the plunger gently, creating gentle suction, until fluid appears in the syringe. Only

a small amount of fluid is required, 0.5–1mL, to confirm the position of the NG tube using the pH indicator strips.

19 If no fluid is obtained, try changing the child's position and aspirating again. Give the child a small drink if it is safe to do so and the child is not fasting.

20 If it is still difficult to obtain an aspirate, the tube may need to be withdrawn a little or passed further in order to obtain an acidic aspirate. It may be necessary to obtain an X-ray to determine the position of the tube.[21]

21 When satisfied the tube is in the correct position, remove the guide wire if one has been used.

22 Close off end of tube with a spigot or attach to feeding equipment.

23 Document the date and time of insertion and the type of tube used in the child's nursing care plan or clinical notes.

### Checking the position of a nasogastric tube

It is very important to check the position of the NG tube prior to administering any medications or nutrition. The tube can become dislodged by coughing or vomiting and there is a risk that the medicine or feed could go into the patient's lungs instead of their stomach.[25] It is important to check if the child is receiving any medication that could alter the pH of the aspirate giving a false reading. The most reliable bedside check to confirm the position of an NG tube is to measure the pH (acidity/alkalinity) of the patient's stomach contents using pH indicator strips or paper.[25,26]

### Procedure for checking gastric pH aspirate

1 Wash hands, dry and put on plastic apron to prevent cross-infection.

2 Remove the cap or disconnect the tube from feeding equipment.

3 Attach a syringe containing air (1–5 mL for infants and children) into the feeding tube to remove any water or feed from the tube.

4 Draw back the syringe to obtain contents from the stomach (aspirating the tube).

5 Take the pH strip/paper and place a few drops of the stomach contents onto it

6 Match the colour change of the strip/paper with the colour code on the box to identify the pH of the stomach contents

7 A pH reading of 5.5 or 5 indicates an acid reaction, which means the tube is correctly positioned in the stomach.[25,26]

8 If an aspirate is not obtained after following the above directions it may be necessary to reposition the patient on to their side. If the patient can drink, offer a drink, wait a few minutes then try the procedure again.

9 If an aspirate is still not available the tube may need to be repositioned or repassed. An X-ray to confirm position prior to feeding may be necessary.

If at any stage during the feed the child becomes distressed, e.g. difficulty with breathing, stop the feed and check the position of the NG tube. Medical assistance will be required.[11] Document all procedures in the child's nursing and clinical notes. The NG tube position should always be checked following insertion and before administering medication or enteral feed. Tube position should also be checked at least once daily during continuous feeds.[25] The NG tube should be flushed well with sterile water following feeding and administration of each drug to help keep the tube clear and prevent blockage.[21] The enteral feed should be prepared, checked and administered in a similar way to any medication, i.e. checked independently by two nurses, at least one a registered nurse.[22] Check local policy regarding procedures to follow when administering enteral feed in your hospital. Enteral feeds are usually administered through a pump, so preparation and checking of equipment prior to administration of the feed is necessary. Again two nurses, at least one a registered nurse, should check the rate and duration of the enteral feed to be administered via a pump.[21]

## Orogastric feeding

Orogastric feeding may be selected over nasogastric feeding for some infants and preterm infants. Coordination of sucking and swallowing and coordination of breathing is not well established before 35 weeks' gestation.[14] Therefore tube feeding rather than breast- or bottle feeding is advocated in preterm infants. Infants use only their nose to breath so a tube in their nose could partially block air entry. Therefore an orogastric tube rather than an NG tube may be more appropriate for preterm infants who are ventilated or receiving oxygen nasally. Introducing feeds especially expressed breastmilk via the gastrointestinal tract rather than parenteral feeding has shown to be advantageous and may reduce the incidence of bowel complications in newborns, e.g. necrotising enterocolitis.[14] The care and management of an infant with an orogastric tube for feeding is very similar to the care and management of a child with an NG tube. However, the orogastric tube is difficult to secure in position as babies can chew and suck on it, displacing it from the stomach.[14]

## Nasojejunal feeding

Nasojejunal feeding may be indicated for children at high risk for regurgitation or aspiration such as those on ventilation or suffering from brain injury.[27] It is also a method of introducing early milk feeds to low birthweight babies to enhance their weight gain.[14] Diminished gastric motility in critically ill children means NG or oral feeding is usually poorly tolerated.[28] Insertion of a nasoduodenal or nasojejunal tube is usually carried out by a doctor because of the risk of bowel perforation at insertion as it involves using a stylet to help introduce the nasojejunal tube.[27] Confirmation of correct nasojejunal tube placement is by X-ray. A nasojejunal tube is passed via the nose into the stomach and time is allowed for gastric emptying to enable the tube to pass through the pylorus. Confirmation of tube position at the bedside prior to feeding or administering any medications is similar to obtaining confirmation of NG tube position. Aspirate from a nasojejunal tube is alkaline and therefore gives a pH reading of between 6 and 8. It is important to check if the child is receiving any medication that could alter the pH of the aspirate. Complications of nasojejunal tube feeding include abdominal pain and diarrhoea from bolus feeding because the stomach's natural reservoir and anti-infective properties are bypassed.[21]

## Gastrostomy feeding

Gastrostomy feeding is used for children who require long-term administration of enteral feeds either as a supplement, e.g. children with cystic fibrosis, or for full nutritional requirements, e.g. children with an absent gag reflex.[1] Insertion of a gastrostomy tube is a surgical technique requiring the child to undergo a general anaesthetic, or percutaneous procedure using an endoscope under local anaesthetic. There are many different types of gastrostomy tubes that can be inserted through the child's abdominal wall, giving direct access to the stomach for enteral feeding. The two main types are balloon catheters and button devices.

### Balloon catheters

Balloon catheters have a balloon at the distal end, which is inflated with water and pulled up against the wall of the stomach thus maintaining its position as well as preventing leakage of gastric contents.[1] The sterile water in the balloon should be changed weekly. Some gastrostomy tubes have a securing device that lies against the skin to prevent excessive traction on the tube causing soreness or widening of the opening. Some tubes may need to be taped to the body. The disadvantage to having a balloon catheter-type gastrostomy tube is that the tube can be seen on the child's body surface all of the time. However a balloon catheter gastrostomy tube can be changed to a button device at a later stage (Figure 13.5).

### Button device

A button device (Figure 13.6) can be inserted after a balloon catheter gastrostomy, once an established tract has been created.[1] A button device is inserted via percutaneous endoscopic gastrostomy (PEG) under local anesthetic. The advantage of a button device is that it can't be easily seen on a child's body because it is positioned at skin level. Another advantage is that a one-way valve built into the button device prevents leakage even when the button is opened.

### General care and management

Reference to local policy or guidelines regarding the care and management of children requiring gastrostomy feeding is required.

The following information is a guide only for the general care and management of a child with a gastrostomy.

#### Site cleansing

- Following initial insertion (24 hours) of the gastrostomy tube/button, cleanse the stoma site gently with warm soapy water as per normal hygiene needs daily.[2]

**Figure 13.5** A balloon catheter gastrostomy tube. PEG, percutaneous endoscopic gastrostomy.

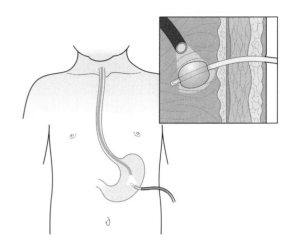

**Figure 13.6 (a)** A button device and **(b)** its appearance on the body surface.

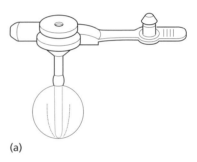

(a)

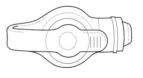

(b)

#### Balloon care

- Check and change the fluid in the balloon weekly or as per instructions.
- Deflate the balloon by aspirating the fluid with an empty syringe. Usually 5–10 mL of sterile water is sufficient to ensure correct reinflation of the balloon.

### Tube/button care

- Following the initial period of insertion and removal of anchoring suture (approx. 2 weeks after insertion). rotate the tubing or button 360° daily to prevent pressure sore development.[2,7]

### Feeding

1 Check and confirm position of the gastrostomy tube/button prior to administering any medications or feed. Similar to checking/confirming position of an NG tube, gastrostomy tube aspirate is acidic so therefore gastric aspirate should read below 5.5 on pH paper.
2 It is important to flush the tube well after each medication and feed to prevent blockage and to ensure all the contents reach the stomach as intended.[2]
3 The dietician is responsible for the calorific requirements and the number of feeds required for each child. Therefore liaise with the dietician and consult the notes for each child requiring gastrostomy feeding.
4 Bolus or continuous feeds can be prescribed. Night feeds are commonly prescribed for children with cystic fibrosis who require supplementation. However, night feeds can deter from a normal daily eating pattern so sometimes bolus feeds during the day time and a rest period at night time is better for children only requiring supplemental feeds.[7] Continuous feeds are often tolerated better by infants with rest periods during the day to allow for some activity. It is important to listen to each child's and parent's needs when planning a feeding regime.
5 Most gastrostomy feeds are delivered through a feeding pump such as a kangaroo. However, gravity feeding is also performed. If gravity feeding is used, it might be necessary to give a gentle push with a plunger to allow feed to flow into the stomach initially. If using a pump, check that the rate of administration is set correctly and monitor it closely.
6 Document amount infused on fluid balance or feeding charts.
7 Change administration tubing and feeding bags every 24 hours or according to local policy.
8 Pour feed into syringe or feeding bag and prime tubing before connecting to the patient for administration. If gravity feeding via a syringe, clamp tube when filling the syringe to avoid air entering the stomach.

### Potential complications of a gastrostomy

- *Choking*: Always supervise a child or infant receiving a gravity feed and monitor closely a child receiving a feed through a pump. A feeding tube can inadvertently become misplaced during feeding causing the feed to reflux or be administered into the lungs. Stop the feed immediately if the child experiences any difficulties such as coughing, cyanosis or respiratory distress.
- *Infection*: Observe for any signs of gastrostomy site infection such as inflammation, redness, swelling, pain or discharge. Report and document any signs of infection to the surgical team.
- *Tolerance of feeds*: An infant or child should always be monitored regarding their tolerance of feeds. Assess for any signs of diarrhoea. Possible causes of diarrhoea include infection, high osmolar feeds or medications. Be careful to administer feeds at room temperature, i.e. not cold, and to administer feeds slowly to avoid 'dumping syndrome'.[2]
- *Discomfort*: Abdominal distension may be relieved temporarily by aspirating air via the gastrostomy or venting the tube. Note the amount and colour of aspirates. Any abnormal aspirate such as bile or blood must be reported to the doctor immediately.
- *Blockage*: This is best avoided by flushing the tube well after feed and medications or 4–6 hourly during continuous feeding. Ensure only liquid medications are administered via gastrostomy if at all possible. If a tube does become blocked, administration of some warm water or a fizzy fluid such as 7-Up should help unblock tubing. If not seek medical assistance.
- *Over-granulation*: This can sometimes occur at stoma site. Skin will appear red, raised and lumpy. Silver nitrate sticks maybe prescribed as treatment.
- *Dislodgement*: Accidental dislodgement can occur in children! If a tube is pulled out, insert a replacement tube into the stoma as soon as possible to avoid closure of the tract.

## TOTAL PARENTERAL NUTRITION

Total parenteral nutrition (TPN) consists of nutrients in liquid form, such as amino acids, glucose, electrolytes, vitamins, minerals, trace elements and lipids. TPN is delivered to the child through a central or peripheral catheter. Line selection is dependent on the composition of the solution. Peripheral administration of TPN may not be greater than 10% of dextrose concentration because of the risk of vein sclerosis or burns if extravasation occurs.[21] Therefore administration of TPN is more commonly infused via a central vein cannula with a dedicated line for TPN.[1] TPN is made to order by pharmacy staff under strict asepsis. It is the most expensive and complex form of artificial nutrition.[14]

TPN is used to maintain nutrition for those unable to use the gastrointestinal tract for feeding such as children with short bowel syndrome. TPN can be used temporarily to rest the bowel during the incidence of necrotising enterocolitis (NEC) or Crohn's disease. The main complications of TPN are cholestatic jaundice and catheter-related sepsis.[14] Prevention of complications can be minimised by careful monitoring and management of a child on TPN. In particular it is important to prevent infection, vascular injury and electrolyte and glucose imbalance.[18]

## General principles regarding the care of a child prescribed TPN

1 Leave bag of TPN at room temperature for at least 30 minutes prior to administration

2 The contents of the TPN bag should be checked carefully against the prescription prior to preparation and administration.

3 Checking should be carried out by two nurses, one of whom should be a registered nurse. Cross-checking the bag content against the prescription, patient details, expiry date and that the bag is fully intact is important to avoid any mistakes or contamination risk.

4 Wash and dry hands using aseptic technique and put on sterile gloves to prevent cross-infection.

5 Clean the bag connection site well with an alcohol wipe and allow it to dry prior to spiking it with the administration set.

6 Prime all tubing with the TPN or lipid solutions. Lipids are often given separately because of the child's ability to metabolise fats and because of the risk of fat embolism.[1] Sometimes lipids can't be given for medical reasons such as sepsis,

jaundice or respiratory distress.

7 Administer TPN though a pump, taking care to set the correct rate of administration. TPN should be stopped only gradually, i.e. by reducing the rate for an hour or two before stopping it altogether. This is to prevent hypoglycaemia.

8 The TPN bag should be covered to protect it from sunlight as additives can degrade in sunlight.[21]

9 The child should be monitored closely while receiving TPN. There should be hourly observation of the cannula site and rate of administration; 4-hourly observations of temperature, pulse and respirations; and 6-hourly monitoring of blood glucose via a glucometer to detect any possible complications. Daily urinalysis for glucose, ketones and pH is recommended.

10 Routine blood tests for urea and electrolytes and lipid index are carried out daily initially, then twice weekly to ensure correct prescription for child's needs. A full blood count should be taken weekly to detect any signs of infection. Careful monitoring of the child's liver function (LFTs) is also required so that staff can be alerted to any risk of failing liver function associated with long-term TPN administration.

11 TPN bag, lipids and administration sets should be changed every 24 hours to prevent infection.

12 Remember to offer mouth care and encourage teeth brushing, especially for infants or children nil by mouth. A pacifier may help to encourage oro-motor skills development in infants.[21]

13 TPN is often delivered during the night with a break scheduled during the day time to allow for some activity.

## PH STUDIES

A pH study involves the insertion of a pH probe by a doctor or appropriately trained nurse. pH studies detect acid gastric juices with the help of a digitrapper, which records the frequency and duration of any gastro-oesophageal reflux (GOR) present. The role of the children's nurse on the ward is to ensure that the child and parent/guardian have been appropriately prepared for the procedure. The children's nurse can also explain to the parent/guardian how to document relevant information on the activity record sheet.

A pH study lasts 16–24 hours and its primary purpose is to confirm the presence or absence of GOR and to determine its severity.[18,29] GOR is the involuntary passage of gastric contents into the oesophagus. Other reasons for carrying out pH studies may include the following:[29]

- symptoms of GOR, i.e. vomiting, regurgitation, failure to thrive or feeding difficulties;
- recurrent chest infections;
- recurrent wheeze;
- apnoea (episodes of non-breathing);
- prior to nissen fundoplication (asurgical procedure to correct GOR).

The children's nurse can assist in the care and management of a child undergoing a pH study by considering the following needs.[18,29]

- Nursing assessment of the child upon admission or presentation to a clinic should include a description of their clinical symptoms and difficulties.
- Information about their normal feeding pattern at home should be documented.
- Checking when the child last received anything to eat or drink. The child may need to fast for a period (usually 2 hours) prior to commencing the study.
- Observing the child's weight, height, temperature, pulse and respiratory rate.
- Checking when the child last received any medications. Medications such as omeprazole should not be administered for up to 10 days prior to carrying out a pH study because it will interfere with the results.
- Checking local guidelines or policy regarding what food and drink a child is permitted during the study. Milk tends to neutralise stomach contents so it might be discouraged during the study as it could interfere with the results. Apple juice can increase the acidity so drinking this might be encouraged during the study to help detect if GOR is occurring.
- Documenting the time the pH probe is inserted and when the study is commenced. Documenting how the child tolerated the procedure. Also documenting the time the study ends.
- Checking that all equipment is intact and appears to be functioning during the pH study.
- Helping the child and parent/guardian to complete the activity sheet as part of the study. If the child complains of any symptoms such as heartburn or vomits, note the time it occurred and what the child was doing when it occurred, i.e. resting or playing.
- Informing the doctor or specialist nurse immediately if there are any concerns about the child's condition during the study.

## CONCLUSION

This chapter has outlined the main components of infant and child feeding applicable to children's nurses. Nutrional assessment is routinely carried out by nurses during the admission stage when a child presents to hospital. Therefore children's nurses must be familiar with the expected normal diet of an infant/child in their care. The principles involved in caring for children requiring enteral or parenteral nutrition have been discussed. Further practice and experience in aspects of care will be required.

Appropriate referral of children to the relevant community personnel such as the community nurse should be considered for children due to be discharged home on enteral or parenteral feeding.

 Go to the website to find the PowerPoint presentation for this chapter and MCQs to test your knowledge. **www.hodderplus.com/childnursingskills**

# REFERENCES

1   Moules T, Ramsay J (2008) *The textbook of children's and young people's nursing*, 2nd Edition. Oxford: Blackwell Publishing.

2   Ferguson D (2008) *Clinical assessment and monitoring in children*. Oxford: Blackwell Publishing.

3   Coben D, Atere-Roberts E (2005) *Calculations for nursing and healthcare*, 2nd edition. China: Palgrave Macmillan.

4   National Children's Hospital Clinical Guidelines Committee (2006) *Guideline on IV fluids for children*. Unpublished document.

5   Advanced Life Support Group (2005) *Advanced paediatric life support: the practical approach*, 4th edition. Oxford: BMJ Books.

6   Hoey H, Tanner J, Cox L (1986) *Irish clinical growth standards*. Hertford: Castlemead Publications.

7   Hockenberry M, Wilson D, Winkelstein M, *et al.* (2003) *Wong's nursing care of infants and children*, 7th edition. St Louis: Mosby.

8   World Health Organization (2002) *WHO Global strategy for infant and young child feeding, the optimal duration of breastfeeding*. 55th World Health Assembly, May 2002. (www.who.int/child-adolescent-health/NUTRITION/complementary.htm).

9   Health Service Executive (2008) *The evidence for breastfeeding: factsheet 01*. www.hse.ie (accessed September 2008).

10  National Children's Hospital (2008) *Nursing care plan: supporting breastfeeding relationship between mother child*. Dublin: AMNCH (unpublished).

11  Dunne T, Farrell P, Kelly, V (2008) *Feed your child well: a handbook for parents in Ireland*. Dublin: A. A. Farmar.

12  UNICEF UK Baby Friendly Initiative (2005) *Sterilising baby feeding equipment*. London: UNICEF.

13  UNICEF UK Baby Friendly Initiative (2005) *Preparing a bottle feed using baby milk powder*. London: UNICEF.

14  Yeo, H (1998) *Nursing the neonate*. Oxford: Blackwell Science.

15  Health Services Executive (2006) *Starting to spoonfeed your baby*. Dublin: HSE.

16  Food Standards Agency (2008) *Feeding your baby in the first year*. www.eatwell.gov.uk/yourbaby (accessed 30 July 2008).

17  Health Services Executive (2006) *Food for young children*. Dublin: HSE.

18  Bowden VR, Greenberg CS (2003) *Pediatric nursing procedures*. London: Lippincott Williams Wilkins.

19  Hunt F (2007) Changing from oral to enteral feeding: impact on families of children with disabilities. *Paediatric Nursing* **19**(7): 30–32.

20  Koen FM, Hulst JM. Hulst, J (2008) Prevalence of malnutrition in pediatric hospital patients. *Current Opinion in Pediatrics* **20**(5): 590–596.

21  Trigg E, Mohammed TA (2006) *Practices in children's nursing: guidelines for hospital and community*, 2nd edition. London: Churchill Livingstone.

22  National Children's Hospital (AMNCH) (2008) *Guidelines on the insertion of and feeding through nasogastric tubes in children*. Unpublished.

23  Wikipedia (2007) *Nasogastric intubation*. http//en.wikipedia.org/wiki/Nasogastric_intubation (accessed 29 May 2007).

24  Kids Health Info for Parents (2006) Royal Children's Hospital, Melbourne. www.rch.org.au/kidsinfo/factsheets.cfm?doc_id=9766 (accessed 26 May 2009).

25  National Patient Safety Agency (2005) *Patient and carer briefing: checking the position of nasogastric feeding tubes*. London: NHS

26  Wilkes-Holmes C (2006) Safe placement of nasogastric tubes in children. *Paediatric Nursing* **18**(9): 14–17.

27  Wilson D, Hockenberry MJ (2008) *Wong's clinical manual of pediatric nursing*, 7th edition. St Louis: Mosby Elsevier.

28  McDermott A, Tomkins N, Lasonbys, G (2007) Nasojejunal tube placement in paediatric intensive care. *Paediatric Nursing* **19**(2): 26–28.

29  National Children's Hospital (2008) Guidelines on the management of the child who requires pH studies to be performed at the National Children's Hospital. Unpublished.

# FURTHER READING

Bradford and Airedale Teaching Primary Care Trust NHS (2007) Community children's team nasogastric feeding policy and procedure. www.bradfordairedale-pct.nhs.uk/NR/rdonlyes/D5A63A4C-87E6–42BC-A8DO-2BA0222412BE/60470/NGPolicy2008.doc (accessed 17 October 2008).

Lang, S (2003) *Breastfeeding special care babies*, 2nd edition. London: Baillière Tindall.

# Promoting children's continence

## A) Enuresis

Diane Atwill, Mary Booy and Lubna Ezad

## LEARNING OUTCOMES

*Upon completion of the chapter, the reader should be able to accomplish the following:*

1 Understand the definition of enuresis
2 Identify key factors of childhood incontinence
3 Undertake an assessment of incontinence using appropriate questioning techniques
4 Gain knowledge of management and appropriate treatment options
5 Become aware of the psychosocial effects of incontinence on the child and family

## CHAPTER OVERVIEW

The negative impact of bedwetting on the lives of children and their families cannot be underestimated. The condition is not openly discussed and children feel low self-esteem, and parents experience embarrassment and despair. Research has shown that many children feel 'different' and fear being 'discovered' by others.[1]

Parents become frustrated and feel helpless too; these pressures can lead to an increase in the risk of emotional and physical abuse.[2]

Continence problems are extremely common in childhood, and it is estimated that about 500 000 children and young people over 7 years of age in the UK regularly wet the bed.[3] A significant number of these children have a daytime wetting problem. It is clear that early intervention, using the right treatment approach, not only reduces the risks to the child but also is a cost-effective solution to what could become a long-term problem. With no intervention, the rate of natural resolution is slow; each year only one in seven or eight children (of all ages) will find that their bedwetting naturally resolves.[4]

A community-based enuresis service can and does play a key role in treating these children and supporting their families; it is in this environment that specialist nurse-led treatment and counselling makes a major impact on the condition. Although the child is seen as an individual, the whole family

## Definition

**Enuresis:** in the absence of congenital or acquired defects of the nervous system or urinary tract, an involuntary discharge of urine by day or night, or both, in a child aged 5 years or older.

**Nocturnal enuresis** (bedwetting): a lack of night time bladder control. This condition can be subdivided into primary nocturnal enuresis, which affects those children who have never achieved dryness, or secondary nocturnal enuresis, which is loss of control after a significant period of being dry, usually one year or more.

**Diurnal enuresis:** lack of daytime bladder control.

is dealt with, all members taking some responsibility for the management of the bedwetting problem.

## PHYSIOLOGY OF ACHIEVING CONTINENCE

A variety of skills are required to achieve total continence. To understand enuresis, we must look at normal bladder function and how bladder control is achieved.

In a baby the bladder is controlled by a simple reflex arc: as the bladder fills the stretch receptors in the bladder wall (detrusor muscle) send messages to the spinal cord (sacral bladder centre) which return to the detrusor to ensure it stays relaxed and to the sphincter so it remains tightly closed. When the bladder reaches its capacity, messages to contract are relayed along the spinal cord to the detrusor, the sphincter relaxes and the bladder empties.

For a child to achieve control a sequence of events must take place.

The child will

- be aware of wetting;
- become aware of the sensations just before he or she wets;
- understand that other people want them to communicate this in some way;
- inhibit the relaxation of his or her sphincter long enough to reach a potty/toilet;
- relax his or her sphincter when on the potty/toilet.

The nerve pathways are developed at around 18 months of age, but the emotional maturity to link the processes together does not often come before 20 months.

Achieving night continence requires either the child to learn to wake to a full bladder, or develop a bladder that has a large enough capacity to hold properly concentrated urine overnight and until the child wakes in the morning.

## CAUSES OF CHILDHOOD INCONTINENCE

- Any disruption to bladder and urinary anatomy or bladder nerve supply will prevent the

development of the normal bladder cycle and lead to wetting, for example spina bifida.
- Any child with a learning or physical disability may have delay or inability to achieve continence.
- Medical causes predisposing/contributing to incontinence include diabetes, recurrent urinary tract infection (UTI) and constipation
- Some children with incontinence have overactive bladders. Here the detrusor muscle contracts involuntarily at low volumes or urine in the bladder, leading to sphincter relaxation and urinary leakage.
- Recognised inheritance patterns and gene markers in children with night wetting are being discovered for primary nocturnal enuresis (PNE, chromosomes 4, 8,12,13, and 22). Studies show that there is a 40 per cent likelihood of a child wetting the bed if one parent did, rising to 77 per cent where it is both parents.

## ASSESSMENT OF INCONTINENCE USING APPROPRIATE QUESTIONING TECHNIQUES

Assessment is the key to deciding what management or treatment programme to use. The following questions will help in the assessment process. (Table 14.1)

### Examination

A full neurological, abdominal examination and general examination, including blood pressure, needs to be done to ensure no underlying cause has been missed, such as spina bifida occulta, renal disease or constipation.

## MANAGEMENT AND APPROPRIATE TREATMENT OPTIONS

The model most widely used to help identify and diagnose bedwetting is Richard Butler's *Three systems approach* (Table 14.2).[7]

This is a useful way of understanding nocturnal enuresis by envisaging it as a problem in one or more of the following systems:

- lack of vasopressin release;
- a problem of bladder stability;

**Table 14.1** Assessing incontinence

| Questions | Rationale |
| --- | --- |
| 1 The age when first seen with a continence problem | How long has the child had the problem? |
| 2 Who makes up the family | What are the family dynamics? |
| 3 Family history of enuresis | 77 per cent chance of having nocturnal enuresis if both parents previously suffered and 40 per cent chance if one parent did |
| 4 Medical history, general health, developmental history | Child's ability to be continent |
| 5 Any stressful events, school problems, family circumstances | Psychological influence on continence |
| 6 Child's view of their condition | Is the child keen and motivated to take an active part in the treatment? |
| 7 What re the parents' view and attitude to their child's condition | Are the parents supportive or potentially intolerant? This can change the outcome and choice of treatment |
| 8 Toilet facilities both at home and at school | An important factor which can subconsciously affect the child's willingness to use the toilet |
| 9 Fluid intake: what they drink; how much and when | Any drink containing caffeine should be avoided as it is a diuretic. Some fizzy drinks and blackcurrant drinks can irritate the bladder. A child or young person should be drinking around seven to eight glasses of fluid daily. The fluid intake should be spread evenly through the day, and not be upped just before bedtime |
| 10 Voiding pattern | To look at frequency, urgency and voided volumes |
| 11 Bowel pattern | Constipation plays a big part in a child's ability to empty their bladder completely; constipation irritates the bladder, and predisposes to urinary tract infections |
| 12 What previous management methods have been tried | If something has been done before and has been unsuccessful it can put the child and parent off trying it again |
| **Investigation** | **Rationale** |
| • Urine test or diabetes | Used to exclude infection, renal pathology, |
| • Renal tract ultrasound scan Gauge bladder capacity and post-micturition residue | Used to look for any renal or bladder pathology |
| • Other renal imaging | As clinically indicated |

- an inability to wake from sleep to full bladder sensations.

A child needs only to wake to void when either of the two other systems are ineffective. Parents and children can believe that night wetting occurs because the child sleeps deeply. Sleep patterns are no different from those of children who do not have enuresis. Bedwetting can occur at all stages of sleep. Wetting episodes appear independent of the sleep stage because of the child's inability to arouse from sleep when the bladder is full.

## Selecting treatment interventions

Before engaging in treatment a range of issues should be considered. They include parental intolerance, goal setting, motivation and preferences.

**Table 14.2** The clinical benefits of the Three systems approach

---

- Provides an explanation for children and parents. This is often the first time that the ongoing problem begins to make sense to them

- Helps the assessment process. The model generates questions and a focus on clinical signs that highlight which aspect or part of the system is failing to function effectively

- Following the assessment, the model enables the appropriate treatment interventions to be selected to address the child's difficulty

- [a] Having an understanding as to why a particular treatment might be advocated improves the family's compliance with treatment

- Because the model emphasises the child's difficulty in acquiring processes that are outside his or her control it avoids any blame being attached to the child

**System 1: Lack of vasopressin release[8]**

Arginine vasopressin (AVP) is produced in the hypothalamus and stored in the posterior pituitary. Normally when a child is asleep the pituitary gland releases more AVP, which acts directly on the kidney to reduce the amount of urine produced at night. Children producing insufficient AVP produce excess urine and the bladder capacity may be exceeded and the child may wet

*Clinical signs of low AVP:*
- Wetting soon after going to sleep
- Consistently large wet patches
- Dry nights occur only when the child wakes for the toilet

**System 2: Bladder instability and low voiding volumes[9]**

In order to function appropriately, the bladder needs to be stable while filling (by keeping the detrusor muscle relaxed) and have a reasonably large capacity. Research has indicated that about one-third of children with nocturnal enuresis had uninhibited contractions during the filling phase, resulting in wetting before the bladder was full[19]

*Clinical signs of bladder instability:*
- Frequent day time voiding (more than seven times a day)
- A sense of urgency
- Unsuccessful holding manoeuvres
- Low or variable functional bladder capacity
- Small voiding volume
- Multiple wetting at night
- Variable size of wet patch
- Waking after wetting

**System 3: An inability to arouse from sleep to full bladder sensations[10]**

Children who wet the bed find it very difficult to wake up to bladder signals

*Degrees of arousability can be determined clinically by:*
- How often the child wakes from sleep and voids in the toilet
- How often the child wakes to external signals (sounds) or internal signals (self-instructions, anxiety or excitement
- The child's own comments can provide an indication of rousability or reluctance to wake

---

## General advice

- Adequate fluid intake throughout the day. Increasing the fluid intake dilutes the urine. This helps reduce the incidence of urinary tract infections and improves bladder function.
- Keep the perineum clean and dry, avoid bubbles in the bath and apply barrier cream as necessary; this will help to avoid stinging when voiding. The child is then more likely to know when to use the toilet.
- Treating constipation by dietary advice and medication prevents irregular bowel actions that can irritate the bladder and increase day time frequency and urgency.
- Establishing a regular toilet routine. This should include set toilet times and discourage holding. A vibrating wristwatch alarm or a reminder on a mobile phone can prompt regular voiding.

The recommended intakes of water for children are shown in Table 14.3. Higher levels of total intakes of water would be required for children who are physically active or exposed to hot environments.

**Table 14.2** Recommended adequate intake of water: children[14]

|  | Age (years) | Total water intake per day (including water contained in food) (L) | Water obtained from drinks per day (L) |
|---|---|---|---|
| Children | 1–3 | 1.3 | 0.9 |
| Children | 4–8 | 1.7 | 1.2 |
| Boys | 9–13 | 2.4 | 1.8 |
| Girls | 9–13 | 2.1 | 1.6 |
| Boys | 14–18 | 3.3 | 2.6 |
| Girls | 14–18 | 2.3 | 1.8 |

## Lack of vasopressin release

Children who clinically show low levels of AVP can be prescribed oral desmopressin (Desmotab® or Desmomelt®). Desmopressin is an analogue of the natural form of arginine vasopressin. It has an antidiuretic action, decreases urine production and increases urine concentration.

## Bladder instability

A treatment programme designed to reduce bladder instability includes

- increasing day time fluid intake;
- learning to void immediately once the sensation occurs;
- voiding every 2–3 hours, or at break times when at school. This establishes cognitive control over voiding;
- using anticholinergic drugs, e.g. oxybutynin, relaxes the detrusor muscle in the bladder and enables the bladder to become stable, to function appropriately and have a reasonable functional capacity;
- treating constipation: this will remove pressure and irritation to the bladder.

Methods used to encourage waking if there is an inability to arouse from sleep to full bladder sensations are listed below.

- Enuresis alarm: this alarm can be used as bed or body alarm. It works by the child awaking to the noise or vibration of the alarm sensor as the child begins to urinate. This helps the child wake up and hold on. Signs of improvement are that the wet patches become smaller and smaller and the child eventually wakes before wetting or sleeps through the night.
- Practising using the alarm before sleeping by lying on the bed, imagining sleeping, the alarm going off and the child waking up and going to the toilet.
- Positive self-reminders to stay dry before sleeping. The child should never think wet.
- A child should not rely on being taken to the toilet in the night (lifting), although it may result in a dry bed. This may delay the child's ability to develop control, as a child does not learn to associate waking up with the feeling of a full bladder.

Other medications are listed below.

- Antibiotics are used to treat urinary tract infections. Prophylactic antibiotics (a small daily dose of antibiotic) are occasionally used for the child who is prone to frequent urinary tract infections.
- Laxatives are used to treat constipation.
- Anticholinergic medication can be used to relax the detrusor muscle in the bladder; oxybutynin is usually recommended as it helps decrease detrusor hyperactivity and increases functional bladder capacity, by relaxing the bladder muscle, as the bladder fills with urine.

## Benefits of a dry bed

- Self-esteem and confidence improve and children feel more inclined to join in with social activities.[11]

- Parents also feel the benefit, not just in reduced laundry and financial savings but also in their own emotional state.[12]
- A reduction in parental intolerance has been shown to occur when children overcome their night wetting.

Treatment is considered successful if:[13]

- initially an achievement of 14 consecutive dry nights within a 16-week treatment period;

- relapse is more than two wet nights in a 2-week period;
- continued success: no relapse in the 6 months following initial success;
- complete success: a 2-year period with no relapse after initial success.

Figure 14.1 shows the information above as a diagram.

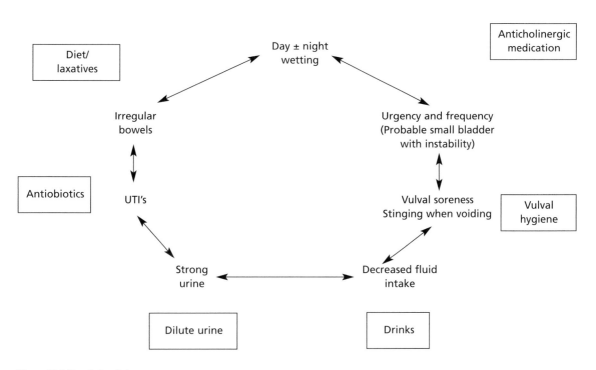

**Figure 14.1** The circle of change.

## Referral to tertiary services

At any stage through the assessment process, from the initial interview when the child's medical history is taken and at each stage of the care plan, if it appears that it is not appropriate for treatment and support to take place within the community setting, then immediate referral to tertiary intervention is an option. This referral can take a variety of forms: from a one-off meeting with a consultant for reassurance and return to the community to one of shared care between consultant and community; to an assumption of total care, perhaps because the condition is so complex, by a consultant urologist or nephrologist.

# PSYCHOSOCIAL EFFECTS OF INCONTINENCE ON THE CHILD AND FAMILY

Bedwetting is one of the commonest and most frustrating disorders of childhood.

Negative psychosocial consequences are common among children being secondary to the impact the condition has on family members and others. The child with wetting problems may be at increased risk for emotional or even physical abuse from family members and may experience stress related to fear of detection by peers.[15] These factors contribute to the loss of self-esteem that the child often experiences.

The effect of enuresis on a family is major, and research has shown that bedwetting is the second most commonly stated reason, after persistent crying, for non-accidental injury in children.[16]

It is interesting to note that stressful early life events can trigger bedwetting; however, most children who are incontinent of urine do not present with more emotional problems than non-bedwetters, and any differences seen may be the result, not the cause, of the wetting problem.[17]

There is no doubt, however, that the levels of stress and anxiety within the family unit are high and get higher as the condition worsens. As the condition escalates the child spirals down towards an emotional low, with parents feeling frustrated, helpless and financially penalised: it has been estimated that laundry bills associated with a child who wets the bed every night costs a family an extra £26 a week.

It is vitally important before embarking on a care plan that the following issues should be considered:

- the child's motivation
- parent/carer motivation
- the child's preferences
- parent/carer preferences
- parental/carer intolerance (It may be that parents are more concerned about themselves than the child, or that the bedwetting is caused by the child's behaviour or that the bedwetting is controllable and that the child is lazy or doesn't care and that a parent is prepared to punish a child.)
- tasks that are achievable set against realistic goals[18].

Motivation steers and very much guides behaviour in certain directions rather than others. For example, a choice might have to be made about eating food if hungry against finding shelter if one is cold and wet. Similarly, a child with enuresis has to deal with a motive that is essentially unlearned, i.e. a desire to become dry at night, and which relates to that individual alone.

A fundamental action for the healthcare professional who is introducing a care plan is to identify the child's motivational issues and, indeed, those of the parent/carer when considering its implementation.

A close look at how parents are coping with the condition is one of the first steps on the road to dryness. It is important that both parents are in harmony about the way they are dealing with the condition at home. It is not sufficient for one parent to be supportive and caring towards the child while the other is harbouring aggression, anxiety and other negative attitudes towards the child's behaviour. The feelings and views of the extended family are also vital if success is to be achieved. How a sibling deals with, and understands, a brother or sister who is regularly wetting the bed can have a big impact on how that child copes with the condition. For example, siblings who do not understand the outcome of telling friends at school about a bedwetting brother or sister cannot themselves grasp the notion of fear, low self-esteem and shame that disclosure of this nature could cause. A survey in 1989 described the third most stressful event for a child, coming only behind losing a parent and going blind, was the revelation of diurnal enuresis.[19]

Likewise, an understanding of parental intolerance should be sought, as this will help show what their true feelings are towards the child and bedwetting. Disclosure about arguments and disagreements about how to deal with the condition, and feelings of depression, are common when talking to parents. Often they will punish the child by smacking, shouting or through verbal abuse. It has been shown that punishment will not resolve the situation in any way and will only make the child feel even worse about the problem and thus lower his or her self-esteem.

The journey towards dryness can be long and winding, sometimes beset by obstacle after obstacle, and there is no quick-fix for success. For each child, for every parent and for every family, the road they travel along is unique to them, with treatments, interventions, support and guidance that have been tailored for their individual needs.

Experience in the field, however, suggests that there are some common components that lead to a successful outcome in the end. They are: a willingness on the part of the child, and family, to engage with every facet of the individual care plan; to want to be dry; to support each other; to talk about the problem and its solution; to drink more fluids; to take the medicine as directed.

The successful result that is being sought by the healthcare professionals, the child and the family is the final discharge from the children's continence clinic, and a life free from bedwetting and all the psychosocial and physiological impacts the condition imposes on family life.

This can only be achieved by being non-judgemental and through a tailored and closely managed care plan that is delivered via various channels such as telephone support; setting of realistic goals in a realistic time frame; bite-sized pieces of work and achievable tasks (for instance, working on an adequate fluid intake spread evenly throughout the day); regular contact and support with and from specialist nurses and doctors; continuing education and information about the condition throughout the duration of the care plan and referral; empathetic and sympathetic engagement with the child and family, combined with high levels of approachability.

## CONCLUSION

The negative impact of bedwetting on the lives of children and their families cannot be underestimated.

There is no easy solution to bedwetting and the underlying problems that go with it. The main reason for this is that each child is unique and comes with a unique set of circumstances that require a non-judgemental and tailored approach to care and treatment.

Successful treatment and management of the condition makes an enormous difference to family relationships, the child's self-esteem and confidence.

Dealing with enuresis through the *Three Systems Approach*[20] to managing the condition, by sharing ideas and techniques between professionals, by devising an individual treatment programme, and the creation of a support network, gives children the best possible chance to overcome their bedwetting problem.

 Go to the website to find the PowerPoint presentation for this chapter and MCQs to test your knowledge. **www.hodderplus.com/childnursingskills**

## REFERENCES

1  Butler RJ (1994) *Nocturnal enuresis: the child's experience.* Oxford: Butterworth Heinemann.

2  Warzak WJ (1993) Psychological implications of nocturnal enuresis. *Clinical Paediatrics* **32**: 38–40.

3  ERIC (2001). *A compilation from the Europa World Year Book 1998, using the statistics from a survey in Great Britain, Holland, New Zealand, and Ireland* Butler (1998)

4  Forsythe WI, Redmond A (1974) Enuresis and spontaneous cure rate: study of 1129 enuretics. *Archives of Diseases in Childhood* **49**: 259–263.

5  Bakwin H (1971) Enuresis in twins. *American Journal of Diseases of Children* **121**: 222–225.

6  Butler RJ, Holland P (2000) The three systems: a conceptual way of understanding nocturnal enuresis.

*Scandinavian Journal of Urology and Nephrology* **34**(4): 270–277.

7  Devitt H. Holland P, Butler RJ, *et al.* (1999) Plasma vasopressin and response to treatment in primary nocturnal enuresis. *Archives of Diseases in Childhood* **80**: 448–451.

8  Watanabe H (1995b) Sleep patterns in children with nocturnal enuresis. *Scandinavian Journal of Urology and Nephrology* (Suppl.) **173**: 55–57.

9  Norgaard JP, Rittig S, Djurhuus JC (1989) Nocturnal enuresis: an approach to treatment based on pathogenesis. *Journal of Paediatrics* **114**: 705–710.

10  Hagglof B, Andren O, Bergstrom E, *et al.* (1997) Self-esteem before and after treatment in children

with nocturnal enuresis and urinary incontinence. *Scandinavian Journal of Urology and Nephrology* **183**(Suppl.): 79–82.

11  Butler R J, McKenna S (2002) Overcoming parental intolerance in childhood nocturnal enuresis: a survey of professional opinion. *British Journal of Urology International* **89**: 295–297.

12  Butler R J (1991) Establishment of working definitions in nocturnal enuresis. *Archives of Diseases in Childhood* **66**: 267–271.

13  Valtin, H (2002) Drink at least eight glasses of water a day. Really? Is there scientific evidence for "8 × 8"? *American Journal of Physiology. Regulatory, Integrative and Comparative Physiology* **283**: R993–R1004.

14  Butler RJ (1994) *Nocturnal enuresis: the child's experience*. Oxford: Butterworth Heinemann.

15  Bakwin H (1971). Enuresis in twins. *American Journal of Diseases of Children* **121**: 222–225.

16  Eiditz-Markus T, Shapura A, Amir J. (2000) Secondary enuresis: post-traumatic stress disorder in children after car accidents. *Israel Medical Association Journal* **2**: 135–137.

17  Butler R J, Holland P (2000) The three systems: a conceptual way of understanding nocturnal enuresis. *Scandinavian Journal of Urology and Nephrology* (4): 270–277.

18  Ollendick TH, King NH, Frary R (1989) Fears in children and adolescents. Behavioural research and therapy. **27**: 19–26.

19  Wantanabe H (1995) Sleep patterns in children with nocturnal enuresis. *Scandinavian Journal of Urology and Nephrology* **173**(Suppl.): 55–58.

# Promoting children's continence

## B) Childhood constipation

Susan Slater-Smith

## LEARNING OUTCOMES

*Upon completion of this chapter, the reader should be able to accomplish the following:*

1 Define constipation
2 Describe the basic structure and function of the gastrointestinal tract
3 Discuss causes of constipation, signs and symptoms of constipation and explain them to the child/family
4 Discuss effective prevention and management of constipation
5 Explain preferred treatments and rationale for their preference to meet the child's and family's lifestyle needs
6 Develop in collaboration with child/parents/carers a care plan to encourage and manage childhood constipation

## CHAPTER OVERVIEW

Continence and defecation are two essential functions in humans. Any alteration resulting in anal incontinence, soiling and/or constipation can severely impair a child's quality of life. It presents a management problem for healthcare practitioners, and parental concern is often high. Although, constipation is the most common digestive complaint in the UK,[1,2] it is NOT a normal part of childhood! Constipation that is not recognised or treated effectively may result in faecal impaction; faecal retention caused by tears in the wall of the anus, known as fissures, with consequent bleeding and worsening pain on defecation; incontinence of faeces and urine, vomiting, abdominal pain; depression, social withdrawal and school-related problems; effects on nutrition and growth and other physical and psychological effects; continued constipation persisting into adulthood.[3] Families find these problems shameful and difficult to manage, and, in addition, they are often a source of conflict between children and parents due to common misconceptions about the aetiology of the problem. A unique feature of faecal incontinence is the isolation that children and families experience: they typically report knowing no one else with this problem.[4]

This chapter aims to provide the reader with an understanding of what constipation is and the background knowledge in order to promote effective care in the prevention and management of constipation through developing best practice. This chapter does not deal with the management of childhood constipation that may result from organic causes. This chapter is intended for children's nurses who are not specialists in the management of constipation or enuresis.

## KEY WORDS

Adolescence    Childhood    Constipation
Faecal incontinence    Non-retentive

## DEFINITION OF ENURESIS

A review of the literature showed there has been and continues to be a lack of an agreed set of definitions for constipation and terms associated with it. However, this chapter will use the terminology recommended by PaCCT Group[5] (see below).

The terms soiling and encopresis were often used interchangeably and both have now been replaced by the general term faecal incontinence (FI) to define the passage of stools in an inappropriate place. FI can be either organic (less than 5 per cent), as a result of neurological damage through trauma or congenital conditions such as anal sphincter abnormalities, or functional in origin. However, it is reported that 95 per cent of children who are incontinent of faeces have functional constipation with overflow.[6]

FI is subdivided into constipation-associated faecal incontinence (CAFI) and non-retentive faecal incontinence (NRFI). Chronic constipation is diagnosed if two or more of the following symptoms are present for 8 weeks:[5]

- fewer than three bowel movements per week;
- more than one episode of faecal incontinence per week;
- presence of large stools in the rectum or palpable on abdominal examination;
- production of large stools that obstruct the toilet;
- indications in the child's posture and behaviour

that they are withholding stools;
- painful defecation.

With regards to NRFI, emotional factors such as anxiety trigger the accidents and the child is unaware when this happens,[7] or it might be that the child has simply never achieved toilet training for the bowel and there is no underlying emotional cause. There are some children who deliberately pass faeces in an inappropriate place. They require a specialised behavioural approach, perhaps through referral to the child and adolescent mental health service. In the past, this was referred to as 'true encopresis'.[11] A recent study that analysed data from 8000 parents and children found significantly higher rates of behaviour and emotional problems, bullying and antisocial activities in children who have the problem compared with those who do not.[8] FI is sometimes perceived as being a behavioural problem, leading to parents and children feeling that they are somehow to blame. The associated shame and embarrassment can lead to avoidance of social situations and feelings of isolation, often for the whole family.

Factors that predispose a child to constipation are listed in Table 14.4 below.

**Table 14.4** Factors that predispose children to constipation

| Factor | Definition |
|---|---|
| Withholding | Ability of a child to hold on to and prevent the passing of a stool often initiated by passage of large/painful stool, delay in passage of normal stool, anal fissure, group 'A' haemolytic streptococcal anal infection, toilet phobias/fears, sexual abuse |
| Anal phobia | The child does not like the feeling of faeces passing through the rectum and wilfully prevents a stool from being passed |
| Toilet phobia/refusal | The child perceives toileting as a to-be-avoided frightening event. These children view bowel movement as an extension of themselves to be swept away down in the toilet. Some avoid using the toilet, sometimes due to poor facilities at school, or the fear of bullying |
| Absent toilet routine | Lack of a toilet routine (some children have such busy lives that it can be difficult to find time to sit on the toilet) |
| Low-fibre diet | Children may not consume sufficient dietary fibre |
| Low fluid intake | Children may not drink enough during the day particularly at school, and the resulting dehydration contributes to continence problems |
| Sedentary/immobility | Lack of physical exercise or physical disability, e.g. wheelchair bound |
| Medication | For example anticonvulsants and antihistamines can cause constipation, |
| Psychological factors | Anxiety/emotional upset due to a threatening event, e.g. seeing birth of a sibling, sexual assault |
| Learning disability | Some toddlers and older children are too distracted to evacuate, e.g. ADHD |

## Definitions[5]

**Constipation:** Defecation that is unsatisfactory because of infrequent stools, difficult stool passage, or seemingly incomplete defecation. Stools are often dry and hard, and may be abnormally large or abnormally small.

**Faecal incontinence (FI):** The passage of stools in an inappropriate place.

**Constipation-associated faecal incontinence (CAFI):** The result of prolonged constipation leading to stretched muscles in the bowel which cannot send messages reliably to the brain and cannot contract reliably (retention and overflow). Previously referred to as 'soiling.'

**Non-retentive faecal incontinence (NRFI):** The passage of stools in an inappropriate place by a child with a mental age of 4 years and older, with no evidence of constipation by history and/or examination. Previously referred to as 'encopresis'.

**Faecal impaction:** No adequate passing of faeces for several days or weeks. Faeces become compacted in the rectum and colon, causing abdominal distension. Mega stools are eventually passed with pain and difficulty.

# INCIDENCE: NON-ORGANIC CONSTIPATION

Difficulty in defecation, with or without soiling, accounts for about 25 per cent of a paediatric gastroenterologist's work and is one of the 10 most common problems seen by general paediatricians.[12] Constipation can affect children at any time throughout childhood, regardless of race, gender, culture or social class. It is estimated that up to 10 per cent of children suffer from constipation at any one time[1] and is most common in children between the ages of 2 and 4 years when they are potty training.[2] The rates are even higher for infants and children with disabilities and learning difficulties and are nearly ubiquitous in children with spina bifida and spinal cord injuries because of the impact on anorectal function. Seventy-four per cent of children with cerebral palsy have chronic constipation. Fifty per cent of children with severe developmental delay have chronic constipation, e.g. Down's syndrome.[3,11]

Adolescence is recognised as a time of physical and emotional change that can be confusing and challenging for young people and their families. There are additional anxieties for 11- to 19-year-olds who have continence problems. There are very few data about constipation in adolescents, but a prevalence of 1.2 per cent in girls and 0.3 per cent in boys aged 10–12 years has been recorded.[7] A longitudinal study of children with constipation showed that one-third of children followed up beyond puberty continued to have the condition.[9] This suggests a number of teenagers will have bowel management issues, with or without FI.

There is a social stigma attached to FI that can cause young people to fear ridicule from their peers and even bullying if their problem is discovered.[8] This can be a barrier to the young person seeking help.[10] Young people may also believe that nothing can be done, feel different or even fear that there may be something wrong with them 'mentally'. Indeed, FI, especially in older children and teenagers, is sometimes incorrectly associated with laziness or a lack of discipline, and the child and the family can experience a negative response from teachers and youth workers and even some healthcare professionals because of this. Recent research has indicated that FI itself contributes to behavioural problems.[8]

## PHYSIOLOGY OF DEFECATION

The understanding of normal physiology of continence and defecation *facilitates* a systematic approach to *nursing* assessment and management.

The lower alimentary tract is divisible into two distinct functional units:

1 the colon
2 the rectum.

Both are regulated by the autonomic nervous system. However, the external anal sphincter (EAS) usually comes under voluntary control later as a consequence of toilet training.[12] Normal continence is maintained by the resting tonicity of the internal anal sphincter (IAS). It can be enhanced by contraction of the puborectalis muscle.

When a volume of stool enters the normal rectum, stretch receptors and nerves in the intramural plexus are activated. Inhibitory interneurons decrease the resting tone in the involuntary smooth muscle of the IAS. Relaxation of the IAS allows the stool to reach the EAS and the urge to defecate is signalled. If the child relaxes the EAS, squats/sits on a toilet or potty, the anorectal angle is increased, that is a funnel is formed with the outlet at the top on the anal canal. This in turn increases intra-abdominal pressure, which is directed down the funnelled rectum on the faecal bolus, expelling it.[4] The rectum is evacuated of stool.

Once initiated, defecation is either a continuous process or passed in bits preceded by periodic straining. The pattern is influenced by stool consistency and size as well as by individual habit.[13] Upon completion, a closing reflex occurs. The IAS and puborectalis muscles transiently contract and restore the anorectal angle.[4] This allows the IAS to recover its tone, thus closing the anal canal (Figure 14.2).

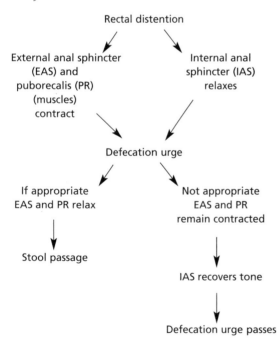

Figure 14.2 Physiology of defecation.

In a socially inconvenient situation, defecation can be voluntarily deferred by contraction of the puborectalis and EAS. The contents in the upper anal canal are returned to the rectum. Passive accommodation in the rectum keeps the pressure low and cortical pathways suppress the urge to defecate. If, however, the child tightens the EAS and the gluteal muscles, the faecal mass is pushed back into the rectal vault and the urge to defecate subsides.[13] Repetitive denial of evacuation leads to stretching of the rectum and eventually of the lower colon, producing a reduction in muscle tone and retention of stool (Figure 14.3, page 233). The longer the stool remains in the rectum, the more water is removed, and the harder the stool becomes to the point of impaction. This can result in the child passing large stools very infrequently, causing further pain and even anal tears; there may also be overflow diarrhoea as a result of watery faeces leaking around the harder stools. The child has no control over this and will often be unaware that they have soiled. This can happen up to 10 times a day and it can be difficult for parents to accept that there is an underlying constipation when stools appear so loose.

The large bowel or colon acts as a 'waste processor', receiving semi-liquid stool from the small intestine and gradually re-absorbing fluid, resulting in formed stool. There is continuous mixing and churning of matter in the colon, with occasional 'mass movements', when waves of peristalsis propel stool large distances along the colon. Typically these mass movements are triggered by eating or drinking known as the gastrocolic response. Food ingestion stimulates evacuation of the colon, which is most active after the first meal of the day in the morning. This is why 15–30 minutes after breakfast is the most common time for defecation.[14] Once the phase of toilet training is passed, the urge to defecate is felt once rectal filling passes a threshold volume, but this urge should not be desperately urgent and can easily be resisted until a toilet is found to empty the bowel.

Straining with the passage of soft stool is normal in neonates and infants. It is related to their inability to coordinate pelvic floor relaxation with increased abdominal pressure (push down) manoeuvre and to straighten the anorectal canal when lying down. Once a week, may be still normal for some infants.

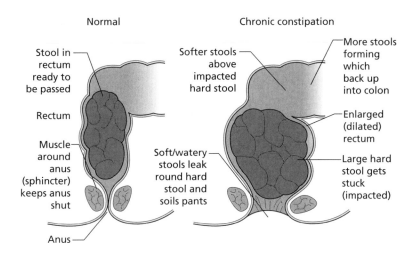

Normal          Chronic constipation

Stool in rectum ready to be passed

Rectum

Muscle around anus (sphincter) keeps anus shut

Anus

Soft/watery stools leak round hard stool and soils pants

Softer stools above impacted hard stool

More stools forming which back up into colon

Enlarged (dilated) rectum

Large hard stool gets stuck (impacted)

**Figure 14.3** Continence mechanism

Normal frequency (Table 14.5) and consistency of stool changes during early childhood up until the age of 10 years and then it is as for an adult. A newborn infant's first stool is black–dark green and sticky. This is known as 'meconium'. Most (99.2 per cent) healthy newborn babies will pass this within the first 48 hours of birth.[14] The frequency of stools in most children decreases from a mean of four per day in the first week of life to 1.7 per day by the age of 2 years, although breastfed infants pass significantly more stools than the formula-fed infants. Over this interval, stool volume increases more than 10-fold while maintaining consistent water content of approximately 75 per cent. Intestinal transit time from mouth to rectum increases from 8 hours in the first month of life to 16 hours by 2 years of age to 26 hours by the age 10.[14]

There is a wide individual variability, but stools are normally passed anywhere between three stools/day to three stools/week.[11] In addition to the frequency, there is also a wide variation in consistency. Changes in consistency towards either extreme can stress the mechanisms of continence, e.g. if small hard pellets of stools are introduced into

**KEY POINTS**

To achieve continence a child needs:
- Normal rectal and anal anatomy
- Normal nerve supply
- Soft consistency of stools
- Normal frequency of stools from three per day to alternate days[2]
- To be cognitively developed to achieve continence
- Motivated to achieve continence

**Table 14.5** Normal frequency of bowel movements (BM)[15]

| Age | BM per week | BM per day |
|---|---|---|
| 0–3 months | | |
| breast milk | 5–40 | 2.9 |
| formula | 5–28 | 2.0 |
| 6–12 months | 5–28 | 1.8 |
| 1–3 years old | 4–21 | 1.4 |
| >3 years old | 3–14 | 1.0 |

The nature of stool, not frequency, is the basis for nursing diagnosis

the rectum slowly, the perception of rectal contents may be delayed till relatively severe distension of the rectum occurs.[13] Liquid stools, on the other hand, introduced rapidly into the rectum can overcome the continence mechanisms, even in healthy individuals. Therefore, passing large deformable stools is easier and less straining is required than with small hard pellets. Semi-solid stools are also more completely evacuated than solid or liquid stools. Therefore, it is logical that manipulation of stool consistency and volume be the first line in the management of children with FI.

## PRINCIPLES OF MANAGEMENT

Historically the management of children with constipation was based purely on clinicians' experience and 'custom and practice'. It is now recognised that this is no longer sufficient to provide optimum levels of care.[16] However, there is

little research available to inform practice. In its absence, it is recommended that the management of children with constipation should follow evidence-based algorithms and care pathways written by expert panels. The IMPACT pathway was developed by a multidisciplinary group of practitioners from around the UK who were actively involved in the management and treatment of children with bowel problems.[17] Following a 6-month pilot, final changes were made and the IMPACT resource was launched in 2005. The IMPACT paediatric bowel care pathway should be adapted to local policies which support the ERIC minimum standards[18] which endorse a holistic approach to care. Copies of the IMPACT paediatric bowel care pathway (2005) are available from mss@norgine.com.

There are many things that can be done by a registered children's nurse to treat constipation before a clinic appointment to seek assistance from a medical practitioner or specialist nurse is sought.

### The procedural goal is to

- identify children and young people with bowel dysfunction and ensure that they receive age-appropriate care.

## PROCEDURE: Management of childhood constipation

| Procedural steps | Evidence-based rationale |
| --- | --- |
| 1 Refer children over 4-years-old to a medical practitioner to exclude any underlying contributory factors, such as infection, constipation or signs of renal problems. It will also exclude rarer neurological conditions, such as sacral cord tethering, that very occasionally present in adolescence, although most abnormalities of the bowel would have been diagnosed at an earlier age | A medical examination is recommended before assessing and treating constipation and/or soiling in children over 4 years |
| 2 Before commencing an assessment, carefully consider the child/young person's age and/or cognitive ability<br>Children with special physical needs or learning disabilities can take longer to achieve bowel control. The incidence of unusual toileting behaviour, including stool holding, is known to be higher in children with neurodevelopmental disorders, e.g. autistic spectrum disorders. | Professional judgement is required regarding issues of obtaining informed consent and child protection<br>Educational or physical needs affecting the child, such as learning difficulties or mobility problems are ubiquitous with constipation with/without soiling |

## PROCEDURE: Management of childhood constipation (continued)

| | |
|---|---|
| Occasionally the toileting problem is the first indication of an underlying condition which requires follow-up | |
| 3 Obtain a thorough medical history:<br>• time after birth until first bowel motion (BM)<br>• family/child's definition of constipation<br>• length of time the condition has been present<br>• medication use<br>• fluid and fibre intake<br>It may be necessary to defer assessment until the family/child has recorded whether stools have been passed in the toilet or soiled pants, using the Paediatric Bristol stool chart[19] for 1 week prior to assessment | A full history and a careful analysis of all factors is paramount to successful treatment and will enable prompt referral to the medical team if there is a possibility of an organic cause<br>A shared definition of constipation will help to ensure attainment of an accurate and reliable history |
| 4 Obtain a thorough BM history:<br>*Bowel profile*<br>• Check passage of meconium<br>• Description of stools; frequency, consistency, size, may utilise Bristol Stool Form Chart<br>• Any pain /discomfort/blood/mucus<br>• Feelings of the child and psychological issues, such as anxiety about using the toilet or fear of pain<br>*Constipation symptoms*<br>• Begin after first year<br>• Passage of enormous stools<br>• Increasing faecal loading:<br>  • soiling/irritability/abdominal pain/anorexia<br>  • resolve on passage of stool<br>• Seemingly irrational coping skill behaviour<br>• Nonchalant attitude/hiding underwear<br>• Use of toilet/potty<br>• Any previous treatments/interventions | Providing valid and reliable information about the frequency and nature of the problem will direct an effective care plan<br>Amount, size, circumference and density of the stool can give an indication of the capacity of the rectum and therefore the degree of the faecal impaction<br>To ascertain whether the child has ever been successfully toilet trained. If successful, this would help to rule out an organic cause for the constipation<br>There are many things that can be done to treat constipation before a clinic appointment for assistance from a medical practitioner or specialist nurse is sought<br>Bristol Stool Chart for Children:<br>www.childhoodconstipation.com/About/Normal.aspx |
| 5 Toilet training profile (if appropriate):<br>• Age toilet training commenced<br>• Age acquired bladder control<br>• Age acquired bowel control<br>• Any significant changes/problems/events occurring at this time | To help determine the underlying primary cause(s) of functional constipation, e.g. hiding behaviour may indicate withholding constipation, blood on toilet tissue may indicate an anal fissure and will direct the plan of care and its evaluation |
| 6 Obtain a thorough family and school profile:<br>• Family, social and environmental factors<br>• Fear/anxiety<br>• Precipitating family stress<br>• Learned behaviour<br>• ? Coercive potty training<br>• 'Cry' for help<br>• School attitudes and availability of quality toilet facilities and access to palatable drinking water | Do parents have realistic expectations? A child is usually able to begin bowel control after the age of 20 months and achieve continence by age 4 years<br>Children frequently report poor toilet facilities, lack of privacy and the problems associated with bullying in their schools. Dirty toilet seats encourage children to crouch rather than sit and crouching may inhibit the anorectal angle required to assist defecation |
| 7 Conduct a focused nursing physical assessment of the child:<br>• General physical appearance | Helps determine level of hydration and nutrition. Childhood is an important time to promote a healthy lifestyle. Children's nurses have an important |

## PROCEDURE: Management of childhood constipation (continued)

| | |
|---|---|
| • Distended abdomen<br>• Skin colour, e.g. pallor<br>• Baseline weight | and positive role to play in health education |
| 8 'Red flags' found on nursing assessment/observation require prompt referral to a medical practitioner. 'Red flag' symptoms include:<br>• >48 hours before passing meconium as a neonate<br>• Abdominal distension especially if failing to thrive (see item below)<br>• Evidence of poor growth and/or development<br>• Infrequent small or ribbon stools<br>• Constant leaking, especially if linked with urinary leaking too<br>• Failed management with appropriate standard intervention (with compliance) | To enable prompt referral to medical team if there is a possibility of an organic cause<br>Medical practitioner may need to investigate, e.g. possible failure to thrive, or neglect<br>Organic causes need to be excluded: general malaise or other systemic signs such as weight loss, nausea/vomiting, and blood in the stools or abdominal distension |
| 9 Review your nursing assessment and report the following red flags to a medical practitioner immediately:<br>• Onset < 12 months<br>• Delayed passage of meconium<br>• No stool withholding<br>• No soiling<br>• Intermittent diarrhoea explosive stools<br>• Failure to thrive<br>• No response to constipation treatment<br>• Malaise, lethargy not improved with treatment. | Maintain child's safety and facilitate access to timely and appropriate medical care |

**KEY POINT**

Dispel blame from the child. It is imperative that parents fully and accurately understand the cause and effect of constipation and that their child is not deliberately soiling

## Nursing management

### *Procedural aims*

1 Education
2 Evacuation
3 Restore
4 Maintenance

## PROCEDURE: Nursing management of childhood constipation

| Procedural steps | Evidence-based rationale |
|---|---|
| 1 **Education**<br>Work collaboratively and informatively with child and family to demystify understandings and correct misconception of toilet training, constipation and FI. Ensure that the child and family are aware of:<br>• normal variation in bowel habits<br>• protracted course of treatment | Parental persistence, consistence and the child's compliance is required. The success of each depends on the cooperation and understanding of the parent and, when possible, the child |

## PROCEDURE: Nursing managment of childhood constipation (continued)

| | |
|---|---|
| • common relapses<br>• long-term laxatives often being required, only to be topped on advice<br>• symptoms getting worse initially | |
| **2 Education**<br>Augment demystification with written information (available from ERIC, NELH Treatment notes, perhaps locally from bowel clinic). This will include information regarding:<br>• structured toileting programme<br>• consistent scheduled toileting<br>• positive reinforcement<br>• diet/fluid adjustment<br>• oral laxatives<br>*Suppositories/enemas are used as very last only resort and if tolerated by child*<br>Setting up a written individual care plan with the child, family and teaching staff can help the school manage a toileting and changing routine, in line with school policies on health and safety and equal opportunities | Treatment for constipation and faecal soiling may include dietary changes, an increase in fluid intake, oral and or rectal medication and behavioural training. Education of the child and parent or carer is an essential part of the treatment programme.<br>Need to take into account 'whole child' approach<br>How the child perceives the problem important<br>Family dynamics need to be taken into account<br>Need to be aware of external factors, e.g. access to a 'suitable' toilet facilities at school<br>It is important that the school staff have an awareness of the principles of treatment and the individual needs of the child. They also need to understand that FI is outside the child's control. The school nurse and head of pastoral care need to ensure that the child is supported in a discreet and confidential way, with good access to toilet and drinking facilities and a changing bag containing clothing, wipes and disposal bags provided from home |
| **3 Education: reward systems**<br>Give reward for sitting on the toilet (as is age appropriate to the child). Note that a child who is constipated cannot earn a sticker for doing a 'poo'<br>Families often perceive the main problem is the 'soiling'. Constipation secondary issue. Emphasis needs to be made on 'poos' in the toilet not clean pants | Engaging the child to sit on the toilet and perform often most difficult part of treatment<br>Use, for example, ERIC Incentive Charts to encourage and motivate a child<br>All approaches emphasise importance of:<br>• no undue pressure, calm, matter of fact approach<br>• minimal attention and no negativity about mistakes<br>• positive attention for success (praise, maybe stickers)<br>• remember age of child: tends to be oppositional! |
| **4 Education: fluid intake**<br>Ensure adequate fluid intake, e.g. a 4-year-old weighing 16 kg needs 85 mL/kg = 1360 mL. Therefore, aim for six to eight cups throughout the day (Table 14.6, page 239)<br>Encourage water-based drinks | Between six and eight drinks a day will help to maintain regular bowel function. The young person will need ongoing support and encouragement to ensure that they adhere to this |
| **5 Education: fibre intake**<br>Ensure adequate fibre intake<br>There are no 'DRA' for fibre for children. The daily recommended intake is the amount required to produce a soft stool. Suggested daily intake is 'age + 5 g of fibre'[18]<br>Encourage regular meal times with an appropriate healthy balance of foods which includes minimum of five portions of fruit and vegetables per day | A varied diet will help to maintain regular bowel function. The young person will need ongoing support and encouragement to ensure that they adhere to this<br>High-fibre foods include fruit, vegetables and cereals. Bulking agents, such as wheat bran, help make stools softer and easier to pass |
| **6 Education: exercise**<br>Encourage regular daily exercise; at least 30 minutes per day | This will encourage regular filling and emptying of the rectum |

## PROCEDURE: Nursing managment of childhood constipation (continued)

| | |
|---|---|
| **7 Education: practical toiletting**<br>Encourage the child to pass stool daily. Encourage to defecate, approximately 30 minutes after each meal. Older children should be encouraged to sit on the toilet for 5–10 minutes<br>Make sure the child in a position with physiological advantage for defecation and of comfort while on the toilet. A toilet-training or foot stool seat may be required<br>Bubbles or balloons can be blown<br>Encourage parents to keep a diary; 'pooper snoopers'. It should note stool consistency and volume, pain on defecation and excessive straining and satisfaction ('empty'?)<br>Encourage parents to make the toilet a nice place to visit, e.g. posters, books, colouring books, etc. | Take advantage of natural gastrocolic reflex. A routine of sitting on the toilet for 5–10 minutes after meals (after waiting for about 15–20 minutes) will help to encourage regular bowel movements. In time the signals of a full bowel will be recognised by the child as the bowel regains tone but this may take many months or even longer<br>To achieve the advantage of an anorectal angle, the knees need to be just above the hips. This makes it easier to relax the pelvic floor and release stool. The feet should be flat for stability<br>To assist in relaxing the pelvic floor<br>Bowel actions should be recorded using the Bristol Stool Scale so that dosages can be adapted to maintain a normal easy-to-pass stool |
| **8 Evacuation**<br>Single step approach: disimpaction<br>Movicol Paediatric Plain: start with minimum number of sachets for age and increase every other day until evacuation complete (usually within 7 days):<br>    2–4 years: 2–8 sachets<br>    5–11 years: 4–12 sachets<br>Movicol: Adult dose 8 sachets per day for 3 days<br>Sachets can be taken in divided doses but total daily dose should be taken within 12 hours.<br>Suppositories, enemas and manual removal of faeces are not considered appropriate for children<br>Following the introduction of Movicol Paediatric Plain the majority of children can undergo single-line treatment with appropriate dose titration | Treatment often needs to start with evacuation of accumulated stool. Local protocol may suggest what medication to use, what dose and when specialist advice should be sought<br>Traditionally, softened stools first using osmotic laxative, e.g. lactulose, then a stimulant was introduced, e.g. senna. Sodium picosulphate or similar was then added to the regimen if poor result. Finally an enema or manual evacuation under anaesthetic was used if all of the above failed. Problems can occur with the above as there is often poor compliance and may involve protracted treatment time<br>Eliminates need for powerful stimulants and use of enemas. Children find enemas very distressing and therefore should only be given to children as a very last resort |
| **9 Restore**<br>Laxative dosage:<br>• Lactulose: <1 year, 2.5 mL bd; 1–5 years, 5 mL bd; 5–10 years, 10 mL bd; adult 15 mL bd<br>• Senna (syrup): 2–6 years, 2.5–5ml in morning, over 6 years, 5–10 mL; adult, 10–20 mL usually at bedtime<br>• Movicol Paediatric Plain: 2–6 years, 1–4 sachets; 7–11 years, 2–4 sachets per day (titrate dose as necessary)<br>• Movicol: adults 1–3 sachets per day | Aim to achieve regular defecation; soft stool with a diameter no greater than a 50 pence piece without pain/difficulty, defecation 1–3 times daily (not to be confused with overflow) and no evidence of soiling<br>Using a single or combination of treatments at an early stage can prevent long-term psychological and physiological problems[20] |
| **10 Maintenance therapy**<br>• Ongoing advice and support<br>• Continue with diet/fluid advice<br>• Long-term laxative therapy<br>• Consider cautious reduction 6 monthly with medical team<br>• Behaviour modification (if appropriate) | Aim to prevent relapse<br>A maintenance dose established to keep stools soft and easy to pass.<br>May need to use a combination of stool softener/bulking agent and bowel stimulant (e.g. lactulose and senna) or Movicol Paediatric Plain<br>Will need at least 6 months' treatment and often |

## PROCEDURE: Nursing managment of childhood constipation (continued)

| | |
|---|---|
| • Use adequate doses to pass stool one every 1–2 days | much longer to learn/re-learn bowel habit<br>Referral to Child and Adolescent Mental Health Services may be required if there are any associated emotional or behavioural problems |
| **11 Finishing treatment**<br>• Gradual reduction, do not stop suddenly<br>• Reduce bowel stimulant (if using) first<br>• Treat early if relapse<br>• Give ongoing support | Further referral and the need for specialist hospital appointments is greatly reduced if there is an effective programme with ongoing contact and support from the community nurse<br>There may be setbacks, so it is vital that the nurse is there to give encouragement to continue with the programme and avoid the 'cycle' of recurring constipation that leads to the problem starting all over again |
| **12** A very small number of children will not respond to conservative treatment and, until recently, surgery, such as formation of a colostomy or antegrade continence enema, was often considered to be the only option. Rectal irrigation is recommended for these children.[21]<br>Indications for use:<br>• Neurogenic bowel dysfunction<br>• Faecal incontinence associated with congenital abnormality | The Peristeen system consists of a rectal catheter that is passed into the rectum and is retained by a balloon that is inflated while the patient is sitting on the toilet. Warm irrigation fluid from a reservoir is slowly pumped in to the rectum using a hand-held pump. Once the fluid has been pumped in, the balloon is deflated and the rectum is emptied. The whole process can take up to 45 minutes, but this is adjusted to suit the child. It is recommended that the procedure is carried out every day for a few weeks then, depending on the result, the frequency can then be reduced to every other or every third day |

**Table 14.6** Recommended fluid intake per day[19]

| Age | mL/kg/day |
|---|---|
| 0–3 months | 150 |
| 4–6 months | 130 |
| 7–9 months | 120 |
| 10–12 months | 110 |
| 1–3 years | 95 |
| 4–6 years | 85 |
| 7–10 years | 75 |
| 11–14 years | 55 |
| 15–18 years | 50 |

## CONCLUSION

Achieving continence is an important milestone in a child's development. It helps them to socialise independently with their peers and enables them to participate in normal childhood activities. Failure to achieve continence beyond the toddler stage may restrict social and psychological development. NICE has published guidelines on the management of faecal incontinence in adults, stating that: 'People who report or are reported to have faecal incontinence should be offered care to be managed by healthcare professionals who have the relevant skills, training and experience and who work within an integrated continence service'.[22] Based on this philosophy, NICE is currently working on guidance (due 2011) on the management of faecal incontinence in children and young people. However, the guidance will follow a 'whole child approach' as adults and children function differently.

Children need a relational model of interaction and communication cannot be ignored. In the meantime, ERIC (Education and Resources for Improving Childhood Continence) offers support and information on all aspects of childhood continence; interactive websites eric.org.uk and trusteric.org (for young people).

 Go to the website to find the PowerPoint presentation for this chapter and MCQs to test your knowledge. **www.hodderplus.com/childnursingskills**

## REFERENCES

1  Loening-Baucke V. (2007) Prevalence rates for constipation and faecal and urinary incontinence. *Archives of Disease in Childhood* **92**: 486–489.

2  NHS Institute for Innovation and Improvement (2008) *Constipation*. www.cks.library.nhs.uk/constipation/management/ quickanswers/scenarioconstipation_ infantsandchildren#-320518

3  Farrell M, Holmes G, Coldicutt P (2003) Management of childhood constipation: patients' experiences. *Journal of Advanced Nursing* **44**: 479–489.

4  Pijpers MAM, Tabbers MM, Benninga MA (2009) Currently recommended treatments of childhood constipation are not evidence based: a systematic literature review on the effect of laxative treatment and dietary measures. *Archives of Disease in Childhood* **94**: 117–131.

5  Benninga M, Candy DC, Catto-Smith AG (2005). The Paris Consensus on Childhood Constipation Terminology (PACCT) Group. *Journal of Pediatric Gastroenterology and Nutrition* **40**: 273–275.

6  Price KJ, Elliott TM. (2001) Stimulant laxatives for constipation and soiling in children. *Cochrane Database of Systematic reviews* **3**: CD002040.

7  Bonner L (2003) Children who soil: guidelines for good practice. *Journal of Family Healthcare* **13**: 2–32.

8  Joinson, C, Heron J, Butler U (2006) Psychological differences between children with and without soiling problems (ALSPAC study). *Pediatrics* **117**: 1575–1584.

9  Van Ginkel R Johannes B, Büller RHA (2003) Childhood constipation: longitudinal follow-up beyond puberty. *Gastroenterology* **125**: 357–363.

10 Weaver A, Jacques E (2008) Encouraging adolescents to seek continence help. *Nursing Times* **104**(46): 46–48.

11 Voskuijl WP, Heijmans J, Heijmans HS (2004). Use of Rome II criteria in childhood defecation disorders: applicability in clinical and research practice. *Journal of Pediatrics* **145**: 213–217.

12 Rubin G, Dale A (2006) Clinical review: chronic constipation in children. *British Medical Journal*, 333: 1051–1055.

13 Cerdan C, Cerdan J, Jimenez F (2005) Anatomy and physiology of continence and defecation. *Cirugia Espanola*, **78**(Suppl 3): 2–7.

14 Clayden G, Wright A (2007) Constipation and incontinence in childhood: two sides of the same coin? *Archives of Disease in Childhood* **92**: 472–474.

15 Fontana M, Bianchi C, Cataldo F (2008) Bowel frequency in healthy children. *Acta Paediatrica*, 78: 682–684.

16 Schattner A, Fletcher RH. (2003) Research

evidence and the individual patient. *Quarterly Journal of Medicine* **96**: 1–5.

17 Rogers J (2008) An integrated paediatric continence service. *Nursing Times* **104**(13): 70–71.

18 ERIC (2006) *Managing bowel and bladder problems in schools and early years settings: guidelines for good practice.* www.promocon.co.uk/Promocon Booklet.pdf (Accessed 26 March 2009).

19 Bracey J (2002) *Solving children's soiling problems: a handbook for health professionals.* London: Churchill Livingstone.

20 Clayden G, Wright A (2007) Constipation and incontinence in childhood: two sides of the same coin? *Archives of Disease in Childhood* **92**: 472–474.

21 Bohr C (2009) Using rectal irrigation for faecal incontinence in children. *Nursing Times* **105**(7): 42–44.

22 NICE (2007) *Faecal incontinence: the management of faecal incontinence in adults. NICE Clinical Guideline 49.* London: NICE.

## CHAPTER 15

# Delivery pre- and postoperative care

Des Cawley and John Larkin

## LEARNING OUTCOMES

*Upon completion of this chapter, the reader should be able to accomplish the following:*

1 Define the terms, pre-operative, peri-operative and postoperative care
2 Demonstrate an understanding of the needs of a child undergoing surgery
3 Discuss the nurse's responsibility in ensuring the safe transfer of a child from the ward to the operating department
4 Describe the nurse's role in caring for child in the peri-operative environment, including the care provided in the post-anaesthetic care unit
5 Discuss the postoperative nursing care of a child who has undergone a surgical procedure
6 Outline the complications which may develop in the postoperative phase of care, either as a result of anaesthesia or surgery

## CHAPTER OVERVIEW

Approximately 450 000 children aged 0–16 years undergo a surgical procedure in England each year. The type and acuity of surgery is patient and centre dependent; it is essential that all children's nurses have an awareness of the essential nursing care that a child and his/her family will require while the child is in hospital.

This chapter provides an overview of the essential elements of care which a child undergoing surgery might require. It describes the care to be provided in each distinctive phase of operative care, from admission to hospital through to the preparation for discharge home from hospital following a surgical procedure. In addition, it provides an overview of care that may be required in the peri-operative phase and reinforces the need for family-centred care in each phase of care.

## KEY WORDS

Pre-operative    Peri-operative    Postoperative    Family-centred care    Induction    Post-anaesthetic care unit

## Definitions

**Pre-operative care:** the preparation and multidisciplinary management of a patient prior to surgery. It should be holistic, taking cognisance of the biopsychosocial and spiritual needs of the patient.

**Peri-operative care:** the multidisciplinary management of the anaesthetic and surgical environment, including the comprehensive planning and provision of care for the patient within this environment.

**Postoperative care:** the multidisciplinary management of patient care after surgery. This includes care given during the immediate postoperative period in the operating theatre and recovery room/post-anaesthesia care unit (PACU) and on day(s) following surgery when the patient returns to the ward.

# BACKGROUND

In 2005, 444 059 children aged 0–16 years underwent surgical procedures in England.[1] These procedures varied from minor surgery performed in general hospitals to major specialist surgery performed in tertiary centres.[1] It is important to note that while the hospitals in which certain surgical procedures are carried out have changed over the last number two decades, classification of surgical procedure and frequency remains unchanged.[1,2]

Based on the 2005 figures, general and specialist paediatric surgery accounted for 28 per cent of children admitted to hospital to undergo a surgical procedure. A further 27 per cent of children were admitted for ear, nose and throat (ENT) surgery, with other surgical categories including trauma and orthopaedics, oral surgery and plastics accounting for 20 per cent, 10 per cent and 9 per cent of the surgical workload respectively. The remaining admissions were classified in sub-specialties such as ophthalmic, urological, neurological and cardio-thoracic surgeries and are usually carried out in a tertiary centre of specialist care.[1]

While details of the hospital site and type of surgery performed on a child provides important epidemiological data, it is important to recognise the provision of patient care as paramount. It is also important that the nurse who provides care for a child before, during or after a surgical procedure recognises that child as an individual. This implies that all care provided to a child awaiting or undergoing a surgical procedure should be child and family focused, meeting the child's physical and emotional needs but also allowing healthcare professionals to provide care in a safe and effective manner. The provision of this care should be in partnership with all the key stakeholders, i.e. child, family and health professionals, to ensure that all participants in care are fully informed,[2] which may reduce child and parental anxiety[3,4] and assist the recovery process.[5]

It is therefore vital that all aspects of the child's care include family members and significant others (where appropriate) and not just parents. The premise of this argument relates to the variance in age among children admitted to hospital for surgical procedures.[1] This variance requires nurses and all healthcare professionals to be cognisant of age-dependent need and adapt the care which he/she is providing accordingly. Having due regard for current trends and best practice it is essential that each nurse involved in the care of a child undergoing a surgical procedure must display competency in provision of care with due regard for professional guidelines.

# PRE-OPERATIVE CARE

Children regardless of age need to be properly prepared for theatre.[6] Children experiencing surgical procedures require both physical and psychological preparation.[7] It is important to recognise that the entire family is undergoing anaesthesia and the surgical procedure, in the sense that anxiety felt by parents will be transmitted to the child.[7] Parents who are fully informed and involved are confident and competent partners in the hospitalisation and recovery process of their child and on discharge.[8] Research has highlighted that pre-surgical preparation benefits children by preventing or reducing their negative responses to surgery.[9]

The pre-operative preparation of a child for surgery can be divided into two categories: pre-immediate and immediate (day of surgery). Pre-immediate preparation can be described as the care that both child and parents receive prior to the day of surgery.

## Maintaining a safe environment

On admission to the unit the parents and child are orientated to the environment, including unit layout, toilet facilities, meal times, call bell, other children and personnel.[3] It is important to ensure that the environment is age appropriate, i.e. cots, small beds, larger beds. Facilities may be provided that allow parents to stay in the hospital. Ensure that identification band/s are correctly labelled (including patient full name, surname, date of birth, hospital number) and placed on the patient in accordance with hospital policy.

## Communication

The nurse must assess the child's and parent's comprehension of the pending surgery. All preparation and support must be based upon the child's age, developmental stage and level; personality; past history and experience with health professionals and hospitals; background, including socioeconomic status, religion, culture and family attitudes.[10] It is important to assess what information the child has previously received, what his/her understanding is and what is expected.

Age-appropriate preparation is essential.[6] Children have different attention spans and their ability to absorb information and make sense of it may be limited. It may be more suitable to direct most of the educational efforts towards the parents. On the other hand, older children are seeking answers; knowledge gives them a sense of control and the capability to cooperate. Prepare the child using age-appropriate language (simple non-medical terminology). Give explanations slowly and clearly and provide both child and parents opportunities to express concerns and ask questions. Providing honest answers helps to buildup trust. Prepare the child with what to expect; reason for surgery, pre-operative procedures, time of surgery, where parents can wait for child, room to which child will return and postoperative care and routines (e.g. nil orally, intravenous fluids, nasogastric tubing, and wound drains if indicated, wound care and pain management). The involvement of play specialist and theatre staff (anaesthetist, theatre nurse, recovery nurse) may help alleviate anxiety. The parents should be encouraged to bring the child's own toys/comforters Through the medium of play children learn about their world and about themselves operating within that world: what they can do, how to relate to things and situations, and how to adapt themselves to the strains that society puts on them.[7] If it is appropriate for the child based on age and if they so wish, they may visit (in line with hospital policy) the anaesthetic room, recovery and intensive care unit to familiarise themselves with location, equipment and personal.

It is vital that that the patient/client (child/guardian) be given adequate information so that they are able to make a meaningful and informed decision regarding their care.[11] Healthcare workers are required by law to attain consent from their patients before they commence any type of care or treatment.[12] Consent of patients/clients under 16 years is complex; nurses must be aware of local policies and legislation, and professional body advice that affect the care of this client group.[11]

## Breathing and circulation and body temperature

It is important to perform a head to toe assessment of the child. This again will be age specific and condition specific. Record temperature, pulse, respiratory rate and blood pressure. Identify any unusual patterns or values outside the norm for the particular age group; deviations in these vital signs may indicate changes in patient status.[13] Elevated temperature may indicate fever. If appropriate the importance of sitting upright, deep-breathing exercises and wound support should be taught to the child in preparation to aid the postoperative recovery. Physiotherapist involvement and the use of play, such as blowing bubbles and wind instruments, can assisted in this regard,[7] as this facilitates good inflation of the lungs.[14]

## Eating and drinking

The child's normal diet and nutritional status will be assessed on admission. Make a note of likes/ dislikes, and any special dietary requirements. Refer the child to a dietician if indicated. An accurate weight and height will be recorded as per hospital policy. Height and weight recordings are used to determine drug dosages, blood volume and fluid requirements.[13] Ensure that the child has nothing by mouth (NPO) (from the Latin nil per os) as per hospital policy/anaesthetist instructions.[10,13] Research has identified that prolonged periods of fasting reduce blood glucose and increase the risk of dehydration.[14] A review of literature with regard to children found that drinking clear fluids up to a few hours before surgery did not increase the risk of regurgitation during or after surgery, and also had the added benefit of a more comfortable pre-operative experience with regards to hunger and thirst.[15] A minimum of a fasting period of 2 hours for clear fluids prior to surgery/procedures in children may be sufficient.[16] Therefore, there is no requirement for excessive periods of fasting before elective procedures in any paediatric patient.[8] Provide the underlying rationale to the parents and child that is required to prevent aspiration of gastric contents during anaesthesia.[7] Place fasting sign over child's bed/cot; in older toddlers it may be necessary to remove drinks, sweets, etc., and ensure parental supervision to ensure adherence to fasting. It is also important to monitor hydration status, particularly in younger infants, infants with certain medical conditions or those at risk of dehydration. It may be necessary to commence an intravenous infusion.

## Mobility

Assess child's mobility on admission, i.e. crawling, walking, etc. Depending on type of surgery it may be necessary to highlight any restrictions to movement afterwards, e.g. short-term bed rest, limb elevation. Involvement of the physiotherapist, play specialist and occupational therapist may be indicated.

## Personal cleansing and dressing

Encourage/assist the child to bath/shower the evening prior to or morning of the surgery if time permits. Adhere to local policy with regard to standards for cleansing or shaving of operative skin.[13] This is necessary to minimise the risk of postoperative infection.[14] However, research into the use of antiseptic preparations in baths and showers and the removal of body hair has produced contradictory findings.[14] The child's vaccination history and any recent contact with infectious children should be noted and reported to the doctor. While fasting, perform or assist with oral hygiene.

## Sleeping

The child's normal sleeping pattern is established and maintained in the hospital as much as is possible. Locate the child in a quiet room with minimum distraction to promote relaxation and facilitate sleep.[7] Identify if child has a favourite toy or comforter, music or video games that may assist

with relaxation. Parent(s) may be offered the opportunity to 'room in' with the child, or parent's accommodation may be available in the hospital.

## Elimination

Obtain the child's normal bowel and urination pattern. Encourage the child to void prior to surgery and note and document any unusual appearance or changes.[13] Perform a urinalysis to detect any abnormalities which must be reported. If the child is going to have abdominal surgery it may be necessary for the child to have an empty bowel; therefore, administer appropriate bowel preparation as prescribed by the surgeon and note the effect.

## PRE-OPERATIVE CHECKS

### Immediate (day of surgery)

On the day of surgery the nurse must reinforce the psychological preparation of the child and complete a pre-operative checklist in line with hospital policy.

### *Equipment[13]*

Identification band for child
Surgical gown
Stethoscope
Thermometer
Blood pressure monitor
Pulse oximetry monitor
Scale
Pre-operative checklist
Pre-operative medications (if prescribed)

## PROCEDURE: Paediatric pre-surgical check procedure

| Procedural steps | Evidence-based rationale |
|---|---|
| 1 Confirm that identification band is secure, legible and corroborates with patient/family statement and matches chart documentation (patient's name, date of birth and hospital number) | To ensure identification is correct and to prevent possible misidentification[17] |
| 2 Ensure that all necessary consents are completed, with dates, procedure identified, parent/guardian signature and signature of witnesses | This is done to comply with legal requirements and hospital policy[13,14]<br>To ensure that the patient (parents, those with parental responsibility) understand the surgical procedure[11] |
| 3 Ensure that the child is fasting as requested by the doctor and in accordance with hospital policy | To prevent aspiration of gastric contents during anaesthesia[7] |

## PROCEDURE: Paediatric pre-surgical check procedure (continued)

| | |
|---|---|
| **4** Ensure that the child has had a bath or shower as close to the planned time of surgery as possible[18] | This is necessary to minimise the risk of postoperative infection[14] |
| **5** Remove any make-up from the face and nail polish from fingers and toes | This allows the anaesthetist to examine for signs of hypoxia[14] |
| **6** Dress the child with surgical gown as per hospital policy. Some hospitals allow the child to wear underwear to theatre in order to reduce anxiety<br>Small babies/neonates may need to wear a hat | To minimise the risk of postoperative infection[14]<br><br>To prevent heat loss through the scalp[6] |
| **7** Record the temperature, pulse, respiratory rate, blood pressure, oxygen saturation (if indicated) | To give base line recordings with which to compare postoperative observations[14] |
| **8** Record and document current weight and height in line with hospital policy | Height and weight recordings are used to determine drug dosages, blood volume and fluid requirements[13] |
| **9** Note any known or suspected allergies to food or medication in the chart | This decreases the risk of adverse reaction[7] |
| **10** Check that laboratory and X-ray results are in the patient's chart. Assess laboratory results and report results outside normal range to doctor | |
| **11** Remove any jewellery, hairpins (note older children may have body piercings). Tape rings that cannot be removed. Also remove contact lenses, spectacles, hearing aids and orthodontic devices (retainers)<br>Document on pre-operative checklist any piercings/jewellery and whether taped/untaped<br>Hearing aids or spectacles may be removed in the anaesthetic room at the last moment in accordance with hospital policy<br>Label personal items. Give items to parents for safekeeping or record and store in hospital safe as per policy[14] | Metal or other materials may be a risk factor for burns from the cautery used in surgery or may contribute to pressure sore development during prolonged surgery[13]<br><br>This allows for continuation of communication thus reducing anxiety.<br><br>To prevent loss[7] |
| **12** Examine the mouth and inquire about potential loose teeth/fillings, caps, crowns<br>Remove any dentures or plates<br>Document and report to the anaesthetist[6] | There is a risk of accidental damage or accidental ingestion/inhalation during the operation[18] |
| **13** Encourage the child to void before surgery or make sure there is a clean nappy on prior to giving a pre-medication<br>Ensure that urinalysis is performed and documented<br>Record time of last voiding or if unable to void | The child may not get an opportunity to void in the operating theatre, and will also receive considerable amounts of intravenous fluids intraoperatively[1]<br><br>A full bladder is more prone to be damaged during abdominal surgery[14] |
| **14** Check that operation site if previously marked by surgical staff is still visible[6] | To ensure that patient undergoes the correct surgery[17]<br>Chief Executive Officers are required to ensure that surgical safety checklists including correct surgery site identifiction are undertaken within their organisation.[19] |
| **15** Check that the patient has undergone pre-anaesthetic<br>anaesthetic review by the anaesthetist | To ensure that any special requirements for<br><br>have been highlighted[17] |

## PROCEDURE:  Paediatric pre-surgical check procedure (continued)

| | |
|---|---|
| 16 Administer any pre-operative medication as prescribed and at the correct time[6] Allow enough time to achieve desired effect and monitor patient for any adverse reactions[13] Apply a topical anaesthetic (e.g. EMLA, an eutectic mix of lidocaine and prilocaine) to the chosen intravenous site/s 60 minutes before the insertion of the intravenous cannula[20] as prescribed by the doctor and in line with local policy At this stage patient should not be left alone, it may be necessary to put up bed rails, cot sides as patient may become drowsy. Parents are encouraged to stay with the child[7] | This helps to promote relaxation and reduce anxiety[13] To reduce the risk of falls following the administration of a sedative[14] |
| 17 The pre-operative checklist should be completed directly prior to the child going to theatre[6] as per hospital policy and await confirmation that theatre is ready to accept the child | |
| 18 It is also important that medical notes, nursing documentation, prescription and fluid balance chart accompany the child to theatre | |
| 19 Once contacted by theatre the child is transported to theatre in line with hospital policy. When the porter from the theatre reception area arrives to collect the patient, accompany the child to the theatre reception area and hand over to the care of the theatre nurse | To ensure continuity of care and to maintain the safety of the patient by ensuring that all relevant information is exchanged using patients records and the pre-operative checklist[17] |
| 20 The child may travel to theatre on a hospital bed or padded theatre trolley in accordance with hospital policy. Parents are encouraged to accompany child as far as possible[7] | Parents may be permitted to remain with the child until induction; this is dependent on hospital policy |

## PERI-OPERATIVE CARE

The provision of safe and effective care to all children in the peri-operative setting is essential and requires a family-centred approach. This approach can be facilitated in the peri-operative environment by ensuring effective communication in the pre-operative phase of care (specifically relating to the peri-operative phase) and ensuring that care is managed a competent manner from induction in the anaesthetic room through to discharge from the PACU/recovery room.

### Effective communication

1 An information leaflet about the operative environment (including the surgical procedure) should be provided. This leaflet should be age specific to meet the needs of both child and parents, detailing information about the theatre team providing care, parental involvement in the peri-operative phase and facilities available to parents while their child is in surgery. This information can be invaluable to parents whose child is undergoing emergency surgery and may reduce parental anxiety.[3]

2 If surgery is elective a pre-operative visit from an operating department nurse is advocated, which provides both parent and child with an opportunity to ask questions about the operative environment. Where appropriate a visit to operating department should be arranged, which may allow both parent and child to familiarise

themselves and reduce their anxiety.[21]

3 Parents should be encouraged to accompany their child to the operating department (OD) (they should not feel pressurised) and in line with local policy may be allowed to accompany their child to the anaesthetic room, which may provide reassurance to the child undergoing surgery.[22–24]

## Care of the child in the peri-operative environment

1 Parents and children should be welcomed in a warm and friendly manner to the OD by nursing staff. This welcome should incorporate a detailed hand over from the ward nurse, including an introduction of both child and parents to the OD nurse, which may help reduce child/parental anxiety.[23, 24] This handover should detail any specific religious or cultural beliefs which may have to be adhered to in the peri-operative phase, e.g. jewellery or items of clothing which may have to remain on the child's person. Where possible the nurse receiving the parents and child to the operating department should have previously visited the family on the ward, which will ensure familiarity and may also reduce anxiety.

2 The peri-operative environment should be child friendly and decorated appropriately with bright colour schemes, murals/action characters on the walls and ceilings. This may provide distraction to younger children, and where appropriate the child's favourite music or familiar toy may be used to provide distraction.

3 The nursing staff and other members of the OD team should wear brightly coloured/decorative theatre hats and shoes.

## Care of the child in the anaesthetic room

1 Where possible a parent should remain with his/her child until induction is complete or in line with anaesthetist's requests, as clinical situations or patient condition may not always allow for parental presence in the anaesthetic room. This should be discussed with the parent as part of pre-operative care.[23–24]

2 Where possible, non-essential clinical equipment should be removed from the child's view prior to his/her arrival in the anaesthetic room. However,

safety is a priority and to ensure safe anaesthetic induction the following equipment will be required in the anaesthetic room:[25]

- a theatre trolley which is height adjustable, with protective sides and has a head tilt facility;
- oxygen and suction (fully functional);
- monitoring equipment: cardiac monitor, non-invasive blood pressure monitor, pulse oximetry and thermometer;
- cannulation equipment and intravenous fluids;
- intubation equipment including a variety of sizes of endotracheal tubes, oxygen masks, oral/nasal airways and anaesthetic machine;
- emergency resuscitative equipment including defibrillator and emergency drugs.

This list is generic in nature and may be altered depending on patient-specific or anaesthetist requirements. Also note that neonatal induction is usually carried out in the operating theatre.

3 The induction procedure should be performed in a calm environment with emotional support provided to child and parents throughout as both may become upset, and it is essential that the nurse remains with both to ensure patient safety.[11] It is also essential that a second anaesthetic nurse assists the anaesthetist(s) with the induction procedure. Note that neonatal induction is usually carried out in the operating theatre.

4 Parental involvement at this time may reduce the child's anxiety and can help.

5 All monitoring equipment should be attached to the child prior to commencement of induction to assist in establishing baseline vital signs and to facilitate continuous observation throughout surgery. All equipment should be size appropriate for the specific patient, checked and in working order prior to the procedure commencing.[18]

6 When the child is asleep the parent should be escorted to the waiting area or ward according to institutional policy and ensure that the parent is aware of the possible duration of the surgery (approximate times are recommended as complications or procedural delays may occur).

7 When the child is deemed medically stable he/she is transferred from the anaesthetic room to the operating room.

## Care of the child in the operating room

1 The optimum goal of care is to ensure the safety of the child throughout the operative procedure. Key or central to this goal is ensuring that the environmental temperature is constant at a minimum of 24–25°C. However, it should be considered that some children such as neonates, infants or children undergoing long surgical procedures may be at increased risk of hypothermia for a number of reasons:[25]

- exposure;
- impaired shivering ability (particularly in infants and neonates);
- poikilothermia, i.e. all patients under anaesthetic are at risk of assuming room temperature.

It is therefore essential that steps are taken to reduce the risk of patient cooling (unless surgically warranted) by covering the child's head and exposed extremities. A warming mattress or warm air blanket may also be used to maintain the child's body temperature. These steps may reduce the need to increase the room temperature therefore maintaining a constant temperature for all peri-operative personnel.

2 The child will need to be transferred from the theatre trolley to the operating room bed. This transfer will require a number of staff (the exact number is dependent on child age and size); but staff need to be familiar with the techniques of moving and handling and follow local policies and procedures. The team will be coordinated by the anaesthetist who will manage the child's airway and all staff should be aware of the risk of injury to themselves and others and thus use effective moving and handling techniques with patient transfer.

Following safe transfer of the child on to the theatre bed, he/she will be positioned in accordance with the surgical procedure being performed, e.g. prone positioning (lying face down; head to one side and pillows used to support the chest, abdomen and legs) may be used in spinal surgery. Other common positions include supine, lithotomy, lateral and Trendelenburg.

3 The correct positioning of a child undergoing surgery is an important part of the role of the operating room nurse, but within this role a number of other aspects of care also need to be considered, i.e. pressure area care and electrosurgery (diathermy) plate position.

It is clear that any patient undergoing surgery is at increased risk of developing a pressure sore,[26] which is particularly evident in the case of hypothermic infants and neonates, who may shunt blood from the peripheries because of catecholamine release.[25] This possibility reiterates the need to prevent hypothermia in children undergoing surgery, but also highlights the need for a thorough assessment of pressure areas prior to surgery commencing. This assessment may be carried out when transferring the patient on to the theatre bed, and steps should be taken to prevent pressure sore development with the use of pressure-relieving devices such as head rings and heel pads. A further assessment of pressure areas should be carried out on transfer from the operating bed at the end of surgery and any alteration in skin condition should be documented in the peri-operative care plan.

Electrosurgery is one of the most frequently used pieces of equipment in the operating room[27] and the plate which facilitates its use is usually put in place by an operating room nurse or member of the interdisciplinary team. To ensure the safe use of this electrical equipment and reduce the risk of injury to the child, the nurse should be aware of the risks of injury from using this device and ensure that all policies and procedures are adhered to within the operating room.

4 The invasive nature of surgical procedures performed in the operating room increases the risk of infection for the child undergoing any these procedures; it is therefore essential that all members of the surgical team adhere to best practice[28] as outlined below:

- hand washing, i.e. using an antiseptic surgical solution and cleaning nails with a single-use nailbrush;
- wearing sterile gowns by all members of the operative team;
- washing hands between each surgical procedure;
- preparing incision site using an antiseptic solution just prior to surgical incision: solutions include povidone–iodine or chlorhexidine.

All surgical equipment used as part of an operative procedure should be sterile and sterility should be maintained throughout surgery in order to prevent or reduce the risk of infection.

5 The nurse 'scrubbed in' as part of the operative team is usually responsible for accounting for items used throughout the operation.[29] The items accounted for usually include all sharps, ties, clips, surgical instruments and swabs (Raytec). The method of accounting for these items can vary from hospital to hospital but each nurse should be aware of and adhere to local policy in this matter. This checking usually occurs at fixed times throughout the procedure and provides a mechanism to ensure that no foreign bodies are retained in the child. All equipment used should be documented as part of the peri-operative care plan.

6 A plan of care may be initiated by the operating room nurse who visits the child in the ward prior to surgery; this may address the fears and anxiety of both child and parent, e.g. parental wishes, etc. The care plan is continued on the day of surgery and care is usually divided under the subheadings outlined above right up to discharge from the PACU. It is the responsibility of all peri-operative nurses to ensure that all aspects of each child's care plan is completed while in the peri-operative environment. Additional documentation should be completed to facilitate the organisation and management of care, i.e. operating register or any other documentation in line with local policy. Implicit in all aspects of care provided to a child undergoing surgery should be the nurse as advocate, and rights of the child should be respected.

## Care of the child in the PACU/recovery room

The child is transferred to the PACU after the surgical procedure, anaesthesia reversal and extubation (if it is necessary). The amount of time the patient spends in the PACU depends on the length of surgery, type of surgery, status of regional anaesthesia (e.g. spinal anaesthesia), and the patient's level of consciousness. The care of the child in the PACU usually entails the following.

1 The PACU should operate on a one-to-one nurse-to-child ratio, with all appropriate monitoring, oxygen and emergency equipment available.[25] The monitoring of the child will be continuous to deal with any postoperative complications that may arise. These complications can be anaesthetic related, i.e. laryngospasm or bronchospasm, or procedural related, such as haemorrhage.[25] It is therefore essential that the operating room nurse give a detailed handover of the child's status, from induction through to surgery completion. This detail should be documented and include:

- induction and any difficulties with same;
- cardiovascular status since admission to operative suite, including surgery;
- blood loss during surgery;
- surgical incision, wound and vacuum drains;
- medications and intravenous fluids administered;
- specific surgical and anaesthetic requirements;
- specific nursing requirements, including parental involvement.

2 On arrival in the PACU, initially the primary concern for the nurse must be airway management, and in the initial period this may have to be supported manually with an artificial (Guedel) airway. Oxygen will be administered as prescribed by the anaesthetist and titrated in accordance with child's condition and in line with local policy as some units have standing orders in this regard.

3 The nurse should remain with the child, continuously observing his/her respiratory pattern for signs of distress or complications such as bronchospasm after extubation. Respirations are documented every 15 minutes or more frequently as necessary, monitoring the rate, depth and rhythm, including symmetry of chest rise. As the effects of anaesthesia wear off, the child's ability to cough out the artificial airway (if one is in place) and maintain his/her own will be enhanced. Breathing and the effort required may be reduced by sitting the child upright, as the condition allows.

4 One of the greatest risks with surgery is haemorrhage, and constant monitoring is required in the immediate postoperative period to assess the child for signs of this. Vital signs are documented every 15 minutes and these include:

- heart rate and pulse, which will usually increase when bleeding occurs due to hypovolaemia; the depth of pulse should also be monitored as this can be used to indicate the alteration of haemodynamic status;
- blood pressure: a drop in pressure usually indicates bleeding, which may or may not be directly evident;
- temperature may initially be low following surgery and warming should be gradual; the temperature will remain low and decrease if haemorrhage is evident due to catecholamine release;
- other indicators of haemorrhage in the absence of visible blood maybe pallor or reduced urinary output.

5 The child's wound site will be covered with a sterile dressing; the area surrounding this dressing should be observed for redness, swelling, bruising or increased tension, all indicators of fluid accumulation or haemorrhage. There may also be increased pain at the site and if a surgical or wound drain is in place, there may be visible blood loss in this also. If haemorrhage is evident, steps to remediate this should be immediate; inform surgeons and apply pressure dressings.

6 As the child wakes he/she may become more active and irritable; this irritability may be as a result pain or parental separation.[30,31] It is therefore essential that parents are encouraged to come and stay with their child in recovery as the condition allows and to reduce anxiety for both. Parents know their child best and can therefore help staff in establishing a child's normal responses when assessing awakeness. The parents may also assist staff in assessing the child's pain levels, i.e. own terminology, pain scales or other appropriate tools may be used and documented. Analgesia should be administered as prescribed and providing the child is comfortable and vital signs stable he/she can be transferred back to the ward.

7 Children returning to the recovery room will have an IV cannula in place, which is usually sited in a peripheral vein on the non-dominant arm[30] (site and type of intravenous access used is patient and condition dependent). The child will have intravenous fluids in place on transfer to the PACU; these fluids should be administered as prescribed in accordance with medical prescription and the child's body weight. The patency of IV cannula should be accessed, observing site for signs of tissue infiltration, i.e. redness, pain and swelling around the cannula site.[30,31] The IV cannula should be securely fastened and observed frequently for the previously cited reasons. In addition, all intravenous fluids should be administered via an infusion pump with the hourly rate documented and an accurate fluid balance maintained while the child is in the PACU.

8 In order to facilitate this transfer, a detailed plan of care should be completed with all aspects of care documented. Specific postoperative instructions with a complete peri-operative profile of care should be provided to the ward nurse detailing the information previously outlined in point 1.

## POSTOPERATIVE CARE

This is described as the nursing care given to the patient during the postoperative period after discharge from the recovery room to the ward, and is directed towards the prevention of potential complications resulting from surgery and anaesthesia which might be expected to develop over a longer period of time.[18]

### *Equipment*

Postoperative bed/cot
Clean linen/sheets folded back
Oxygen/suction (both checked and working)
Nil-by-mouth sign over bed
Oral hygiene tray
Emesis bowl (if indicated, older child)
Intravenous stand and infusion pumps
Extra blankets or a warming device
Stethoscope
Thermometer
Blood pressure monitor
Pulse oximetry monitor

Equipment that may be required postoperatively should be tested and ready when the child is transferred back to the ward.[32,35]

Based on the age of child, type of surgery and any other medical issues it may be necessary to locate the child's bed/cot in a room close to the nurses' station to facilitate closer observation by nursing staff.[35] Also ensure that there is a call bell at the bed space and check that it is working correctly. Once the child is stable and satisfies the discharge requirements of the recovery room, he/she is ready to be transferred back to the wards.[36] The ward staff can be contacted and the child is transferred back to ward in accordance with hospital policy. The child may be transported to the ward in their own bed/cot, otherwise transfer from hospital trolley to bed/cot using techniques appropriate to type of surgery to prevent injury.[7] A plan of care is implemented that is patient specific and supportive of condition.

## PROCEDURE: Postoperative care

| Procedural steps | Evidence-based rationale |
|---|---|
| 1 When receiving the patient back to the ward the immediate priority is to assess and maintain a patent airway<br><br>It may be necessary to position child on his side or abdomen<br>Otherwise place the child in a comfortable position and safety in accord with the surgeon's orders[7] | The patient is usually conscious before leaving the recovery room; however, if he/she is heavily sedated, the tongue may slip back and cause airway obstruction[14]<br>To allow secretions to drain and prevent tongue from obstructing pharynx[10] |
| 2 Observe general condition and vital signs as indicated by child's condition, as per doctor's instructions, and in accordance with hospital policy[7,10,13,35] | The frequency of routine postoperative observations may vary and is dependent on the condition of the child[35] |
| 3 Observe respirations (rate and depth), oxygen saturations, colour, conscious level of the child, pulse and blood pressure | The initial findings of the nurse become the baseline for comparison of postoperative changes. Vital signs are evaluated in terms of side-effects from anaesthesia, pain and signs of potential shock or respiratory compromise[13,34]<br>Signs of shock may be indicated by pallor, coldness, restlessness, increased pulse and irregular respirations, decreased blood pressure. Respiratory depression may be a side-effect of opiates, or may indicate pain[13] |
| 4 Encourage the child to sit up well in bed (unless contraindicated: age, type of surgery, clinical status) well supported with pillows[14] | To facilitate optimum lung expansion[18] |
| 5 If oxygen is to be administered, ensure that the mask is securely positioned and that oxygen is delivered at the prescribed rate[35] | |
| 6 Document, report any changes or concerns to the doctor | |
| 7 Record temperature as indicated by child's condition | If elevated, this may indicate an infection[18]<br>Patients who have undergone long periods of surgery or where large amounts of blood or replacement fluids have been administered are at a high risk of hyperthermia<br>Extra blankets or Bair Hugger® blankets may by required[18] |
| 8 As discussed in the pre-operative preparation, age-appropriate communication is vital and is reinforced in the postoperative period | To alleviate anxiety, provide reassurance and gain the patients cooperation and confidence[18] |

## PROCEDURE: Postoperative care (continued)

| | |
|---|---|
| Reorientate the child to time, place, environment and circumstances as often as required<br>Explain procedures and other activities before carrying them out, using age-appropriate language<br>Encourage the child to talk about the operation and ask questions<br>Provide support for the parents and facilitate parental involvement as soon as possible<br>Give encouragement and positive feedback to the child for involvement in care, e.g. praise | To increase the child's degree of comfort in unfamiliar situations and promote trust with parents[13] |
| 9 Assess the child's pain level using a pain assessment tool relevant to the child's age and development level to identify the need for analgesia[35]<br>In addition to the pain assessment tool observe the child's behaviour, cues and vital signs for indicators that suggest pain[36]<br>Provide the child with education and information about pain control, including non-pharmacological options:[13]<br>• relaxation: soft music, massage<br>• distraction: quiet play, favourite story telling<br>• physical contact: soft touch, cuddles from parents<br>• involvement of play specialist<br>• ensure a position of comfort unless contra-indicated<br>• move child smoothly and gently<br>• support the wound with a pillow, soft toy when moving, deep breathing<br>Administer analgesics as prescribed and monitor the effect<br>Do not wait until the child experiences severe pain before intervening in order to prevent pain occurring<br>Before performing nursing activities such as (mobilisation, deep-breathing, dressing change, removing drains) administer analgesia[7,10,13,35]<br>If intravenous analgesia is prescribed, i.e. PCA, maintain it at the prescribed rate and monitor the effect[35]<br>Monitor the pulse and respiratory rate every hour<br>Inform the anaesthetist and the pain control specialist if significant relief of pain is not achieved[18] | All postoperative patients should have their pain assessed, recorded and treated, and where possible patients should have an active role in the process[38]<br>Unrelieved pain has a number of undesirable psychological and physical consequences that may delay and complicate the postoperative recovery of children[36]<br><br><br><br><br><br><br><br><br><br>To promote comfort and minimise pain[13]<br><br><br><br><br>Routine administration of IV analgesia, patient-controlled analgesia (PCA) and epidural infusions, rather than as needed (prn), provide excellent analgesia in paediatric patients postoperatively[34]<br>Some opiates may cause respiratory depression[35] |
| 10 Observe wound sites and drains at the same time as performing observations to reduce disturbance to the child<br>Monitor wound site at regular intervals for signs of leakage, mark as necessary<br>Change dressings or add additional pressure padding as required<br>Observe and record output from any drains, | To assess and monitor for signs of leakage, haemorrhage or haematoma[14] |

## PROCEDURE:  Postoperative care (continued)

| | |
|---|---|
| noting the characteristics of the fluid, e.g. haemoserous fluid<br>Report any excessive leakage from wounds/ drainage from drains[34,35] | |
| **11** Assess and maintain surgical dressing integrity[7,10,13]<br>• consult with doctor regarding first dressing<br>• adhere to proper hand-washing technique<br>• use sterile dressings and technique during wound care<br>• assess the wound for signs of infection, pain, redness, swelling, heat, purulent drainage and constriction of circulation<br>• keep wound clean and dry; keep nappy below wound if appropriate | The aim is to minimise the risk for infection and detect any early signs of infection[13] |
| Monitor intravenous infusion, ensure it is at the correct rate as prescribed and record the amount infused hourly<br>Check the intravenous site for signs of extravasation or phlebitis<br>Commence fluid balance chart and monitor all intake and output (urine, vomit, wound drainage, nasogastric tube)<br>Oral fluids should be re-introduced once the child is sufficiently awake unless there are contra-indications (complex surgery, decreased bowel sounds, doctor's instructions)<br>In these circumstances increase diet as ordered from clear liquids to full liquids to solids<br>Observe for signs of dehydration:<br>• decreased urine output<br>• sunken eyes<br>• sunken fontanelle (babies)<br>• dry mucous membranes,<br>• poor skin turgor<br>• prolonged periods of vomiting[13,35]<br>Report any abnormalities<br>Losses via nasogastric tube (bile and secretions) if in situ are replaced millilitre for millilitre[33] | To rehydrate the patient, prevent electrolyte imbalance and help restore blood glucose level to within normal limits[13,14] |
| Administer antiemetics as prescribed and monitor effect | Antiemetics may help to reduce nausea and vomiting[35] |
| **12** Provide mouth care while the child is nil orally | To promote comfort |
| **13** Encourage a gradual return to a normal diet, high in protein and vitamins | To promote wound healing[14] |
| **14** Monitor urinary output<br>Assess for urinary retention or incontinence<br>Provide catheter care if urinary catheter in place as per local policy | Anaesthesia can alter muscle tone and may cause difficulty with micturition[14]<br>Accurate monitoring/recording of intake and output helps to assess circulatory and renal function[13] |
| **15** Maintain normal bowel elimination.<br>Monitor bowel movements | Anaesthetic agents may depress peristalsis and normal gastrointestinal motility[13] |

## PROCEDURE: Postoperative care (continued)

|  |  |
|---|---|
| Assess bowel sounds, note signs and symptoms of distension, nausea and vomiting, flatus and abdominal pain |  |
| 16 Once diet and fluids have been established, encourage a diet that contains roughage and a good fluid intake[35] | To prevent constipation |
| 17 Observe and relieve pressure areas frequently Encourage the child to move by themselves where possible It is usual to mobilise as soon as the child's condition permits[35] | To monitor and prevent pressure sores[39] Changing position may also assist in relieving any pain or discomfort the child may have[35] Reduced mobility can also lead to constipation[35] |
| 18 Facilitate coughing and deep breathing using splinting technique and blowing games as discussed in pre-operative care. It may be necessary to involve the physiotherapist | Anaesthesia agents may depress respiratory function because lungs may not be inflated fully during surgery, the cough reflex is suppressed and mucus collects in airway passages[13] |
| 19 Begin planning for discharge from the time of admission whenever possible | Effective discharge planning can reduce any delay once the decision to discharge has been made[35] |
| 20 The discharge plan should include: <br> • any supplies that may be required, e.g. dressings <br> • prescription and specific instructions <br> • when child can resume physical activity and school <br> • information regarding pain relief and observation of wound site <br> • written instructions and contact numbers should problems arise <br> • referral to community services, e.g. general practitioner, district nurse, paediatric community nurse <br> • arrangement for any follow-up outpatient appointments[14,35] | To ensure that the child's home care needs will be met by parents who are completely informed of child's healthcare issues[13] |

The complications which may arise as a result of anaesthetic or surgical intervention may become evident in the peri-operative or postoperative period. These complications have been outlined in Table 15.1, page 256 and possible difficulties or causes of the potential complication have been classified according to operative phase.

**Table 15.1** Possible complications resulting from anaesthetic or surgical intervention

| Complication | Peri-operative period and PACU | postoperative period |
| --- | --- | --- |
| Difficulty in thermoregulation | Malignant hyperthermia, poikilothermia[23] | Hypothermia in immediate postoperative period<br>Pyrexia secondary to infection/ inflammatory process |
| Altered respiratory status | Inability to maintain own airway due to inductive and anaesthetic agents Laryrgospasm or bronchospasm secondary to intubation | Reduced respiratory effort secondary to (1) pain; (2) opiate-based analgesics |
| Altered haemodynamic status | Hypovolaemic shock due blood loss characterised by acute hypotensive episode and tachycardia | Haemorrhage at surgical site: may be due to ligature displacement or normalisation of blood pressure |
| Risk of wound infection | | Can become evident with pyrexia or signs of inflammation at surgical wound site |
| Nausea and vomiting | May be related to (1) anaesthetic agents; (2) surgical procedure; (3) analgesic agents | May be related to (1) anaesthetic agents; (2) surgical procedure; (3) analgesic agents |
| Pain | | |

PACU, post-anaesthesia care unit.

Go to the website to find the PowerPoint presentation for this chapter and MCQs to test your knowledge. **www.hodderplus.com/childnursingskills**

# REFERENCES

1  The Royal College of Surgeons England (2007) *Surgery for children delivering a first class service report of the children's surgical forum*. London: RCS.
2  The Audit Commission for England and Wales (1993) *Children first: a study of hospital services*. London: HMSO.
3  O'Connor-Von S (2000) Preparing children for surgery: an integrative research review. *AORN Journal* **71**: 334–343.
4  Shields L, King S. J (2001) Qualitative analysis of the care of children in hospital in four countries: Part 1. *Journal of Pediatric Nursing* **16**(2): 137–145.
5  Shields L, King SJ (2001b) Qualitative analysis of the care of children in hospital in four countries: Part 2. *Journal of Pediatric Nursing.* **16**(3): 206–213.
6  Lynch F, Tulp S (2006) Preoperative care. In: Trigg E, Mohammad TA (eds) *Practices in children's nursing guidelines for hospital and community*. Edinburgh: Elsevier pp. 315–320.
7  Wong DL (1995) *Whaley & Wong's nursing care of infants and children*, 5th edition. St Louis, Mosby.

8  Cote CJ (1999) Preoperative preparation and premedication. *British Journal of Anaesthesia* **83**(1): 16–28.
9  Darrbyshire P (2003) Mothers' experience of their child's recovery in hospital and home: a qualitative investigation. *Journal of Child Healthcare* **7**(4): 291–312.
10  Brunner LS, Suddarth DS (1991) *The Lippincott manual of paediatric nursing*, 3rd edition. London: Chapman & Hall.
11  Nursing and Midwifery Council (2006) *A–Z advice sheet consent*. London: NMC. www.nmc.org (Accessed 12th October 2008).
12  Department of Health (2001) *Consent: what you have a right to expect. A guide for children and young people*. London: Stationery Office.
13  Bowden VR, Smith Greenberg C (2008) *Pediatric nursing procedures*, 2nd edition. Philadelphia: Lippincott Williams and Wilkins.
14  Jamieson EM, McCall JM, Whyte LA (2002) *Clinical nursing practices*, 4th edition. Edinburgh:

Churchill Livingstone.

15 Brady M, Kinn S, O Rourke K, Randhawa N, Stuart P (2008) Pre-operative fasting for preventing perioperative complications in children. *The Cochrane Collaboration.* http://www.thecochrane library.com

16 Meurling S (2004) Paediatric aspects: no fasting in children? *Scandinavian Journal of Nutrition* 48(2):83.

17 AORN (2000) Recommended practices for safety through identification of potential hazards in the peri-operative environment. *AORN Journal* 72: 690–698.

18 Dougherty L, Lister S (2008) *The Royal Marsden Hospital manual of clinical nursing procedures*, 7th edition. Chichester: Willey-Blackwell.

19 WHO Surgial Patient Safety Checklist (2009) National Patient Safety Agency. http://www.npsa. nhs.uk/alerts-and directives/alerts/safer-surgery-alert/ (accessed 20 June 2009).

20 Wilson D, (2007) Balance and imbalance of body fluids. In: Hockenberry MJ, Wilson D (eds) *Wong's Nursing care of infants and children*, 8th edition. St Louis: Mosby Elsevier, 1140–1179.

21 Wennstrom B, Hallberg LR-M, Bergh I, (2008) Use of peri-operative dialogues with children undergoing day surgery. *Journal of Advanced Nursing* 62(1): 96–106.

22 Glasper A, Powel C (2000) First do no harm: parental exclusion from the anesthetic room. *Paediatric Nurse* 12: 14–17.

23 Kain ZN, Mayes LC, Wang SL, *et al.* (2000) Parental presence and a sedative premedicant for children undergoing surgery: a hierarchical study. *Anesthesiology* 92: 936–946.

24 Wollin SR, Plummer JL, Owen H, *et al.* (2004) Anxiety in children having elective surgery. *Journal of Pediatric Nursing* 19(2), 128–132.

25 Nagelhout JJ, Zaglaniczny KL (2005) *Handbook of nurse anesthesia*, 3rd edition. St Louis: Elsevier Saunders.

26 Waterlow J (1996) Operating table. The root cause of many pressure sores? *British Journal of Theatre Nursing* 6: 19–21.

27 Wicker P (2000) Electrosurgery in peri-operative practice. *British Journal of Theatre Nursing* 10: 221–226.

28 National Institute of Health and Clinical Excellence (2008) *Surgical site infection prevention and treatment of surgical site infection.* London: NICE.

29 Taylor M, Campbell C (1999) The multidisciplinary team in the operating department. *British Journal of Theatre Nursing* 9: 178–183.

30 Fisher S (2000) Postoperative pain management in paediatrics. *British Journal of Peri-operative Nursing* 10(1): 80–84.

31 Kristensson-Hallstorm I (2000) Parental participation in paediatric surgical care. *Paediatric Nursing* 11(3): 37–39.

32 Fitzsimmons R (2001) Intravenous cannulation. *Paediatric Nursing* 13(3): 21–23.

33 Liversley L (1996) Peripheral IV therapy in children. *Paediatric Nursing* 8(6): 29–33.

34 Algren CL, Arnow D (2007) Pediatric variations of nursing interventions. In: Hockenberry MJ, Wilson D (eds) *Wong's nursing care of infants and children*, 8th edition. St Louis: Mosby Elsevier, pp. 1083–1139.

35 Lynch F, Tulp S (2006) Postoperative care. *Practices in children's nursing guidelines for hospital and community.* Trigg E.& Mohammad TA (eds) Elsevier, Edinburgh, 307–313.

36 Sheilds L, Tanner A (2006) Children and surgery. In: Glasper A, Richardson J (eds) *A textbook of children's and young people's nursing.* Edinburgh: Churchill Livingstone, pp. 278–296.

37 Anderson D, De Voll-Zabrocki A, Brown C, *et al.* (2000) Intestinal transplantation in pediatric patients: a nursing challenge. Part 2: Intestinal transplantation and the immediate postoperative period. *Gastroenterology Nursing* 23 (5): 201–209.

38 Quality Improvement Scotland NHS (2004) *Postoperative pain management*, Edinburgh: NHS QIS www.nhshealthquality.org (accessed 21st October 2008)

39 National Institute for Health and Clinical Excellence (2005) *The management of pressure ulcers in primary and secondary care, a clinical practice guideline.* London: NICE.

## FURTHER READING

Action for Sick Children (2002) *Setting standards for children undergoing surgery.* London: Action for Sick Children.

Nursing and Midwifery Council (NMC) (2004) *Guidelines for records and record-keeping.* London: NMC.

Cockett A (2002) A research review to identify the factors contributing to the development of pressure ulcers in paediatric patients. *Journal of Tissue Viability* 12(1): 16–23.

Kelly MM, Adkins L (2003) Ingredients for a successful preoperative care process. *AORN Journal* 77(5): 1006–1011

La Montague L (2000) Children's coping with surgery: a process-oriented perspective. *Journal of Pediatric Nursing* 15(5): 307–312.

Lissauer T, Clayden G (2001) *Illustrated textbook of*

paediatrics. Edinburgh: Mosby

National Health Service Estates (2003) *Standards of cleanliness in the NHS: a framework in which to measure performance outcomes.* Leeds: NHS Estates.

Nikkane E, Kokki H, Touvinen K (1999) Post operative pain after adenoidectomy in children. *British Journal of Anesthesia* **82**: 886–889.

Rodgers J, Irwin K (2003) *Digital rectal examination. Guidance for nurses working with children and young people.* London: RCN.

Royal College of Nursing (RCN) (1993) *Code of Practice for the handling of patients.* London: RCN.

Royal College of Nursing (RCN) (1999) *Clinical practice guidelines. The recognition and assessment of acute pain in children: recommendations.* London: RCN.

Royal College of Nursing (RCN) (2001) *Clinical practice guidelines. The recognition and assessment of acute pain in children: implementation guide.* London: RCN.

Royal College of Nursing (RCN) (2004) *Sheet 3: day surgery information. Children/young people in day surgery.* London: RCN

Royal College of Nursing (RCN) (2005) *Good practice in infection prevention and control.* London: RCN

Rushforth H (1996) Nurse' knowledge of how children view health and illness. *Paediatric Nursing* **8**: 23–27.

Santo A, Purden M, Tanguay K (2008) Developing an information booklet for parents and caregivers of children recovering from spinal fusion surgery. *Journal of Orthopaedic Nursing* (doi:10.1016/j.joon).

Watt S (2003) Safe administration of medicines to children: part 2. *Paediatric Nursing.* **15**(5): 40–44.

Watt S (2003) Safe administration of medicines to children: part 1. *Paediatric Nursing.* **15**(4): 40–44.

Wollin SR, Plummer JL, Owen H, *et al* (2004) Anxiety in children having elective surgery. *Journal of Pediatric Nursing* **19**(4): 128- 132.

## CHAPTER 16

# Elimination: collecting, measuring and testing urine

## Jane Willock

## LEARNING OUTCOMES

*Upon completion of this chapter, the reader should be able to accomplish the following:*

1 Describe the assessment of urine output in infants and children
2 Identify methods of urine collection in infants and children
3 Describe how to carry out urinalysis on a sample of urine, and discuss what test results may signify
4 Describe with rationale how to safely perform urethral catheterisation
5 List the potential complications of urethral catheterisation, and how to avoid them
6 Describe with rationale how to safely remove an indwelling urethral catheter
7 Illustrate the importance of testing urine with reagent strips
8 Describe how to test for pregnancy using a urine sample

## CHAPTER OVERVIEW: PRINCIPLES OF CARE

The assessment of urine output and urine testing are very important nursing skills. The accurate measurement of urine output is vital to accurate fluid balance measurement; this will be covered in more detail in Chapter 27.

Collecting urine specimens can either be done by invasive or non-invasive methods. Urinary tract infections (UTIs) in infants and young children can cause significant morbidity. Treatment of potential urine infections depends on obtaining uncontaminated, quality urine specimens, and the quality of the urine specimen is dependent on the method and skill of collection.

Some methods of urine collection and urine drainage may put the child at additional risk of UTIs; nursing care and skill are important in preventing these.

Near patient urine testing is a quick and useful way of obtaining information about the health of the child. However, the accuracy of the result is dependent on following the instructions provided with the testing equipment.

## ASSESSING URINE OUTPUT

In continent children urine output can be measured by collecting all urine voided and measuring it. If the weight of the empty urine container is known, the amount of urine produced can be calculated by weighing the container with urine in it and subtracting the weight of the container (1 mL of water = 1 g, 1 L of water = 1 kg).

In infants and children in nappies, the nappies can be weighed prior to use and the weight of the nappy documented (for example, by writing it in biro on the nappy). When the child has passed urine, the nappy can be reweighed, the weight of the dry nappy subtracted and the volume of urine documented. If the child has passed faeces, it may be possible to remove this before the nappy is weighed; otherwise, it should be documented that the nappy also contained faeces.

## COLLECTION OF URINE SPECIMENS

- Midstream specimen of urine (MSU)
- Clean catch specimens
- Urine bag
- Urine collection pad
- Catheter specimen of urine (CSU)

Care should be taken in the collection, storage and transport of urine specimens to prevent contamination. Ideally, urine should be cultured within an hour of the specimen being passed. However, this is not always possible and it should be cooled to 4°C in a fridge to prevent contaminating bacteria multiplying before it can be cultured.[1] Bottles containing borate, which prevents bacterial multiplication, are available commercially for transporting urine specimens. However, borate can inhibit growth on the culture medium giving rise to false-negative results. Dipslides coated with agar and cysteine–lactose-

depleted media are also available and enable the urine to be plated immediately.

Before a urine specimen is collected, wash the perineal and genital area with warm tap water and ordinary soap in infants and young children or if there may have been faecal contamination. Antiseptic soaps or solutions must not be used as they will kill bacteria and the sample might be falsely sterile. The perineal area should then be dried with a clean tissue or soft paper towel.

### Obtaining a midstream specimen of urine
#### *Equipment*

Apron
Non-sterile gloves
Plain wipes, mild unscented soap, warm water (if cleansing is necessary)
Sterile bowl or jug
Sterile urine specimen container with secure top
Laboratory request form

## PROCEDURE: Collection of urine specimens

| Procedural steps | Evidence-based rationale |
|---|---|
| 1 Explain to an older child or parent how to obtain a midstream specimen of urine, and what the sample is for | To prevent the child's embarrassment if they are able to perform this procedure themselves or would prefer a parent to help them |
| 2 Wash hands. Put on apron and non-sterile gloves | To reduce cross-contamination and the spread of infection |
| 3 Ask child to thoroughly wash and dry their hands. Ask child or parent to cleanse the child's genital area with soap and warm water and dry, only if there may be contamination with faeces | Contamination rates in adult women were found to be similar with or without cleansing[2] |
| 4 Encourage the child to start passing urine into the toilet, then hold the sterile bowl in the urine stream to collect a sample (10–20 mL is adequate for testing). | The first voided urine may wash some contaminating organisms out of the urethral meatus |
| 5 Allow the child to finish passing urine into the toilet | The child should be comfortable |
| 6 Pour enough urine into the urine container for laboratory investigations (1–5 mL is usually sufficient for microscopy) and put the top on. Urine remaining in the bowl can be tested using reagent strips | To prevent urine spillage<br>To prevent contamination of the urine specimen which is being sent for laboratory analysis |
| 7 Discard any unwanted urine and equipment according to hospital policy<br>Remove gloves and apron and wash hands | To reduce the risk of infection |
| 8 Label the urine sample and transport to the microbiology laboratory immediately.<br>If transport to the laboratory is delayed, the sample should be refrigerated at 4°C, or preserved with boric acid immediately | Urine should be cultured within 4 hours of collection to prevent growth of contaminants[1] |

## Obtaining a clean catch specimen

Urine can be collected directly into a universal container or into a sterile bowl. This is a useful method with young infants who micturate frequently and are relatively immobile, but is very difficult and time consuming with older infants, particularly in the 9–24-month age group.

Of the non-invasive methods of urine collection, this method has the lowest contamination rate with infants and young children and is the recommended method for urine collection.[1] In adult women it has a similar contamination rate to midstream urine collection.[2]

### Equipment

Apron
Non-sterile gloves
Plain wipes, mild unscented soap, warm water (if cleansing is necessary).
Sterile bowl or jug
Clean bath towel (if collecting specimen from an infant)
Clean potty if collecting urine from a toddler
Sterile urine specimen container with secure top
Laboratory request form

## PROCEDURE: Obtaining a clean catch specimen

| Procedural steps | Evidence-based rationale |
| --- | --- |
| 1 Explain to parent how to obtain a clean catch specimen of urine, and what the sample is for | |
| 2 Give the child or infant a drink | To encourage the production of urine |
| 3 Wash hands. Put on apron and non-sterile gloves | To reduce cross-contamination and the spread of infection |
| 4 Cleanse of the genital area with soap and warm water if necessary. Dry with tissue or soft wipe | To reduce the risk of contamination with skin flora |
| 5 Spread the towel on your knee. Sit the infant on the bowl on your knee<br>With toddlers the sterile bowl can be placed in a clean potty, then the toddler can sit on the potty. Alternatively, the toddler can urinate directly into a potty that has been washed well with detergent and hot water | To prevent contamination of clothes<br><br>Improve the comfort of the baby or toddler<br><br>Washing a potty well with detergent and hot water removes potential contaminants making the potty suitable for urine specimen collection |
| 6 When the infant or child has passed urine, wash and dress them as normal | To prevent infant or child getting cold and maintain dignity |
| 7 Pour the enough urine into the urine container for laboratory investigations (1–5 mL is usually sufficient for microscopy) and put the top on. Urine remaining in the bowl can be tested using reagent strips.<br>If a potty is used the urine sample should be aspirated from the potty with a syringe | To prevent urine spillage<br>To prevent contamination of the urine specimen which isbeing sent for laboratory analysis<br><br>If urine is poured out of the potty, it may become contaminated where the toddler has been sitting on the rim of the potty |
| 8 Discard any unwanted urine and equipment according to hospital policy<br>Remove gloves and wash hands | To reduce the risk of infection |
| 9 Label the specimen and request form, and ensure it reaches the microbiology laboratory as soon as possible (ideally within 1 hour of taking the specimen), or store it in a refrigerator at 2–8°C until it can be transported to the laboratory | To prevent cell lysis and growth of contaminating bacteria |

*Adhesive urine bags* may be applied over the genital area after washing and drying. However, these appear uncomfortable, are prone to leakage and falling off, and may cause further damage if skin is already broken. The contamination rate for this method is high, and direct microscopy and white cell count are more reliable than colony count.

Before using this method, ensure that the infant has not had any previous sensitivity reactions to skin adhesive.

If the infant has a rash, broken skin, excoriation or other skin lesions around the genital area or perineum, this method should not be used as it will increase discomfort and exacerbate the skin condition.

### Equipment

Non-sterile gloves
Plain wipes, simple soap, warm water
Adhesive urine bag
Urine container with secure top

## PROCEDURE: Using adhesive urine bags

| Procedural steps | Evidence-based rationale |
|---|---|
| 1 Explain to an older child or parent how to obtain a specimen of urine with an adhesive bag, and what the sample is for | |
| 2 Give the child or infant a drink | To encourage the production of urine |
| 3 Wash hands. Put on non-sterile gloves | To reduce cross-contamination and the spread of infection |
| 4 Cleanse the genital area with normal soap and warm water. Dry with tissue or soft wipe | To reduce the risk of contamination with skin flora |
| 5 With boy infants, using a male urine collection bag of appropriate size, put the penis through the hole in the bag so that urine will flow into the bag. Peel off the protective film and stick the adhesive evenly to the skin so that there are no creases.<br>With girl infants, using a female urine collection bag of appropriate size, start to peel off the protective film from the centre of the adhesive and stick this to the perineum (in between the anus and the vulva) first. Then remove the remaining protective film while sticking the adhesive evenly to the skin around the vulva, so that there are no creases<br>The infant's nappy can be put on loosely. Check the urine bag about every 15–20 minutes | To minimise leakage of urine |
| 6 When the infant or child has passed urine, put on non-sterile gloves and gently remove the urine bag avoiding any spills. Wash and dress the infant as normal | To reduce the risk of infection<br>To maintain dignity |
| 7 Hold the urine bag over a sterile container. Cut the corner of the urine bag with clean scissors or remove tab in the corner of the urine bag. Pour enough urine into the urine container for laboratory investigations (1–5 mL is usually sufficient for microscopy) and put the top on | To prevent urine spillage<br>To prevent contamination of the urine specimen which is being sent for laboratory analysis |

## PROCEDURE: Using adhesive urine bags (continued)

| | |
|---|---|
| **8** Discard any unwanted urine and equipment according to hospital policy<br>Remove gloves and wash hands | To reduce the risk of infection |
| **9** Label the specimen and request form, and ensure it reaches the microbiology laboratory as soon as possible (ideally within 1 hour of taking the specimen), or store it in a refrigerator at 2–8°C until it can be transported to the laboratory | To prevent cell lysis and growth of contaminating bacteria |

*Urine collection pads* are similar to sterile sanitary pads, and can be placed in a clean nappy after washing and drying the perineal and genital area. Urine specimens collected with urine pads may have a lower contamination rate than those collected by the bag method, but higher than the clean catch method.[3] Ideally, they should be renewed every 30–45 minutes to reduce contamination of the urine sample.[4]

### Equipment

Non-sterile gloves
Plain wipes, simple soap, warm water
Urine collection pad
Urine container with secure top

## PROCEDURE: Using urine collection pads

| Procedural steps | Evidence-based rationale |
|---|---|
| **1** Explain to an older child or parent how to obtain a specimen of urine using a urine collection pad, and what the sample is for | |
| **2** Give the child or infant a drink | To encourage the production of urine |
| **3** Wash hands. Put on non-sterile gloves | To reduce cross-contamination and the spread of infection |
| **4** Cleanse the genital area with normal soap and warm water. Dry with tissue or soft wipe | To reduce the risk of contamination with skin flora |
| **5** Place the infant's or child's buttocks on a clean nappy. Hold the sterile urine collection pad by the edges, remove the adhesive strip, and position the non-adhesive side over the infant's or child's genital area. Continue to put the nappy on the infant or child so that the adhesive sticks to the nappy and the urine collection pad is in maximum contact with the genital area. Check the pad every 15–20 minutes. Change the pad for a new one if the child has not passed urine within 45 minutes | |
| **6** When the infant or child has passed urine, put on non-sterile gloves and remove the nappy containing the urine collection pad avoiding any spills. Wash and dress the infant as normal | To feduce the risk of infection<br>To maintain dignity |

## PROCEDURE:  Using urine collection pads (continued)

| | |
|---|---|
| 7 Wear non-sterile gloves. Aspirate some urine from the pad using a syringe. Alternatively, carefully tear the surface covering of the urine collection pad and put some urine-soaked fibres into the barrel of a sterile 10 mL syringe, replace the plunger and squeeze enough urine into a sterile urine container for laboratory investigations (1–5 mL is usually sufficient for microscopy) and put the top on | Tp prevent urine spillage<br>To prevent contamination of the urine specimen which is being sent for laboratory analysis |
| 8 Discard any unwanted urine and equipment according to hospital policy<br>Remove gloves and wash hands | To reduce the risk of infection |
| 9 Label the specimen and request form, and ensure it reaches the microbiology laboratory as soon as possible (ideally within 1 hour of taking the specimen), or store it in a refrigerator at 2–8°C until it can be transported to the laboratory | To prevent cell lysis and growth of contaminating bacteria |

## Obtaining a catheter specimen of urine

A urine sample for microbiology must never be taken from the urine bag. It is important that this procedure is carried out aseptically, as infection can be introduced when the sample is taken.[5]

*Equipment*

Apron
Gloves
Alcohol swabs
Hypodermic needle
Syringe
Sterile sample container
Sharps container

## PROCEDURE:  Obtaining a catheter specimen

| Procedural steps | Evidence-based rationale |
|---|---|
| 1 Check the identity of the child with the request form<br>Explain to the child and carer why you need to collect a sample of urine and what you are going to do | To ensure that the correct child's specimen is sent to the laboratory<br><br>To maintain privacy and dignity |
| 2 Wash and dry your hands well. Use alcohol hand gel | To prevent cross-infection |
| 3 Put on apron and gloves<br>Clean the sampling port on the catheter bag tubing with the alcohol swab, allow to dry for 30 seconds making sure that nothing touches it before you take the sample | Prevent cross-infection<br>The action of the alcohol drying denatures cell proteins and kills microbes[6] |
| 4 Put the needle and syringe together | |
| 5 Pierce the cleaned sample port with the needle<br>Withdraw the plunger to draw back a sample of urine (you may need to wait while some urine drains into the tubing next to the sample port) | |

## PROCEDURE: Obtaining a catheter specimen (continued)

| | |
|---|---|
| Remove the needle from the sampling port (this port is designed to reseal after withdrawal of the needle) | |
| **6** Put the urine sample into the sterile urine specimen container | |
| **7** Discard equipment safely. Wash hands | To prevent cross-infection |
| **8** Ensure the child is comfortable | To maintain dignity |
| **9** Label the specimen and request form, and ensure it reaches the microbiology laboratory as soon as possible (ideally within 1 hour of taking the specimen), or store it in a refrigerator at 2–8°C until it can be transported to the laboratory | To prevent cell lysis and growth of contaminating bacteria |

## URETHRAL CATHETERISATION

Urethral catheterisation is the introduction of a tube (catheter) into the bladder through the urethra. Urinary catheterisation should be contemplated only as a last resort,[7] when absolutely necessary, and the catheter must not be left in situ longer than necessary as the risk of UTI with an indwelling catheter is reported to increase by 5 per cent per day.[8] Of patients with a UTI, 1–4 per cent develop bacteraemia and of these 13–30 per cent die. The six most common organisms causing UTI in European hospitals in 2001 were *Escherichia coli*, *Enterococcus* sp., *Candida* sp., *Klebsiella* sp., and *Pseudomonas aeruginosa*, and 63 per cent of these are urinary catheter related. Apart from UTIs, urinary catheterisation has other complications.[9] The insertion of a urethral catheter is a common cause of urethral damage and stricture formation in males.

There are two types of urethral catheterisation.

1 *Short-term intermittent catheterisation* is used when the catheter needs only to stay in the bladder long enough to empty the bladder of urine. Short-term intermittent catheters have only one lumen. Catheterisation can be done several times a day, and the procedure is usually done by the child or a carer. This procedure is used for children with neuropathic bladder problems or when the bladder does not completely empty. It can also be used to measure residual urine volume. Intermittent catheterisation can be carried out almost anywhere.

2 *Indwelling catheterisation* is used when the catheter needs to be left in the bladder. Indwelling catheters have two lumens and ports: one to attach a syringe to inflate a balloon with water (this keeps it in the bladder), and one to attach to a urine drainage bag.

Short-term catheters (up to about 14 days) are used for the drainage of urine postoperatively (for example after urology, anal or rectal surgery), accurate monitoring of urinary output during an acute illness, and management of short-term urinary retention.[10]

Long-term indwelling catheters should be considered only if all other options are ineffective. Children who need long-term bladder drainage because they are not able to completely empty their bladders, may be able to manage with clean intermittent catheterisation via the urethral route or via a Mitrofanoff (a type of continent vesicostomy).

Ensure that the catheter chosen is suitable for the intended use and that it is used in accordance with the manufacturer's instructions.[11,12] There are reports of the use of feeding tubes as urinary catheters, which have become knotted in the child's or infant's bladder, and could not be withdrawn, so had to be surgically removed.[13,14]

### Catheter material

Catheters need to be comfortable, easy to insert and remove, and must minimise problems such as colonisation by micro-organisms, encrustation and tissue inflammation. The material they are made of must conform to British Standards to minimise toxicity to tissues.

Short-term catheters are relatively cheap and made from materials such as polyvinylchloride (PVC). They can be rigid and inflexible and may cause urethral spasm. Uncoated latex catheters tend to have a high surface friction that may cause discomfort and tissue trauma. Latex catheters coated with silicone elastomer or hydrogel cause the least tissue inflammation. Hydrogels and polymers used to coat catheters absorb water and produce a slippery surface making insertion easier and reducing trauma. Individuals with a history of atopy or allergies to bananas, avocado, kiwi or chestnuts may cross-react with latex, and catheters containing latex should not be used with these children. Pure silicone catheters are latex free and have a slightly wider lumen for their size than latex catheters as they have thinner walls. They are reported to be more biocompatible with urethral tissue than latex leading to a reduced incidence of urethritis and possibly urethral strictures, and are less likely to allow bacterial adherence than latex catheters.[14] However, pure silicone catheters are not as soft as latex catheters, and silicone balloons have been reported to deflate in situ in long-term use because of diffusion of water out of the balloon, but this may not be a problem for short-term use. Antibiotic-impregnated catheters may reduce urine infection in the short term.[15] Silver-coated catheters are reported to delay the onset of bacturia[15] over a period of less than 14 days.

## Catheter and balloon size

The most common indwelling urinary catheter is the Foley catheter. This is a flexible catheter with a side channel leading to a balloon near the tip of the catheter. The balloon is inflated with water when the catheter is in position, and helps to retain the catheter in the correct position.

The external diameter of a catheter is measured in Charriere (Ch) or French gauge (Fg). A diameter of 1 Fg or Ch is equivalent to 1/3 mm; therefore, a 6-Fg catheter will have an external diameter of 2 mm. Balloon sizes range from 1 mm to 10 mm for paediatric catheters. The smallest catheter and balloon for the function of the catheter should be used, as large catheters and balloons are associated with increased bladder irritability, resulting in painful spasms and leakage, blockage of the urethral glands or ulceration of the bladder neck and urethral wall caused by pressure. Larger balloon sizes are associated with leakage of urine around the catheter. However, very small catheters must not be used in larger children as the tips can curl over in the urethra as the catheter is advanced (especially in boys) making the catheter very difficult to remove, traumatic and painful. As a rough guide 6 Fg can be used for infants, 8 Fg for toddlers and early school age, 12–14 Fg for later school age and adolescents (see Table 16.1).

Table 16.1 Guide to sizes of urethral catheters for girls and boys

| Age of child | Boys | | Girls | |
| --- | --- | --- | --- | --- |
| | Catheter size (Fg) | Insertion length (cm) | Catheter size (Fg) | Insertion length (cm) |
| 0–5 months (3–6 kg) | 6 | 4 ± 2 | 6 | 1.5–2 |
| 6–12 months (4–9 kg) | 6 | 6 ± 2 | 6–8 | 1.5–2 |
| 1–3 years (10–15 kg) | 8 | 8 ± 2 | 8 | 1.5–3 |
| 4–7 years (16–20 kg) | 10 | 10 ± 2 | 10–12 | 2–6 |
| 8–12 years (21–40 kg) | 12 | 12 ± 2 | 12 | 3–6 |
| Over 13 years | 12–14 | 14–22 | 12–14 | 4–8 |

## Drainage equipment

Urine collection must be into a closed system to prevent the entry of infective organisms. It may incorporate a measuring device and a drainage bag. The catheter bag should ideally incorporate a valve to prevent any back flow of urine, and a drainage tap so that the bag does not have to be disconnected for emptying. The connection between the catheter and the urine collection device must not be disconnected unless it is absolutely necessary, as this can increase the risk of infection. The catheter bag or tubing should not be raised above the level of the child's bladder, as this can enable potentially colonised urine to flow back up the tubing and catheter and increase the risk of infection. The catheter bag must hang on a stand so that it does not touch the floor, as this can be a source of contamination. The urine drainage bag should be emptied frequently enough to maintain urine flow and prevent reflux.[16]

## Procedure for insertion of a Foley indwelling urethral catheter[5]

Urethral catheterisation can be an uncomfortable and distressing procedure; the child may benefit from play preparation and distraction as well as the presence of a parent.

Catheters must be inserted using an aseptic technique, by people trained and assessed as competent to carry out the procedure.

Catheter balloons must be inflated and deflated only once, as recommended by the catheter manufacturer, so if a problem occurs after the balloon has been inflated it is safer to change the catheter than to deflate the balloon and try to reposition it.

Two nurses are needed for this procedure: one nurse to assist and comfort the child, one nurse to insert the catheter

### Equipment

Alcohol hand rub
Clean trolley or surface
Catheter pack or three large sterile towels (check packaging is intact, expiry date)
Plastic apron
Two pairs of sterile gloves
Sterile aqueous chlorhexidine, iodine or saline solution for washing
Sterile gallipot
Two packs sterile gauze swabs
Sterile bowl
Foley catheter of correct size and type to suit the child and reason for catheterising (plus spare catheter) (check packaging is intact, expiry date, manufacturer's instructions)
Sterile lubricant (aqueous gel)
Lignocaine and chlorhexidine gel or sterile lignocaine gel
Ampoule of sterile water
Sterile syringe (appropriate size for filling balloon) and needle
Urine drainage system
Urine specimen container
Catheter bag stand

## PROCEDURE: Insertion of a Foley catheter

| Procedural steps | Evidence-based rationale |
|---|---|
| **1** Identify why urinary catheterisation is necessary | Avoid unnecessary catheterisation |
| **2** Check that the child does not have any anatomical abnormalities that may make urethral catheterisation difficult or increase risk | Some children may require an experienced professional to carry out the catheterisation. Some children may require antibiotic prophylaxis |
| **3** Explain the procedure to the child and carer and gain consent. Child and parents may request healthcare professional of specific gender to perform procedure | The child and carer will be prepared for the procedure |
| **4** Check that the child does not have any allergies to soap, antiseptic solution, latex or foods that may predispose to latex allergy | To prevent allergic reaction |

## PROCEDURE: Inserting of a Foley catheter (continued)

| | |
|---|---|
| **5** Close doors and or curtains | To ensure privacy |
| **6** Put on plastic apron | To prevent cross-infection |
| **7** Wash the child's perineal and genital area gently with mild soap and water and dry well (the child or parent can do this) | To clean the perineal and genital area and reduce skin flora and risk of infection |
| **8** Wash hands well, dry and use alcohol hand rub | To prevent cross-infection |
| **9** Clean work surface | To prevent infection |
| **10** Put on one pair of sterile gloves | To maintain asepsis, prevent cross-infection |
| **11** Spread sterile towel over trolley to make a sterile field on the trolley | To maintain asepsis |
| **12** Tip the gallipot, gauze swabs, the second pair of sterile gloves, the two remaining sterile towels, the sterile bowl, sterile tube of lignocaine gel (or put a large blob of gel onto a gauze swab), Foley catheter (in its sterile plastic sleeve), needle and syringe on to the sterile field | |
| **13** Pour the chlorhexidine, iodine or saline solution into the gallipot | |
| **14** Squeeze some lignocaine gel lubricant onto a gauze swab so that it can be applied to the catheter Attach the applicator nozzle to the lignocaine gel (if necessary) | |
| **15** Tear the end of the end of the plastic sleeve on the Foley catheter so that the tip of the catheter is exposed | The Foley catheter is ready for use |
| **16** Cover the tip of the catheter in the lubricating lignocaine gel. Wrap the end of the catheter loosely in the gauze swab | The catheter needs to be lubricated to prevent urethral trauma |
| **17** Place the whole catheter in the sterile bowl | To prevent contamination of the catheter |
| **18** Draw up the correct amount of sterile water into the syringe to fill the balloon and remove the needle from the syringe | The balloon must be filled with the amount of sterile water indicated by the manufacturer. If the balloon is underfilled it may not inflate evenly |
| **19** Assist the child to get into a comfortable position lying down with legs slightly apart, ensuring that the child's dignity and privacy are maintained as much as possible<br>Place sterile towels underneath child's thighs and over abdomen, to create a sterile field | |
| **20** In a boy, hold the penis with a gauze swab with one hand and, clean the glans penis with gauze swabs soaked in washing solution with your other hand (do not try to retract the foreskin fully in infants and young boys as this can cause damage)<br>In a girl, hold the labia slightly apart with a gauze swab in one hand so that the urethral orifice is visible, and clean the area from front to back with the washing solution, using a new gauze swab for each stroke | Although Pratt et al.[8] stated that expert opinion indicates there is no advantage in using antiseptic solutions for cleansing the urethral meatus prior to catheterisation, Panknin and Althaus[17] recommend the use of an antiseptic solution, as 22 per cent of catheter-associated UTIs have been shown to occur during catheter insertion |

## PROCEDURE:  Inserting of a Foley catheter (continued)

| | |
|---|---|
| 21 Using the applicator nozzle, apply some anaesthetic gel to the urethral meatus (in older children with larger urethras, the anaesthetic gel can be squeezed inside the urethral meatus, and in boys it can be massaged into the urethra)<br>Wait for 3–5 minutes for the lignocaine gel to act | No lower age limit was found for the use of lignocaine gel for urethral catheterisation. Bendixen *et al.*[18] used lignocaine gel for the lubrication of intranasal and endotracheal tubes in premature neonates and did not observe toxic plasma concentrations of lignocaine or its metabolite, monoethylglycinxylidin with the use of 0.3 mL/kg lignocaine gel 20 mg/mL<br>Girls as well as boys benefit from the use of lignocaine gel to relieve the discomfort of urethral catheterisation and reduce the risk of trauma[5] |
| 22 Remove gloves<br>Put on second pair of sterile gloves | These are now contaminated.<br>Gloves must be sterile for catherisation |
| 23 Put the sterile bowl containing the catheter between the child's legs<br>Hold the labia apart with sterile gauze, or hold the end of the penis with sterile gauze<br>Insert the catheter into the urethra ensuring that it does not come into contact with the surrounding area. As the catheter is advanced, make sure that the end to be connected to the drainage bag stays in the plastic sleeve and in the sterile bowl to avoid contamination | Catheter in sterile bowl should be as close to the child as possible for ease of use and to prevent accidental contamination<br>If the catheter comes into contact with the child's skin it could become contaminated with microbes and introduce infection into the bladder |
| 24 If the catheter is accidentally inserted into the vagina, leave this in place to prevent it happening again, and use a new catheter. Once the catheter is in the bladder, the first catheter can be removed | |
| 25 When urine starts to flow down the catheter, advance the catheter a further 2–4 cm<br>Attach the syringe to the balloon inflation port and inject the amount of water specified by the manufacturer, then remove the syringe. The catheter can then be gently drawn back until slight resistance is felt | Urine will flow down the catheter when the opening at the tip is in the bladder. At this point the balloon is still in the urethra and will cause trauma to the neck of the bladder if inflated. Advancing the catheter more than the length of the balloon will ensure that the balloon in well inside the bladder<br>Only sterile water for injections must be used to inflate the balloon. Air must not be used as the balloon will float. If sodium chloride or tap water is used, deposits will form in the balloon and prevent it deflating<br>It is important to use the correct amount of water in the balloon to prevent distortion of the balloon |
| 26 Attach the catheter to the urine drainage system ensuring that the end of the catheter and the end of the urine drainage tubing remain sterile | Contamination with microbes in any part of the urine drainage system could result in a UTI |
| 27 Secure the catheter to the child's upper thigh, or abdomen (whichever is most comfortable for the child) ensuring that there is a small loop of catheter so that it will not exert any tension on the catheter in the bladder when the child moves | If the catheter does pull at all, it will exert pressure on the urethra and on the trigone and may cause pressure damage and scarring; it may also cause trauma to the urethral meatus |
| 28 If the foreskin has been retracted, this must be gently pushed back into place | To prevent paraphimosis |

## PROCEDURE: Inserting of a Foley catheter (continued)

| | |
|---|---|
| 29 Pour a small amount of urine that initially drained out of the catheter into the sterile urine specimen container. This can be tested and sent for microscopy, culture and sensitivities if necessary | |
| 30 Hang the urine drainage bag or system on the urine bag stand so that it does not touch the floor | Contact with the floor can potentially contaminate the urine drainage port allowing microbes to enter the drainage system |
| 31 The date and time of insertion of the catheter, its type and size, the catheter details (manufacturer, type, batch number, expiry date), the balloon capacity and volume used to fill it must be documented in the patient's records | In case of any adverse reactions, or other problems with the catheter
When the balloon is deflated, it is important to know the amount of water used to fill it |

## CATHETER CARE AND PREVENTION OF COMPLICATIONS

### Infection

Micro-organisms can enter the bladder during catheterisation, up the lumen of the catheter from the tubing or bag, or up the urethra around the outside of the catheter. Micro-organisms can form a biofilm on the surface of the catheter; this may create a barrier and protect them from antibiotics.

In susceptible children, such as those with vesicoureteric reflux, micro-organisms can ascend the ureters and infect the kidney tissue causing pyelonephritis, renal scarring, and can potentially lead to chronic renal failure or hypertension in later life. UTI can also lead to septicaemia.

The urethral meatus should be washed daily with soap and water.[16] Washing more frequently than this may increase the risk of infection,[8] and using antiseptic solutions for meatal cleansing is not recommended. Cleaning of the catheter itself should be directed away from the insertion site or urethral meatus. Talcs, creams and strongly perfumed soaps should be avoided.

If appropriate, encourage oral fluids to achieve a urine output of 1–4 mL/kg/hour.

Signs and symptoms of UTI may be:

- cloudy, foul smelling urine
- blood, protein, leucocytes and/or nitrites in the urine
- urine bypassing the catheter
- pyrexia
- signs of abdominal discomfort/pain

- lethargy/irritability
- vomiting.

If the child exhibits any of these signs or symptoms, a urine specimen must be taken and sent for microscopy, culture and sensitivity to rule out a symptomatic UTI.

Please see website for potential catheter problems.

### Flushing a urinary catheter

Bladder washout or flushing a catheter should only be done if absolutely necessary and all other options for improving urine flow have been exhausted. It should be done under strict aseptic technique through an indwelling catheter to avoid introducing infection. The solution should be warmed to blood heat, and should be instilled very gently, under gravity if possible by elevating the administration device above bladder height. Exerting even gentle pressure during instillation causes shedding of cells from the bladder endothelium.

### Emptying a catheter bag

Catheter bags should be emptied when they are between half and two-thirds full to avoid them becoming over-full and heavy.

#### *Equipment*

Apron
Gloves
Alcohol swabs
Clean container to empty the urine into (e.g. jug or papier mâché urine bottle)
Paper towel

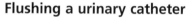

## PROCEDURE: Emptying a catheter bag

| Procedural steps | Evidence-based rationale |
|---|---|
| 1 Explain to the child and carer what you are going to do | The child and carer will be prepared for the procedure |
| 2 Wash and dry your hands well. Put on apron and gloves | To prevent infection |
| 3 Clean the catheter bag drainage valve or tap inside and outside with an alcohol swab. Allow the alcohol to dry | The drying action of alcohol kills microbes |
| 4 Open the drainage tap and completely empty the urine bag into a clean container, ensuring that the end of the catheter tap does not touch anything | To reduce contamination |
| 5 Close the catheter valve or tap and clean it inside and out as before with a sterile alcohol swab | |
| 6 Cover the container with a paper towel | To reduce the risk of cross-infection |
| 7 Measure the urine if necessary | |
| 8 Dispose of the urine and container in the dirty utility room according to hospital policy | |
| 9 Dispose of gloves and apron Wash hands well | To reduce the risk of cross-infection |
| 10 Record the urine volume in the child's records if necessary | |

 Please see the website for carrying out a timed urine collection.

### Urethral Foley catheter removal

*Equipment*

Apron
Non-sterile gloves

Syringe
Receiver
Paper towel or tissues

## PROCEDURE: Foley catheter removal

| Procedural steps | Evidence-based rationale |
|---|---|
| 1 Explain to the child and family what you are going to do | The child and carer will be prepared for the procedure |
| 2 Remove any tape securing the catheter to the child's leg or abdomen. Ensure that there is no tension on the catheter | If the catheter pulls it can cause trauma to the urethra and bladder neck |
| 3 Wash and dry your hands well Put on gloves and apron | To prevent cross-infection |

## PROCEDURE:  Foley catheter removal (continued)

| | |
|---|---|
| **4** Loosen the syringe plunger by pulling it out slightly in the barrel. Attach the syringe to the balloon valve securely and allow the water from the balloon to enter the syringe<br>The amount of water retrieved from the balloon should be almost the same as the amount used to inflate the balloon. Detach the syringe | Do not exert force to draw the water out of the balloon as cuffing of the balloon will occur. The deflated balloon can form ridges, creases or cuffs which increase the diameter of the catheter and form a rough uneven surface that scrapes the inside of the urethra when the catheter is withdrawn[19] this can cause urethral trauma and pain. Semjonow et al.[20] suggested reinserting 0.5 mL of water into the balloon of adult catheters following deflation to remove the creases and ridges and act as cushioning as the catheter is withdrawn. However, catheter inflation valves are designed for single inflation and deflation, and Robinson.[19] does not recommend this practice<br>Some water may diffuse out of the balloon over a period of time, so the amount in the balloon when it is deflated may be slightly less than was used to fill it |
| **5** Place paper towel or tissues and receiver under the catheter in between the child's legs<br>Pull the catheter out gently and place in the receiver. Inspect the catheter for blood or pus and ensure it is intact. Report any abnormalities to medical or senior staff<br>Make sure the child is dressed and comfortable | The paper towel or tissues will prevent any urine still in the catheter from dripping on to the child's bed |
| **6** Dispose of the urine and catheter in the sluice<br>Remove gloves and apron<br>Wash hands | |
| **7** Document | |
| **8** Inform the child and parents that the child may experience urgency, frequency and some discomfort passing urine for the first 24 hours after the catheter has been removed, and that urine should be inspected and measured during this time<br>If the child is unable to pass urine within 4 hours, try sitting them in a warm bath and allowing them to pass urine in the bath. Inform medical staff if the child cannot pass urine or complains of abdominal pain | A warm bath may help the child to feel relaxed and reduce the discomfort of passing urine<br>Abdominal pain may be an indication of UTI |

Please see the website for more information on catheter care.

## Screening methods: observation of urine

Infected urine is usually cloudy or slightly hazy. If you hold a specimen up to the light, and it is absolutely crystal clear, it is unlikely (but not impossible) that the child has a urine infection (Table 16.2).

**Table 16.2** Appearance and smell of urine

| Appearance of urine | Possible reason |
| --- | --- |
| Colourless to pale yellow, crystal clear | Normal |
| Dark yellow | Concentrated urine, may indicate dehydration |
| Yellow, cloudy or hazy, sediment | Bacteria, blood cells, pus[21] |
| Red/brown | Fresh blood/old blood, haemoglobin, myoglobin21 |
| Smoky red | Intact red cells |
| Yellow, froths when shaken | Protein/albumin |
| Brown/green or dark yellow, froths when shaken | Bilirubin[21] |
| Brown/black | Inborn error of metabolism such as porphyria |
| Dark yellow/black | Metronidazole excretion |
| Brown | Paracetamol overdose |
| Reddish orange | Rifampicin |
| Amber | Carrots |
| Red/pink | Beetroot[21] |
| *Smell of urine* | *Possible reason* |
| • Ammonia/fishy | • Infection |
| • Acetone/pear drops | • Ketones |

# URINALYSIS: TESTING WITH REAGENT STRIPS

Reagent strips that detect leucocyte esterase, nitrites, protein and blood are useful in screening for UTI.

Urine testing (Table 16.3) should be carried out in a 'dirty utility' room to prevent spread of infection.

## Equipment

Bottle of reagent strips
Non-sterile gloves
Apron

**Table 16.3** Urine testing

| Urine test result | Indication |
| --- | --- |
| Specific gravity less than 1.001 | Dilute urine. Excessive fluid intake, diabetes insipidus or hypercalcaemia |
| Specific gravity more than 1.035 | Concentrated urine. Child may be dehydrated or urine may contain large amounts of dissolved substances such as glucose |
| PH 5.0 to 8.0 | Normal range |
| Glucose | Blood sugar greater than 10 mmol/L. Diabetes mellitus, steroid therapy, pregnancy. Blood sugar should also be checked |
| Protein | Renal damage, UTI, nephrotic syndrome |
| Ketones | Breakdown of fat to use as energy source. May occur in fasting, starvation, prolonged vomiting, or diabetes mellitus. Captopril and other drugs may give false positive |
| Blood | Renal damage, trauma to any part of renal system, UTI. |
| Bilirubin | Liver disease or biliary obstruction |
| Urobilinogen | Elevated levels may indicate liver damage or abnormal breakdown of red blood cells |

**Table 16.3** Urine testing (continued)

| Urine test result | Indication |
| --- | --- |
| Leucocytes | UTI, general febrile illness, inflammation or irritation in the renal system. The leucocyte esterase test is very specific for intact and lysed leucocytes, and may be positive when microscopy is negative. False negative results may occur in the presence of high glucose, ketone or protein concentrations, or in the presence of cephalexin, cephalotin, nitrofurantoin, tetracycline and tobramycin |
| Nitrite | Some bacteria such as Escherichia coli, Klebsiella, Pseudomonas reduce nitrates in the urine to nitrites. The presence of nitrite is detected on the reagent strip. This test is very specific for nitrate reducing bacteria, but will not detect non-nitrate reducers such as some Pseudomonas, Staphylococcus and Streptococcus species. False negative tests may also occur in alkaline urine, when the stay in the bladder is too short, and if the urinary nitrite concentration is too low |

## PROCEDURE:  Urinalysis

| Procedural steps | Evidence-based rationale |
| --- | --- |
| 1 Obtain a urine sample from the child by an appropriate method | False results can occur if the urine sample is not freshly voided |
| 2 Wash hands. Put on gloves and apron | To prevent spread of infection |
| 3 Ensure a clean level work area is available. Check the testing kit has been stored correctly Check packaging is intact. Check expiry date | To ensure that test results will be as accurate as as possible |
| 4 Dip the testing strip in the urine briefly, or apply the urine to the testing strip with a syringe if the sample is small | To ensure all reagent pads are soaked with urine |
| 5 Read the testing strip after the designated time according to the manufacturer's instructions | Reagents may take different times to react with the urine constituents |
| 6 Dispose of urine, equipment, gloves and apron according to local policy | To prevent spread of infection |
| 7 Wash hands | To prevent spread of infection |
| 8 Record procedure and observations in child's records | Other staff will be aware of findings |

If leucocyte esterase, nitrite or blood is detected, antibiotic treatment should be commenced immediately. If the child has not improved in 48 hours, or the culture results indicate that the organism is resistant to the chosen antibiotic, the treatment can be changed.

Please see website for urine microscopy.

## PREGNANCY TESTING

Pregnancy testing can be offered to teenage girls who have reached menarche and have missed a period following intercourse and pregnancy is suspected.[22] A urine or venous blood sample may be sent for laboratory testing for human chorionic gonadotrophin (hCG) levels. Alternatively, 'near patient' testing may be carried out using a urine sample and commercially prepared kits. Testing the urine with urine-testing kits will give a positive or negative result depending on whether hCG is detected. It is advisable to wait at least 19 days after unprotected sex before testing. If pregnancy testing is done before the fetus has implanted it will be negative, and if pregnancy is strongly suspected it should be repeated 3–7 days later.

Please refer to the website for further information on pregnancy testing.

## PROCEDURE: Pregnancy testing

| Procedural steps | Evidence-based rationale |
|---|---|
| 1 Ask the girl in confidence whether she has considered the possible implications of a pregnancy test, whether she is aware of sexually transmitted diseases, and establish whether the act of sexual intercourse was consensual | Maintain confidentiality as far as possible<br>Protect the patient from sexually transmitted diseases<br>Establish whether child protection measures are required |
| 2 Ensure a clean level work area is available<br>Check the testing kit has been stored correctly<br>Check packaging is intact. Check expiry date | To ensure that test results will be as accurate as possible |
| 3 Ask the girl to collect a urine sample (preferably early morning sample) in a clean dry container<br>Maintain patient privacy and confidentiality | Early morning samples of urine are more concentrated and contain higher levels of hCG than samples collected later in the day |
| 4 Wash hands. Put on protective apron and non-sterile gloves | To prevent cross-infection. Personal protection |
| 5 Follow the manufacturer's guidance on using the pregnancy testing kit. Use a timer to ensure that urine is in contact with the reagent for the specified period of time. Ensure that the control line is present | To ensure that test results will be as accurate as possible |
| 6 Dispose of the kit in clinical waste bag according to hospital policy<br>Dispose of gloves and apron. Wash hands | To prevent cross-infection |
| 7 Advise the girl of the result of the test<br>Discuss what to do next<br>Discuss contraception if appropriate.<br>Complete appropriate documentation | To ensure that the girl has appropriate support and protection |

Go to the website to find the PowerPoint presentation for this chapter and MCQs to test your knowledge. **www.hodderplus.com/childnursingskills**

# REFERENCES

1  National Institute for Health and Clinical Excellence (2007) *Urinary tract infection in children*. NICE Clinical Guideline 54. London: NICE.

2  Lifshitz E, Kramer L (2000) Outpatient urine culture: does collection technique matter? *Archives of Internal Medicine* **160**: 2537–2540.

3  Liaw LC, Nayar DM, Pedler SJ, Coulthard MG (2000) Home collection of urine for culture from infants by three methods: survey of parents' preferences and bacterial contamination rates. *British Medical Journal*, **320**: 1312–1313.

4  Rao S, Bhatt J, Houghton C, Macfarlane P (2004) An improved urine collection pad method: a randomised clinical trial. *Archive of Diseases in Childhood* **89**: 773–775.

5  Bissett L (2005) Reducing the risk of catheter-related urinary tract infection. *Nursing Times* **101**(12): 64–67.

6  Inwood S (2007) Skin antisepsis: using 2% chlorhexidine gluconate in 70% isopropyl alcohol. *British Journal of Nursing*, **16**: 1390–1394.

7  Pellowe C (2001) Preventing infections from short-term indwelling catheters. *Nursing Times* **97**(14): 34–35.

8  Pratt RJ, Pellowe C, Loveday HP, *et al.* (2001) The epic project: developing national evidence-based

guidelines for preventing healthcare associated infections. *Journal of Hospital Infection* **47**(Suppl.): S1–S82.

9   Hart S (2008) Urinary catheterisation. *Nursing Standard* **22**(27): 44–48.

10   Cropper J (2003) postoperative retention of urine in children. *Paediatric Nursing* **15**(7):15–18.

11   MHRA (2001) SN 2001(02): Problems removing urinary catheters. http://devices.mhra.gov.uk/ (Accessed 22 May 2009).

12   Sanders C (2002) Choosing continence products for children. *Nursing Standard* **16**(32): 39–43.

13   Sujijantararat P (2007) Intravesical knotting of a feeding tube used as a urinary catheter. *Journal of the Medical Association of Thailand* **90**: 1231–1233.

14   Smith L (2003) Which Catheter? Criteria for the selection of urinary catheters for children. *Paediatric Nursing* **15**(3): 14–18.

15   Schumm K, Lam TBL (2008) Types of urethral catheters for management of short-term voiding problems in hospitalised adults. *Cochrane Database of Systematic Reviews* **2**:CD004013.

16   National Institute for Clinical Excellence (2003) *Clinical Guideline 2. Infection control: prevention of healthcare-associated infection in primary and community care*. London: NICE.

17   Panknin HT, Althaus P (2001) Guidelines for preventing infections associated with the insertion and maintenance of short-term indwelling urethral catheters in acute care. *Journal of Hospital Infections* **49**(2): 146–147.

18   Bendixen D, Halvorsen A-C, Hjelt K, Flachs H (1994) Lignocaine gel used for lubrication of intranasal and endotracheal tubes in premature infants. *Acta Paediatrica* **83**: 493–497.

19   Robinson J (2003) Deflation of a Foley catheter balloon. *Nursing Standard* **19**(17): 33–38.

20   Semjonow A, Roth S, Hertle L (1995) Reducing trauma whilst removing long-term indwelling balloon catheters. *British Journal of Urology* **75**(2): 241

21   Steggall MJ (2007) Urine samples and urinalysis. *Nursing Standard* **22**(14–16): 42–45.

22   Kraszewski S (2007) Procedure for pregnancy testing. *Nursing Standard*, **22**(12): 45–48.

## CHAPTER 17

# Pain assessment and management

Lizzie Dickin and Helen Green

## LEARNING OUTCOMES

*Upon completion of this chapter, the reader should be able to accomplish the following:*

1 Discuss how children and young people perceive pain
2 Define the rationale for using pain assessment and the choice of tools used
3 Discuss the potential options for pain management, both pharmacological and non-pharmacological, and what may influence the choice of management techniques
4 Describe the preparation of children prior to any procedures including surgery in relation to their pain management
5 Discuss specific aspects of postoperative nursing care that can influence pain management

## CHAPTER OVERVIEW

Many children who are in hospital will have the potential to, experience pain. This ranges from blood tests through to major surgery. Every child has the right to expect their pain to be managed to a level that ensures they can perform the tasks and activities that will enhance their recovery without side-effects and psychological trauma.

Unrelieved pain can have significant detrimental effects on all body systems and on the child's health and wellbeing in the short and long term. We must look holistically at the child and consider both pharmacological and non-pharmacological techniques and approaches. All options should be considered and every child regarded on an individual basis.

The focus of this chapter is to address how and why we perform pain assessment and as a result of that pain assessment how we manage acute pain in children. Children of all ages will be considered. The care of neonates, children in intensive care and those with chronic pain is not covered in this chapter.

## WHAT IS PAIN?

There are many definitions of pain, encompassing physiological and psychological aspects. Each has something specific to say about pain and the person who experiences pain.

From a physiological point of view and in its simplest form pain is related to the sensory nervous system. Pain is the sensation felt when particular nerve cells in the cortex of the brain are stimulated. These cells are linked to certain types of sensory receptor called nociceptors. Stimulation of nociceptors gives the sensation of pain, just as stimulation of other specific sensory receptors creates the sensations of touch, heat, smell, taste and sight.

The complex sensation of pain involves the affective (arouses emotion), autonomic (accompanied increase in vital signs) and motor (pain is usually accompanied by a reflex response) components of the nervous system.

Two definitions of pain commonly used look at pain from different viewpoints:

*Pain is whatever the experiencing person says it is and exists whenever he says it does.*[1]

and

*Pain is an unpleasant sensory and emotional experience associated with actual or potential damage described in terms of such damage.*[2]

Pain itself has not changed. What has changed is our understanding of pain and the methods used to treat it.

## Perception of pain

Pain perception is present in the first stages of development and fundamentally acts as a signal for potential or actual tissue damage. Management of pain was previously guided by the fact that this damage was directly proportional to pain experience. However, as stated by the International Association for the Study of Pain:[2]

*Pain is always subjective; each individual learns the application of the word through experiences related to injury in early life.*

As the child develops, the perception of pain concurrently develops, drawing on experiences and adapting their responses to pain. In addition, as the child gets older these experiences change and become more frequent, thus manipulating perception once again. This highlights how subjective and personal perception is, as each child will be exposed to differing experiences throughout life.

## PAIN ASSESSMENT

The first step to providing effective pain relief is to identify how much pain a child has and therefore pain assessment is the fundamental component of pain management.[3] Pain assessment can never be entirely objective as it is an experience individual to that child, and can be influenced by a vast array of factors. The current Royal College of Nursing clinical guidelines[4] on the recognition and assessment of acute pain in children highlights these dimensions, including:

- cognitive
- sensory
- physiological
- behavioural
- affective
- sociocultural
- environmental.

Consequently, responses to pain are subjective and assessment must be individual.

## Why do we assess pain?

As pain is a personal experience, pain assessment can be a challenge. In spite of this, assessment of the acuity and effect of pain is fundamental to the diagnosis, treatment and management of the child in pain. Pain can have a huge debilitating effect on sufferers and, if not recognised appropriately, can become established and difficult to manage. Under the declaration of the Rights of the Child distributed by the United Nations General Assembly,[5] it is now recognised that 'children should in all circumstances be among the first to receive protection and relief, and should be protected from all forms of neglect, cruelty and exploitation'. Pain management is an ethical imperative in the care of children. Systematic assessment of pain is vital in order to achieve this and to fulfil an adequate duty of care as outlined by the Nursing and Midwifery Council.[6]

## Effects of unrelieved pain

The prolonged stress response triggered by acute pain can prolong hospitalisation, cause significant morbidity and increase the risk of mortality in the critically ill.[7] Misdiagnosis and under-treatment of acute pain leads to long-term and severe physiological and psychological adverse effects. The catabolic state induced by acute pain may also be more detrimental in infants and children because of higher metabolic rates and reduced nutritional reserves than adults. In addition, mechanisms to dampen or inhibit nociception are immature at birth, leading to hypersensitivity to pain. Please see the website for further information on pain hypersensitivity.

## How should we assess pain?

It is often useful to adopt an approach that involves the use of a framework that can assist in the development of a plan of comprehensive, individualised care. One such framework is QUESTT.[8]

- Q – Question the child starting at the admission, find out any pain history or experiences. Ask the child specifically about their pain. Where is it, what words describe the pain?
- U – use the pain assessment tools.
- E – evaluate behavioural and physiological changes.
- S – secure the parents input.
- T – take into account the cause of the pain; look at the whole picture – this may not always be what you think.
- T – take action.

## PAIN ASSESSMENT TOOLS

Many tools are now available assisting nurses to acquire perspective and assessment of children's pain experiences. They involve the documentation of a pain score relative to the child's experience. Pain assessment tools should be used only in conjunction with a holistic assessment of the child's complex experience.

Most children, provided with the right technique can communicate the intensity of their pain and therefore the challenge lies in identifying the correct means of assessment for that child. Pain scales are required to be reliable, consistent, easy to understand, appropriate to the setting and type of pain. If possible, the child should be allowed to develop or choose a scale for themselves based on those currently available. In order to achieve effective pain management, there is a requirement to achieve consistency of pain assessment, integrated into daily clinical practice.

### Self-report tools

The use of a self-report tool allows a more subjective and systematic assessment of pain in children, and is classed as the gold standard in current practice. Selection of the most appropriate tool is based on the child's age, cognitive ability and clinical condition, and thus they are excluded for use in cognitively impaired, pre-verbal or non-verbal children. They may be used for a vast range of children, adapted to the child's stage of development and vocabulary. Self-reporting can be made as simple or as complicated as required for the individual child in order to gain the most accurate assessment.

Self-report tools on the whole provide anchors (represented by numbers, colours and words for example) at each end of the scale denoting the extremes against which the child can rate their pain. Please see the website for further information on those most commonly used in practice; these are also documented in the RCN guidelines governing current clinical practice.[4]

### Behavioural assessment

The use of children's behavioural cues can act as a proxy for self-report in those children who are unable to communicate their experiences effectively. This assessment evaluates changes in the child's behavioural patterns in order to estimate their pain intensity. In babies, infants and non-verbal children, this method is valuable in order to gain insight into their experience. However, as the child develops this may become limited due to withdrawal and concealing pain as a means of protection. Again these should not be assessed in isolation and a combination of pain tools may be required. Please see the website for some non-verbal cues.

### Physiological assessment

In the very young infant or critically ill child, including the ventilated or sedated patient, physiological cues may be the only means of pain assessment. These include:

- heart rate
- respiratory rate
- blood pressure
- $O_2$ dependency
- skin colour
- pallor/sweating
- muscle spasm
- vomiting
- dilated pupils.

These signs are open to interpretation. First, although sensitive to changes in pain intensity, physiological measures also reflect a global response to stress-related situations and underlying conditions; thus changes may not strictly be as a result of pain. Second, if pain persists, the child cannot sustain this response and as a consequence physiological signs will return to normal (adaptation) making this an unreliable means of review in the long-term assessment of pain.

## Behavioural/physiological assessment tools

These tools should be used only when the child is unable to self-report because of their limitations. Even though behavioural cues and physiological measures can be observed separately, in order to obtain a systematic pain assessment they must not be analysed in isolation.

 Please see the website for those most commonly used in practice and they are also documented in the RCN guidelines governing current clinical practice.[4]

## When should pain be assessed?

Pain assessment must be regular and systematic in order to judge the value of interventions and to promote effective healthcare. It should start on admission to hospital, whether this is an elective or trauma presentation, and continue until the child is discharged from the nurse's care. In elective situations prior to surgery/medical intervention, a detailed pain assessment, including previous experiences, expectations and current coping strategies, can be outlined and used as a baseline for further assessment and evaluation (Table 17.1). However, in emergency situations this is not possible. The British Pain Society cited in McGann[9] advocates continuous assessment of pain as the fifth vital sign, along with blood pressure, heart rate, temperature and respiratory rate in order to provide an evidence base for intervention and to optimise pain control. Documentation of assessment not only formalises the cyclic nature of pain management, but promotes multidisciplinary communication and meets legal implications.

## Assessment of the cognitively impaired child

Currently we do not know whether children with cognitive impairment, irrespective of the cause, experience pain acuity and sensation in the same way as the child without impairment. Studies have suggested that children with physical and learning disabilities show higher pain thresholds than those with no impairment. Derangement in their autonomic, motor and sensory systems may have an effect on pain experience, with much research concluding that they have reduced sensitivity to pain.[13] However, we cannot exclude the possibility that this is due to impaired communication. Therefore, systematic and accurate pain assessment in children unable to communicate because of cognitive/physical impairment is even more crucial.

**Table 17.1** What should be assessed?

| Enquiry | Outcome |
| --- | --- |
| Previous pain experience | Identifies experience, expectation and current coping mechanisms |
| Location and radiation | Key to enabling diagnosis of the cause |
| Identify singular or multiple source of pain | |
| Description | Description of the quality of pain to enable diagnosis of the cause (i.e. somatic, visceral or neuropathic pain) |
| Intensity | Used to determine the type of intervention required |
| Frequency and duration | Aids diagnosis and planning of intervention |
| Aggravating and relieving strategies | Aids planning of intervention<br>Factors that cause/increase pain (i.e. positioning/ physiotherapy)<br>Factors that aid relief or coping (i.e. analgesia/ deep breathing) |

## Parental involvement in assessment

Parents can have a positive influence on the whole process and are especially valuable in pain assessment as they 'know their child' the best and can provide vital information about their child's normal behaviours. This is extremely beneficial and can assist in distinguishing pain behaviours from others associated with anger, hunger or fatigue. This is especially important in the child with cognitive impairment, as the range of behavioural response may vary dramatically. However, it is essential to also assess the parent's ability to do this reliably, ruling out parental anxiety and fear which may influence the child's behaviour. This is especially important in the intensive care unit (ICU), which can evoke huge stresses on the parents affecting their coping and thus proving counter-productive. Consequently, while parental participation complies with the philosophy of family-centred care, the nurse must ensure that this is appropriate under particular circumstances. Once again this is a vast area of research which is under continuing development and investigation.

## PAIN MANAGEMENT

Pain management in children can be a challenge. A combination of both pharmacological and non-pharmacological approaches should be used. Good pain management provides the potential for children to have a positive experience in their hospital journey.

Pain management should be pre-emptive (anticipating what pain the child may experience and acting accordingly) rather than reactive. It is a lot simpler to prevent a child experiencing high levels of pain than reducing that pain once experienced.

Be aware of what is potentially going to be painful without making assumptions about how the child has experienced pain in the past or their pain threshold. Children should not be told that they will be completely pain free. Our aim is for the child's pain to be controlled to enable them to perform activities such as deep breathing and moving in the bed.

This section of the chapter will be split into a number of sections:

- preparation
- procedural pain management
- postoperative care
- pharmacological pain management
- non-pharmacological pain management.

## Preparation

The preparation of children prior to procedures and surgery is an important component to the success of those procedures and in the postoperative recovery period. Preparing children for the pain they may experience emphasises the management of that pain rather than the pain itself.

This preparation should include the following.

- Introducing pain assessment tools and ensuring the child's understanding of the tool; getting them to practice after you have explained it to them.
- Discussing the potential options that may be used to control their pain. These will depend on the range available on your unit, the procedure intended and the child and family. For surgical patients clarify if an anaesthetist has already discussed the options and if a decision has been made; if so concentrate on that technique.
- Using information booklets or sheets to explain and answer any questions on specific techniques.
- Demonstrating any machinery to be used, i.e. Entonox and PCA (patient-controlled analgesia).
- Allowing the handling of any equipment as appropriate to aid understanding of how the equipment works.
- Discussing potential side-effects and risks.

Please refer to Chapter 7 on play.

## Procedural pain management

The goal of procedural pain management is to ensure the procedure is carried out successfully in such a way that the child feels comfortable, knows what is going to happen to them (if they are of an age that this can be explained and understood), is cooperative and experiences as little pain as possible.

The main influences on the choice of strategy for managing procedural pain are the child, the procedure and the experience and expertise of the care team (Table 17.2).

**Table 17.2** Pain-relieving options in procedural pain management

| Treatment option | Advantages | Disadvantages |
| --- | --- | --- |
| Topically anaesthetising creams, e.g. EMLA, Ametop | Some creams effective for 4–6 hours after removed. | Needs time to work. Not always placed exactly where blood test performed |
| | Useful for venepuncture and cannulation and possibly lumbar puncture | Some creams cause vasoconstriction |
| Ethyl chloride | Instant effect | Very cold – can cause burns if not used properly. Very short acting |
| Distraction | Parents can assist | |
| | Often effective with younger children especially if creams used also. Numerous tools that can be used, bubbles, TV, books, videos, games, etc. | |
| Relaxation and guided imagery (a therapeutic technique allowing two people to communicate on a reality that the child has chosen to describe through imaging) | Can be extremely effective if patient receptive | Need to be trained for guided imagery, basic techniques |
| Entonox | Inhalation self-administered; short acting and effective | See page 291 for more details |
| Sedatives from drugs | May not have analgesic properties but helps the child to forget | Need time to wear off. Not always effective. |
| | Useful for longer and more complicated procedures for inpatients | The use of anxiolytics and sedatives can reduce anxiety and dampen the pain behaviour response but without relieving pain |

Factors to consider in procedural pain management include:

- age and cognitive ability of the child;
- parental support;
- preparation;
- technique options depending on age, condition, procedure and experiences of the child;
- what the procedure is and where will it take place;
- who is available to assist, who is performing the procedure;
- timing of the procedure with drugs and other activities;
- communication between all concerned so that everyone knows who is doing what.

Whichever method is used, the level of potential pain the procedure itself may cause needs to be considered. Does the child need a longer lasting analgesic to ensure that any pain caused by the procedure is controlled?

# Postoperative pain management

Sometimes the most basic of interventions can create the greatest pain relief. In any situation where there is pain the source of that pain should be explored.

Consider the following:

*Positioning*
- Any injured limb or surgery site should be well supported. A folded towel or cloth can be used as a pad to hold against any surgical wound to add support when coughing.
- Sources of potential pressure should be eliminated and pressure areas checked and relieved frequently.
- The child's position should be changed as appropriate for their condition and as the surgery or injury allows.
- Position the child in their preferred position whenever possible.

- There may be attachments that can be added to the bed to enable the child to help themselves gain the best position.
- There are specific mattresses that can be used to allow better positioning and general comfort for the sick child.

*Tubes and drains*

- Tubes and drains are often the source of many high pain scores. Some children will feel more discomfort from these than major surgical wounds. They should therefore be considered carefully when assessing a child's pain.
- For example, urine catheters should be taped to the child's abdomen and not the leg to reduce movement of the catheter when the leg moves, causing irritation. Remember to check potential pressure areas under drains.
- Are drains and tubes secure or is the child holding themselves tense with anxiety that the tubes are going to fall out?
- Explain to the child what the drains and tubes are for and what they can do to help reduce any discomfort from them, i.e. making sure they are supported when moving.
- Do not tape drains to the bed as they may be forgotten when moved. Allow slack on any tubes to allow freedom of movement.

*Hygiene*

- Make sure that the child's hygiene needs are met. There may be some argument that to give a child a wash may be more painful than the consequences of not having a wash but even a simple wash may make the child feel better. It provides a normal activity in an abnormal situation.
- Give mouth care by cleaning teeth or using mouthwashes and rinses.
- Catheter care should be performed to reduce irritation.
- Use appropriate loose clothing to avoid any restriction of movement or pressure on tubes or drains.
- Change sheets and ensure no crumbs or creases are producing points of pressure or irritation.

*Environment*

- Is the ward area chaotic or calm?
- Lack of sleep affects us in different ways but generally we feel less able to cope with situations when we are tired. The perception of pain may be heightened when we are tired.
- Make sure lights are turned off and noise is controlled when appropriate. Provide periods when the child can sleep; this can be negotiated with the child and carers.

*Fears and anxieties*

- Give explanations at a level that the child can understand.
- Explore any fears the child and family may have and relieve where possible.
- Find out what expectations the child and family had prior to surgery with regard to the outcome of the surgery and the level of pain they expected to experience. Have these expectations been fulfilled or are they disappointed at the level of pain they or their child are experiencing and do they understand what is causing their pain?
- Explain any symptoms they may have and what they may mean, or request explanations from medical staff.

*Visitors*

- Visitors can have a positive and negative effect on a child's pain. Be aware of which effect visitors are having on the children in your care.
- Parents are a great source of comfort for children but can often be the target of any expression of fear and anxiety. Encourage parents to use distraction and cuddles where appropriate, which will help reduce a child's pain.
- Siblings can also be a great resource in distracting and providing comfort.
- Be aware of how visitors may be making the child tired or upset.

*Multidisciplinary team*

- Ensure you have an understanding of the child's condition and what may be causing the pain. Parents and children need to feel confident in the care they are receiving. If you are not sure of anything refer to more experienced staff.
- Know what the usual pattern of pain for the procedure is; ask for a review if pain is unexpectedly high.
- Encourage a team approach so that nurses, physiotherapists and medical staff are all working together.

- Time care, treatment and procedures so there is minimal disturbance to the child and maximum benefit from any pain relief that has been given. Negotiate with the child and professionals to ensure this can be achieved.

# PHARMACOLOGICAL PAIN MANAGEMENT

Medicines inevitably play a large role in paediatric pain management. This section of the chapter will discuss some basic pharmacology. There are legal restrictions on the use of drugs in children. This is due to an understandable reluctance to carry out research in this age group. As a result much treatment is based on adult research or clinical experience. The main source of information for drugs used in children is the British National Formulary for children.[11] Some specialist centres may have their own formularies that are specific to the specialty.

## Which drugs should be used for children?

We start with simple analgesics such as paracetamol and ibuprofen, and progress to mild opioids if the pain persists or is increasing. If pain continues to persist or increases in intensity or is very severe, then stronger opioids will be started, such as morphine. The simple analgesics will be continued as there is often a combined effect, which can reduce the amount of strong opioids required. Some drugs work well together and provide a synergistic effect so their combined effect is more effective than their single benefit.

Adjuvant analgesics are added in at any stage to enhance pain control. This includes drugs that assist the action of another drug. Diazepam is an example when used for muscle spasm.

Titration of analgesia is the reduction and increasing of medicines in controlled stages and assessing the effect of each change before moving on to the next stage.

The practice of regular analgesic administration in established pain is also widely felt to be beneficial. This practice enables a proactive and pre-emptive approach by not allowing the child's pain to escalate to the point where pain control is lost and allowing therapeutic drug levels to be maintained. The alternative is to give pain relief 'when required'. This may lead to pain relief not being given until the child is in a lot of pain or with long gaps between administration of drugs, which allows therapeutic drug levels to drop causing a peak and trough effect rather than a steady state effect.

## Which route should be used to administer pain relief?

The main routes of administration are:

- oral
- rectal
- intravenous
- topical
- epidural.

Other less frequently used routes are:

- subcutaneous
- intrathecal
- inhalation.

The choice of route will depend on:

- pain: the degree of pain, the location and character of the pain;
- patient: contraindications caused by their condition and potential allergies; experience of pain and preparation;
- staff: staff availability and experience;
- environment: the higher the technical environment the more likely will be the ability to use high-tech delivery systems.

### Oral

The route of choice for children is the oral route. There are many preparations of drugs and delivery devices that are designed for children and for easier administration. Do not assume older children can take tablets. There are different types of tablets that are designed to make them palatable and easier to swallow. These include caplets, capsules, melts (dissolve on tongue, saliva is swallowed and absorption occurs in the stomach), dissolvable tablets and various liquids.

Potential contraindications with the oral route:

- inability to swallow;
- may be nil by mouth pre- or post surgery;
- non-compliance;
- nausea and vomiting;

- inability to absorb due to disease process or surgery delayed recovery.

Some of these problems may be overcome by the presence of a nasogastric tube, the use of antiemetics, preparation and distraction.

## Rectal

When the oral route cannot be used the next choice would be the rectal route, usually prescribed as PR or per rectum on drug charts.

Factors that have to be taken into account when considering this route:

- the dose may change for the rectal route, usually increases;
- may be traumatic for the child;
- the effectiveness of the drug may take longer to achieve.

Potential contraindications for the rectal route:

- rectal surgery;
- disease process: the child may have a low platelet or neutrophil count due to treatment or the disease process; this route would then be discouraged due to the risk of potential trauma causing increased risk of infection or bleeding;
- non-compliance;
- no consent from parents;
- some drugs are not available in rectal preparations, e.g. ibuprofen. Some drugs may require a special order to be made for the rectal route.

## Intravenous

When oral and rectal routes are not possible the next route of choice in most cases would be the IV (intravenous) route. This allows for direct administration of stronger analgesics such as morphine. The IV route can be used as either intermittent bolus doses or as a continuous infusion. The former is generally seen in very acute circumstances and is ideally administered in controlled situations with adequate monitoring to detect early complications of the drug, which are seen more rapidly when administered via this route.

The IV route is generally used where there is severe pain and stronger analgesia is required. The main drugs used are opioids, but not solely. Paracetamol is now available intravenously and is very effective via this route. Diclofenac is also available intravenously, but is not frequently used in children.

Techniques that use the IV route include:

- bolus administration
- continuous infusions
- patient-controlled analgesia (PCA).

PCA and continuous infusions are described in more detail later in the chapter.

When the IV route is used the primary concern is the observation of the child. It is a route that allows the rapid effect of stronger drugs, and these need to be monitored.

## ADVANCED TECHNIQUES FOR ADMINISTERING PHARMACOLOGICAL PAIN RELIEF

As technology and advances in medicine have progressed over the years, techniques and machines have been developed that enable us to deliver analgesia to children in more complex but effective ways where previously this was not possible. There are many types and makes of machines on the market and each clinical centre will have their own preferences.

The principles of the techniques are the same however. This section briefly covers these principles for the more common techniques used.

### Continuous infusions

This is a technique that is primarily used for severe pain that cannot be controlled effectively with oral or rectal preparations. There are several reasons why oral or rectal preparations cannot be used, such as being nil by mouth, nausea, compliance and consent, and physiological reasons. Continuous infusions may be over a small number of hours or continuously for 24 hours a day, and for as long as is required.

A continuous infusion is generally thought of as an IV infusion but can also include the subcutaneous, wound infiltration, epidural and extrapleural routes. Analgesic drugs in continuous infusions are generally but not exclusively opioids. The most common ones are morphine infusions, but fentanyl, pethidine and diamorphine can also be given as infusions, but are used more frequently in the adult patient population.

The nursing aspects are predominantly based around the drug that is used for the infusion and the route chosen.

## Patient-controlled analgesia

PCA describes the mechanism of patients administering their own analgesia, through a variety of routes including the oral (PO), IM or IV routes. However, in current practice this commonly refers to the administration of IV opioids via an infusion pump. The rationale behind PCA devices, first described by Sechzer,[12] was to provide individualised pain management, and to promote independence and give the patient control of their own pain relief.

## Individualised pain management

Analgesics have limited effects if the plasma concentration fails to achieve a particular threshold, and this can vary between individuals. Thus requirements for analgesia differ greatly between patients, especially in children where factors such as age, development and weight are influential. The use of a PCA device can assist in overcoming this interpatient variation.

Initially the patient can titrate the amount of dose delivered against pain intensity over time, providing flexibility and predictability for acute pain stimuli, such as physiotherapy. Second, the ability of the child to adjust their opioid consumption in relation to pain experience may also aid in minimising the potential adverse effects associated with the use of opioids. Subsequently, this achieves maximum pain relief with minimal severity of side-effects.

## Patient independence

It is well established in the literature that people who can exert control over their individual experiences are better able to deal with stressors and are more tolerable to changing situations.[13] This is especially relevant to children, and, as Morton[14] highlighted, the child who has established control over their pain management gains vast psychological advantages in relation to pain perception. This relates directly to the knowledge that patients have immediate access to pain relief, thus they can administer analgesia as required. Pain memories in children are extremely influential on future experiences and therefore by using PCA, they lose their fear that future pain will go unrelieved (Table 17.3).

**Table 17.3** Patient-controlled analgesia (PCA) programme terminology

| Terminology | Outline |
|---|---|
| Opioid solution | Concentration of the opioid solution in the syringe for delivery<br>Calculated and prescribed in relation to the individual child |
| Loading dose | One-off dose administered on commencing the programme |
| Bolus dose | The amount of opioid delivered on activation of the button by the child |
| Dose duration | The rate at which the PCA delivers the bolus dose |
| Lockout Interval | Time elapsed between the delivery of one dose to the time the pump will respond to another demand<br>Allows the opioid to achieve peak effect before another dose can be administered, thus gaining maximum analgesia without the risk of increasing adverse effects |
| Demands/tries | The amount of times the button has been activated by the child |
| Good demands/tries | The amount of times the button has been activated resulting in the administration of a bolus dose |

## Opioids used

Morphine sulphate is the mainstay of opioids used in acute postoperative pain management and in IV PCA.[9] It is inexpensive, widely available and overall is the standard against which all other opioids are measured in clinical trials. Fentanyl is a useful alternative when morphine is contraindicated, although is more widely used in epidural pain management. However, the choice of opioid is chiefly down to the avoidance of adverse effects and the selection of the PCA programme and parameters, such as bolus dose, are more critical for adequate and safe pain management.

## Naloxone

- Opioids are agonists and naloxone is a pure antagonist, binding to the opioid receptors without stimulation and reversing the effects of the opioid.
- Each patient should have naloxone prescribed when starting an opioid infusion.
- Naloxone can be titrated to reverse side-effects while retaining analgesic cover.
- Naloxone has a shorter half-life (1 hour) than most opioids (morphine 2–3 hours) so if required to antagonise the effects of the opioid completely, repeated doses or an infusion may be needed.

## Side-effects

Opioid compounds act directly on the central nervous system in order to produce an analgesic effect; as a consequence, the incidence of side-effects associated with their IV use is unfortunately quite high. Sensitivity to these effects is variable between patients and it is essential to balance the use of opioids in relation to adverse effects and analgesic benefit.

### Respiratory depression

- Respiratory depression is the most serious concern of opioid use, although clinical incidence is reported as low.[13]
- Monitoring the respiratory rate, sedation levels and oxygen saturation and the correlation between these signs provides the most accurate clinical picture and the earliest detection of depression.
- Management of severe respiratory depression starts with ABC (airway, breathing, circulation) and includes oxygen therapy to treat the hypoxaemia, naloxone to reverse the effects of the opioid and stopping the infusion to prevent further complication.

### Sedation

- Sedation is the best clinical indicator of respiratory depression and is often a precursor to this potentially fatal effect.
- This highlights the need for close monitoring of sedation levels throughout opioid use. The sedation score is outlined in Table 17.4.[15]
- The use of PCA with a bolus dose-only programme has a built-in safety component as the child can only administer the dose when sedation allows, thus not sedating further.
- Extreme care should be taken if a background infusion is being used because the opioid is being continuously infused.

### Nausea and vomiting

- Nausea and vomiting have the highest clinical incidence associated with opioid use.[9]
- Movement and sudden administration of opioid boluses can exaggerate these effects.
- Administer regular antiemetics alongside the PCA to reduce these effects; however, some antiemetics have a sedative component, so careful consideration is required.

### Urinary retention and gastrointestinal symptoms

- Opioids alter smooth muscle activity, thus inhibiting gastric emptying, bowel motility and urinary retention.
- Low-dose naloxone administration may ease these effects.
- Urine catheterisation is sometimes performed in surgery or may be performed postoperatively if retention is suspected.

### Pruritis

- Opioids cause the release of histamine from mast cells, and as a result cause localised pruritis or severe urticaria.

**Table 17.4** Sedation score

| Score | Sedation |
|-------|----------|
| 0 | Eyes open spontaneously |
| 1 | Eyes open to speech |
| 2 | Eyes open when roused |
| 3 | Unrousable |

**Table 17.5** Monitoring

| Physiological observations | Equipment monitoring |
| --- | --- |
| Pulse | Volume of opioid administered |
| Respiratory rate | Patient-controlled analgesia programme |
| Oxygen saturation | Usage patterns (demands/tries ratio) |
| Incidence of nausea/vomiting | Site of infusion |
| Sedation score (refer to sedation score shown previously) | |
| Pain score (refer to tools for assessment) | |

- Pruritis can be effectively treated with antihistamines; however, care must be taken because of their sedative effects.
- Ondansetron has been found to be effective in treating pruritis.
- Alternatively, low-dose naloxone may assist in severe cases.

## Monitoring

Observation of the child receiving opioids comprises checking the equipment, actively monitoring for adverse effects and monitoring the efficacy of analgesia (Table 17.5, page 288). Consequently, hourly observation enables closer titration of the child's response to the opioid analgesia in use.

## Considerations

In the past, concerns have been raised about paediatric patients having the ability to use PCA safely and effectively in pain management. However, over recent years PCA has been successfully used in children, with positive feedback.[7] Before consideration, it must be established whether the child wishes to be actively involved in their own management. Also, the patient must be able to understand the theory and technique behind PCA and physically operate the equipment.

## EPIDURALS

An epidural infusion is used for moderate to severe pain using local anaesthetic to spinal nerves via a fine catheter. It is almost always inserted while the child is anaesthetised in the operating theatre.

## Epidural/extradural space

The brain and the spinal cord are covered by 3 layers of connective tissue called the meninges pia mater, arachnoid and dura mater. The epidural space is found outside the dura mater. It contains fat, connective tissue, nerves and blood vessels. Entry to this space in children is at thoracic, lumbar, sacral and caudal levels. A catheter is threaded up to the desired level (Figure 17.1, page 289).

The local anaesthetic is administered into the epidural space at the appropriate dermatome level to cover the operation site. e.g. T10 for hip surgery, L3–T6 for intestinal surgery.

## Single doses

Bupivacaine can be used alone as a bolus prior to and during surgery. It is important to ensure adequate analgesia is timed to be given before the bupivacaine wears off.

## Caudal epidurals

Babies and small children have a flatter sacrum which makes injection or insertion of a catheter in this area easier. The catheter is inserted at the sacral hiatus just above the coccyx and can be threaded up to the level needed, even as far as the thoracic region.

## Spinal (or subarachnoid block)

A spinal is different from an epidural. Local anaesthetic is injected into the subarachnoid space, containing cerebrospinal fluid (CSF). The block is often more profound and reliable than from an epidural and this technique is often chosen for surgery without a general anaesthetic.

**Figure 17.1** Epidural catheter placement.

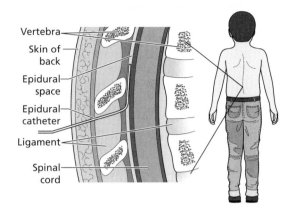

Vertebra
Skin of back
Epidural space
Epidural catheter
Ligament
Spinal cord

## Epidural infusions

These are safer and more convenient than a bolus injection using a mix of local anaesthetic and opioid. Usually a low dose of Bupivacaine and an opioid, such as Fentanyl, is infused through the epidural catheter. Infusions of a local anaesthetic alone may not be ideal in young children. The use of an opioid can enhance analgesia and provide some sedation. Smaller doses of each agent will be needed with less risk of toxicity.

## Local anaesthetic

Local anaesthetics prevent transmission of the nerve impulses along the axons of nerves, this reduces sensation (afferent nerves) and also muscle power (efferent nerves). Weak concentrations of local anaesthetics will only block the smaller nerve fibres, so analgesia can be achieved, but the child will usually still have some sensation and be able to move their legs. Local anaesthetic toxicity will occur if given intravenously or in prolonged high doses.

## Signs of local anaesthetic toxicity

- Tingling of mouth, tongue, and lips
- Increased irritability or anxiety
- Sedation
- Nausea
- Hypotension
- Respiratory distress
- Cardiac arrhythmias
- Convulsions

## Management of local anaesthetic toxicity

- Be alert to the signs of toxicity.
- Hypotension is rarely seen in children of 6 and younger, due to their cardiovascular stability.
- If hypotension occurs do not tip head down. This can potentially cause sensation block to rise too high compromising cardiac and respiratory effort.
- Young children are less likely to report tingling etc.
- Treatment is symptomatic, e.g. airway management.

## Opioids

Opioids given via an epidural will bind to the opiate receptors in the dorsal horn, blocking pain transmission. They will also diffuse across into the CSF and vascular system. If CSF levels are high the opioid may reach higher centres in the brainstem, depressing respiration. This is rare with lipid soluble opioids such as fentanyl and diamorphine.

## Monitoring for safety

Frequent observations are essential:

- to detect and *treat* any complications at an early stage;
- to ensure effective pain management.

The frequency and nature of observations should be dictated by the condition of the patient. In general it may be possible to reduce the frequency as the child's overall condition improves. However, increasing the frequency should be considered if the infusion rate is increased or a supplemental bolus is administered to improve the quality of analgesia. This is particularly important in older children who may experience hypotension due to peripheral vasodilatation below the level of the block.

Detecting the level of sensation in children can be difficult. It is vital to know that the child can feel below T4 (nipple height). If the block rises too high sympathetic nerves supplying the heart will be affected, leading to bradycardia and hypotension. With a thoracic epidural the intercostal muscles could be weakened mainly affecting the ability to cough.

The cold test is useful for detecting the level and any problems with the block, for example a unilateral block, described below. Different centres will have their own methods of checking sensation and block levels.

## Procedure for testing the level of sensation block

- Spray the child in a place where the epidural will not be affecting them (i.e. shoulder) so that they know how cold the spray is.
- Spray at intervals from the foot to above the level that needs to be covered by the epidural.
- Ask the child where the spray feels as cold as on the shoulder.
- For younger and non-verbal children you need to look for a reaction and need to limit the area sprayed.
- Spray both sides of the body to check for a patchy or unilateral block
- Record the dermatome level at which the sensation block appeared to be (this may be different for each side).

Potential problems for assessing sensation level.

- The child has a dressing or plaster cast in situ.
- The child has a physical disability with impaired sensation.
- The child is non-verbal or has special needs.

With these patients the priority is to ensure that the block is not too high and that the epidural is maintaining pain control. The main aim is to elicit a response to the cold spray at a level of T4 or below.

## Complications of epidural infusions

It is advisable to have intravenous access maintained throughout the epidural infusion and for approximately 4 hours after discontinuation. This is required for emergency treatment of complications such as hypotension; in the event of an unsuccessful epidural infusion, alternative pain management can be commenced.

## Unsatisfactory block

- *Ineffective block indicated by pain*: the child should be reviewed, as they may need a bolus, increased rate or change in position. Consider adding an opioid into the infusion.
- *Unilateral block* (one-sided block) the child may need to have their position changed to allow a more even spread and/or given a bolus, or increased rate of infusion. Consider adding opioid into the infusion.

- *Block too dense* (no movement of limbs at all): the child may be at risk of developing pressure sores=. The infusion rate or concentration of local anaesthetic may be reduced. Consider stopping the infusion temporarily to check for movement and to ensure no nerve damage has occurred.

## Epidural catheter problems

- *Leakage*

Observe the site frequently, and if the child is showing signs of pain. Some leakage is not uncommon. It is not considered a problem as long as the dressing remains in situ and pain is controlled. It is best to put a new occlusive dressing on top, rather than removing the old one and risk displacing the catheter.

- *Infection*

Check entry site frequently and particularly when the child has pyrexia of unknown origin. If there is any suspicion of infection, seek advice from medical staff or pain service; the catheter will probably have to be removed.

- *Disconnection*

Weak points are where the catheter and bacterial filter are connected. If disconnection occurs seek advice. The site of the disconnection will dictate the action taken.

- *Occlusion*

As the epidural catheter is very narrow, it can be easily kinked. Sometimes repositioning the patient can help with a catheter kink just under the skin.

## Urinary retention

Some children will return from theatre with a urinary catheter in situ. For uncatheterised children who have not passed urine for a significant amount of time after surgery:

- assess if child is hydrated or not;
- check for palpable bladder;
- consider gentle suprapubic pressure (if not at surgery site);
- catheterise as required.

## Opioid side-effects

See the section on PCA.

## Discontinuation of epidural infusions

The infusion is delivered within a prescribed range. The rate required to provide analgesia without side-effects is normally continued throughout the infusion.

A period of assessment is required to verify that the child is comfortable without the epidural infusion, usually 4–6 hours. Epidurals are rarely weaned down.

## Removal of epidural catheter

The catheter is removed using a non-touch technique. It is advisable to help the patient back into the position in which the catheter was inserted (usually the fetal position); the child with a hip spica in situ can be turned prone.

Children with potential bleeding problems *must* have a platelet count/INR (international normalised ratio) check. If on enoxaparine (clexane) do not remove the catheter until at least 6 hours after the last dose or 2 hours before the next dose.

The catheter should be removed easily without force. If you feel resistance, seek help from the pain service or anaesthetist. *Do not pull hard.*

Check that the tip of the catheter is present. If the entry site is inflamed on removing the catheter, swab it and send with the catheter tip for microscopy. Document removal of the intact catheter.

## ENTONOX

Entonox is a 1:1 mixture of nitrous oxide and oxygen. In the UK it is provided in cylinders that are blue with blue and white quartered shoulders. Nitrous oxide is a colourless and odourless gas that is a useful analgesic and is safer when pre-mixed with oxygen.

The specific mechanisms of action are unclear; the analgesic, sedative and anxiolytic effects of nitrous oxide are thought to be derived from its action at opioid receptors in the dorsal horn of the spinal cord. Nitrous oxide is absorbed into the bloodstream from the lungs and reaches the brain very quickly, allowing a very rapid onset of action. Its action is rapidly terminated as it is breathed out after discontinuing administration.

Entonox is usually self-administered via a facemask or mouthpiece using a demand valve system. Continuous flow is used in some centres but may cause deep sedation.

## When to use Entonox

Entonox is best used for short-term pain relief, primarily for procedural pain but it may also be used for acute pain relief until longer acting analgesia is established.

Please see the website for more in-depth information of Entonox uses and contraindications.

## Administering Entonox

### Preparation

- Explain how the demand system works; let the child practise before the procedure to ensure they can master the technique of mouth-only breathing.
- Select mouthpiece or mask.
- Check a suitable environment is available for the procedure and administration of Entonox, i.e. there is adequate ventilation to reduce occupational exposure and avoiding disruptions for the child during the procedure.
- Check oxygen and suction and resuscitation equipment.
- Explain procedure and use of Entonox to the child and check they understand and obtain consent; the preparatory explanation should explore fears and reassure the child.
- Check Entonox equipment is in working order and a spare cylinder is available should it be needed.
- Ensure the drug has been prescribed; some areas will have PGDs (patient group directives) in place or may not require the gas to be prescribed.
- Ensure the Entonox is going to be administered by an appropriately trained professional.

### Administration

- Encourage parent to be present to aid with distraction and encourage use of the Entonox.
- Instruct the child to take slow and steady breaths.
- Ensure that the demand valve is being activated, listening for the appropriate sounds.
- Allow 2 minutes for the gas to start taking effect before starting the procedure.
- Stay with the child, encouraging and supporting them through the procedure.
- Observe for side-effects.
- When finished, turn off cylinder, purge system and store in a lockable cupboard.
- Child should sit quietly for 10–20 minutes after using Entonox for the effects to wear off.

## Advantages and disadvantages of using Entonox

### Advantages

- Very quick acting
- Minimal side-effects
- Self-administration therefore child has control
- Wears off quickly if patient dislikes the sensation.

### Disadvantages

- Limited to age and understanding of patients for self-administration
- Side-effects can be disliked
- Staff may need to be trained to competent standard before administering to children in some centres.

# NON-PHARMACOLOGICAL PAIN MANAGEMENT

Non-pharmacological intervention provides a complementary and integrative approach to pain management, considering psychological, emotional and social components that influence pain perception.[16]

The aim of non-pharmacological intervention is to provide effective coping strategies for painful experiences and stimuli, reducing anxiety and stress, which in turn can exacerbate pain. However, there is little evidence to support that these techniques actually reduce pain intensity and merely provide the child and family with more control over the situation, aiming to make pain more tolerable. On the whole this is not a negative conclusion, but as healthcare professionals we should strive to provide actual therapeutic pain relief and thus non-pharmacological techniques must be used in conjunction with analgesic drugs. The benefit of combination therapy reduces the need for pharmacological intervention and thus decreases the incidence of adverse effects.

The multidisciplinary team is vital in providing optimum non-pharmacological therapy, as much of these approaches are specialised fields of practice. Play specialists and clinical psychologists are but a few who hold vital roles in the implementation of complementary therapies. This knowledge is essential, as overstimulation and sensory overload can in fact increase the pain response. Many techniques can be facilitated by the nurses/specialist to enable the use of such techniques safely by the child and family on future occasions providing continuation of care.

## Mainstay techniques

*Distraction/play therapy*
- Refer to Chapter 7

*Feeding (milk/sucrose)*
- Feeding a baby or infant can induce relaxation or settled sleep by the stimulation of natural endogenous opioids, thus having analgesic and sedative effects.
- The use of sucrose solution has been developed for children <12 weeks of age.[17]

*Massage/touch*
- Promotes blood circulation, production of natural endogenous opioids and relaxation.
- This links directly with the more specialist use of physiotherapy (refer to specialist techniques).
- Physical touch and the desire to have contact are present at birth and continually develop with the child. It is therefore one of the most effective methods of relaxation, communication and empathy.

*Relaxation*
- States of relaxation and anxiety cannot coexist.[18]
- Relaxation aims to provide freedom from physical and mental tension, thus subduing anxiety, fear and negativity and, in painful situations, the child's perception of pain.
- Techniques such as deep breathing, blowing bubbles and rhythmical exercise can aid in relaxation.

*TENS (transcutaneous electrical nerve stimulation)*
- A non-invasive technique that is effective in the relief of localised acute pain by increasing endorphin levels and decreasing the nerve conduction to pain mediators.
- Acts by delivering rapid impulses of controlled, low-voltage electrical current via electrodes attached to the skin.
- Effective immediately.

*Psychological support*
- Centred on information giving, reassurance and providing the child and family with a sense of choice and control over their pain management.

- Fear of the unknown can alter a child's perception of pain, and heighten responses to such pain.
- Informing the child of the experience and possible management strategies not only allows them some control over the situation and enhances compliance, but may assist in developing a less negative perception of pain in the future.

*Parental involvement*
- Parents provide instinctive therapeutic touch, comfort, distraction and continuing care for their child and can therefore provide essential assistance with all non-pharmacological therapies.
- However, the cooperation of the parents with the healthcare professional is fundamental so as not to escalate distress and anxiety.
- Educating the parents about such situations is essential in order to rule out any negativity transmitted from the parents to the child, thus proving to be counteractive.
- Once again it is highlighted that nurse–child–family relationships are key to successful practice.

## SPECIALIST COMPLEMENTARY TECHNIQUES

These techniques should only be undertaken by a trained practitioner.

*Acupuncture*
- A traditional Chinese therapy aiming to correct the abnormal flow of life forces around the pain, i.e. pain signal transmission.
- Stimulates the production of natural endorphins (opioid compounds).

*Aromatherapy*
- Holistic form of healing using essential oils used as a means of relaxation.

*Guided imagery*
- Engagement of the child's imagination and concentration on a specific event individual to

the child, and the development of this journey throughout the painful experience.
- Use of pleasant sensory images as a substitute to pain, in which the climax of the journey should coincide with the acute pain experience to achieve maximum effect, i.e. scoring a goal, diving underwater.

*Hypnosis*
- Creates an altered state of consciousness, focusing attention away from pain and the child's perception of pain.

*Physiotherapy*
- Physical therapy reduces pain by stimulating non-nociceptor fibres (those that do not transmit pain signals) which in turn inhibits the transmission of pain signals.

## CONCLUSION

To ensure effective pain management for children we need to be assessing their pain from admission to discharge and in any potential painful procedure or situation. It should be based on a robust model of assessment, which will then lead to a proactive, effective approach to pain management where all options are explored and appropriate techniques are applied safely and effectively to cause no harm and maximum relief to our patients.

This chapter has covered the basic principles of pain management and explored some of the options: it cannot cover all the information that you require but will have enabled you to look at what is available and what approaches may work for the young patients in our care. It must be borne in mind that each clinical centre will have their own policies and procedures relating to this subject.

We must constantly re-evaluate and reassess the actions that we perform to ensure that these actions have been effective. We must look at each child as an individual who behaves and interacts and expresses themselves in their own manner consequently ensuring that we treat each child's pain on that individuality.

Go to the website to find the PowerPoint presentation for this chapter and MCQs to test your knowledge. **www.hodderplus.com/childnursingskills**

# REFERENCES

1  McCaffery M (1983). *Nursing Management of the patient in pain*. Philadelphia: JB Lippincott.
2  International Association for the Study of Pain (1979) Pain terms: a list with definitions and notes on usage. *Pain*; **6**: 249–252.
3  Glasper EA, Richardson J (eds) (2006) A *textbook of children's and young people's nursing*. London: Churchill Livingstone.
4  Royal College of Nursing (2000) *Clinical guidelines for the recognition and assessment of acute pain in children: technical report*. London: RCN Publishing.
5  United Nations General Assembly (1989) *Convention on the rights of the child*. New York: United Nations.
6  Nursing and Midwifery Council (2008) *The code: standards of conduct, performance and ethics for nurses and midwives*. London: NMC.
7  Frank LS (2003) Nursing management of children's pain: current evidence and future directions for research. *Nursing Times Research* **8**: 330–353.
8  Baker C, Wong D (1987) QUESTT: a process of pain assessment in children. *Orthopaedic Nursing* **6**(1): 11–21.
9  McGann K (2007) *Fundamental aspects of pain assessment and management*. London; Quay Books Division.
10  Coniam S, Mendham J (2006) *Principles of pain management for anaesthetists*. London: Hodder Arnold.
11  British National Formulary for children (BNFc) www.rcpch.ac.uk/Publications/bnfc (accessed 1 June 2009)
12  Sechzer PH (1968) Objective measurement of pain. *Anaesthesiology* **29**: 209–210.
13  McDonald AJ, Cooper MG (2001) Patient-controlled analgesia: an appropriate method of pain control in children. *Paediatric Drugs* **3**(4): 273–284.
14  Morton NS (1998) *Acute paediatric pain management: a practical guide*. London: Saunders.
15.  Yildiz K, Tercan E, Dogru K, *et al.* (2003) Comparison of patient-controlled analgesia with and without a background infusion after appendicectomy in children. *Paediatric Anaesthesia* **13**: 427–431.
16  Royal College of Nursing (RCN). *Clinical practice guidelines: the recognition and assessment of acute pain in children – recommendations*. London: RCN Publishing, 1999.
17  Cignacco E, Hamers JPH, Stoffel L, *et al.* (2007) The efficacy of non-pharmacological interventions in the management of procedural pain in preterm and term neonates: a systematic review. *European Journal of Pain* **11**: 139–152.
18  Wilkinson R (1996) A non-pharmacological approach to pain relief. *Professional Nurse* **11**(4): 222–224.

# FURTHER READING

Welchew E (1995) *Patient controlled analgesia*. London: BMJ publishing group.

## CHAPTER 18

# Administration of blood and blood products

Diana Agacy-Cowell

## LEARNING OUTCOMES

*Upon completion of this chapter, the reader should be able to accomplish the following:*

1 Define the purpose of a red cell transfusion, platelet transfusion and a fresh frozen plasma transfusion

2 Demonstrate a basic knowledge of the ABO and the Rh D blood groups

3 Identify the various stages of the blood transfusion process

4 Identify the difference between a group and screen sample and a cross-match sample, and the correct process of labelling these samples

5 Identify the correct procedure of collection and transportation of blood components

6 Identify the equipment required for a blood transfusion

7 Explain the safe process for the administration of different blood components

8 Discuss the care of a child receiving a blood transfusion and rationalise your answers

9 Discuss potential adverse reactions to a blood transfusion

10 Discuss the risks of blood transfusion and identify the biggest risk of transfusion. Explain how this risk can be completely eliminated

*A glossary of terminology is provided on page 309.*

## CHAPTER OVERVIEW

In an acute hospital setting the transfusion of blood components and blood products is an integral part of everyday life; however, it is a finite commodity as we rely on voluntary donors for its supply. The National Haemovigilance Office states that blood components and products are life saving and when used appropriately they will improve the quality of life in a large range of clinical conditions. However, it is also widely recognised that, as in any other clinical intervention, there are a number of risks associated with this therapy: transfusion-transmitted infections (TTIs) and human error. The quality of blood has been given precedence over that of human error because of the impact of hepatitis, human immunodeficiency virus (HIV) and more recently variant Creutzfeldt–Jakob disease (vCJD). However, in the last decade the Serious Hazards of Transfusion (SHOT) scheme[1] has attributed most major incidents to human error.

Safe transfusion practice relies on collaborative teamwork, as blood transfusion is a complex, high-risk and multistep procedure. The transfusion process crosses several professional boundaries and involves many individuals. There are at least 23 stages between taking a pre-transfusion compatibility blood sample, the recipient receiving their transfusion and the completion of the transfusion.[2] Six different professional groups intervene at different stages of the process, and with each stage there is the potential of error.

In 2005 when the European directive for blood was transcribed into British criminal law as the Blood Safety and Quality Regulation,[3] it became a legal requirement that every unit issued for transfusion had to be fully traceable from donor to recipient, vein-to-vein traceability. The health professional responsible for communicating the final fate of every unit in the clinical area is the responsibility of the nurse, as they are invariably the ones who administer the transfusions on the wards. To make this process easier most hospitals, if they have not already done so, are in the process of implementing an electronic tracking system to meet the above requirements. The laborious paper systems, which might be still in use in some hospitals, are unreliable and few have achieved 100 per cent traceability as they rely heavily on the health professional remembering to sign, date and return the traceability slip. Despite this change from paper to electronic systems, the transfusion process will remain the same and the same safety steps will need to be followed.

With the transcription of the EU Directive on Blood Safety and Quality Regulations to British criminal law also came a new haemovigilance scheme, monitored by the MHRA (Medicines and Healthcare Products Regulatory Agency), known as SABRE (Serious Adverse Blood Reactions & Events). This new scheme works alongside SHOT.

## SAFE TRANSFUSION PRACTICE

Paediatric patients should not be exposed unnecessarily to blood components and products as there is always the potential risk of TTIs, those that we are aware of and those yet to be discovered. Therefore, it is important to check the most recent haemoglobin result and assess the patient for signs of anaemia. If the patient is not actively bleeding, infection free and haemodynamically stable, query the transfusion: protect your patient. Remember the use of blood requires a conservative approach, as the safest transfusion is the one not given.

It is important to follow procedure even though at times it can be quite prescriptive, but the evidence demonstrates that when we disregard procedure errors occur. In 2005 SHOT[4] produced a paediatric report as they were worried about the

increasing incidents in paediatrics. The 2007 SHOT[1] reported a paediatric death directly related to a human error which resulted in an 'over-transfusion'. The error was attributed to the misunderstanding of a verbal prescription of the rate and volume of a transfusion of platelets.

Children are a particularly vulnerable age group; apart from having many special requirements there are other concerns.[4]

- Neonates are particularly susceptible to infective and toxic effects of transfusion owing to their immature immune and metabolic systems while they are still undergoing rapid neurodevelopment.
- Consideration must be given to long-term side-effects of transfusion as the majority of children have decades of life ahead of them.
- The acute side-effects of transfusion may be greater in children than in adults, as a single unit may represent a much greater proportion of their blood volume.
- In general, transfusions are rare on paediatric wards; therefore, there is less awareness of transfusion-related hazards.

## ANATOMY AND PHYSIOLOGY OF BLOOD

Blood is a highly specialised circulating tissue consisting of several different types of cells suspended in a straw-coloured fluid called plasma (Table 18.1, page 297).[5]

The main components transfused are red blood cells (RBCs), platelets, plasma (non-cellular) and cryoprecipitate (non-cellular). In this chapter we will focus on the first three as they are the most commonly used components.

Please refer to the website for illustrations of blood components.

All components and products are derived from whole blood. The National Blood Service (NBS), part of the National Health Service Blood and Transplant (NHSBT) take whole blood from voluntary donors. These voluntary donations are then processed, to provide us with the components we see in hospital (Figure 18.1).[5]

### Red blood cells

Red cells are prescribed to treat anaemia and haemorrhage.

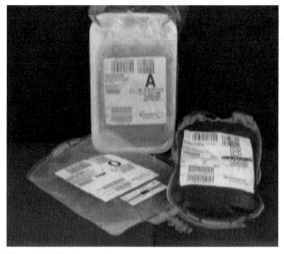

**Figure 18.1** Blood components.

## Causes of anaemia

- Iron deficiency
- Vitamin B12 deficiency
- Folate deficiency
- Bone marrow failure
- Secondary to chemotherapy
- Slow bleeding, especially from the gastro-intestinal tract

The diagnostic test used to detect anaemia is the full blood count (FBC).

One of the indices measured by this diagnostic test is the level of haemoglobin (Hb) (Table 18.2) and it is this Hb level that is used to quantitate the degree of anaemia.

The FBC is a valuable test for the diagnosis of anaemia as it provides other valuable data which haematologists use to differentiate between types of anaemia.

Red cells are stored in refrigerators in the blood transfusion laboratory (BTL) or in designated refrigerators, away from the BTL. The temperature of these refrigerators is strictly monitored in order to preserve the quality of red cells. It is important to maintain red cells at 2–6°C. Therefore under *no* circumstances should red cells ever be stored, even for a short period, in the ward refrigerator

## Platelets and fresh frozen plasma

Platelets and fresh frozen plasma (FFP) are prescribed to treat a coagulopathy; that is, to stop excessive internal or external bleeding or in some circumstances to prevent bleeding.

The FBC provides us with the number of circulating platelets (Table 18.2), while the

**Table 18.1** Components of blood

| Cellular constituents | Function |
| --- | --- |
| Red cells or erythrocytes | Carry respiratory gases and give it its red colour because they contain haemoglobin, an iron containing protein that binds to oxygen in the lungs and transports it to the tissues in the body |
| White cells or leucocytes | Fight infection |
| Platelets or thrombocytes | Play an important part in the clotting of blood |

**Table 18.2** Normal paediatric haematology values

| Haemoglobin (Hb) | g/dL |
| --- | --- |
| Infant (2–6 month) | 10–15 |
| Child (1–12 years) | 11–16 |
| Adolescent: male | 13–16 |
| Adolescent: Female | 12–16 |
| Critical values | <5 or >20 |
| **Platelet/thrombocyte count** | **× $10^9$/L** |
| Infant/child/youth | 150–450 |
| Critical values | <30 or >7100 |

**Table 18.3** Normal coagulation screen values

| International Normalised Ratio (INR) | |
|---|---|
| Infant (2–6 month) | 0.9 –1.2 |
| Child (1–12 years) | 0.9 –1.2 |
| Adolescent: male | 0.9 –1.2 |
| Adolescent: female | 0.9 –1.2 |
| Critical values | >5 |

diagnostic test coagulation screen (CS) will indicate if FFP is required, depending on the international normalised ratio (INR) (Table 18.3).

- FFP is stored frozen, hence the name, in the BTL and is defrosted before it is sent to the clinical area.
- Platelets are stored in an incubator at approximately 22°C on a 'rocker'. The gentle motion of the rocker prevents the platelets from aggregating.
- Platelets should never be stored in a refrigerator.
- Platelets and FFP are ordered on a named patient basis.

## Patients born after January 1996[7]

In order to minimise the risk of transmitting new variant CJD these patients should receive pathogen-reduced FFP sourced from outside the UK. This would either be methylene blue or solvent detergent-treated FFP (Octaplas). Cryopreciptate, produced from plasma, is also now available.

## Blood groups

There are many blood group systems along with their subgroups, but at this stage we will limit our attention to the two most clinically significant blood groups, the ABO and the Rh D blood systems. All blood groups are inherited and there are two ways of reporting the ABO blood group:

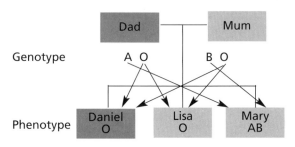

**Figure 18.2** ABO gene inheritance (Mendelian inheritance)

the genotype or the phenotype. The latter is the most common of the two (Figure 18.2).

Table 18.4 shows which blood group each recipient is compatible or suitable with depending on the component they need.

This choice is dictated by a substance that is present or absent on the red cells of the recipient.

- People who are blood group A have an 'A' substance (*antigen*) on their red cell membrane. This 'A' substance stimulates the production of *anti-B antibodies* that will circulate in plasma. The function of these antibodies is to defend the body from B antigens, which are present on the surface of B red cells and AB red cells
- People who are blood group B have a 'B' substance (*antigen*) on their red cell membrane. This 'B' substance stimulates the production of

**Table 18.4** Blood group compatibility

| Recipient/patient ABO blood group | Donor red cells compatible with | Donor FFP compatible with | Donor platelets compatible with |
|---|---|---|---|
| A | A or O | A or AB | A or B or O |
| B | B or O | B or AB | B or A or O |
| AB | AB, A, B, O | AB | A or B or O |
| O | O | O, A, B, AB | O or A or B |

FFP, fresh frozen plasma.

*anti-A antibodies* that will circulate in plasma. The function of these antibodies is to defend the body from A antigens, which are present on the surface of A red cells and AB red cells

- People who are blood group AB have both the 'A' and 'B' substances (*antigens*) on their red cells. The presence of both the substances prevents the stimulation and therefore the production of *antibodies* in plasma.
- People who are blood group O do not have 'A' or 'B' substance (*antigens*). Hence they produce *A, B antibodies* in plasma.

The rationale for producing the specific antibodies is to defend the body from what is foreign to it. For example:

- Elizabeth is blood group A and needs a red cell transfusion.
- John is blood group B and wants to donate blood to give to Elizabeth.
- However, if John's red cells are transfused to Elizabeth the anti-B antibodies in Elizabeth's plasma will destroy John's donated B red cells causing haemolysis.
- This will make Elizabeth very ill and can be fatal.
- Elizabeth can only receive type A or O red cells.
- The absence of AB antigens on O red cells make them safe to transfuse to A, B or AB recipients.

## Rh D blood group

In the past, though you will still hear the term used, this blood group was referred to as the Rhesus blood group. However, the term Rhesus refers to the species of monkey in which a similar antibody to that of the human version was discovered. Using the previous example both blood groups would be reported as:

- Elizabeth is 'A negative' or 'A Rh D negative';
- John is 'B positive' or 'B Rh D positive'.

Negative means the *absence* of the Rh D factor on the surface of the red cell membrane. Those that have this factor on their red cells are said to be Rh D positive.

However, unlike the ABO antigens, the antibodies against the Rh factor are developed either through placental sensitisation or transfusion; that is, a person who has never been exposed to the Rh D antigen will not posses the Rh D antibody (Figure 18.3)

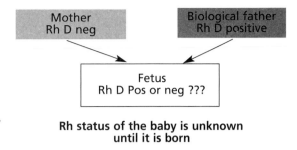

Rh status of the baby is unknown until it is born

**Figure 18.3** Haemolytic disease of the newborn.

If the fetus is Rh D negative like the mother there is no problem, but if the fetus is Rh D positive there could be a problem. Usually if it is the first pregnancy the child is born without any problems; however, the risk increases with future pregnancies. The problem occurs when the baby's blood (RH D positive) crosses the placenta into the mother's circulation. When this occurs the mother can become sensitised and her immune system will produce Rh D antibodies. These Rh D antibodies will attack an Rh D-positive fetus causing haemolytic disease of the fetus and of the newborn (Figure 18.4).

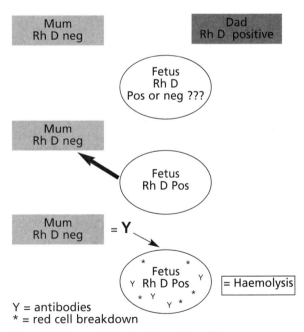

Y = antibodies
* = red cell breakdown

**Figure 18.4** How red cell antibodies are formed in prenancy. Y, antibodies; asterisks, red blood cells

Some cases may warrant an intrauterine transfusion. If the baby is born with a high bilirubin count caused by haemolysis, the baby will require an exchange transfusion. In order to avoid this Rh D-negative pregnant women are offered preventative treatment with anti-D immuno-globulin; however, as it is a blood product some women refuse this treatment.

Therefore, it is important to always transfuse the right Rh D blood group. If a child or adolescent is Rh D negative they must always receive Rh D-negative red cells and platelets. There can be exceptions to this rule during a major incident or severe donor blood shortage; however, this is beyond the scope of this chapter.

The Rh D status does not affect the transfusion of FFP or cryoprecipitate.

## THE TRANSFUSION PROCESS

### Sample taking

The transfusion process begins the moment a pre-transfusion sample is taken. For this purpose a request form indicating the nature of the test required must completed. Please see the website for illustration of request form.

A group and screen/save is required for the transfusion of all components.

For a cross-match the time, date and number of units required must be specified on the request form. This test is requested when a patient requires a red cell transfusion.

Before taking a blood sample the person taking the sample must first obtain the patient's or carer's consent to take the sample and inform them of the purpose of the test.

Use an open-ended question to identify the patient.

- Are you Tommy Smith? X
- Is this Tommy Smith? X
- Can you tell me your full name and date of birth? ✓

- Can you tell me this boy's full name and date of birth? ✓

All blood samples for the BTL must have the following information.

Patient's
- forename
- surname
- date of birth (DoB)
- hospital number or NHS number
- gender.

The person taking the sample *must* sign, date and time the sample tube as well.

The sample label must be completed by the person taking the sample before leaving the patient's side or in outpatient clinics before the patient leaves the room.

The labelling of blood transfusion samples in the event of a major incident or for unknown/unconscious patients vary at different hospitals. The reader is advised to find out what the local policy is for these situations.

Once all of the above has been completed, send the sample to the BTL.

### Pre-collection checklist

1  Patient is ready for the transfusion
2  Prescription and concomitant drugs are prescribed
3  *Identification wristband* in situ
4  Cannula in and patent
5  Baseline observations carried out
6  Equipment required for the transfusion (Appendix 1):
   - transfusion-giving set
   - pump (see hospital policy)
   - protective equipment, usually just gloves and apron, as per hospital policy
   - 0.9 per cent saline flush for intravenous access.

## PROCEDURE: Preparing for a transfusion

| Procedural steps | Evidence-based rationale |
|---|---|
| **1** Consent<br>• Formally identify the patient. Explain the procedure to the patient/parents/carers<br>• Assess for any history of reactions<br>• Obtain verbal consent from the patient/parent/carer for the transfusion to take place<br>• Document in transfusion record (TR) or in patient's medical notes<br>• Give information to the patient/parent/carer and the need to report problems, about the potential side-effects of transfusion such as anaphylaxis, which may present as shivering, flushing, shortness of breath, pain in loins or feelings of agitation | To establish positive identification<br><br>To prevent any reactions<br>Give patient/parent/carer information leaflet to read to enable them to have a full understanding of the procedure[8]<br><br>Patient/parent/carer informed about potential hazards of transfusions and report early indications or reactions |
| **2** Medication preparation<br>• Under no circumstances are drugs to be added to any blood component/product<br>• The doctor must prescribe transfusion cover – paracetamol and/or chlorphenamine and/or hydrocortisone, which must be given prior to commencement of transfusion<br>• If a reaction occurs during a transfusion, either insert another cannula or flush the exsisting cannula with at least 10 ml normal saline 0.9% before administering the above drugs only<br>• Check that the component/product has been prescribed on the transfusion record to ensure correct transfusion of blood products<br>• Do not prime giving sets with normal saline 0.9 per cent. Do not flush giving sets post transfusion with normal saline 0.9 per cent<br>• Blood must be prescribed on a prescription chart or TR that contains the patient's ID number, surname, first name and date of birth<br>• The prescription must state the name of the blood component/product to be transfused, the volume to be transfused, rate of transfusion.<br>• A unit of red cells is usually given over a minimum of 1 hour and a maximum of 4 hours<br>• A unit of platelets or FFP is given over 30 minutes | To comply with professional standards of practice<br><br>To avoid reactions in patients who have had reactions in the past<br><br><br>To avoid drug-induced haemolysis or coagulation<br><br><br>To ensure correct transfusion given<br><br><br>It is unnecessary to prime the blood transfusion set and increases the risk of priming with the wrong solution. The only solution that is compatible with blood is normal saline 0.9 per cent. Dextrose solutions can cause haemolysis while Ringer lactate solution may cause clotting of the transfused substance in the tubing[5] |
| **3** Cannulation or central venous access<br>• Cannulate the patient according to the cannulation policy. Ensure cannula is patent<br>• The choice of cannula used for the procedure should be depend on the individual and the desired rate of infusion<br>• Assess the need to flush the cannula (using a pulsating flush) according to policy, prior to | <br><br><br>To ensure appropriate cannula is used and individual patient needs addressed<br><br>To keep cannula patent and therefore stop blocking |

## PROCEDURE: The transfusion process (continued)

| | |
|---|---|
| transfusion and following procedure<br>• Secure with non-allergic tape or intravenous (IV) dressing depending on choice of cannula<br>• Ensure cannula is well secured | To reduce the need for extra trauma to the patients<br><br>To avoid blood wastage if access unobtainable |
| 4 Baseline observations<br>• Take the patient's temperature, pulse, respiratory rate and/oxygen saturation and blood pressure prior to transfusion commencing<br>• Document on observation chart or specific TR. If using ordinary observation chart highlight that the vital signs correspond to those recorded during a blood transfusion | To have baseline vital signs recorded and ensure that the patient is fit for transfusion |
| 5 Collection or receipt of blood component<br>• To collect any blood component the person doing the collection must take four points of patient identification (PID):<br>  • forename<br>  • surname<br>  • DoB<br>  • hospital number/NHS number<br>• The nurse requesting the collection must provide the person delegated to collect the component with the four points of patient identification | |

## Collection and transport of blood components

All blood components must be transferred from the site of collection, e.g. BTL, satellite blood bank, etc., to the clinical area in a box or non-transparent bag. Blood components must be transferred directly from the collection point to the clinical area and the person who receives the unit on the ward should take it directly to the patient's side in order to begin the transfusion immediately. Blood components should be collected or requested only for delivery when the patient is ready for the transfusion in order to avoid wastage.

To collect any blood component the person doing the collection must take four points of patient identification (PID):

1 forename
2 surname
3 DoB
4 hospital number/NHS number

## PROCEDURE: Checking the blood component

| Procedural steps | Evidence-based rationale |
|---|---|
| 1 Formally identify the patient and ensure that the information matches the TR | |
| 2 Check that the 14 digit number on the bar-coded National Blood Service (NBS) label matches the compatibility tag (CT) (luggage tag label attached to the bag) | The correct unit of blood will be given |

## PROCEDURE: Checking the blood component (continued)

| | |
|---|---|
| **3** Start time of unit must be recorded on peel off section of CT, once the first few millilitres have been transfused | |
| **4** The third section of CT needs to be torn off and completed once the transfusion has started ideally when doing the 15 minutes' observation after commencement | |
| **5** The third section must be returned to the blood transfusion lab. This is a legal requirement under the Blood Safety and Quality Regulations 2005 | Vein-to-vein traceability |
| **6** Fill in the time of arrival of blood component/ product in clinical area | Tracking of blood from blood bank to recipient |
| **7** Each blood component/product must be inspected for defects prior to their infusion. Particular attention should be paid to the following <br> • integrity of pack <br> • discolouration <br> • presence of clots | Faulty products will not be infused |

### Receipt of blood components in the clinical area

Best practice is for the nurse who is going to administer the blood transfusion to go and collect the blood component. However, sometimes the collection is delegated to a porter, healthcare assistant or another nurse. The nurse requesting the collection must provide the person delegated to collect the component with the four points of patient identification.

If it is a porter who is delivering the blood, it is best practice for the nurse who requested the collection to sign the receipt of delivery. The receipt slip should include PID and the time of collection and delivery to the clinical area. It is important for patient safety and therefore the responsibility of the nurse to check that the blood component being delivered is the right one for the right patient.

The blood component must never be left unattended. On delivery to the clinical area it should be checked and the transfusion should begin immediately.

In some hospitals a single registered nurse may check and administer the component. While in other hospitals two registered nurses are required for the checking process, but each must check the details individually and then sign the relevant paperwork.

## ADMINISTRATION OF BLOOD COMPONENTS[6]

### 'Final bedside check'

**Step 1:** Check 14-digit donation number on the NBS unit label to the Unit Identification Label; if they match

**Step 2:** Check patient information on unit to identification label to patient's ID wristband; if the information matches

**Step 3:** Prime the line with the blood component at the patient's bedside/side and commence the transfusion.

### Transfusion rate

Red cells: for non-emergency transfusions the transfusion of red cells must finish within 4 hours from the time the unit was taken out of the fridge. Most red cell transfusions can be prescribed over 2–3 hours

platelets over 30 minutes

FFP over 30 minutes.

### Care of patient being transfused[9]

#### Observations required for a blood transfusion

*One unit*

• Baseline observations

- At 15 minutes following start
- At end of transfusion (this will form the baseline observations for second unit etc.)

*Two units and more*

- Baseline observations (taken at the end of transfusion of previous unit).
- At 15 minutes following start of each unit.
- At the end of each unit.
- Further observations will depend on the clinical condition of the patient or if the patient becomes unwell or shows signs of an adverse reaction to the transfusion.
- Unconscious patients can be difficult to assess for signs of adverse reaction to the transfusion and must be closely monitored during the first 15 minutes of each unit for any visual or vital sign changes.
- It is good practice to remain with the patient for the first 15 minutes of every unit transfused as this is when the majority of reactions occur. This is why some textbooks recommend that the rate

of transfusion during the first 15 minutes should be slower than the prescribed rate. Once the 15-minute vital signs have been checked and no change has been observed from the baseline then the rate can be increased to the prescribed rate.

- It is important to physically observe the patient at regular intervals during the blood transfusion and to warn the patient or parents/carers to inform a member of staff immediately should the patient become agitated or develop a rash, etc. (Appendix 2).

### End of transfusion: disposal of empty packs

- Empty packs should be kept on the ward until the current transfusion episode (one or more units in one session) is complete. If the patient's observations have remained stable and there have been no signs of an adverse reaction the empty packs may be disposed of in ward clinical waste or return to the BTL as per hospital policy.

## PROCEDURE: Transfusion of platelets

| Procedural steps | Evidence-based rationale |
|---|---|
| 1 Transfusion of platelets should be commenced as soon as possible following collection/receipt in the clinical area | This component is used to stop bleeding |
| 2 Always administer platelets before a red cell transfusion | Platelets are given first in the blood transfusion process as they act to stop bleeding. |
| 3 Platelets are stored at room temperature (ideally 22°C but can be between 20 and 24°C). Platelets should never be stored in a refrigerator | To preserve the maximum activity of platelets |
| 4 If possible use a platelet giving set | These giving sets are shorter and it maximises the volume infused, therefore there will a better increment and it is more cost effective |
| 5 Agitate platelets before administering. | To prevent clumping |
| 6 Platelets are administered rapidly over 30 minutes. Carry out visual observation for rashes, level of consciousness and change in respiratory rate. Monitor temperature, pulse and blood pressure as for blood transfusion | As platelets are delivered rapidly, a reaction is possible |
| 7 Proceed as for blood transfusion | Platelets are more likely to react than red cells because of the temperature at which they are stored |

## PROCEDURE: Transfusion of fresh frozen plasma

| Procedural steps | Evidence-based rationale |
|---|---|
| 1 Transfusion of FFP should be commenced as soon as possible following collection/receipt in the clinical area | This component is used to stop or avoid bleeding by correcting the INR |
| 2 Always administer FFP before a red cell transfusion | FFP is given first in the blood transfusion process as they act to stop bleeding |
| 3 FFP should be returned to the BTL within 30 minutes if it is not going to be transfused | Preserve FFP up to 24 hours, reduces wastage |
| 4 Use blood component giving set | It has the correct filter |
| 5 FFP is administered rapidly over 30 minutes. Carry out visual observation for rashes, level of consciousness and change in respiratory rate. Monitor temperature, pulse and blood pressure as for blood transfusion | As FFP is delivered rapidly, a reaction is possible |
| 6 Proceed as for blood transfusion | FFP is more likely to give an allergic reaction owing to plasma proteins |

## PROCEDURE: Transfusion of red cells

| Procedural steps | Evidence-based rationale |
|---|---|
| 1 Transfusion should commence within 30 minutes delivery. If start of transfusion is delayed, contact BTL or see local policy | Maximum time of transfusion 4 hours from time out of fridge<br>Avoid wastage |
| 2 The red cells can be used only for the person who is named on the compatibility tag | |
| 3 If time out of the refrigerator is uncertain it must not be transfused but returned to the BTL and the staff informed | Risk of bacterial contamination |
| 4 All blood components/product must be transfused through a sterile blood product giving set which has a 170–200 µm filter | To filter micro-aggregates and prevent the accumulation of clots in the filter. This is why a giving set must never be flushed after transfusion. It increases the risk of clots and adverse reactions |
| 5 The first 15 minutes of a red cell transfusion should be transfused at a slower rate (approximately 20 drops per minute) than the prescribed rate | Most moderate to severe reactions will occur in the first 15 minutes of a transfusion |
| 6 Set the rate of the transfusion to 30–40 drops per minute for 1 unit of blood to be administered over 2 hours | To ensure correct delivery rate |

## PROCEDURE: Patient monitoring

| Procedural steps | Evidence-based rationale |
|---|---|
| 1 Patients who receive transfusion should be monitored throughout the whole process[6] | To avoid risk of reactions |
| 2 Ensure that the patient is in a setting where they can be closely observed and they can access the nurse call bell | |
| 3 Advise and encourage your patient to notify you immediately if they begin to feel anxious, or if they become aware of any adverse reactions such as shivering, flushing, pain or shortness of breath | |
| 4 Monitor the patient's temperature, pulse respiratory rate and blood pressure 15 minutes after you begin the transfusion of each unit, and record them on the transfusion record | Care of patient being transfused |
| 5 Once transfusion is completed record post-transfusion observations immediately after taking down empty bag | |
| 6 Discard bag and line as per local policy | Safe disposal of waste |
| 7 Discard the blood bag in this way unless there has been a reaction.<br>If there has been a reaction do not discard the pack (see Procedure following reactions) | |
| 8 Complete documentation recording the date and time transfusion ended | Good record keeping is the mark of a skilled practitioner.[9]<br>Continue patient observation |

## REPORTING ADVERSE REACTIONS

An acute haemolytic transfusion reaction is almost always due to ABO incompatibility. The most likely cause of such an incompatibility is patient misidentification by people involved in the transfusion process.

## PROCEDURE: Action for all suspected reactions *always*

| Procedural steps | Evidence-based rationale |
|---|---|
| 1 Stop transfusion immediately | To prevent further reaction. |
| 2 Check the patient's identity (verbally and/or ID wristband) to the compatibility tag attached to the unit. | To ensure right blood right patient |
| 3 Check unit label to compatibility tag | To ensure right blood right patient |
| 4 Get prompt medical evaluation | To assess patient |

## PROCEDURE: Types of reactions

| Procedural steps | Evidence-based rationale |
|---|---|
| **1 Reactions mild (Acute)**<br>Signs and symptoms<br>Usually occur within the first 15 minutes of each unit<br>A. *temperature*: a rise of 1.5°C above a patient's baseline is identified as pyrexial<br>Give Paracetamol: dose should be calculated on the patient's weight to be effective<br>Encourage patient to drink cold fluids. Keep cool, sponge down as necessary.<br>B. *urticaria rash (hives)*<br>Contact the Medical Practitioner<br>Chlorphenamine Should be administered. Dose will depend on the age of the child | *Stop transfusion*<br>Get prompt medical assessment<br>To reduce severity of reactions<br>If signs and symptoms subside or do not get any worse, restart transfusion at a slower rate but continue to monitor/observe patient closely |
| **2 Moderate to severe (acute)**<br>Burning sensation along the vein, while blood is being transfused<br>Shock<br>A feeling of faintness, loss of consciousness, hypotension, chest pain, loin pain, bronchospasm and breathlessness.<br>A rise in temperature, urticaria, tachycardia, rigors and haematuria<br>*Leave cannula in for venous access.*<br>Give adrenalline (epinephrine) dose will be age dependent (see local anaphylaxis protocol)<br>Check airway, breathing and circulation<br>Commence CPR if indicated | *Stop transfusion*<br>Get prompt medical assessment<br><br><br><br><br><br><br>For fluid infusion |
| **3 Infective shock (moderate to severe: acute)**<br>Bacterial contamination of Platelets or, less likely, red blood cells. Usually occurs with the first 100 mL of contaminated pack<br>*Signs and symptoms:*<br>• Myalgia<br>• Shocked patient<br>• Hypotension<br>• Rapid pulse<br>• Raised temperature<br>• Rigors<br>• Possible wheeze/dyspnoea<br>*Action*<br>• Stop transfusion immediately<br>• Inform medical practitioner<br>• Treat for shock<br>• Administer 100 per cent oxygen via a re-breathe bag.<br>• Treatment includes prompt medical attention for septicaemia | *Stop transfusion* |

## PROCEDURE: Types of reactions (continued)

| | |
|---|---|
| **4 Transfusion-related lung injury**<br>• This occurs when donor plasma contains antibodies to the patient's white cells<br>• Extremely rare but may be life threatening<br>• Occurs during or soon after transfusion<br>*Signs and symptoms*<br>• Acute respiratory reaction with fever, cough, wheeze/dyspnoea<br>• Pyrexia<br>• Tachypnoea<br>*Action*<br>• Stop transfusion<br>• Aim to keep patient relaxed<br>• Inform medical practitioner<br>• Treat as per shock patient | *Stop infusion*<br>Patient will require intubation |

## PROCEDURE: Procedure following reactions

| Procedural steps | Evidence-based rationale |
|---|---|
| • Re-check transfusion documentation and inform BTL | To establish any errors in patient identification |
| • Return blood bag and giving set to BTL plus any empty bags already used | To alert BTL of the possibility of another patient being involved in the mismatch. |
| • Return all unused units to ensure no further blood component is transfused | Blood is required by BTL for re-analysis, if possible |
| • Blood samples will need to be taken from the patient:<br>  • 1 cross-match sample<br>  • 1 EDTA<br>  • 1 Sodium citrate<br>  • 1 Heparin<br>  • 1 clotted | Take appropriate blood samples from patient |
| • Cultures if there is pyrexia | |
| • Ensure that the adverse reaction part of the transfusion record is completed and return a photocopy of the transfusion record along with<br>• If a transfusion record is not used the following information must documented and sent to the BTL.<br>  • Vital signs before and after incident<br>  • Rate of transfusion<br>  • Patient's clinical diagnosis | Information required for investigation |

 Go to the website to find the PowerPoint presentation for this chapter and MCQs to test your knowledge. **www.hodderplus.com/childnursingskills**

# REFERENCES

1 Serious Hazards of Transfusion (SHOT) (2007) *10th Annual report*. Manchester. www.shotuk.org

2 Southampton University Hospitals Trust Blood Transfusion Policy, 2006.

3 Department of Health (2005) The Blood safety and quality regulation (No. 50). www.opsi.gov.uk

4 Serious Hazards of Transfusion (SHOT) (2005) *8th Annual Report*. Manchester. www.shotuk.org

5 McClelland DBL (ed.) *Handbook of transfusion medicine*, 4th edition. United Kingdom Blood Services www.transfusionguidelines.org.uk

6 British Committee for Standards in Haematology (1999) Guidelines for the administration of blood and blood components and the management of the transfused patient. *Transfusion Medicine* 9(3): 227–238. www.bcshguidelines.com

7 British Committee for Standards in Haematology (2004) *Transfusion guidelines for neonates and older children*. www.bcshguidelines.com/

8 Department of Health (2001) *Essence of care*. London: HMSO.

9 Nursing and Midwifery Council (2002) *The code of professional conduct*. London: NMC.

# GLOSSARY

*Blood component:* red cells, platelets, fresh frozen plasma, cryoprecipitate, white cells.

*Blood product:* any therapeutic product derived from human whole blood or plasma donations.

*BSE:* a neurological disease of cattle which is generally thought to have caused the incidence of vCJD in humans.

*CJD:* A neurological disease that targets the brain, which can be fatal.

*Cross-match:* laboratory test used to find compatible or suitable allogenic blood (donor blood) for transfusion to a patient/recipient.

*Febrile non-haemolytic:* Fever or rigors during red cell or platelet transfusion affect 1–2 per cent of recipients, mainly multitransfused or previously pregnant patients, although these reactions are probably less frequent with leucodepleted components. Features are fever (>1°C above baseline) usually with shivering and general discomfort occurring towards the end of the transfusion or up to 2 hours after it has been completed. Most febrile reactions can be managed by slowing or stopping the transfusion and giving an antipyretic, e.g. paracetamol (not aspirin). These reactions are unpleasant but not life-threatening.

*Group and screen:* laboratory test to identify the patient's ABO and Rh D blood group and screen for antibodies.

*Haemoglobin count:* Laboratory diagnostic test to identify the amount of haemoglobin in a person's blood.

*Satellite blood bank:* a refrigerator that stores cross-matched blood but is situated away from the BT laboratory, e.g. by theatres or in the Emergency Department.

*Serious adverse events:* any untoward occurrence associated with the collection, testing, processing, storage and distribution of blood and blood components that might lead to the death or life-threatening, disabling or incapacitating conditions for patients or which results in, or prolongs, hospitalisation or morbidity.

*Serious adverse reactions:* any unintended response in a donor or recipient that is associated with the collection, testing, processing, storage and distribution of blood and blood components that is fatal, life-threatening, disabling or incapacitating conditions for patients or which results in, or prolongs, hospitalisation or morbidity.

*SHOT:* a voluntary, confidential, anonymous reporting scheme for the notification of serious sequelae of transfusion of blood components or blood products.

*Traceability:* means the ability to trace each individual unit of blood or blood component derived thereof from the donor to its final destination, whether this is a recipient, a manufacturer of medicinal products or disposal, and vice versa

*Transfusion transmitted infection (TTI):* blood-borne infections, e.g. human immunodeficiency virus (HIV), hepatitis C and B, syphilis, etc., that can be transmitted from donor to recipient via a blood transfusion.

*Variant Creutzfeldt–Jakob disease (vCJD):* a fatal disease which may be transmissible through prions transferred during transfusion of blood products from an infected donor. It is believed to be linked to bovine spongiform encephalopathy (BSE) and affects much younger adults than Creutzfeldt–Jakob disease (CJD).

# APPENDIX 1: EQUIPMENT REQUIRED FOR TRANSFUSION[5]

## Cannulae/venous access devices

Any size cannula can be used for transfusing blood products but choice must depend on the size of the vein and the speed at which the product is to be given.

### Recommendations

- The needle diameter for transfusion of blood in adults is 18–19 gauge.
- Needles as small as 23 gauge can be used in paediatric practice.

## Blood giving sets/blood administration sets

- Do not prime the giving set with sodium chloride 0.9 per cent.
- If platelets and red cells are to be transfused give platelets first.
- Do not transfuse platelets through a giving set that has previously been used for red cells or other blood component as this may cause aggregation and retention of platelets in the line.
- It is strongly recommended that platelet-giving sets be used because they are shorter and fewer platelets are left in the line at the end of a transfusion.
- Red cells and FFP *must* be transfused through a sterile giving set designed for this procedure with integral mesh filter 170–200 µm pore size.
- A screen filter should be used for paediatric patients if the transfusion is being administered by syringe. The filter (170 µm pore size) is placed between the product bag and the syringe.
- Giving sets with burettes should not be used for the transfusion of blood components/products.
- All giving sets should be primed with the blood product being transfused.
- If there is another red cell unit to follow of the same ABO group the same giving set can be used.
- If blood of a different ABO group is to follow, the giving set must be changed.
- For patients requiring ongoing transfusion, the giving set should be changed at least every 12 hours.
- On completion of the transfusion take down the giving set. Do not flush the giving set with sodium chloride 0.9 per cent.

- A new giving set should be used if any other type of IV infusion is to continue after the blood transfusion.
- The cannula or central venous line must be flushed with sodium chloride 0.9 per cent prior to commencing any further infusions.

## Infusion pumps

Infusion pumps can be used to achieve optimal flow rate.

- All paediatric red cell and FFP transfusions are administered via a volumetric infusion pump.
- When any pump is used t is important to ensure that the giving set is compatible with the volumetric pump.

## Pressure devices

In large volume transfusions, the use of a pressure device is recommended. The maximum pressure that should be applied to a blood transfusion pack is 300 mmHg (40 kPa).

## Blood warmers

Blood should only be warmed using a specifically designed commercial device with a visible thermometer and audible warning alarm. The manufacturers instructions must be followed.

*Blood must not, under any circumstances, be warmed using any other measures.*

Blood warmers are indicated if:

- the flow rate is >15 mL/kg/hour for children and for exchange transfusion in infants;
- the patient has severe cold agglutinin disease where cold agglutinins may be clinically significant.

Note that for intrauterine transfusions (IUT), blood is drawn into 20-mL syringes using a filter or via a blood component giving set, which already has an incorporated filter, and allowed to reach room temperature for 30 minutes before infusion. A specific blood warmer is not used.

# APPENDIX 2: ADVERSE REACTIONS TO A BLOOD TRANSFUSION[5]

If a transfusion reaction is suspected the transfusion must be stopped immediately and the patient assessed.

## Action for all suspected reactions:

1 Stop the transfusion.
2 Check the patient's identity (verbally and/or ID wristband) to the compatibility tag attached to the unit.
3 Check the 14-digit donor number on the unit label to the 14-digit number on the compatibility tag. They should be identical.
4 Get prompt medical evaluation.

## Recognition of an acute adverse reactions

Acute adverse reactions occur during the transfusion commonly within the first 15 minutes from commencement of *any* unit.

### Types of acute reactions

*Mild (not life threatening):* there can be signs of urticarial rash and/or a temperature rise of less than 1.5°C above baseline.
- To treat the urticarial rash give 10 mg of chlorphenamine as a slow intravenous bolus.
- To treat the temperature give paracetamol.

If the patient does not get any worse or symptoms subside the transfusion can be recommended but at a slower rate of infusion. It is important to monitor the patient more frequently. The reaction must be documented in the patient's medical notes.

*Moderate to severe:* those that compromise the patient's condition and require immediate attention.

1 ABO incompatibility or haemolytic reaction (OHR)
- *Signs and symptoms*: Chills, restlessness/agitation; pain at infusion site, muscle in abdo/chest/lumbar region; oliguria and anuria (reduced or no urine output), haemoglubinuria.
- *Treatment*: Give furosemide if urine output falls/absent. Treat DIC with appropriate blood components.

2 Severe allergic reactions
- *Signs and symptoms*: Bronchospasm, angioedema, abdominal pain, hypotension, oedema – general/local, uticaria rash, facial flushing, dyspnoea.
- *Treatment*: Give chlorphenamine (the dose will depend on the child's age). Commence $O_2$ and Salbutamol nebuliser if necessary. If severe hypotension give adrenaline (epinephrine) (the dose will depend on the child's age).

3 Bacterial contamination
- *Signs and symptoms*: Pyrexia, nausea and vomiting, urticarial rash, facial flushing, tachycardia, hypo/hypertension.
- *Treatment*: Oxygen, fluid support (IV), commence broad-spectrum antibiotics.

4 TRALI (transfusion-related acute lung injury)
- *Signs and symptoms*: Dyspnoea, severe SOB.
- *Treatment*: Give 100 per cent oxygen and ventilate if hypoxic.

5 Fluid overload
- *Signs and symptoms*: Pulmonary oedema, SOB, hypertension, generalised oedema.
- *Treatment*: Give furosemide and reduce fluids.

# Skin health care
## A) Normal skin function and managing common skin conditions

Di Keeton

## LEARNING OUTCOMES

*Upon completion of this chapter, the reader should be able to:*

1 Have an understanding of the normal structure of healthy skin
2 Be able to identify the skin's functions
3 Be able to correctly describe the condition of skin
4 Understand the importance of skin integrity and identify different methods and treatments that enable integrity to be maintained
5 Have a broad understanding of eczema
6 Understand how and when to apply topical treatment and occlusive dressings for children suffering from eczema
7 Understand the need for clear and detailed education of corers to optimise skin care
8 Understanding of some other common skin infections

## CHAPTER OVERVIEW

Skin is multifunctional and is the largest organ of the body, both by area and weight. It plays an important role in both overall physical and psychological health: tough enough to act as a shield against injury and function as a barrier to protect the body from the environment yet supple enough to permit movement and growth. It is a highly developed immune organ, able to detect and fight infection. It is a temperature regulator and a senso-organ able to detect temperature, touch and vibration, and it is a visible sign for social communication. When any of these functions fails there can be serious consequences for the individual.[1,2]

The condition of the skin is affected by both disease and the external environment and is one of the most important windows into a person's health and wellbeing. Many people with a skin disease that won't cause seriously harm, can have their lives ruined by rejection from others because of their changed appearance. The effects of damaged or abnormal looking skin can be as devastating to a child as to an adult. Knowledge of normal skin function and the maintenance of healthy skin are a good basis for understanding skin conditions and complaints and how different treatments can aid healing and improve skin integrity.

The information in this chapter aims to clarify the structure and main functions of healthy skin. To inform nurses how to help keep skin healthy and able to function and offer some guidelines to treatments for skin conditions that commonly affect children.

## KEY WORDS

Structure   Function   Barrier   Integrity
Cleansing   Emollients   Eczema   Topical steroids
Dressings

# SKIN STRUCTURE

The average adult has 2 m² of skin weighing 3.2 kg and has approximately 300 million skin cells. Each square half-inch of skin contains approximately

- 10 hairs
- 15 sebaceous glands
- 100 sweat glands
- 1 metre of blood vessels.

Skin thickness varies. It is thickest on the palms of the hands and soles of the feet and thinnest on the lips and around the eyes. Facial skin is approximately 0.12 mm thick but body skin is 0.6 mm thick.

Skin thickness, condition and sensitivity should be taken into account when you are choosing and applying topical treatments. The young and older people have more sensitive skin because their barrier is less well formed.[1]

Human skin is composed of three layers:

- the epidermis
- the dermis
- the subcutaneous tissue fat layer.

## The epidermis

The epidermis is the almost waterproof outside layer that acts as a barrier (Figure 19.1). It includes the 'stratum corneum' or dead layer made up of cells that are known as corneocytes, which have lost their nucleus. Intercellular lipids bind the corneocytes together. These special oils (cholesterol,

ceramides and free fatty acids) have a natural moisturising factor, which also acts to prevent the evaporation of water. Their function is to produce keratin and melanin. Keratin is the end product of maturation of epidermal cells, whose function is to make the skin waterproof. Melanin or pigment helps to protect the skin form the harmful effects of ultraviolet radiation. If the epidermis is removed, the dermis is completely permeable. This is partly why grazes and burns 'weep'. The epidermis is constantly growing. New skin cells grow from the base of the epidermis and slowly move upwards, losing moisture and flattening out as they rise to form the outer barrier layer, the stratum corneum at the top. In young skin, cells are replaced about every 30 days. This ongoing cycle can take twice as long in older skin but in some skin diseases such as psoriasis and eczema the process is much faster, leading to a breakdown in the natural skin's defences.[1,3]

## The dermis

The bulk of the dermis is made up of connective tissue containing collagen, blood vessels, sebaceous and sweat glands, mast cells, Langerhan cells, nerve cells and hair follicles, providing the physical and nutritional support to the avascular epidermis, which is dependent on a healthy dermis. Sweat and sebum contain substances that are antimicrobial so inhibit the growth of bacteria on the skin surface; sebum maintains the condition and pH of the hair and skin. Fibroblast cells produce collagen, which provides the skin's strength and structure and plays a critical role in wound healing, and elastin, which gives the skin resilience and flexibility (Figure 19.2).

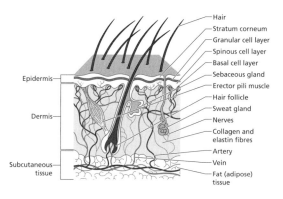

**Figure 19.1** Skin structure.[4]

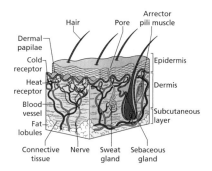

**Figure 19.2** The dermis.

## The subcutaneous adipose tissue layer

This deepest layer acts as an insulator, cushion and shock absorber as well as storing fat as an energy reserve in case extra calories are needed to power the body. It attaches the skin to the underlying tissues and supports the skin. It is missing on parts of the body where the skin is especially thin: the eyelids, nipples genitals and shins. Blood vessels, nerves, lymph vessels and hair follicles also cross through this layer.

## SKIN FUNCTION

### Barrier function

Skin protects us from the outside world and holds us together. In its healthy state it is able to repel water and micro-organisms that can cause us harm while preventing water and electrolyte loss from the internal environment. The natural slight acidity of skin helps to reduce the number of harmful bacteria while protecting the normal bacteria that live on the skin which are essential for healthy skin to function.

### Regulatory function

The skin helps to control and regulate body temperature to protect internal organs. In the cold, blood vessels in the dermis constrict to conserve heat whereas in the heat they dilate to encourage heat loss. Sweating also helps because its evaporation aids skin surface cooling. Excess toxins and salts are also excreted in sweat.

### Sensation

Skin is the largest sensory organ of the body. There are millions of nerve endings that allow the sensation of touch, pressure and temperature as well as the experience of pain and itch. The skin is able to react to and interpret visual or psychological sensations such as the 'goose bump', associated with fear or anxiety, and vasodilatation that occurs when blushing due to embarrassment.

### Immunological function

Immunological cells (Langerhan and mast cells) amass in the dermis and are able to release mediators to defend and protect the body when a foreign body breaches the epidermal skin barrier. This is a positive response to harmful proteins, but in conditions such as atopic eczema and psoriasis it is thought that these responses are triggered unnecessarily, in that the response is against itself, resulting in chronic disease.

### Biochemical reactions

The skin is able to convert 7-dehydrocholesteral into vitamin D, which promotes the natural absorption of calcium and phosphates in the gastrointestinal tract, essential for healthy bone structure.

## DESCRIBING SKIN CONDITIONS

In order to choose appropriate topical treatments, a correct diagnosis is necessary. It is important, therefore, to be able to understand different types of lesions or rashes and to be able to describe their shape, texture, distribution, site, number. Skin conditions are not just a surface rash but can be an indication of underlying disease and, as with any other branch of medicine, diagnosis is reached by taking a full history and physical examination in combination with examining the skin.[18]

| Definitions |
| --- |
| **Skin lesion terminology:** |
| **Abscess or boil** (>1 cm): large collection of pus. |
| **Atrophy:** thinning of tissue, epidermis or dermis of subcutaneous fat. |
| **Blisters:** vesicles and bullae containing clear fluid (serum) – tend to last a few days. |
| **Cyst:** fluctuant papule or nodule lined by epithelium containing fluid, pus or keratin. |
| **Depigmentation:** complete loss of melanin due to loss of melanocytes in the epidermis, as in vitiligo. |
| **Erosion:** result of loss of some or all of the epidermis; may be caused by a blister or trauma and will heal without scarring. |
| **Erythema:** redness due to dilated blood vessels which blanche on pressure. Usually as a result of inflammation or an allergic type reaction. |
| **Exudate:** serum, blood or pus that has accumulated on the surface. |
| **Fissure:** splitting through full thickness of skin due to abnormal keratin, often secondary to eczema or psoriasis. |
| **Hyperkeratotic:** rough uneven surface due to increased formation of keratin; usually seen on palms and soles of feet. |
| **Hyperpigmentation:** increase in melanin |

**Definitions** *continued*

pigmentation. Usually following inflammation in the epidermis, such as in eczema. In coloured skin it may be the first sign of inflammation.

**Hypopigmentation:** partial loss of melanin secondary to inflammation in the epidermis, as in eczema.

**Lichenification:** thickened localised damage of epidermis with increased skin markings due to persistent scratching, as is atopic eczema.

**Macule (<1 cm): Patch (>1 cm):** change in colour only; the surface is always the same as surrounding skin.

**Melanin pigment:** melanin pigment situated deep within dermis, as in malignant melanoma and blue naevus.

**Nodule:** any elevated lesion (>1 cm diameter), palpable between finger and thumb; diameter is equal to thickness.

**Papule:** any solid lesion (>1 cm) raised above the surface or can be felt on palpation.

**Plaque:** any raised lesions (>1 cm) where the diameter is greater than the thickness, i.e. can be felt with the fingertips, such as psoriasis.

**Pruritis:** itchy skin.

**Purpura:** Red, purple or orange due to blood that has leaked out of blood vessels. Purpura does not blanche on pressure and remains the same colour.

**Pustule (<1cm):** pus-filled lesion.

**Scale:** dry/flaky surface.

**Scar:** healed dermal lesion secondary to trauma, surgery, infection or loss of blood supply.

**Telangiectasia:** redness due to individually visible dilated blood vessels.

**Ulcer:** full thickness loss of epidermis and dermis causing surface exudate, crusting or slough and will heal with scar tissue formation.

**Urticaria:** commonly known as **hives** or **nettle rash**, is a disorder in which well circumscribed, itchy wheals erupt over different areas of the body as a result of localised vasodilatation and oedema in the superficial dermis. Allergic urticaria is often associated with type 1 hypersensitivity and can affect any part of the body. It is typically acute in onset following exposure to an allergenic protein. Common allergens in children include dairy, eggs, nuts, fish, aeroallergens, such as cats and pollen, artificial colourings and various medicines.

**Vesicle (<1 cm): Bulla (>1 cm):** fluid-filled lesion/blister.

**Weal:** transient swelling due to dermal oedema as in allergic nettle (urticarial) rash.

# SKIN INTEGRITY

Maintaining skin integrity is an important part of the provision of care and allows the nurse to recognise where potential problems may arise and warns of the need to initiate treatment.

Keeping skin clean is an essential part of ensuring skin integrity. The daily use of topical emollients is a simple and effective way of promoting and maintaining healthy skin and its barrier function. Soap is designed to clean the skin by removing surface dirt but at the same time it also affects the natural pH[6] thus drying the skin, with possible impairment of the natural barrier function. If skin integrity is already compromised by disease or injury, this becomes even more relevant. In the presence of inflammatory dry skin conditions, such as eczema and psoriasis, the external outer skin cells, corneocytes, which contain a natural moisturiser that holds the cells together like the mortar in a brick wall, shrink and separate and the lipid levels decrease, allowing further water loss and evaporation from the epidermis.[2] The dry skin becomes rough and often itchy, and if uncorrected may permit allergens to penetrate the skin and a breakdown of skin integrity (Figure 19.3).

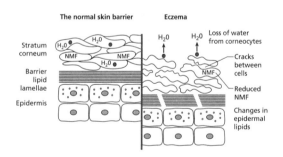

**Figure 19.3** Normal and altered skin barrier in eczematous skin. NMF, natural moisturising factor.

## Causes of skin breakdown

- Prematurity: fragile skin with immature barrier function
- Birth injury
- Skin disease: eczema, nappy rash

- Adhesive use: plasters, dressings
- Burns
- Infections
- Trauma injury
- Surgical wounds
- Pressure: friction, oedema
- Sensitised substances.

## Atopic eczema

Atopy is a syndrome of allergic hyperactivity where there is a genetic tendency and capacity to produce the allergic antibody immunoglobulin (Ig)E and to develop the classic allergic diseases such as eczema, food allergies, asthma or hay fever. Eczema is a chronic inflammatory, dry itchy skin condition. It is a multifactorial disease, affecting up to 15–20 per cent of schoolchildren in the UK (Holm *et al.* 2006). It is not caused by a specific allergy but by a combination of genetic, immunological, environmental and psychological factors.[1] Children with eczema have hypersensitive skin, which may be adversely affected in response to common environmental allergens, such as house dust mite (HDM), animal dander, cigarette smoke, pollens and certain foods. The pattern of reactions is not consistent from one child to the next and may alter as the child ages. The itch is the most distressing and diagnostic symptom. If there is no evidence of pruritis a differential diagnosis should be sought.

Not all atopic children will suffer from all aspects of atopy. There is typically a history of an immediate family member suffering from one or all of these conditions. Eczema is usually the first manifestation of atopic disease and although it may coincide with food allergy, food allergy exacerbates eczema in less than 1 in 10 (BAD 2003). Eczema commonly begins between the ages of 3 and 12 months; asthma at age 3–4 years; and hay fever in the teens. This is known as the 'atopic march'. Allergies can develop hand in hand at any stage, although are not always lifelong.[3,9] In the majority of cases, the eczema will have spontaneously cleared by puberty, and for many it will be significantly less severe by school age.

In infancy, eczema frequently begins on the face and scalp and may or may not spread down the body. The nappy area is characteristically spared. Urea, a natural physiological product derived from the protein metabolism of urine, has a naturally protective action of increasing the capacity of the skin's horny layer to retain moisture. As children grow the eczema tends to localise more to the flexures, but severe cases can affect the whole body.

Although atopic eczema is not thought of as a serious condition, while it is active the constant itching/scratch cycle can be severe enough to result in bleeding excoriations, lichenification and loss of skin integrity. This commonly means restless nights or complete loss of any meaningful sleep for the child and parent, and can have a significant impact of the quality of life for the whole family.[9] Recent studies have suggested that sleep deprivation as a result of severe uncontrolled eczema, can also have a detrimental effect on the child's general growth and impact on everyday activities and psychosocial wellbeing, and may also affect their ability to function properly at school. Following the publication of the National Guidelines in 2007, it is recommended that all children attending secondary care for eczema are monitored for their growth and development. The psychological aspects of having red, rough unpleasant-looking skin can also be devastating (Figure 19.4, page 317). Please see website for illustration of eczema in a 2-year-old.

The mainstay of controlling eczema is optimising emollient therapy, and sometimes this may be all that is needed. The most important intervention in the management of atopic eczema is the time spent listening, explaining its causes, how to avoid irritants and demonstrating topical applications.[20] It is also essential to take a full and detailed family and personal history: although an 'allergy' will not be the cause of eczema, it may be one of a number of possible exacerbating factors that are contributing to the condition and these need to be identified if relief of symptoms is to be achieved. The natural history of eczema is very fluctuant and the cause of sudden 'flare-ups' is often unidentifiable, and parents will frequently request 'allergy testing', hoping to identify an offending product that if removed from the diet will result in an instant cure. This is rarely the case, especially after the first year of life, and there is a genuine risk of dietary insufficiency if dairy or other foods containing essential nutrients are simply removed from the diet without input from a paediatric dietician, especially for the infant. Where there is evidence of a genuine allergy or of specific dietary protein exacerbation, i.e. the sudden onset of

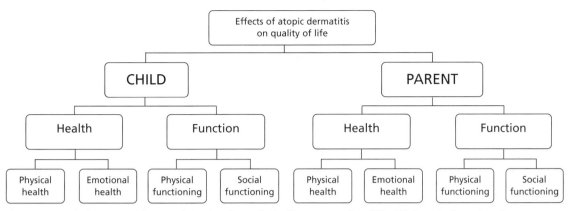

**Figure 19.4** Original conceptual framework for the effects of skin disease on quality of life. This hypothesis was based on a literature review and directed focus
sessions with experts and parents. The constructs addressed by the eight scales of Childhood Atopic Dermatitis Impact Scale are bordered with double lines. (adapted with permission from Daniels[8]).

widespread eczema on weaning from breast milk to formula feeds, and the eczema has not responded to good standard topical treatment, it may indicate the need to switch to a hypoallergenic hydrolysed formula along with optimising topical treatment. Similarly, it is important to identify if there has been an instant reaction with allergic symptoms (urticaria, swelling, severe itch, instant vomiting) as well as an increase in eczematous symptoms the first time a food is introduced into the diet. However, appropriate testing, such as skinprick testing with or without blood tests for allergic antibodies should be undertaken alongside careful assessment, referral to a paediatric allergist and continuing dietician input, which is essential to ensure nutritional input is maintained for healthy growth and development when a child is on any form of exclusion diet to minimise the risk of accidental severe allergic reactions. Approximately 80 per cent of children who are diagnosed with milk and or egg allergy as an infant will have outgrown this by 3–5 years.[10,11] Aeroallergens such as animal dander (especially cats), pollens, HDM, perfumes and detergents can also be very irritant to eczematous skin and for older children are more likely than food stuffs to be the exacerbating factors. All these factors should also be taken into consideration when deciding and advising on treatments. Appropriate reduction of exposure to any identified exacerbating factor, alongside a user-friendly emollient therapy regime, will, in most cases, result in a marked improvement of symptoms

with minimal use of long-term topical steroids. Any product that claims to be a cure for eczema must be treated with scepticism. There is no known cure for the condition, but there are very good tried and tested treatments that can bring long-standing control. Parents often need advice and reassurance about over-the-counter or alternative treatments. Some herbal medicines and ointments, although appearing to work well initially, have been found to contain high levels of steroids.[14]

## MAINTAINING SKIN INTEGRITY

Emollients (or moisturisers), come in many forms and have differing actions. In order to aid in selecting the most suitable product, it is very important to make a full assessment of the skin and be aware of previous treatments tried and any allergies to creams, dressings or medications.[7]

Emollients are the mainstay of controlling eczema and are essential for maintaining skin integrity, no matter which skin disorder is being treated. Table 19.1 (page 318) shows the different types of emollient available and some guidance of best usage is shown in Figure 19.5, page 319.

Emollients help to restore the natural defence barrier by forming an occlusive layer to prevent further transepidermal water loss. (Figure 19.6, page 320) However, it must be remembered that the effects of any emollient therapy is only short lived and to achieve therapeutic results, frequent applications are necessary, at least three or four times.

**Table 19.1** Emollients

| Types of emollients | Uses | Advantages/disadvantages |
|---|---|---|
| **Creams** | | |
| Water-in-oil emulsion (cold creams) | User friendly, especially on face, easy to apply | Many contain lanolin as oil, can cause contact dermatitis |
| Oil-in-water emulsion (milky creams) | User friendly, dries quickly, e.g. aqueous cream | Makes skin drier as high water content evaporates. Contains preservatives (parabens) which can result in allergic dermatitis |
| | | Not generally recommended for dry skin conditions |
| **Lotions** | | |
| Liquid insoluble powder in water, alcohol or propylene gel | Good for wet/weeping rashes Light and cooling Less messy on hair, e.g. potassium permanganate | Cooling effect but liquid evaporates leaving inert powder on skin (calamine), therefore very drying Alcohol base may sting Used as astringent to coagulate protein and dry exudate |
| **Gels** | | |
| Transparent semisolid emulsions in water | Semisolid cold, jelly like on warming, e.g. Doublebase | Good alternative to lotion especially on hairy skin Soothing, antipruritic and cooling |
| **Ointments** | | |
| Contain little or no water Organic hydrocarbons, alcohols and acids White ointments | Greasy and form an impermeable layer over the skin preventing water evaporation, e.g. emulsifying ointment; Epaderm, e.g. Cetraben, Dibrobase, Oilatum, Balnuem Plus | More effective than creams for dry skin as penetrate dry skin well. Soothing and cooling. Greasiness not always user friendly Least likely to cause irritation |
| | | Often the preferred treatment for eczema: the greasier the better if tolerated User friendly: mixture of soft and liquid soft paraffin white creams |
| **Pastes** | | |
| Mixture of powder in an ointment | Thick, messy, stay where you put them Used under occlusive dressings, e.g. Icthopaste zinc oxide/tar bandages Zipzoc stockings Lasser's paste Dithronol | Can stain clothing and be unsightly. Need protective gloves, spatulas to apply Soothes severe chronic lichenified and excoriated eczema. Please see website for illustration of excoriated eczema For psoriasis: use with care as can damage healthy skin |

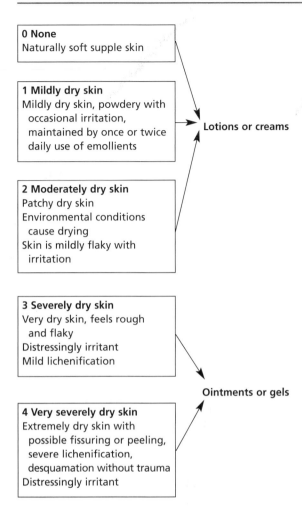

**0 None**
Naturally soft supple skin

**1 Mildly dry skin**
Mildly dry skin, powdery with
occasional irritation,
maintained by once or twice
daily use of emollients

→ **Lotions or creams**

**2 Moderately dry skin**
Patchy dry skin
Environmental conditions
cause drying
Skin is mildly flaky with
irritation

**3 Severely dry skin**
Very dry skin, feels rough
and flaky
Distressingly irritant
Mild lichenification

**Ointments or gels**

**4 Very severely dry skin**
Extremely dry skin with
possible fissuring or peeling,
severe lichenification,
desquamation without trauma
Distressingly irritant

**Figure 19.5** Plymouth hydration flow chart (reproduced with permission from Daniels[8]).

Emollients help to protect against irritants and allergens that can cause or exacerbate skin conditions. The effects of emollient therapy are to soothe, soften and remove scale from the skin, aiding medicinal treatment application and penetration. However, it must be remembered that the effects of emollient therapy is only short lived and, to achieve therapeutic results, frequent applications are necessary, preferably at least three or four times a day. The British Association of Dermatologists and the National Institute of Health and Clinical Excellence (NICE)[9] recommend prescribing minimum quantities of 250 g for toddlers and 500 g for older children a week, for the treatment of widespread chronic skin conditions. Emollients should always be applied by stroking onto the skin in a downward motion, (in the direction of hair growth) and allowed to soak into the skin. This will reduce the chance of folliculitis, and maximise the cooling and soothing effects with minimum irritation. When possible, emollients should be applied approximately 30 minutes after topical steroid therapy, allowing maximum benefit from topical medicinal treatment; following this bandages or garments may be worn. Massaging or rubbing emollients into damaged skin should be avoided as this creates heat, increases irritation, itch and may exacerbate the skin condition. Good communication skills on the part of the practitioner greatly affects the outcome of the consultation[19] and the effectiveness of topical treatments. It must be remembered that the only emollient that works is the one that the patient and carer find user friendly so there must be equal consideration of patient's as well as prescriber choice if compliance with effective treatment is to be achieved. You cannot 'overdose' the skin with emollients; it will only absorb as much as it needs.

Damaged skin is more prone to become infected, and keeping the skin clean is a high priority for good skin management as well as general health. Traditionally, the skin is cleansed to remove dirt, debris, odour and other contaminants but also to remove dry, flaky skin and the build up of emollients. Many over-the-counter soaps or cleansers contain detergent (any products that lather and make bubbles) that can be very drying and irritating and exacerbate existing skin conditions. They also leave an alkaline residue which can strip the skin of natural oils, thus exacerbating dry skin conditions. Using a soap substitute specifically designed to cleanse the skin without irritation will help to maintain normal pH, smooth, soothe and rehydrate the skin, which will enhance absorption of topical treatments.[12,13] Several of these products also have an antimicrobial property which helps protect against staphylococcal infection, although occasionally the added antiseptics may cause irritation and sensitisation resulting in allergic dermatitis.

Some products may be used as both topical emollients and as a soap. This can be very useful, as it reduces the number of products needed to be prescribed and aids compliance.

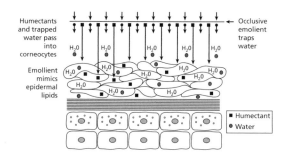

**Figure 19.6** The effects of good emollient therapy repairing the skin's barrier function.

## TOPICAL STEROID USE IN ECZEMA

If used correctly, topical steroid therapy is an effective and safe treatment for eczema flares by calming the inflammation and settling the redness and itching. They are most effective if applied to clean skin, after the evening bath is ideal, prior to and in addition to the regular emollient therapy for short periods (10–14 days). As the steroid molecule persists in the stratum corneum and is slowly absorbed, it is likely that a single application at night will work as well as twice daily and reduce the risk of side-effects. They are not a substitute for emollient therapy. Skin thinning from topical steroids only arises when too strong a steroid has been used for too long a period or in a delicate area where the skin is already thin.[9] Repeated applications of potent topical steroids can also result in a diminished effect (tachyphylaxis), sometimes after only a week of use. Recovery of response will return within a week, but to prevent this happening it is recommended that more potent steroids should be used in 5-day bursts with moisturisers only for the intervening 2 days.[2]

Topical steroids are divided into four main groups according to their potency (Table 19.2, page 321).

Weak to moderate potency steroids are usually sufficient to control childhood eczema and are generally safe when simple principles are followed using the mildest strength necessary to gain the desired effect. Most topical steroids come as a cream or ointment and, as with emollients, it is usually best to go for an ointment, as the greasiness helps it stay where you want it and also aids its absorption. They contain fewer additives and so are less likely to irritate, although they may sting initially if the eczema is very active.

### How much to use

As 15 g of ointment is sufficient to cover the adult body surface, you will therefore need 100 g a week. A useful guide is the 'finger-tip unit' measure. The amount of ointment/cream squeezed onto the index finger from tip to the distal joint is sufficient to cover the area of both palms (Table 19.3, page 321).

## TOPICAL IMMUNE MODULATORS

Use topical immune modulators in children 2 years of age and above.

### 0.3 per cent and 0.1 per cent tacrolimus (Protopic) ointment and 1 per cent primecrolimus (Elidel) ointment

This is an alternative second-line treatment for atopic eczema that has not responded to topical steroids or when topical steroid use is over and above the recommended safe levels to keep the eczema under control. Protopic is as effective as a moderate/potent steroid and Elidel is equivalent to 1 per cent hydrocortisone.

As a topical immune suppressor it works by blocking the molecular mechanisms of inflammation in the skin, inhibiting T-cell activation and inflammatory mediators. They have no effect on collagen synthesis and there is no skin thinning or bruising from long-term use; however, because they may suppress the skin's natural immune defence system, it is recommended that stringent care is taken with sun exposure, and some children may have a minimally increased risk of infections such as *Molluscum contagiosum*. If this occurs, treatment should be halted.

Treatment should be intermittent and not continuous. Treatment should be started twice a

**Table 19.2** Topical steroids

| Group | Strength | Example | Use |
| --- | --- | --- | --- |
| Weak | Hydrocortisone | 1% Hydrocortisone | Face and body |
| Moderate potency | 2.5 × stronger | Eumovate | Body, limited face |
| Potent | 10 × stronger | Elocon/Betnovate | Body only |
| Very potent | 50 × stronger | Dermovate | Not recommended |

**Table 19.3** Finger tip table*

| Age | Number of adult finger-tip units | | | | |
| --- | --- | --- | --- | --- | --- |
| | Face + neck | Arm+ hand | leg+ foot | Trunk (front) | (Back) + buttocks |
| 3-6 months | 1 | 1 | 1.5 | 1 | 1.5 |
| 1–2 years | 1.5 | 1.5 | 2 | 2 | 3 |
| 3–5 years | 1.5 | 2 | 3 | 3 | 3.5 |
| 6–10 years | 2 | 2.5 | 4.5 | 3.5 | 5 |

*Data from Long et al.[15]

day for up to 3 weeks. Afterwards the frequency of application should be reduced to once a day until clear. The greasy ointment should be applied as a thin layer and can be used on any part of the body, including face, neck and flexure areas, but not on mucous membranes. Emollients should not be applied to the same area for about 2 hours after applying Protopic ointment, and it is not recommended for use under occlusion. Some itching and burning may be complained of when first applied; this lasts approximately 15–20 minutes and usually disappears after the first two or three applications.

If no signs of improvement are seen after 2 weeks of treatment, further treatment options should be considered. Protopic can be used for short-term and intermittent long-term treatment. At the first signs of recurrence (flares) of the disease symptoms, treatment should be reinitiated.[3,17]

## OCCLUSIVE DRESSINGS

There are occasions when it may be beneficial to apply occlusive dressings to enhance topical treatments. These come in a variety of forms. The simplest are tubular bandages (Comfifast or Tubifast), which come in five colour-coded sizes of

age-specific garments. They are made of a light stretchy breathable fabric, allowing complete freedom of movement. They are patient specific and can be washed and reused a number of times. Their use is to aid the effectiveness of topical treatments, which can be enhanced up to 10-fold because a larger quantity of emollient can be applied to the skin and allowed to soak in over a number of hours rather than evaporate in the air or be rubbed off on to clothing or bedding. The worst damage to the skin often happens at night when the child often scratches continuously, resulting in waking to a sheet covered in skin and blood and sore excoriated skin. Occlusive dressings often, therefore, will be prescribed to be worn after bathing, at night time. This extra dosing of emollients helps to sooth the skin and reduces the itch while the wrap forms an extra protective layer between scratching fingers and the skin, and thus can aid sleep. Many babies and children will wear them by choice during the day when the eczema is particularly troublesome. As the skin is soothed and rested from being scratched, it begins to heal and so the need for topical steroids can be reduced. The use of wet wrapping with one wet layer covered by a second dry layer when the skin is extremely dry and flaky is rarely used now, as it not thought to be any more effective than applying a single layer with an appropriate quantity of emollient, which is much more comfortable for the child.

It should be remembered that topical steroids should be used with great caution beneath occlusive dressings as their potency may also be increased. As a general rule it is recommended that only occasional use of 1 per cent hydrocortisone plus emollients should be used under wraps in the community setting. They are also not recommended if the skin is open and weeping, as there is a risk of sticking to the skin once the emollient has been absorbed, and pain and damage may occur when peeling them off.

## Impregnated occlusive bandages

These impregnated, mainly tar-based products are very effective for aiding healing of eczematous skin that has become severely lichenified and when there is significant excoriations of the arms and legs; they greatly enhance the effects of topical treatments when simple tubular bandages have been insufficient.

*Ichthopaste bandages* are an open-weave cotton bandage impregnated with a mixture of zinc oxide paste and Ichthammol and should be applied over a generous application of the child's regular emollient. They are messy and a bit smelly to apply but this is not noticeable once application is complete. Their advantage is that they may be left in place for 3–5 days, allowing skin softening and healing to take place while being protected from the environment and scratching. During this time the cotton weave constricts as it dries so it is important to apply them in loose folds to avoid risk of constriction and ensure comfort. A tubular bandage (if being applied to a single limb) or tubular garment is worn on top to protect clothing from the paste and to keep the bandages in place. This treatment may be repeated as and when necessary but it is sensible to bathe between applications.

*Zipzoc stockings* are impregnated with a mixture of zinc oxide, white and yellow soft paraffin and are more user friendly and suitable for the slightly older child as they come in packs of 10 for adult-sized lower legs but can be cut to the length desired for use on arms or legs. They are simply pulled on over the prescribed topical treatment and covered with the tubular garments and worn overnight. Each stocking can be used two or three times before discarding. Again this treatment can be used as often as needed.

## INFECTED ECZEMA

If eczematous skin is cracked and open, suddenly becomes more erythematous and itchy, develops pustules or yellow crusting, it may have become infected – commonly with *Staphylococcus aureus*. This is best treated with systemic antibiotics for 10–14 days, rather than topical antibiotics or a steroid–antibiotic mix as they tend to be less effective and may cause allergic contact dermatitis and resistance with resulting recurrent infections.[3] A temporary increase in steroid strength to treat the eczema flare and using an antimicrobial wash may help to reduce infection recurrence. The use of wet or dry wraps should be avoided while the skin is crusty as, once the topical treatment has dried, they can stick to the crusts and result in bleeding and pain on removal.

*Eczema herpticum:* This is an infection caused by the cold sore virus, typically present round the mouth with yellow crusting. The child is often more unwell than you would expect with eczema. The treatment of choice is to give oral Aciclovir while increasing topical eczema treatment. Widespread, more aggressive cases may require hospital admission and intravenous (IV) therapy. If skin around eyes is affected, an ophthalmological opinion should also be sought.

*Molluscum contagiosum:* This is a pox virus infection that is quite common in children, particularly in children suffering from eczema or who have significant immune deficiency. It presents as small white (occasionally pink), 1–5 mm umbilicated papules. The papules can become red and inflamed, and can appear anywhere on the body but most commonly in small groups and less commonly on the face. They do not itch and are harmless and self-limiting and do not leave any scarring. Parents are often very concerned by them as they tend to fade and then recur somewhere else and can take up to 18–24 months to completely resolve. Popping in the bath can speed up resolution. Once resolved, they do not recur. Treatment is only recommended in very severe, extensive cases, usually if the child has immune deficiency.

*Impetigo:* This is a very infectious superficial infection of the epidermis caused by *Staphylococcus aureus*, a group A beta-haemolytic streptococcus, or a mixture of both. Typically it starts as vesicles, rapidly breaking down to honey-coloured crusts.

Because it is a superficial infection it often responds well to topical antibiotics without the need of systemic treatment. The crusts can be softened with arachis or olive oil and Fucidin or Bactroban applied four times a day for 3–4 days. In more severe widespread cases or if the child also has eczema, systemic antibiotics (Flucoxacillin or erythromycin) are the treatment of choice. Children should be excluded from school until clear.[3]

 Go to the website to find the PowerPoint presentation for this chapter and MCQs to test your knowledge. **www.hodderplus.com/childnursingskills**

## REFERENCES

1   British Association of Dermatologists (BAD) 2008.

2   Cork MJ (1997) The importance of skin barrier function. *Journal of Dermatology Treatment* **8**: S7–S13.

3   Ashton R, Leppard B (2006) *Differential diagnosis in dermatology*, 3rd edition. Oxford: Radcliffe publishing.

4   Hughes E (2001) *Skin, its structure and related pathology: dermatology nursing, a practical guide.* Edinburgh, Churchill Livingstone.

5   Pringle F, Penzer R (2002) Normal skin: its function and care. In: Penzer R (ed.*) Nursing care of the skin.* London: Butterworth-Heinemann.

6   Warner RR, Boissy YL (1999). Effects of moisturising lipids on the outer stratum corneum of humans.

7   Flanagan M (1966) A practical framework for wound assessment. 1. Physiological. *British Journal of Nursing* **5**: 1391–1397.

8   Daniels J (2002) Skin care: practical aspects. *Nurse2Nurse* **2**: 26–28.

9   National Institute for Health and Clinical Excellence (2007) *Atopic eczema in children.* Guideline 57. London: NICE.

10  Lawson V, Lewis-Jones MS, Finlay AY, *et al.* (1998) The family impact of childhood atopic dermatitis: The dermatitis family impact questionnaire. *British Journal of Dermatology* **138**: 107–113.

11  Buttriss J (2002) *Adverse reactions to food: report of the British Nutrition Foundation Task Force.* Oxford: British Nutrition Foundation, pp. 2–10.

12  Cuncliffe B (2001) Diseases of the skin and their treatment (3) Eczema. *Pharmaceutical Journal* **267**: 855–856.

13  Buchannan P, Courtney M (2007) Topical treatments for managing patients with eczema. *Nursing Standard* **21**: 45–50.

14  Ramsay HM, W Goddard, S Gill, and C Moss (2003) Herbal creams used for atopic eczema in Birmingham, UK illegally contain potent corticosteroids. *Archives of Disease in Childhood* **88**: 1056–1057.

15  Long CC, Mills CM, Finlay AY (1998) A practical guide to topical therapy in children. *British Journal of Dermatology* **138**: 293–6.

16  Chamlin LS, Cella D, Frieden IJ, *et al.* (2005) Development of the childhood atopic dermatitis impact scale: initial validation of a quality-of-life measure for young children with atopic dermatitis and their families. *Journal of Investigative Dermatology* **125**: 1106–1111.

17  National Institute for Clinical Excellence (2004) *Tacrolimus and pimecrolimus for atopic eczema.* Technology appraisal; no. 82. London: NICE.

18  Lawton S (2004) Atopic eczema, nurse-led care. 1. Making the most of the consultation. *Journal of Family Health Care* **14**: 6.

19  Maquire P, Pitceathly C (2002) Key communication skills and how to acquire them. *British Medical Journal* **235**: 679–700.

20  Cork MJ, Britton J, Butler L, *et al.* (2003). Comparison of parent knowledge, therapy utilization and severity of atopic eczema before and after explanation and demonstration of topical therapies by a specialist dermatology nurse. *British Journal of Dermatologists* **149**: 582–589.

## USEFUL WEBSITES

National Eczema Society: www.eczema.org
British Dermatological Society leaflets: www.bad.org.uk
British Dermatological Nursing Group: www.bdng.org.uk

# Skin health care
## B) Managing pressure ulcer risk in healtchare settings

Jane Willock

## LEARNING OUTCOMES

*Upon completion of this chapter, the reader should be able to accomplish the following:*
1 List the causes of pressure ulcers
2 Describe pressure ulcers according to the European pressure ulcer Advisory Panel classification
3 Understand what a pressure ulcer risk assessment scale is used for
4 Discuss how a pressure ulcer risk assessment scale can be used in clinical practice

## CHAPTER OVERVIEW

Pressure ulcers are skin and tissue lesions caused by pressure, friction and/ or shear forces. They are very painful, can leave scars, may take a considerable time to heal, and can put patients at risk of potentially life threatening infection. The depth and extent of a pressure ulcer can be described using grading scales. Pressure ulcer risk assessment scales are designed to identify which patients are at risk of developing pressure ulcers so that preventative action can be taken.

## THE DEVELOPMENT OF PRESSURE ULCERS

A pressure ulcer is an area of damaged tissue, which has been caused by pressure, shearing forces or friction, or a combination of these factors.[1]

There are thought to be three main forms of mechanical force acting on body tissues that can cause pressure ulcers: compression, shear and friction.

*Compression* is a force exerted perpendicularly over a given area, when underlying tissues are directly compressed, and greater pressures appear to result in greater damage. The duration of pressure is as important as the intensity, and short periods of high pressure such as lying on a hard surface, or medical equipment pressing on the skin can be as damaging as prolonged periods of lower pressure. Pressure on the skin is transmitted through all internal tissues[2] and can lead to an area of deep ischaemia.

*Shear* is the force exerted parallel or at an angle to skin surface causing layers of tissues to move laterally producing severe distortion. This happens especially when patients slide down the bed or are pulled up the bed and the skin moves against the bed sheets. The shearing forces stretch and squeeze the very small vessels leading to capillary, venule and lymphatic disruption, resulting in an area of skin with inadequate blood supply, tissue ischaemia and necrosis.

*Friction* tends to occur when the skin has been allowed to rub against another surface, for example when elbows or heels rub against bed clothes, the epidermis is stripped away to create blisters or shallow ulcers; this is usually superficial but very painful.

In many cases, tissue impairment arising from shear force or friction could be avoided with correct patient-handling techniques, positioning and equipment.[2] Skin tension has a similar effect to shear and can be seen when very sticky adhesive tape is used. When the tape is removed, it pulls on the skin separating the layers and causing blistering.[3]

**Table 19.4** European Pressure Ulcer Advisory Panel classification of pressure ulcers*

| Grade | Short description | Definition |
|---|---|---|
| Grade 1 | Non-blanchable erythema of intact skin | Discolouration of the skin, warmth, oedema, induration or hardness may also be used as indicators, particularly on individuals with darker skin |
| Grade 2 | Abrasion or blister | Partial thickness skin loss involving epidermis, dermis, or both. The ulcer is superficial and presents clinically as an abrasion or blister |
| Grade 3 | Superficial ulcer | Full thickness skin loss involving damage to or necrosis of subcutaneous tissue that may extend down to, but not through, underlying fascia |
| Grade 4 | Deep ulcer | Extensive destruction, tissue necrosis, or damage to muscle, bone, or supporting structures with or without full thickness skin loss |

*Adapted from EPUAP.[16]

## The prevalence of pressure ulcers in children

The prevalence of pressure ulcers in hospitalised children has been estimated between 0.47 per cent and 13.1 per cent.[4–9] and up to 27 per cent in paediatric intensive care units.[10–12] However, there are very few research publications describing the characteristics of children with pressure ulcers.[5,13,14,15]

## Classification of pressure ulcers

The severity of pressure ulcers is classified using grading scales. The European Pressure Ulcer Advisory Panel (EPUAP) classification[16] (Table 19.4) has been developed by a panel of experts and is widely used in Europe; however, evidence for the scale's development and validation appears to be based mainly on adult data.

## Pressure ulcer risk assessment scales

Pressure ulcer risk assessment scales are used to identify patient risk, level of risk and type of risk.

Good standards of care help to identify and prevent pressure ulcers, but patients may not be monitored closely if they are not considered to be in an 'at-risk' category – especially if circumstances change quickly; therefore, patients need to be reassessed at frequent intervals especially if their condition changes.[2]

While more than 200 published pressure ulcer risk factors have been cited,[17] not all characteristics are relevant to all patient groups, and it would be impossible and impractical to incorporate more than a few risk factors into an assessment scale.

Adult pressure ulcer risk assessment scales were initially developed based on patient observation[18,19] and later on literature reviews,[20] which identified factors believed to predispose patients to pressure ulcer development.

Ten published paediatric risk assessment scales have been identified, of which six are modifications of adult risk assessment scales.[21–26] Two risk assessments are based on patient observation,[27,28] one on a review of relevant literature,[29] and one on a multicentre survey, but this was not predictive.[4,30] No published studies were identified using statistical methods to develop a predictive pressure ulcer risk assessment scale directly from patient data.

## The Glamorgan Paediatric Pressure Ulcer Risk Assessment Scale (Glamorgan Scale)

The Glamorgan Scale appears to be the only published paediatric pressure ulcer risk assessment scale that has been developed using statistical analysis of patient data.

Detailed data of patient characteristics were collected on 336 paediatric inpatients (61 had pressure ulcers). The data were analysed using chi square and regression analysis to give a list of patient characteristics significantly associated (P < 0.01) with pressure ulcer presence. This list of characteristics was used as a guide in the development of the Glamorgan scale. Initial validity tests (sensitivity, specificity area under the receiver operating characteristics curve) indicate that the Glamorgan scale has a high sensitivity, specificity and predictive validity. It also appears to predict pressure ulcer risk more accurately than the Braden Q scale.[31]

---

 Go to the website to find the PowerPoint presentation for this chapter and MCQs to test your knowledge. **www.hodderplus.com/childnursingskills**

---

## REFERENCES

1 Dealey C (1991) The size of the pressure-sore problem in a teaching hospital. *Journal of Advanced Nursing* 16: 663–670.
2 Gould D (2001) Pressure ulcer risk assessment. *Primary Health Care* 11(5): 43–49.
3 Davis P (1998) The pressure is on: preventing pressure sores. *Journal of Orthopaedic Nursing* 2(3): 170–176.
4 Waterlow J (1997) Pressure sore risk assessment in children. *Paediatric Nursing* 9(6): 21–24.
5 Willock J, Hughes J, Tickle S, *et al.* (2000) Pressure sores in children – the acute hospital perspective. *Journal of Tissue Viability* 10(2): 59–62.
6 Baldwin KM (2002) Incidence and prevalence of pressure ulcers in children. *Advances in Skin and Wound Care* 15(3): 121–124.
7 Groeneveld A, Anderson M, Allen M, *et al.* (2004) The prevalence of pressure ulcers in a tertiary care pediatric and adult hospital. *Journal of Wound, Ostomy, and Continence Nursing* 31(3): 108–122.
8 McLane KM, Bookout K, McCord S, *et al.* (2004) The 2003 national pediatric pressure ulcer and skin breakdown prevalence survey: a multisite study. *Journal of Wound, Ostomy, and Continence Nursing* 31(4): 168–178.
9 Dixon M, Ratcliff C (2005) Pediatric pressure ulcer prevalence – one hospital's experience. *Ostomy/Wound Management* 51(6): 44–50.
10 Zollo MB, Gostisha ML, Berens RJ, *et al.* (1996) Altered skin integrity in children admitted to a pediatric intensive care unit. *Journal of Nursing Care Quality* 11(2): 62–67.
11 Curley MAQ, Thompson JE, Arnold JH (2000) The effects of early and repeated prone positioning in pediatric patients with acute lung injury. *Chest* 118(1): 156–163.
12 Curley MAQ, Razmus IS, Roberts KE, Wypij D (2003) Predicting pressure ulcer risk in pediatric patients-the Braden Q scale. *Nursing Research* 52(1): 22–31.

13 McCord S, McElvain V, Sachdeva R, *et al.* (2004) Risk factors associated with pressure ulcers in the pediatric intensive care unit. *Journal of Wound, Ostomy, and Continence Nursing* 31(4): 179–183.
14 Willock J, Harris C, Harrison J, Poole C (2005) Identifying the characteristics of children with pressure ulcers: results of a multi-centre survey. *Nursing Times* 101(11): 40–43.
15 Noonan C, Quigley S, Curley MAQ (2006) Skin integrity in hospitalized infants and children. A prevalence survey, *Journal of Pediatric Nursing* 21: 445–453.
16 EPUAP (2005) European Pressure Ulcer Advisory Panel, EPUAP Statement, Pressure Ulcer Classification: Differentiation Between Pressure Ulcers and Moisture Lesions
17 Salzberg CA, Byrne DW, Kabir R, *et al.* (1999) Predicting pressure ulcers during initial hospitalization for acute spinal cord injury. *Wounds: A Compendium of Clinical Research and Practice* 11(2): 45–57.
18 Norton D, Mclaren R, Exton-Smith A (1962) *An investigation of geriatric nursing problems in hospital.* Edinburgh: Churchill Livingstone.
19 Waterlow J (1985) Pressure sores: a risk assessment card. *Nursing Times* 81(48), 49–55.
20 Braden B, Bergstrom N (1987) A conceptual schema for the study of the etiology of pressure sores. *Rehabilitation Nursing* 12(1): 8–12.
21 Quigley SM, Curley MAQ (1996) Skin integrity in the pediatric population: Preventing and managing pressure ulcers. *Journal of the Society of Pediatric Nurses* 1(1): 7–18.
22 Garvin G (1997) Wound and skin care for the PICU. *Critical Care Nursing Quarterly* 20(1): 62–71.
23 Huffines B, Logsdon MC (1997) The neonatal skin risk assessment scale for predicting skin breakdown in neonates. *Issues in Comprehensive Pediatric Nursing* 20(2): 103–114.
24 Pickersgill J (1997) Taking the pressure off.

*Paediatric Nursing* 9(8): 25–27.

25  Samaniego IA (2003) A sore spot in pediatrics: risk factors for pressure ulcers. *Pediatric Nursing* **29**(4): 278–282.

26  Suddaby EC, Barnett S, Facteau L (2005) Practice applications of research. Skin breakdown in acute care pediatrics. *Pediatric Nursing* **31**(2): 132–138, 148.

27  Bedi A (1993) A tool to fill the gap: developing a wound risk assessment chart for children. *Professional Nurse* **9**(2): 112–120.

28  Olding L, Patterson J (1998) Growing concern. *Nursing Times* **94**(38): 74–79.

29  Cockett A (1998) Paediatric pressure sore risk assessment. *Journal of Tissue Viability* **8**(1): 30.

30  Waterlow J (1998) Pressure sores in children: risk assessment. *Paediatric Nursing* **10**(4): 22–23.

31  Willock J, Baharestani MM, Anthony D (2007) The development of the Glamorgan paediatric pressure ulcer risk assessment scale. *Journal of Children's and Young People's Nursing* **1**(5): 211–218.

## FURTHER READING

Anthony D (1996) Issues in research. Receiver operating characteristic analysis: an overview, *Nurse Researcher* **4**(2): 75–88.

Anthony D, Reynolds T, Russell L (2003) A regression analysis of the Waterlow score in pressure ulcer risk assessment. *Clinical Rehabilitation* **17**(2): 216–223.

Baharestani MM, Ratliff C, and the National Pressure Ulcer Advisory Panel (2007) Pressure ulcers in neonates & children: An NPUAP White Paper. *Advances in Skin and Wound Care* **20**(4): 208–220.

Deeks J (1996) Pressure sore prevention: using and evaluating risk assessment tools. *British Journal of Nursing* **5**: 313–320.

DeFloor T, Schoonhoven L, Katrien V, *et al.* (2006) Reliability of the European Pressure Ulcer Advisory Panel classification system. *Journal of Advanced Nursing* **54**(2): 189–198.

EHCB NHS Centre for Reviews and Dissemination (1995) The prevention and treatment of pressure sores. *Effective Health Care Bulletin* **2**(1): 1–16.

Flanagan M (1995) Who is at risk of a pressure sore? A practical review of risk assessment systems, *Professional Nurse* **10**(5): 305–308. http://www.epuap.org/ review6_3/page6.html (accessed 26 June 2009).

NPUAP (2003) National Pressure Ulcer Advisory Panel Staging Report. www.npuap.org/positn6.html (accessed 8 December 2006).

Royal College of Nursing (2001) *Pressure ulcer risk assessment and prevention.* Clinical Practice Guidelines. London: RCN.

Willock J, Baharestani M, Anthony D (2007) A risk assessment scale for pressure ulcers in children. *Nursing Times* **103**(14): 32–33.

## CHAPTER 20

# The management of the child with an allergy

## Rosie King

---

### LEARNING OUTCOMES

*Upon completion of this chapter, the reader should be able to accomplish the following:*

1 Define allergy

2 Describe the basic immunology of allergic disease

3 Define its spectrum of problems: the atopic march

4 Define food allergy and identify IgE-mediated food allergy

5 Describe how food allergy is diagnosed, with specific reference to the role and responsibilities of the nurse, including taking an allergy history and allergy testing: skin prick testing; blood sample for specific IgE; food challenge

6 Explore teaching a family about food allergy: avoidance of the allergen; rescue medicines; food allergy in schools; how to treat an allergic reaction; the use of an adrenaline (epinephrine) auto-injector

---

### KEY WORDS

Allergy    Atopy    Atopic march    Food allergy
Allergy history    Allergy tests    Allergic reaction
Anaphylaxis    Rescue medicine

---

## CHAPTER OVERVIEW

Allergy is a major health concern in the developed world. The prevalence of allergic disease has risen substantially in recent years.[1] Atopy includes four allergic diseases: eczema, food allergy, asthma and rhinitis (hay fever).

This chapter will describe food allergy, its role in the other allergic diseases and how the multidisciplinary team provides a care pathway for a family with a child with food allergy.

Children with food allergy and their families need to be aware of their risk of dietary and environmental exposure and how to recognise and manage potentially life-threatening allergic reactions (anaphylaxis).[2] Food allergy is a far-reaching diagnosis and must be confirmed by appropriately trained health professionals. Many people think that they have an allergy when in reality they do not.[3] Un-diagnosing food allergy is just as important. Once the diagnosis is made, family, friends and schools need to be taught how to control the outside factors, and also to recognise the symptoms and manage the disease. Training is initially done in the allergy clinic but then devolves to school nurses as well as other nurses working in the community, such as health visitors and paediatric community nursing teams.

# INTRODUCTION: WHAT IS ALLERGY?

Allergy is the inappropriate response of the body's immune system to normally harmless substances;[4] these substances are known as *allergens*. They can be typically found in the air, foods, insect stings, drugs and latex rubber. Airborne allergens (aeroallergens) include house dust mite, cat dander, and tree and grass pollens; egg, milk, peanuts and tree nuts are common food allergens. An ever-increasing number of children are allergic to foods: currently about 1 in 50 preschool children in the UK.[1]

# IMMUNOLOGY OF ALLERGIC DISEASE

Immunoglobulin E (IgE) is the class of antibody that causes the symptoms of allergy. It is the antibody formed to combat parasites such as intestinal worms. IgE can also be formed against specific allergens and can prime the immune system to produce an allergic reaction on exposure. IgE is specific to the allergen to which it was raised. For instance egg-specific IgE will recognise and bind to egg protein but not to other substances. Another good example is IgE to birch pollen, which can also bind to fruit proteins found in apples and peaches.[5] Children with birch pollen (spring-time) hay fever may develop a tingling sensation in the mouth when they eat apples, a condition called oral allergy syndrome. People who make specific IgE to allergens in their environment are known as atopic.[6]

IgE is made by antibody-producing B cells in lymph nodes. The IgE coats mast cells in peripheral tissues such as the skin, nose and lung. When these mast cells come into contact with allergen, specific IgE on their surface binds to the allergen causing the mast cell to activate. Activated mast cells rapidly release inflammatory chemicals such as histamine by a process called degranulation.[6]

These chemicals will cause the signs and symptoms of allergy. Depending upon the tissue in which they are released, these include urticarial rashes (hives) or angio-oedema (swelling) in the skin, breathing problems, shortness of breath, wheezing in the lung and swelling of the throat, lips and tongue. If this swelling is widespread throughout the body it can lead to problems with circulation (drop in blood pressure). Severe symptoms involving the respiratory tract or circulation are termed anaphylaxis. This is an extreme and severe allergic reaction; the whole body is affected, often within minutes of exposure to the allergen but sometimes after hours. It may be fatal if left untreated.[7]

Other parts of the immune system can be involved in allergic disease. This is called non-IgE-mediated allergy (also known as intolerance). It involves T lymphocytes that, like IgE, are once again allergen specific. These specific T cells orchestrate an abnormal immune response leading to inflammation and disease.[8] Non-IgE-mediated allergies are important in eczema and infant gut disorders caused by problems with cow's milk.

There has been an exponential rise in the number of children with food allergy over the last 20 years. Peanut allergy was unheard of in the 1980s and now affects nearly 2 per cent of all children. Children who have parents or siblings who have allergies (or are atopic) appear to be more at risk of developing allergy. Allergy runs in families and has a genetic component, but this is not the whole reason for the increase. Some allergists think it is because in today's society we do not encounter microbes that challenge the immune system. Instead, we are exposed to different stimuli, including pollution and indoor allergens. This primes the immune system to become allergic. This is known as the Hygiene Hypothesis:[9] it is not about being too clean at home, but rather that we have conquered some of the major causes of human and childhood mortality such as dysentery (since the introduction of piped sewerage and clean water) and tuberculosis.

# THE ATOPIC MARCH

In children eczema, food allergy, asthma and rhinitis are often related and their progression through childhood is known as the *atopic march* (Figure 20.1).[10] Commonly, eczema and food allergy start in the first years of life: egg and milk allergy often resolve before the child reaches school age, while other food allergies continue into adulthood. Asthma and then rhinitis, associated with aeroallergens, develop later and can continue into adulthood.[10]

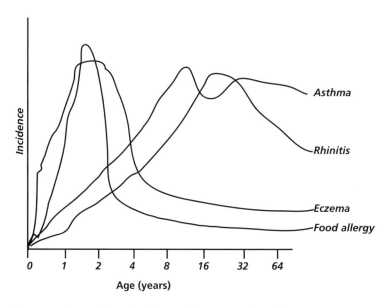

**Figure 20.1** The atopic march redrawn with permission from ref. 6

## Allergy in eczema

Allergic eczema is also known as atopic dermatitis; it is one of the most common skin disorders in young children, and has a prevalence of 10–20 per cent in the first decade of life.[11] The features of eczema include an itchy rash, often confined to flexures of the arms and legs, which can cause extreme discomfort and itching. This in turn can cause disturbed sleep for the child and family, with consequent daytime lethargy. Eczema in infancy can be a precursor to food allergy and asthma (the atopic march). Many children with eczema also have food allergies, especially milk, eggs and peanuts as infants. However, the link between eczema and allergy is not always so straightforward, and infants and young children often follow unnecessary and extensive dietary exclusion, e.g. cow's milk, eggs and wheat. If this is done without proper allergy diagnosis and support it can lead to the risk of malnutrition. Any child with eczema should have an allergy diagnosis made before a food is excluded from the diet. A paediatric dietician should supervise any exclusion to ensure that the diet is adequate in calories, vitamins and minerals.[12]

## Food allergy

Food allergy is common in childhood affecting 6–8 per cent of younger children and 1–2 per cent of

teenagers. In contrast to adults, food allergy resolves in more than 85 per cent of children, especially those with hypersensitivity to eggs and cow's milk.[10] There is no cure for food allergy; management is restricted to constant vigilance: avoiding the implicated food by eliminating it from the diet, and emergency treatment of symptoms caused by accidental exposure with antihistamine and self-injectable adrenaline (epinephrine).

## Allergy in asthma

Severe asthma attacks are the most common reasons for childhood hospital admissions. Children suffering from asthma who also have food allergy are at greater risk of severe allergic reactions, especially if the asthma symptoms are poorly controlled.[13] Asthma alone can lead to disturbance of normal life activities from reduced tolerance of exercise and a disturbed sleep pattern to time off school due to recurrent exacerbation of symptoms. Sudden severe life-threatening attacks with a risk of death can occur. It is important to identify or exclude allergy as part of a multisystem disease and treat it appropriately.

## Allergy in rhinitis (hay fever)

Rhinitis is under-recognised, as are its influences on daily activities, e.g. lethargy and other allergic disease such as asthma. Rhinitis varies from mild to severely disruptive of everyday life. Children suffer from poor sleep, daytime lethargy, and impaired school and examination performance.[5] Symptoms involve the nose and eyes but are often associated with asthma and eczema. Pollen, animals and house dust mite may trigger rhinitis, it may be seasonal or perennial (persistent).

## FOOD ALLERGY

### Classification of adverse reactions to foods

Food allergy is described as an adverse immune response to food proteins;[10] the symptoms can involve the skin, the gastrointestinal tract or the respiratory tract. There are two types: IgE-mediated allergy and non-IgE-mediated reactions (Figure 20.2).

A reaction involving an *IgE-mediated* food allergy usually occurs within 30 minutes of the child having contact with or ingesting the food. This may be followed by a biphasic or late-phase reaction 3–6 hours later.[8]

The onset of symptoms of a T-cell-mediated *non-IgE-mediated* reaction can occur 4–24 hours after contact or ingestion. They can affect the skin, causing eczema, or the gut, causing gastro-oesophageal reflux, colitis, diarrhoea, malabsorption or failure to thrive.[14]

### IgE-mediated food allergy

Food allergy can lead to a spectrum of problems and can affect every area of a child's life. Management is restricted to constant vigilance in avoiding trigger foods and emergency treatment of symptoms caused by accidental exposure.

Although simple, this strategy has wide-ranging consequences for the whole family. Peanut allergy in children is associated with poor quality of life (QoL) and increased anxiety. Children with peanut allergy have been shown to have a poorer QoL than children with insulin-dependent diabetes mellitus, because of threats of potential food hazards within the environment, restriction of activities and worries about being away from home. The mothers of children with peanut allergy report poor QoL and increased stress and anxiety due to their child's peanut allergy.[15,16]

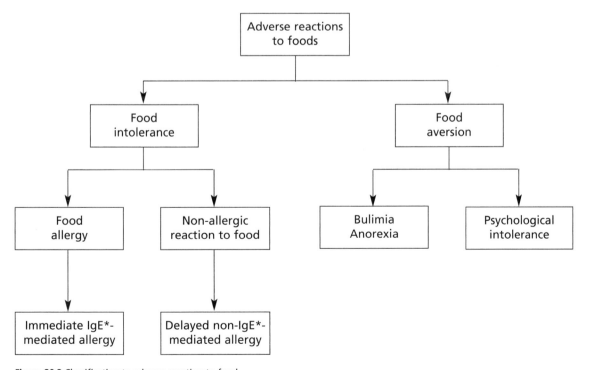

**Figure 20.2** Classification to adverse reaction to food.
*IgE, immunoglobulin E.

Families require careful instruction about which foods to avoid, and how to provide a nutritious and interesting diet. Eating at parties, in restaurants[17] and when abroad on holiday all pose risks for children with food allergy. The advice of a dietician is often required.[12]

Parents and older children should be taught how to recognise an allergic reaction and provide effective first aid. Antihistamines often suffice for milder reactions. Severe reactions should be treated with self-injectable adrenaline (epinephrine). These preloaded syringe devices are called auto-injector pens and deliver a single dose of intramuscular adrenaline to be used before taking the child to the emergency department in hospital. Early treatment with adrenaline can halt an anaphylactic reaction and may save a life.[7]

The final part of the spectrum includes those people, or parents of children, who incorrectly perceive that they have an allergy, usually through self-diagnosis and it is just as important to un-diagnose their allergy as it is to correctly diagnose an allergy. The incorrect management with medication or unnecessary exclusion of foods and a restricted diet[3] can have a detrimental effect on a child's life, and in severe cases lead to malnutrition.[10]

## Causes of systemic reactions to food

The most common foods known to cause IgE-mediated food allergy in the UK are milk, egg, tree nuts, peanuts, soybeans, fish and crustaceans. In children the most common are milk and eggs, which are often outgrown in the early years of life, followed by, peanut, tree nut and fish.[10] Allergy to other foods is not uncommon, for example allergy to kiwi fruit is seen increasingly frequently and can be associated with severe reactions in children.[18]

### Oral allergy syndrome (OAS)

Oral allergy syndrome (OAS) may occur in children who are sensitised to pollens: tree, grass or latex derived from the rubber tree. The pollens cross-react with a wide variety of fresh (raw) fruits and vegetables, e.g. apple, kiwi fruit, nectarine, tomato, potato, peppers. Children with this condition develop itching and swelling in the lips and tongue, and sometimes the throat is affected. Cooking the food usually destroys the allergenicity and prevents the symptoms, as the relevant

proteins causing the cross-reaction are heat labile.[5]

For more information on specific food allergies access the following websites: the Food Standards Agency (www.eatwell.gov.uk); the Anaphylaxis Campaign (www.anaphylaxis.org).

## How food allergy is diagnosed

Diagnosing food allergy is like putting together the pieces of a jigsaw puzzle.

The first step is to take a comprehensive clinical history, from which the clinician decides upon which allergy tests are appropriate, and depending upon the results of the tests whether or not a food challenge is required to confirm the diagnosis.[3] The child and their family should be given information on avoidance of the offending food and instructed in the recognition and management of allergic reactions The use of rescue medicines and an appropriate clinical follow up should be arranged.

Healthcare professionals working in allergy clinics require specialist knowledge. Only those with specific paediatric training should treat children; however, allergy specialist paediatric nurses and doctors are fairly rare and many clinics work in a partnership between allergists and paediatric-trained healthcare professionals.

The clinical allergy team should include:

- specialist allergy consultant (paediatric consultant)
- paediatric allergy nurse specialist
- children's nursing team
- specialist allergy dietician
- clinical psychologist.

### Guidelines for Taking an Allergy History

Allergy is a clinical speciality[3] and being able to take a clear history from parents and the child is a key part of diagnosis and ongoing treatment. Many families are very worried about their child's allergy and a receptive and empathetic approach helps to reassure and develop a shared understanding of the child's condition. In a clinic setting, history taking is undertaken by doctors and allergy nurse specialists. Outside of clinic there will be occasions when a child is admitted to a ward following an allergic reaction, and the nurse admitting the child will need to elicit the facts regarding the episode. Also, on a paediatric ward or day unit prior to surgery, every paediatric nurse should be able to take a basic allergy history and make a baseline assessment of the child's risk factors for allergic reaction. This

would include allergies to drugs and medicines. It is fundamental to their care. The key points are outlined below:

## PROCEDURE: Taking an allergy history

| Procedural steps | Evidence-based rationale |
|---|---|
| 1 Ask the parents and the older child to describe the events of the allergic reaction in their own words without interruption | To establish a clear understanding of events in order to form an accurate allergy history of the reaction |
| 2 Complete a detailed nursing history of any past allergic reactions and other allergic conditions such as eczema, asthma and allergic rhinitis (including seasonal or environmental symptoms) | The clinical allergy history is the corner stone of diagnosing food allergy; its aim is to elicit the likely allergens and to determine the likelihood of severe reaction[10] |
| 3 Examine the child carefully for allergic signs particularly the skin, the eyes and the nose. Assess their breathing and circulatory function (Table 20.1, page 334 ) | To identify current allergic reactions. Note, a child with symptoms of asthma should be assessed for asthma control by having their lung function measured |
| 4 Note any host factors and/or event factors (Table 20.2, page 334). For example a child with asthma is reactions more at risk of having anaphylaxis should they have an accidental exposure to a food to which they are allergic (especially peanut)[13] | The combination of host and/or event factors can help     predict the possible severity of the allergic to foods[19] For example asthma will make their lungs more sensitive and therefore they are more likely to have a reaction involving their airway and breathing – anaphylaxis In addition to Table 20.2 it is important to note that it is not only the amount of food eaten but the manner in which the food is presented that must be considered.[20] For example there are those who cannot eat unadulterated egg or raw egg but can tolerated cooked egg in cakes and biscuits[21] |
| 5 Timing of ingestion and the onset of symptoms are very important | IgE-mediated reactions are often immediate or occur within minutes of ingestion. Non-IgE-mediated reactions may take up to 72 hours to develop[6] |
| 6 Other factors can influence an allergic reaction and should be recorded (Table 20.2) | Attention to detail is paramount |

## SYMPTOMS OF ALLERGIC REACTIONS

The symptoms of IgE-mediated reactions are recorded in Table 20.1. For simplicity they are divided into mild and severe allergic reactions, as they can then guide first aid treatment options for parents.

Non-IgE-mediated reactions are less obvious and are frequently overlooked. They include delayed rashes, vomiting, severe gastro-oesophageal reflux,

infant colic, diarrhoea, abdominal pain and failure to thrive.

### Allergy testing

A suspect history is confirmed by the detection of food-specific IgE antibodies. There are two types of investigations in common use: skin prick testing and a blood test for specific IgE. Skin prick tests require a skilled and trained nurse to conduct the tests, whereas specific IgE blood tests can be taken in a standard way. Skin tests have the advantage of

**Table 20.1** The symptoms of a allergic reaction

| Mild allergic reaction | |
|---|---|
| Eyes | Itchy, runny, swollen |
| Nose | Itchy, runny, congested, sneezing |
| Mouth | Itchy or swollen lips, or mouth |
| Skin | Hives/nettle rash, itchy rash, redness, swelling of the face or other parts of the body |
| Gut | Nausea, abdominal cramps, vomiting or diarrhoea |
| **Severe allergic reaction (anaphylaxis)** | |
| Airway | Tightness or a lump in the throat, hoarse voice, hacking cough |
| Breathing | Short of breath, cough, not able to speak in full sentences, noisy breathing, wheezing |
| Circulation | Feeling faint, weakness or floppiness, glazed expression, unconscious |
| Deterioration | Symptoms getting steadily worse |

**Table 20.2** Factors to be taken into account when recording clinical history. (Based upon Hourihane[19])

| Host factors | Event factors |
|---|---|
| Age | Amount of food involved |
| Associated atopic disease | Food matrix (recipe) |
| Severity of previous reactions | Food form (raw/cooked egg) |
| Family atopy | Allergen stability |
| General health | Season (pollen) |
| Recent infection | Exercise |
| Medication | Alcohol |
| Attitude to risk | Use of rescue medicine |
| Anxiety/panic | Anxiety/panic |

## PROCEDURE: Guidelines for skin prick testing

| Procedural steps | Evidence-based rationale |
|---|---|
| 1 Children should only be skin prick tested by paediatric nurses who are trained to carry out the procedure. Each nurse's technique should be formally validated yearly to ensure gold standard treatment is maintained by demonstrating reproducibility and precision of testing[22] | To maintain child's safety. To ensure the accuracy and reliability of testing |
| 2 The nurse should check this is an appropriate time and method to diagnose food-specific IgE-mediated allergy | There is no lower age limit for skin prick testing.[8] However, if the child is overly distressed, the nurse should enrol the assistance of a play therapist or refer the child back to the clinician for a different form of allergy testing |
| 3 Assemble and check equipment: water-soluble pen, commercially prepared skin prick solutions (within expiry date), single use 1-mm lancets | To ensure a safe environment |

## PROCEDURE: Guidelines for skin prick testing (continued)

| | |
|---|---|
| (one for each allergen), tissues, timer, measuring gauge, results sheet | |
| 4 Ensure the availability at a minimum of the following emergency equipment: oral antihistamine, adrenaline (epinephrine) 1:1000 for intramuscular injection, salbutamol inhaler and spacer | Skin prick testing is considered to be a safe procedure; a small percentage of patients have mild systemic reactions involving itching and a generalised rash, and this can be treated with oral antihistamine. It is recommended that testing for food allergens should be done where treatment for more severe reactions can be rapidly provided[8] |
| 5 The clinician will request that the nurse carries out skin prick testing to detect IgE-mediated allergy | From the detailed clinical history the patient will present with a number of allergens to which they may have a response |
| 6 The nurse should ensure this is the correct child, checking name, date of birth and hospital number | To ensure patient safety |
| 7 The nurse should ensure the child has not taken antihistamine medication. The washout times for each medicine should be available from the hospital pharmacy | The child should not have taken antihistamine medicines before the test, as drugs containing antihistamine prevent histamines attaching to the cells and causing symptoms[3] |
| 8 Prepare the child and parents for the procedure as appropriate and inform them that the results will be immediately available. Inform them that this is considered to be a safe procedure[8] | Informing the child and their family and encouraging their participation has been identified as a strategy to reduce stress and anxiety |
| 9 The nurse must wash her hands according to local infection control policy | To prevent cross-infection |
| 10 The child should be made comfortable, sitting on the parent's lap as appropriate and rest their arm on a pillow. The testing will be on the inner forearm[24] (the volar aspect), which should be uppermost | To reduce stress and anxiety |
| 11 Should the child have active eczema on their arm, the testing can be performed on the back[23] | It is not appropriate to allergy test on broken skin |
| 12 The nurse should use a water-soluble pen to mark on the forearm the initial of each allergen to be used[23] | To ensure each allergen is correctly placed on the arm |
| 13 A negative control (saline) is placed first and a positive control (histamine) is placed last on the arm[23] | To ensure the testing is accurate, the nurse has performed the testing appropriately and the child has not taken antihistamine medication[3] |
| 14 The nurse should place a small drop of each allergen next to the appropriate initial[23] | |
| 15 Using a new 1-mm lancet for each allergen the nurse should press the lancet through the drop at a 90° angle to puncture the skin[23] | To introduce the allergen to the top layer of the child's skin. A new lancet is used for each allergen to prevent cross contamination |
| 16 Using a clean tissue the nurse should carefully blot the drops[3] | To prevent cross-contamination |
| 17 The child should wait for 15 minutes before the results are ready for reading | It takes 15 minutes for the raised white wheal to reach its maximum size[3] |
| 18 After 15 minutes the wheal should be measured | In order to give an accurate wheal size for |

# PROCEDURE:  Guidelines for skin prick testing (continued)

| | |
|---|---|
| using the measuring gauge. Measure the wheal in two planes at 90° to each other and record the mean of the two measurements.[23] | interpretation by the clinician |
| 19 A wheal measuring at least 3mm in size and equal or greater than the positive control is considered to be a positive result | Indicates that the child has IgE antibodies to that allergen.[23] This does not necessarily mean that the child has an allergy to the food. Only a trained doctor or nurse with experience of interpreting the result in the light of the clinical history should discuss the results with the child and family. Further testing may be required to confirm allergy |
| 20 A negative response indicates that the child may not be sensitised to the food[3] | Indicates that the child is unlikely to have allergy. He/she may be they have grown out of the allergy[3] |
| 21 The results of the testing should be accurately recorded in millimetres on the Allergy Testing Results Form and the form signed and dated by the nurse performing the testing[23] | To comply with health and safety and ensure the results are correctly recorded in the child's notes |
| 22 Explain to the child and family that the reaction will usually fade within the hour[3] | To relieve stress and anxiety |
| 23 The test can be carried out with fresh food using the prick-to-prick technique: the lancet is placed into the food and then directly onto the child's skin as described above[3] | If no commercially prepared food allergen is available |

## Blood test for specific IgE

giving an immediate result, while blood tests are delayed by days or weeks. It is important that the specialist has access to well-documented tests.[3] Both tests must be interpreted by an expert, as false positive and false negative results frequently occur.

### Procedural goal is to

• detect of food-specific IgE antibodies.

Blood tests for specific IgE measure the amount of IgE in the blood sample that can bind to specific food allergens. It can be used to aid diagnosis of allergy. If no IgE binds the result is negative.[3] The blood sample must be sent to a specialist laboratory and therefore the results are not immediately available. However, unlike skin prick tests antihistamine does not interfere with the blood test so a child with severe symptoms, e.g. eczema or hay fever, does not have to stop taking their antihistamine medication; the blood test can be used as an alternative.

In the laboratory the blood is brought into contact with the different food allergen extracts and the results are positive depending upon the amount of blood or IgE that binds to the allergens.

False-positive and false-negative results can occur with both skin prick testing and blood tests for specific IgE. A child may have a positive skin prick test but suffer no symptoms when coming into contact with the allergen. One explanation is that the presence of structurally similar allergens to different foods and pollens may in some cases cause IgE to bind to foods to which the child does not react or has never eaten.[24] Children have been known to have a positive clinical history, but negative for both the skin prick test and the blood test, and then go on to have a reaction when challenged to the food itself (false negative). If some allergens are lost or degraded during the preparation of the food allergen extracts, the blood test may not be able to detect a specific food allergy With both skin prick tests and blood tests the reliability is dependent on the quality and stability of the food allergen extracts used. Hospital-based food challenges are the gold standard test for diagnosing food allergy.[24]

## Food challenge

A food challenge is performed when the diagnosis cannot be made by case history and outcome of skin prick testing and blood testing for specific IgE, or when a patient is thought to have outgrown their clinical allergy.[3,24] A challenge should usually be performed in hospital as it carries the risk of anaphylaxis. A challenge involves giving a child increasing doses of the suspected food and allowing time between doses for a response to occur, usually 15–20 minutes. The allergy team closely observe and monitor the child throughout the procedure. If the challenge is negative the food should be reintroduced into the child's diet; if the challenge is positive the child should strictly avoid the food and the family given support and advice on avoidance of the offending food and how to recognise and

manage an allergic reaction.

There are two types of food challenge commonly used to detect food allergy.

1 An *open challenge* is the standard procedure for infants and children. It is used to confirm acute IgE-mediated food allergy with clear objective signs. It is also performed if a negative result is expected, e.g. a child is expected to have grown out of their food allergy. When performing an open food challenge, the doctor, nursing team, child and family are aware of the amount of and type of food given.[24]

2 *Double-blind placebo-controlled food challenge* (DBPCFC) is considered the gold standard. It is an accurate way to establish or rule out an adverse reaction to a food. The challenge food is prepared under the supervision of a dietician and the procedure is carried out over 2 days. On one day the child is given increasing doses of the problem food hidden in a food that they regularly eat, at timed intervals. On the other day the process is repeated using a placebo in the regular food. During this procedure neither the health professionals nor the child or family know which food they are receiving, so no one is able to predict the outcome (the content of the challenge is concealed from both parties – double blind). The challenge is stopped when an objective symptom of an allergic reaction is observed, which is then treated as required. If the child receives all the doses with no evidence of an adverse reaction, it is considered to be a negative challenge and a final open challenge is carried out with a usual serving of food.[24] It is useful where the diagnosis is unclear, or where it might be obscured by anxieties or other problems (such as recurrent urticaria). It is also useful in confirming non-IgE-mediated allergies.[3]

## TEACHING A FAMILY TO LIVE WITH FOOD ALLERGY

Once the diagnosis has been made the hard part begins; there is no cure at present for food allergy, the best treatment is avoidance of the offending food.

It is possible to manage food allergy successfully while allowing the child to participate in common childhood activities.[25] Children with food allergy should be provided with an individual food allergy management plan[2,26] and the family invited to take part in a demonstration of how to use an adrenaline (epinephrine) auto-injector. Verbal, written and visual information should be available to the whole family. The allergy nurse and the allergy dietician give this information and training in the allergy clinic. This is followed up in schools where the school nurse supports the school staff and children.

## Avoidance of the allergen

The only treatment for any type of food allergy is elimination of the problem food. For single exclusion of single foods such as kiwi fruit or strawberries, the elimination is not likely to cause a dietary deficiency. However, for staple foods such as milk, eggs and wheat it is essential that a dietician see the patient. The dietician will give the family a strategy on how to avoid a specific food or foods and what foods are likely to contain the problem food. The dietician will also provide information on all the names that can be used to describe the food and what alternative foods are available. Information should also be given about labelling laws, 'may contain' labelling and food contamination issues.[12]

The allergy nurse should provide children and their families with information on handling situations, such as eating at restaurants, friends' houses and parties; travelling away from home, travelling on aeroplanes;[27] and how to manage their food allergy and medication in a foreign country.

The majority of severe allergic reactions occur when individuals have eaten prepared foods rather than the non-processed food.[20] Children are particularly at risk of a severe reaction if the food is 'hidden' in a high-fat matrix or a highly flavoured food, e.g. nuts in chocolate or curry. A lack of the usual oral 'early-warning signs' that the reaction is developing delays the recognition and management. This increases risk of a severe reaction as more of the offending food is consumed and more allergen present in partially digested food is presented to the mast cells in the gut.[20]

Most severe reactions occur outside the home, when the person preparing the food has little awareness of the individual's allergies.[19,28] This risk can be reduced if the allergic child or their family communicates effectively with the food provider. This is particularly important when those with food allergy eat out in a restaurant, where there is the possibility of cross-contact of foods during preparation and storage. The child and family should inform staff about the food allergy and the risks it carries and ask detailed questions about ingredients used and ask senior waiting staff for advice.[17]

## Rescue medicines

Children and their families need to be able to recognise the early symptoms of allergic reactions and anaphylaxis, so that they are prepared to use their emergency medication and can summon help quickly. They should know they are at risk and be advised to carry antihistamine and an adrenaline (epinephrine) auto-injector with them *at all times*. The whole family should receive training in using the auto-injector and should practise regularly using a suitable training device, so that they will know what to do in an emergency. They should be able to pass on this information to family, friends and schools. The allergy clinic will also provide a written individual Food Allergy Management Plan.[2,29] This is written instructions about what to avoid, and how to recognise and treat an allergic reaction, who to contact and when to phone for an ambulance.

## Food allergy in schools

Children spend a significant amount of their lives in school so it is important that the class teachers and school staff are aware of confirmed food allergies and have the training to recognise and manage allergic symptoms.[30] Every child with food allergy should have available at school a Food Allergy Management Plan and a treatment pack containing prescribed oral antihistamine, an adrenaline (epinephrine) auto-injector and, if they have asthma, an inhaler with a spacer. Children with food allergy should not be excluded from the school dining room, trips or other school activities.[25]

In nurseries and primary schools treatment packs should be kept safely in a central accessible place from which it can be collected at short notice, e.g. the child's classroom or school office.

In secondary schools the older child may carry their antihistamine and adrenaline (epineprhine) auto-injector with them in their schoolbag. The adrenaline auto-injector should be protected in a rigid container and clearly labelled with their name.

## How to treat an allergic reaction

If the child is suspected of having come into contact with or ingested a problem food and has symptoms of a mild allergic reaction involving the eyes, the nose, the mouth, the skin or the gut, he or she should be given oral antihistamine in a syrup or tablet form, appropriate for the age of the child as prescribed by the doctor. They are then advised:

- to rest and take no strenuous exercise of any description, e.g. football, swimming;
- not to eat a heavy meal;
- not to have any form of fizzy drink (adults should also avoid alcohol).

The child should not be left alone and should be observed for 2 or 3 hours; if during this time the condition worsens, the child will require immediate treatment. The symptoms can change very quickly and develop into a severe allergic reaction – anaphylaxis – showing problems with the airway, breathing, circulation or deterioration (see Table 20.1). There are occasions when there are no signs of a mild reaction, and the first signs are of a severe reaction. In either case the following action should be taken:

- Place the person in a comfortable position.
- If the person is conscious and having breathing difficulties, help them to sit up.
- If they are faint or floppy, they should lie flat with their legs raised up.[31]
- Administer intramuscular injectable adrenaline (epinephrine).
- Phone 999 for an ambulance.

## How to use an adrenaline (epinephrine) auto-injector

Immediately administer intramuscular adrenaline via an adrenaline auto injector. In the UK it is available as an Epipen or Anapen; each comes in two strengths. It is prescribed on an individual patient basis.

- Junior: adrenaline 0.15 mg – prescribed for children 15–30 kg
- Adult: adrenaline 0.3 mg – prescribed for persons > 30 kg

Immediately call for medical help – dial 999 for an ambulance.

Adrenaline prevents and relieves laryngeal oedema and circulatory collapse; it causes bronchodilation and reduces the release of histamine. Failure to inject adrenaline promptly increases the risk of a biphasic anaphylactic reaction and death.[29]

> **ACTIVITY**
>
> For manufacturers' instructions on how to use an Epipen and an Anapen access the following websites: www.epipen.co.uk www.anapen.co.uk

Medical help should be sought as soon as possible after developing a severe allergic reaction involving the airway, breathing or circulation, even if after using the adrenaline (epinephrine) auto-injector the child is feeling better. The reaction could return when the effects of the adrenaline have worn off, which is usually between 10–20 minutes.

Immediately call for medical help – dial 999 for an ambulance.

The person making the telephone call should state:

- where to find the child having a reaction;
- that the child is having a severe allergic reaction known as anaphylaxis;
- the name and the age of the child.

If the child has problems with breathing and usually uses an inhaler, give up to 10 puffs of salbutamol (Ventolin) or terbutaline (Bricanyl) with a spacer.

If a second adrenaline (epinephrine) auto-injector has been prescribed, this can be given if there is continued deterioration 5–10 minutes after the first one. Make contact with the child's parents/guardian.

> **KEY POINT**
>
> If an allergic reaction is suspected treat the symptoms immediately:
> - For a mild reaction treat a with oral antihistamine
> - Observe the child for further symptoms
> - If signs of problems with airway, breathing, circulation treat immediately with adrenaline (epinephrine)
> - Call for medical assistance

## SUPPORT ORGANISATIONS FOR PEOPLE WITH ALLERGIC DISEASE

- Anaphylaxis Campaign: www.anaphylaxis.org
- Allergy UK: www.allergyuk.org
- The Food Standards Agency: www.eatwell.gov.uk

These organizations provide valid useful information on food allergy for parents, children, schools and health professionals.

It is recommended that every person who is severely allergic should wear an internationally recognised emergency symbol, such as a Medic Alert bracelet. This ensures that in an emergency, where the cause of collapse is unknown, the necessary information is available to the emergency services. The correct medicine can then be administered and a life saved.

Please refer to the website for a question about peanut allergy.

> **ACTIVITY**
>
> Access www.resus.org for guidelines for healthcare providers treating anaphylaxis in various settings.[32]

> **ACTIVITY**
>
> Access the British Society for Allergy and Clinical Immunology website (www.bsaci.org) to find your nearest children's allergy clinic, contact the nurse in charge and ask for an informal visit to one of the clinics to observe the allergy nurse giving information to a family on the management of allergic reactions and the use of an adrenaline (epinephrine) auto-injector.

## CONCLUSION

The purpose of this chapter has been to provide evidence-based guidance in the care of the child with food allergy. The reader should understand the importance of the correct diagnosis of an allergy so that appropriate measures can be put into place to treat the child. The day-to-day care of the child with food allergy lies with his or her parents, the young person themselves as they grow older, as well as their family, friends and school. Accurate information giving, education in the management of the food allergy and treatment of allergic reactions, as a result of accidental exposure to the food, is vitally important. This falls within the role of the nurse working in the allergy clinic. This nurse must establish a rapport with the child and their family and give them confidence to deal with this disease for which as yet there is no cure.

## ACKNOWLEDGEMENTS

The author thanks the following people for reading and advising on this chapter: Dr Michel Erlewyn-Lajeunesse Consultant Paediatrician and Honorary Senior Lecturer Paediatric Allergy, Immunology & Infectious Diseases at Southampton University Hospital NHS Trust; Dr Jane Lucas Clinical Senior Lecturer/Consultant Paediatrician, Paediatric Allergy and Respiratory Medicine at Southampton University Hospital NHS Trust.

 Go to the website to find the PowerPoint presentation for this chapter and MCQs to test your knowledge. **www.hodderplus.com/childnursingskills**

## REFERENCES

1  Grundy J, Matthews S, Bateman B, *et al.* (2002) Rising prevalence to peanut in children: data from 2 sequential cohorts. *Journal of Allergy and Clinical Immunology* **110**: 784–789.

2  Burks WA (2008) Peanut allergy. *Lancet* **371**: 1538–1546.

3  Asero R, Ballmer-Weber BK, Conti A, *et al.* (2007) IgE mediated food allergy diagnosis: current status and new perspectives. *Molecular Nutrition & Food Research* **51**: 35–147.

4  Macdougall C, Etuwewe O (2005) How dangerous is food allergy? *Current Paediatrics* **15**: 228–232.

5 Scadding GK, Fokkens WJ (2007) Fast facts: rhinitis, 2nd edition. Oxford: Health Press.

6 Durham SR, Church MK (2001) Principles of allergy diagnosis. In: Holgate ST, Church MK, Lichtenstein LM, eds. *Allergy*, 2nd edition. London: Mosby, pp. 3–16.

7 Simons E (2008) Emergency treatment of anaphylaxis. *British Medical Journal* 336: 1141–1142.

8 Host A, Andrae S, Charkin S, *et al.* (200 ) Allergy testing in children: why, who, when and how? *Allergy* 58: 559–569.

9 Strachan DP (2000) Family size infection and atopy: the first decade of the 'hygiene hypothesis'. *Thorax* 55(1): S2–10.

10 Thong BY-H, Hourihane J (2004) Monitoring of IgE-mediated food allergy in childhood. *Acta Paediatrics* 93: 759–764.

11 Krakowski AC, Eichenfield LF, Dohil MA (2008) Management of atopic dermatitis in the pediatric population. *Pediatrics* 122: 812–824.

12 Grimshaw KEC (2007) Expert guide to food allergies. *NHD Magazine* 24(Suppl): 2–4.

13 Roberts G, Patel N, Levi-Schaffer F, *et al.* (2003) Food allergy as a risk factor for life-threatening asthma in childhood: A case controlled study. *Journal of Allergy & Clinical Immunology* 112(1): 168–174.

14 Ahrens B, Beyer K, Wahn U, Niggemann B (2008) Differential diagnosis of food-induced symptoms. *Pediatric Allergy and Immunology* 19: 92–96.

15 Avery NJ, King RM, Knight S, Hourihane JO'B (2003) Assessment of quality of life in children with peanut allergy. *Pediatric Allergy Immunology* 14: 378–382.

16 King RM, Knibb RC, Hourihane J (2009) Impact of peanut allergy on quality of life, stress and anxiety in the family. *Allergy* 64: 461–468.

17 Furlong A, DeSimone J, Sicherer SH (2001) Peanut and tree nut allergic reaction in restaurants and other food establishments. *Journal of Allergy & Clinical Immunology* 108: 867–870.

18 Lucas JSA, Grimshaw KEC, Collins K, *et al.* (2004) Kiwi fruit is a significant allergen and is associated with differing patterns of reactivity in children and adults. *Clinical & Experimental Allergy* 34: 1115–1121.

19 Hourihane JO'B, Knulst AC (2005) Threshold of allergenic proteins in foods. *Toxicology and Applied Pharmacology* 207: S152–S156.

20 Grimshaw KEC, King RM, Nordlee SL, *et al.* (2003) Presentation of allergen in different food preparations affects the nature of the allergic reaction – a case series. *Clinical & Experimental Allergy* 33: 1581–1585.

21 Sampson HA (2004) Update on food allergy. *Journal of Allergy & Clinical Immunology* 113: 805–819.

22 Carr WW (2006) *Allergy skin testing: the nuts and bolts*. Miami: AAAAI.

23 Brydon MJ (2000) *Skin prick testing in clinical practice*. Norwich: NADAAS.

24 Bruijnzeel-Koomen C, Ballmer-Weber BK, Bengtsson U, *et al.* (2004) Standardisation of food challenges in patients with immediate reactions to foods – position paper from the European Academy of Allergology and Clinical Immunology. *Allergy* 59: 690–697.

25 Furlong A (2003) Daily coping strategies for patients and their families. *Paediatrics* 111: 1654–1661.

26 Crespo JF, James JM, Fernandez-Rodriguiz C, Rodriguez J (2006) Food allergy: nuts and tree nuts. *British Journal of Nutrition* 96(Suppl 2) S95–S102.

27 Comstock SS, DeMera R, Vaga LC, *et al.* (2008) Allergic reactions to peanuts, tree nuts and seeds aboard commercial airliners. *Annals Allergy Asthma Immunology* 101: 51–56.

28 Leitch IS, Walker MJ, Davey R (2005) Food allergy: Gambling your life on a take-away meal. *International Journal of Environmental Health Research* 15(2): 79–87.

29 Simons E (2004) First-aid treatment of anaphylaxis to food: focus on epinephrine. *Journal of Allergy & Clinical Immunology* 113: 837–844.

30 Forster D, Bryant J (2004) Risk of anaphylaxis: improving care at school. *Paediatric Nursing* 16: 29–31.

31 Sicherer SH, Leung DYM (2004) Advances in allergic skin disease, anaphylaxis and hypersensitivity reactions to foods, drugs & insect stings. *Journal of Allergy & Clinical Immunology* 114: 118–124.

33 Working Group of the Resuscitation Council (UK) (2008) Emergency treatment of anaphylactic reactions. Guidelines for healthcare providers. The Resuscitation Council (UK) www.resus.org.uk (accessed 29 May 2009).

## FURTHER READING

32 Eriksson NE, Moller C, Werner S, *et al.* (2003) The hazards of kissing when you are food allergic. *Journal of Investigational Allergology & Clinical Immunology* 13(3): 149–154.

# Non-invasive respiratory therapy
## A) Aerosol therapy

Marion Aylott

## LEARNING OUTCOMES

*Upon completion of this chapter, the reader should be able to accomplish the following:*

1 Identify three methods of aerosol administration
2 Correctly identify different types of aerosol delivery systems
3 Describe safe methods of aerosol device administration with reference to flow rate (where appropriate), delivery system, service user monitoring and response
4 Discuss with rationale the recommended techniques for administering a nebuliser
5 Discuss with rationale the recommended cleaning method used for a inhaler spacer and nebulisation system

## KEY WORDS

Respiration therapy    Aerosol    Nebuliser
Inhaler device    Pressurised metered dose inhaler
Dry powder

## CHAPTER OVERVIEW

Research highlights the importance of evaluating inhalation and nebulisation techniques and providing appropriate education to parents and children, especially before commencing and increasing dosage and adding other medication.[1] This research, measured the speed of inhalation among doctors, nurses, pharmacists and other specialists involved in respiratory medicine, and showed that just 6 per cent were inhaling in a way that maximised the dose reaching the lungs and minimised the risk of side-effects. Therefore, it is imperative that those actively involved in administering, teaching and checking children's inhaler and nebulisation technique have adequate knowledge, understanding and skill for optimising the technique. Learning to use an inhaler and/or nebulisation correctly is a key part of optimising treatment.

This chapter will introduce you to inhaler and nebulisation devices and how they work followed by evidence-based guidelines for best practice.

## WHAT IS AN AEROSOL?

Medication, delivered by aerosol is most commonly used for emergency and domiciliary treatment of many respiratory diseases. Indications for aerosol use include the management of exacerbations and long-term treatment of chronic respiratory disease, e.g. management of cystic fibrosis, asthma, bronchiectasis, HIV/AIDS and symptomatic relief in palliative care.

An aerosol comprises solid or liquid particles suspended in a gas. Aerosols are broadly classified into two groups:[2]

- bland: heated or cool sterile water/saline;
- medicated: bronchodilators, steroids, mucokinetic agents (drugs that destroy or break down mucus), antibiotics, anti-allergic agents.

| Definitions |
|---|

**Aerosol:** solid or liquid particles suspended in a gas

**Pressurised metered dose inhaler (pMDI):** a pressurised aerosol inhaler/puffer device for delivering a metered dose of medicine directly into the lungs

**Dry powder inhaler (DPI):** an non-pressurised aerosol inhaler/puffer device for delivering medicine directly into the lungs powered by inspiratory flow

**Actuated MDI:** a pMDI containing a mechanism which automatically releases the medicine once sufficient inspiratory flow is achieved

**Spacer:** non-static holding chamber made of polyamide material

**Nebuliser:** turns an aqueous solution of drug into fine mist

The depth or penetration of aerosol delivery is influenced by many variables such as:

- size and physical characteristics of the aerosol: particle size decreases the depth of penetration as the respiratory tract increases:[3]
  - <1 μm are deposited by in the alveoli; (note that 3 μm is an important size, because gravity begins to lose its influence[3] (Table 21.1))
  - 1–8 μm is deposited by gravity to all of respiratory tract to the alveoli;
  - 8–10 μm are deposited in the upper airway;
- amount of aerosol;
- anatomy and geometry of the airway;
- breathing pattern: slow deep breaths will allow deeper deposition.

# BACKGROUND PHYSIOLOGY

When it comes to aerosol delivery, infants and small children are not simply small adults, and might require different methods, doses and devices. The delivery of inhaled therapy to infants and young children is associated with unique challenges due to anatomy, physiology and cognitive development in this patient population as follows:[3]

- small tidal volume
- small airways
- rapid respiration
- inability to hold breath with inhaled medication
- nose breathing
- aversion to masks
- cognitive ability
- fussiness and crying.

**Table 21.1** Particle size and airway deposition of aerosols[3]

| Size (NMAD) | Site | |
|---|---|---|
| <0.5 μm | No deposition | No clinical effect<br>Systemic absorption |
| 0.5–2 μm | Alveoli | Clinical effect |
| 2–5 μm | Bronchi and bronchioles | |
| 5–100 μm | Mouth, nose and upper airway | No clinical effect<br>Systemic absorption if swallowed |
| >100 μm | Filtered by upper respiratory tract | |

The size of a child, including lungs and airways and thus inspiratory flows, breathing patterns and lung volumes change with growth and development, especially and most dramatically in the first years of life. In the first year of life, a tidal volume of approximately 7 mL per kg results in a 300 per cent increase in tidal volume over the course of that year. Inspiratory flow increases with vital capacity. Resting respiratory rate decreases with age, as tidal volume and minute ventilation increase. The combination of low tidal volume, low vital capacity, low functional residual capacity and a short respiratory cycle provides a short residence time for aerosol in the airways, reducing pulmonary deposition.[3]

The primary job of the upper airways is to filter out particulates from the air. The smaller the airway then the more efficient the filtering system and the lower the drug deposition rate. Therefore, the smaller diameter of the airways in infants and children results in a greater percentage of particles being deposited in the upper airways.[4] In addition, preferential nose breathing filters the aerosolised drug in the nose, reducing drug deposition in the lungs.

## METHODS OF AEROSOL DELIVERY

### Aerosol delivery systems

The three principle types of devices widely used are

- pMDI: pressurised metered dose inhaler
- DPI: dry powder inhaler
- nebuliser.

There are basically two types: those that make the aerosol for the child, i.e. the nebuliser, and others that use the energy of inhalation when they breathe in, i.e. inhalers, which require coordination of timing of inhalation and breathing (flow rate).

## INHALER DEVICES

Children under the age of 3 years are usually unable to form a good seal on a mouthpiece and inhale when requested.[5] For these toddlers, it is best that medications be delivered using a device, such as a nebuliser or a pMDI with a valved holding chamber known as a 'Babyhaler' or 'Spacer'. These are non-static holding chambers, which are attached to a pMDI and combined with a tight fitting face mask to enhance drug delivery. Use of a spacer eliminates the need to coordinate pressing the canister with inspiration. They work by capturing the aerosol cloud as it leaves the pMDI, and holding it ready for the child to inhale at their own rate. The device also allows more time for evaporation of the propellant so that the resulting

aerosol is better suited to being inhaled and travelling deep into the lung.[5] Spacers have also been shown to reduce local adverse effects from inhaled corticosteroids[6].

Aerosols are best given to infants and children during relaxed breathing. The crying and struggling child or infant has very short inhalations and high flows, combined with a long exhalation. This pattern decreases the amount of medication deposited in the lower respiratory tract by as much as 90 per cent.[7] Therefore, aerosol medication should not be given to a child who is upset, fighting the delivery device or crying. Medication should never be given by the blow-by or 'wafting' method as virtually no medication is delivered.[3] Older children are usually able to place the mouthpiece directly in their mouths. When aerosols are given using a mouthpiece, it is important for the child to breathe in slowly and deeply.[5] Recommendations made by the Global Initiative for Asthma[8] and the British Thoracic Society,[9] are shown below.

### Age-related guide to choice of aerosol delivery device[8,9]

<3 years: pMDI + Babyhaler/spacer + mask or nebulisers

3–5 years: pMDI + spacer ± mask/mouthpiece or nebulisers

5–8 years: pMDI + spacer ± mouthpiece or nebulisers

>8 years: DPI or pMDI ± spacer ± mouthpiece or nebulisers

---

**KEY POINTS**
- Blow-by method not recommended
- Masks: Infants to 3-years-olds
- Mouthpieces can be used in children >3 years of age
- DPI: Children > 6years

---

The aim with all inhalers is to try to maximise the dose that can be inhaled (quantity of drug), and produce the right size particles, that is quality of aerosol. Table 21.2 demonstrates how pMDI and DPI inhalers work in very different ways.

**KEY POINT**

To ensure optimal inhaler technique, consideration should be given to the whole process of using an inhaler, from the initial choice of medication and the delivery device through to periodic review

**Table 21.2** Characteristics of pressurised metered dose inhalers (pMDIs) compared with dry powder inhalers (DPIs)[5]

| Type of device | Description | Recommendations |
| --- | --- | --- |
| **pMDI**<br>Many are colour-coded to help identify the medication contained within, although there is no international standard on colours | Comprises a pressurised metal container (the 'canister') within a plastic holder (the 'inhaler actuator' or 'boot'). The inhaler boot is normally made of plastic – the shape may vary slightly depending on which company manufactured it (traditionally, white inhaler 'boots' normally signify a training device, or 'placebo' which contains no active drug)<br>The canister contains a mix of aerosol propellant, and medication suspension. Usually, the canister can hold a reservoir of propellant/medication mixture that is sufficient for about 200 'actuations' or doses. Those with dose counters are recommended<br>Several manufacturers have developed 'breath-actuated' MDI inhalers, which automatically press the canister (so creating an aerosol) only when the child has started to inhale, e.g. Easibreathe, Autohaler. These help users avoid the problem of pressing the canister at the wrong time | Child requires good hand-breathing coordination. Breath activated MDIs are becoming increasingly available and 'spacers' are recommended for improved deposition<br>The unadapted MDI may be difficult for some children to use if they cannot coordinate pressing the canister and inhaling at the same time |
| **DPI**<br>e.g. Rotahaler; Spinhaler; Turbohaler; Diskhaler (Accuhaler) | Activated by inhalation, these devices create an aerosol cloud of small particles without the need for a propellant gas. A wide range of different designs is available. They range from single-dose units that need refilling between inhalations, through to multi-dose versions that contain up to 200 doses | Child's own inspiratory effort (high inspiration flow >28 litres/min) to form aerosol as powder is delivered only when the child inhales. DPI requires faster inhalation than MDI. Generally recommended for use by children above 6 years of age |

The laws of physics help explain why breathing in too quickly is not helpful; particles in moving air will follow the path that the air takes until a change in direction occurs, at which time they will try to continue to move in the same direction they were travelling, that is maintain their 'momentum'. If the change in direction is more than small, there is a risk of the particles impacting on the airway wall. The risk of impaction increases as the particles get larger, and also as the speed of the air increases.

In summary, breathing in too quickly through a device that needs a slow inhalation (or vice versa) not only reduces the amount of medication reaching the lungs, it also increases the risk of side-effects due to unwanted drug deposition in the mouth, throat and upper airways. Several manufacturers have developed 'breath-actuated' pMDI inhalers, which automatically press the canister (so creating an aerosol) only when the child has started to inhale. These devices help users avoid the problem of pressing the canister at the wrong time. Also, some spacers have a training whistle, which sounds as a warning to the user that they are inhaling the aerosol too quickly.

---

**KEY POINTS**

Inhaling too fast means much of the aerosol cannot travel round the sharp bends in the throat, resulting in:
- less of the drug reaching the lungs
- more of the medication hitting the back of the throat, increasing the risk of side-effects.

Inhaling too slowly means the aerosol is not inhaled into the lungs, and it rebounds off the sides of the mouth and throat, resulting in:
- less of the drug reaching the lungs
- more of the medication remaining in the mouth, increasing the risk of side-effects.

Inhaling at the right speed reduces the amount of aerosol that impacts on the rear of the throat, resulting in:
- maximum amount of medication reaching the lungs
- minimum deposition of medication in the mouth and throat.

---

The speed of inhalation required has important implications if an inhaler is being used in an acute asthma attack. During an attack it may be more difficult for the asthmatic to inhale through their inhaler (most important if they are using DPI). In this situation, an anxious child may rush the use of their device because they want to get relief from their inhaler as quickly as possible. At this time when optimum drug delivery would benefit the asthmatic most, correct use of the inhaler may not occur due to panic – unless the child has learnt how to get the technique right previously, and can remember each of the recommended steps. Practising scenarios with the child and family will help this.

Whichever technique is used, it is important to get all the steps right – failing to complete any one properly can significantly reduce the dose that gets to the lungs. Encouraging a child to practise in front of a mirror is helpful. If aerosol or 'mist' can be seen leaking out from the top of the inhaler or from either side of the mouth, then more help is required in order to improve overall inhaler technique.[6]

## DEVICE SELECTION AND COMPLIANCE

The most common reasons for not responding to treatment are:

- being given an inappropriate inhaler;
- not using the inhaler device properly;
- failing to take the medication as directed.

Over recent years, more health professionals have received specialist training on respiratory medicine, but unless the differences between devices are fully understood by all healthcare professionals involved, there is a risk that children may not be given the delivery device best suited to their needs and abilities. 'Poor knowledge of how drugs and inhalers work, coupled with complex prescribing regimes, are contributory factors in up to half of the 1,400 fatal cases of asthma in the UK each year.'[4]

Whenever possible, a child should use only one type of aerosol-generating device for all their inhalation therapy. The technique for using each device is different, and repeated instruction is necessary to ensure that the child (± parents) uses the device appropriately. The use of different devices for inhalation can be confusing and may decrease compliance with therapy.

To improve compliance, regularly scheduled aerosol therapy should be administered along with some easily remembered activity. For twice-daily administration, medications can be kept with the toothbrush and inhaled just before brushing the teeth. This approach helps to reduce corticosteroid levels in the mouth and hypopharynx.[12]

The availability of rescue medication at the child's nursery school, or home must be ensured. Written guidelines for medication use must be distributed to all the places where the child stays. The child's embarrassment and the inconvenience may significantly reduce compliance. Encourage the child/child's parents and other caregivers to keep a diary of medication use. It is important to know how regularly drugs are administered for both scheduled and as-needed medications.

<table>
<tr><td rowspan="1" style="writing-mode: vertical-rl">VIGNETTE</td><td>**Problem:** One of the children in your care does not seem to be responding to their inhaled medication.

**Discussion:** A lack of response to inhaled medication can be related to a number of factors. Poor education of the care provider or child (with the resulting inability to operate the nebuliser or inhaler properly) is a frequent problem. Poor device selection can result in mismatching of the child, drug, and device. If the inhaler has no dose counter, a child may be unwittingly inhaling from empty canisters of medication.[20] In addition, failure to take preventive medications as prescribed, changes in the child's environment, and misdiagnosis also have been identified as problems.</td></tr>
</table>

Inhaled drug aerosol, in the treatment of many lung diseases, has numerous advantages over drugs, which are taken systemically. The onset of action is quicker, the therapeutic dose lower, therefore minimising side-effects, and the drug is better targeted.[5]

### The procedural goal is to

- maximise the dose that can be inhaled (quantity of drug)
- produce the right size particles that is quality of aerosol
- reduce the risk of side-effects due to unwanted drug deposition in the mouth, throat and upper airways.

### Equipment

Inhaler (±) spacer as prescribed
Hand-washing/cleansing facilities

## PROCEDURE: Procedure for using an inhaler (± spacer device)

| Procedural steps | Evidence-based rationale |
|---|---|
| **1** A child's ability to correctly use equipment must be assessed before use<br>Consider use of spacer for child <8 years | In collaboration with medical colleagues, it is important to select an inhaler pMDI ± spacer or DPI that is most likely to achieve maximum deposition of medication (see page 350) |
| **2** Read the equipment instructions completely before use | Read the instructions and ensure that the specific steps and the recommended technique for a particular device are followed.[10] This website provides informative video animations of how to use each type of inhaler correctly<br>www.asthma.org.uk/using_your.html |
| **3** Explain the procedure to child and parents as appropriate, including the importance of good inhaler technique or '5 breath technique' if using a spacer[17] as described below | The difference between good and bad inhaler technique means:<br>• increased drug deposition in the lungs<br>• increased effect from the medication taken<br>• reduced deposition in the throat<br>• lower risk of side-effects<br>• more consistent dosing<br>• less waste |
| **4** Wash your hands thoroughly and teach parents and child to do likewise before procedure | Infection control |
| **5** Remove inhaler cap; check mouthpiece and spacer (if used) is clean | Only use inhaler if cap has been kept in place. Dirty equipment carries the potential for infection in already vulnerable children |

## PROCEDURE: Procedure for using an inhaler (± spacer device) (continued)

| | |
|---|---|
| 6 Shake inhaler well[11]<br>If the inhaler is new or it has not been used for a week or more 'prime' the device; after shaking it well, hold it upright and release one puff into the air | The medication suspension is usually a combination of an inert liquid and the active drug, but the fact that it is a 'suspension' is important; like oil and vinegar salad dressing, it can separate out if left to stand<br>Correctly priming a dry powder inhaler is very important – some DPIs do not measure out a full dose if they are primed in the wrong orientation (e.g. horizontal), as they rely on a 'gravity feed' system to measure the next dose from a hopper reservoir. Read the instructions from the manufacturer carefully |
| 7 If using an autohaler device, push the lever up ('on') before each dose | When the canister is pressed, a measuring system at the base of the canister releases a precise volume of liquid into the inhaler's nozzle, which then rapidly evaporates to produce the aerosol cloud or 'mist'. If the contents of the canister (propellant and medication) are not mixed thoroughly, then too much or too little of one component will be released |
| 8 Hold inhaler upright with thumb on base, below mouthpiece<br>*Using a spacer device*<br>Insert the inhaler into the holder of the spacer in an upright position. | This method prevents accidental blockage of air holes on the top of the device with fingers |
| 9 Holding the inhaler in an upright position, place it in the child's mouth and ask them to grip gently between teeth while ensuring that the tongue is underneath the inhaler; then seal lips around mouthpiece. Take care not to block the air holes on the top of the inhaler device[9] | Placing the mouthpiece directly in the mouth (closed mouth technique) means that all the aerosol created is ready to be inhaled: there is no risk that any misses the mouth |
| 10 Gently breathe out while keeping the inhaler upright[9] | Breathing out fully (or as much as is comfortable), reduces the amount or air in the small airways, and increases space available for air from the next breath. The result is a deeper than normal inhalation, that can last longer, maximising the opportunity to carry all of the aerosol 'cloud' created by the inhaler to where it is needed[12] |
| 11 Instruct the child to then 'press and breathe in deeply at the same time'<br><br><br><br><br>If using a pMDI<br>Instruct the child to then hold their breath for a count of 5–10 (or as long as is comfortable)[12]<br>If using an autohaler (actuated) device tell the child to not stop inhaling until the inhaler 'clicks' and continue taking a deep breathe. Do not rush! | Pressing the canister needs to be coordinated with inhaling to ensure maximum delivery of medication<br>By inhaling, an aerosol cloud is created. Inhaling deeply maximises the opportunity for the aerosol particles to reach the furthest parts of the lungs, where they have maximum effect<br>Holding the breath after inhaling, allows time for gravity to pull more of the drug particles into the airways<br>By keeping the air still for a few seconds, a greater number of particles will fall onto the airways wall (due to gravity). It has been found that 10 seconds breath hold is ideal, but even if this is not possible, many can benefit from holding their breath for as |

## PROCEDURE: Procedure for using an inhaler (± spacer device) (continued)

| | |
|---|---|
| *Using a DPI*<br>Instruct the child to inhale forcefully and deeply | long as is comfortable after inhaling<br>To view animation of this closed mouth technique<br>'and how pressing the canister needs to be<br>coordinated with inhaling go to<br>www.2tonetrainer.net/How_they_should_be_used.htm<br>DPIs generally have a higher resistance to airflow than<br>pMDIs. Like leaves on the ground and wind in<br>autumn, fast moving air will pick up more of the dry<br>powder than slow moving air. Above a certain speed,<br>nearly all the dry powder will be picked up, leaving<br>very little behind in the device. The energy of fast<br>moving air also helps to break up the powder into<br>small particles.<br>To view animation showing airflow through a pMDI<br>and DPI; go to www.2tonetrainer.net/<br>Aerosol_inhalers.htm |
| *Using a Babyhaler/spacer*<br>Place the face mask gently and securely over the<br>infant's nose and mouth and hold at a 45° angle<br>Encourage the child to breathe out, or as the<br>infant breathes out, encourage the child to<br>press down on the canister once to release<br>a 'puff' of medication into the spacer reservoir<br>Keep the spacer in place while the infant/child<br>takes at least five breaths in and out, each<br>inhalation being slow and deep until the 'lungs<br>feel full' (or as long as is comfortable) | Encourage the child to breathe in slowly so gravity can<br>pull more of the drug particles into the airways |
| **12** Breathe normally | To enable accurate and reliable assessment of<br>respiratory status between 'puffs' |
| **13** If another dose is required; 30 seconds<br>between puffs[12] | • The creation of an aerosol from the rapidly<br>  evaporating liquid results in cooling of the canister.<br>  This cooling can, in theory, mean the inhaler does<br>  not perform properly (they work best at room<br>  temperature). A 30-second delay allows the canister<br>  to warm back up to room temperature<br>• Fast-acting drugs that relieve bronchospasm can<br>  help open up the airways very quickly, allowing a<br>  second dose (if needed) to reach the furthest parts<br>  of the lung more easily |
| **14** Before administering another dose ('puff'), remove<br>the inhaler from the mouth, or remove the face<br>mask and remove the canister from the inhaler/<br>spacer device; shake it well before reinserting for<br>the second dose ('puff'). Repeat the actions as<br>above for subsequent doses ('puffs') | The medication suspension is usually a combination of<br>an inert liquid and the active drug; it can<br>separate even in the short period between 'puffs' |
| **15** After use, hold the inhaler upright and immediately<br>close the cap. If using an autohaler device; push<br>the lever down ('off') afterwards | To prevent inadvertent loss (leakage) of drug |
| **16** Always cleanse a child's face after using a steroid | To prevent oral candidiasis[11] |

## PROCEDURE: Procedure for using an inhaler (± spacer device) (continued)

| | |
|---|---|
| inhaler with mask. The older child placing the inhaler device directly between their teeth must be taught and encouraged to take a drink or brush their teeth after using a steroid inhaler[13] | |
| 17 Keep the inhaler (± spacer) close at hand at all times but out of direct sunlight<br>Store the inhaler away from children, dust and excesses of heat and moisture. If an inhaler/spacer becomes damaged, it should be discarded and a replacement obtained[14] | An inhaler is designed for 'single-patient use'[10] device. For hygienic reasons, encourage the child not to loan to others |
| 18 Clean inhaler at least once a month and spacer daily[14]<br><br>• Immerse in warm (but not hot) mild detergent solution for 2–3 minutes, but for no longer than 5 minutes. Agitate in the water<br>Do not insert any object into the inhaler during cleaning. The external surfaces of the device can be wiped with a cloth, if required<br>• Rinse thoroughly in clean warm water, and then shake repeatedly to remove any excess water from the inside of the unit<br>• Allow to air-dry naturally before using again. | For infection control. To reduce static electricity in spacer which pulls medicine to sides of the container leading to loss of dosage[15]<br>To ensure thorough cleaning<br><br>To avoid damage to the mechanism |

---

**KEY POINT**

Corticosteroid inhalers[13]
• Child should rinse mouth with water after using these inhalers to prevent oral candidiasis
• Child should be taught how to correctly use these medications

## NEBULISATION DEVICES

A nebuliser is a device that converts liquid into aerosol droplets suitable for inhalation.[1] Nebulisers use oxygen, compressed air or ultrasonic power to break up medication solutions[2] and deliver a therapeutic dose of aerosol particles directly to the lungs.[3] Nebulisers are used for emergency and domiciliary treatment of many respiratory diseases. Indications for nebuliser use include the management of exacerbations and long-term treatment of chronic respiratory disease, e.g. management of cystic fibrosis and asthma.[6] The use of nebulisers in the community is declining.[16] The 2008 British Guideline[9] no longer recommends nebulised therapy for the majority of asthma care. It cites evidence suggesting that a spacer and pMDI combination can be as effective, if not more effective, in many situations in which nebulisers were formally used. This includes both acute and stable asthma. However, they may still be useful in certain clinical situations, because

• the drug will be inhaled with normal respiration;
• medication reaches lower airways more effectively.

Nebulisers are highly inefficient and many deliver only 10 per cent of the prescribed drug dose to the lungs.[4] Much of the drug is caught on the internal apparatus or wasted during exhalation.

Nebuliser machines have three main parts: a cup that holds the medication, a mouthpiece or mask attached to a T-elbow, and a thin, plastic tube that connects the mouthpiece to the compressor. There are home and hospital models of nebuliser breathing machines, as well as portable nebuliser machines.

Nebulisers can be driven by either

- a jet nebuliser, e.g. OMRON, CompAir, Elite and PARI TREK
- an ultrasonic nebuliser, e.g. Aeroneb, GoMicropump and MicroAir NE-U22V.

When a jet nebuliser is used, in order to produce small enough particles from solution in 5–10 minutes, gas flow rates of at least 6 litres/min are usually necessary. Ultrasonic nebulisers use a rapidly vibrating piezoelectric crystal to produce aerosol particles and are not suitable for viscous solutions; they may damage certain drugs. Suspensions and highly viscous solutions decrease the propagation of ultrasonic sound waves, thus decreasing effective output from ultrasonic nebulisers.[17]

Nebulisers are either disposable or non-disposable. Disposable nebulisers are typically used only for a few weeks because they are subject to breaking and the particle size is affected. The particle size of the mist is important because it determines where in the lung the medication will be deposited. Non-disposable nebulisers last from 6 months to a year without changing the particle size in the mist.

## Hazards of aerosol therapy[18]

- Bronchospasm
- Infection
- Airway obstruction (sputum induction in child with poor cough reflex)
- Over-hydration (infants)
- Thermal injury (heated aerosols)
- Device malfunction

## PROCEDURE FOR ADMINISTRATION OF A NEBULISER

### The procedural goal is to

- maximise the dose that can be inhaled (quantity of drug),
- produce the right size particles that is quality of aerosol
- reduce the risk of side-effects due to unwanted drug deposition in the mouth, throat and upper airways.

### Equipment

Compatible nebuliser system and compressor/gas cylinder
Medication as prescribed
Hand washing/cleansing facilities

## PROCEDURE: Administration of a nebuliser

| Procedural steps | Evidence-based rationale |
|---|---|
| 1 Prepare the child (± parents) as appropriate. Use the help of a play specialist and use distraction and play techniques as required to keep child relaxed and breath as required[19] | The child must be relaxed with regular relaxed breathing and take the occasional deep breath to ensure optimal delivery of drug to the lungs |
| 2 Read the equipment instructions completely before you use a nebuliser. Ensure that compressor, nebulising equipment and drug to be nebulised are compatible<br>If you are using a gas supply to nebulise a drug, set gas flow rate at least 6 litres/min | Studies indicate that mismatched compressor and nebulising equipment can cause problems: they must be compatible to guarantee correct dose delivery, e.g. only jet nebulisation is established as safe and efficacious for Pulmozyme therapy[17]<br>At least 6 litres/min required to produce small enough particles from solution in 5–10 minutes |
| 3 Check condition and servicing date of compressor and condition and change date of disposable for wear and tear. Replace as required | Compressors require annual servicing by manufacturer or local service provider.[11] Disposable components such as the mouthpiece, mask, tubing and nebuliser chamber should be changed every 3–4 months[11] |
| 4 Place nebuliser compressor on a firm flat service, not the floor | |

## PROCEDURE: Administration of a nebuliser (continued)

| | |
|---|---|
| 5 Wash your hands thoroughly and make sure that the nebuliser equipment is clean | For infection control |
| 6 Connect the mouthpiece, or mask, to the T-shaped elbow. Fasten the unit to the cup and connect the nebuliser tubing to the port on the compressor. Before reuse, run the nebuliser for a few seconds before adding medications | To ensure that the entire system is functioning correctly |
| 7 If using a multi-dose glass bottle of medicine when you use a nebuliser, use a blue needle and syringe to draw up and administer the correct dosage of medication as prescribed into the cup with saline solution. If the medicine is in single-use vials, twist the top off the plastic vial and squeeze the contents into the nebuliser cup | Only use medications made specifically for nebulisers. These agents are sterile, contain no contaminants or unwanted particles, and are mixed in exact proportions Ideally nebulisers are prescribed to be delivered in 2.5–5 mL volume. To achieve a 2.5 mL volume, normal saline 0.9 per cent may be prescribed. Never add water; this will cause bronchospasm |
| 8 *Mouthpiece or mask* Use a nebuliser mask for infants and child under 2 years of age. Ensure that the mask fits snugly over the child's face being sure it fits well so the mist does not get in the eyes. If the child becomes distressed; a parent/carer can hold the nebuliser mask on the child's face If developmentally/physiologically appropriate, use a mouthpiece for children over 2 years. Ask the child to place the mouthpiece between their teeth and close their lips around it | To maximise the efficiency of aerosol delivery from a nebuliser. Do not use a 'blow-by' method. This is when the parent/carer directs the flow of the vapour from the nebuliser toward the child. Studies have shown that this method is ineffective[5] as most of the medicine evaporates into the air A mouthpiece will deliver more medication than a mask[20] |
| 9 Place the child in a comfortable upright position, with the nebuliser in a horizontal position if possible | To achieve optimal administration and prevent spillage and ensure correct dose is administered |
| 10 Turn the compressor on and check the nebuliser for misting. When using a finger valve, cover the air hole to force air into the nebuliser. If you are not using a finger valve, the nebuliser will mist continually. | Ensure that the compressor is nebulising the drug effectively. If there is no mist; turn the compressor off and examine the system for leaks usually due to loose connections |
| 11 Tap the nebuliser intermittently during operation | To help the medication drop to where it can be misted and ensure that all the medication is expelled |
| 12 Encourage the child to take slow tidal breaths with occasional deep breaths (over 3–5 seconds) or use distraction and/or play therapy to achieve this | Maximises the efficiency of aerosol delivery from a nebuliser. Deep breaths help the medication time to deposit in the airway |
| 13 Run the compressor/gas until the nebuliser is complete. This is termed 'nebuliser dryness' and is defined as the point in time when the nebuliser was perceived to be no longer producing aerosol by distinctive changes in sound; usually described as a 'hiss' or 'spit'. Usually a 2.5–5 mL nebuliser takes 10 minutes | To terminate uncomfortable treatment when appropriate. Note that a small amount of residual liquid will be left in the chamber If nebuliser times are slow, the equipment should be cleaned and treatment tried again. If it remains slow, a spare nebuliser should be used |
| 14 Ensure that the child rinses their mouth out with water after nebulisation is finished | To prevent thrush from forming from medication left in the mouth. Also, the child is more likely to cooperate with treatment in the future since many drugs leave a bad taste in the mouth |
| 15 Following each use, wash the nebuliser mask in hot water with mild detergent, rinse with warm water and allow to air dry. Store the nebuliser and supplies in a clean, dry, and dust-free location | Neglecting to do so will promote bacteria growth |

## PROCEDURE: Administration of a nebuliser (continued)

| | |
|---|---|
| **16** Dispose of nebuliser tubing that becomes cloudy or retains moisture | To prevent bacteria or mould growth in the unit |
| **17** Replace disposable parts, tubing, and filters according to manufacturer's instructions | Using equipment longer than indicated will result in slower, less efficient delivery of medication |
| **18** Disposable components such as the mouthpiece, mask, tubing and nebuliser chamber should be changed every 3–4 months <br> Compressors require annual servicing by manufacturer or local service provider | To prevent bacteria or mould growth in the unit <br> Promote continued efficient delivery of medication and prolong life of equipment |

## CLEANING THE NEBULISER SYSTEM

Dirty nebulising equipment carries the potential for infection in the already vulnerable child.

### The procedural goal is to

* Keep the equipment from clogging and help it last longer

* Help prevent germs and bacteria that can cause respiratory infection.

Follow the manufacturer's instructions for cleaning and storage of the nebuliser machine. Not all nebuliser machine parts are dishwasher safe. Follow the procedure below.

## PROCEDURE: Cleaning the nebuliser system

| Procedural steps | Evidence-based rationale |
|---|---|
| **1** Remove the mask or mouthpiece and T-shaped elbow from the cup of the nebuliser machine. Remove the tubing and set it aside | The tubing should not be washed or rinsed |
| **2** Wash the mask or mouthpiece and T-shaped elbow with a mild dishwashing soap and warm water | To remove dirt particles and bacteria |
| **3** Rinse the mask or mouthpiece and T-shaped elbow in warm, running water for 30 seconds. Use cooled boiled water or sterile water for rinsing, if possible | To remove all remnants of detergent |
| **4** Shake off excess water and air dry on a clean cloth or paper towel | Air dry to reduce static which will reduce drug availability (static attracts drug to stick to sides of plastic) |
| **5** Put the mask or mouthpiece and T-shaped elbow, cup, and tubing back together, and connect the device to the compressor. Run the nebuliser machine for 10 to 20 seconds | To thoroughly dry the inside of it |
| **6** Disconnect the tubing from the compressor. Make sure the nebuliser is completely dry before storing it in a sealed plastic bag | To prevent growth of bacteria and mould |
| **7** Clean the surface of the compressor with a well-wrung, soapy cloth or sponge or clean with a 70 per cent alcohol disinfectant wipe. Never put the compressor in water | Use the leansing direction as advised by most manufacturers. Water and electricity are a dangerous mix: electricshock! |
| **8** Place a cover over the compressor. Keep in cool dry place | To prevent growth of bacteria and mould |

## USING A PEAK FLOW METER

A peak flow meter is a useful tool for objectively measuring the severity of asthma. The value obtained is called a peak expiratory flow rate (PEFR). The PEFR indirectly shows the degree of airway obstruction or narrowing

### The procedural goal is to

- assess severity of illness/disease
- determine course of therapy.

### Equipment

Peak flow meter
Disposable mouth piece
PEFR chart (Figure 21.2)

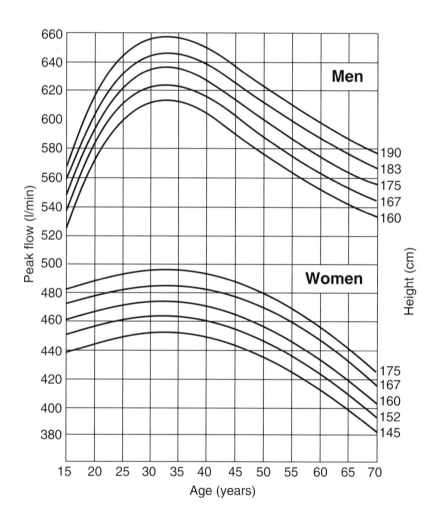

**Figure 21.2** Example of a PEFR normogram (reprinted with permission of Asthma, UK).

## PROCEDURE: Using a peak flow meter

| Procedural steps | Evidence-based rationale |
|---|---|
| 1 In order to obtain accurate results you need to fully inform and involve the child in this procedure. Therefore take time to explain:<br>• the purpose of the test<br>• the technique<br>The test may need repeated up to three times Usually it is worth well demonstrating the technique to the child by performing your own PEFR measurement. Ensure that the child understands your instructions and is willing to carry out the procedure | A peak flow meter can be used by most children over 6 years of age. Children under 6 years of age are not usually prescribed them because they tend to have difficulty in using a peak flow meter. It is more important to concentrate on getting a child to take their medication effectively and gauge asthma control by their symptoms than focus on PEFR measurement |
| 2 Collect appropriate size PEFR meter and check the serviceability of the PEFR meter. Check PERF meter is compliant with EN 13826 | Standard low-range peak flow meters are designed for children, or those with impaired function of their lungs<br>To use a correctly calibrated PEFR meter |
| 3 Wash your hands and encourage the child to do so and attach new disposable mouth piece to the meter | For infection control |
| 4 Before each use, make sure the sliding pointer on the peak flow meter is reset to the 'zero' mark[9] | To obtain accurate reading with 'no cheating' |
| 5 Ask the child to stand and hold the peak flow in a horizontal position while taking care not to place their fingers over the scale | To obtain most reliable result |
| 6 Instruct the child to take a deep breath filling their lungs completely and make a tight seal with their lips around the mouth piece. Observe the child closely making sure their tongue is not in the way | To ensure a reliable and accurate reading |
| 7 Ask the child to blow out as hard and as fast as they can. Observe the child making sure that their cheeks are not puffed out as they blow. Also, if the child coughs; they will need to do an additional blow | To ensure a reliable and accurate reading – a 'fast blast' is better than a 'slow blow'[9] |
| 8 Record the number that appears on the meter. Note the number where the sliding pointer has stopped on the scale. | |
| 9 Reset the pointer to 'zero'. Repeat these steps three times and record the highest of the three readings in an asthma diary | If the technique is done correctly, the three readings will be close together. The best reading is considered the best PEFR standard[17] |
| 10 Record PEFR pre and post treatment and compare to 'personal best' as described on page 356 | Random peak flow may not identify intermittent bronchospasm |

 Go to the website to find the PowerPoint presentation for this chapter and MCQs to test your knowledge. **www.hodderplus.com/childnursingskills**

**VIGNETTE**

**Problem:** How do I help a child to find their 'personal best' (PB) PEFR

**Discussion:** The 'personal best' (PB) PEFR is the highest reading that the child can achieve over a 2- to 3-week period. The PB is the number to which all other PEFR readings can be compared. To obtain a PB the child takes and records their PERF twice a day for 2–3 weeks at the same time in the morning and in the evening and before taking a short-acting B$_2$-agonist for quick relief (if taken). It is important to note that a child's PB can be less than their predicted PEFR value and still be completely normal. There are three asthma zones: the Green zone, the Yellow zone and the Red zone.[5]

Green zone: asthma is well-controlled. PEFR is 80–100 per cent of personal best.

Yellow zone: asthma is flaring up or is poorly controlled. PEFR is 50–80 per cent of personal best.

Red zone: asthma is severe; requires emergency care. PEFR is less than 50 per cent of personal best.

Predicted PEFs based on age, height, and gender are available (see Figure 21.2). These resources might be helpful, but the most important number is the child's own personal best PEFR

# REFERENCES

1   Bell J (2007). Resistance to resistance. Presentation 91. *Primary care: delivering the goods: inhaled therapies symposium.* ERS Annual Scientific Meeting, Stockholm.

2   Rees J (2005) Methods of delivering drugs. *British Medical Journal* 3: 504–6.

3   Everard ML (2003) Infant aerosol holding chambers face masks: not all are born equal. *Advanced Drug Delivery Review* 55: 869–878.

4   Asthma UK (2009) *Using your inhaler.* http://www.asthma.org.uk/using_your.html (accessed 14 March 2009).

5   Rubin BK, Fink JB (2003) The delivery of inhaled medication to the young child. *Pediatric Clinics of North America* 50: 1–15.

6   Dolovich MB, Ahrens RC, Hess DR (2005) Device selection and outcomes of aerosol therapy: evidence-based guidelines. *Chest* 127: 335–371.

7   Iles R, Lister P, Edmunds AT (1999) Crying significantly reduces absorption of aerosolised drug in infants. *Archives of Disease in Childhood* 81: 163–165.

8   Global Initiative for Asthma (2003) *Global strategy for asthma management and prevention.* Bethesda, MD: NIH

9   British Thoracic Society and SIGN (2008) *British guideline on the management of asthma.* London: BTS and SIGN www.brit-thoracic.org.uk/Portals/0/Clinical%cent20Information/Asthma/Guidelines/asthma_final2008.pdf (accessed 14 March 2009).

10  Education for Health (2006) *Simply devices: a practical pocket book.* Education for Health, Warwick.

11  Kamin WES, Genz T, Roeder S, *et al.* (2002) Mass output and particle size distribution of glucocorticosteroids emitted from different inhalation devices depending on various inspiratory parameters. *Journal of Aerosol Medicine* 15: 65–73.

12  National Institute for Health and Clinical Excellence (2005) *Inhaler devices for routine treatment of chronic asthma in older children (aged 5–15 years).* Technology Appraisal Guidance No. 38. London: NICE. http://guidance.nice.org.uk/TA38 (accessed 14 March 2009).

13  National Institute for Health and Clinical Excellence (2007) *Inhaled corticosteroids for the treatment of chronic asthma in children under the age of 12 years.* Technology Appraisal Guidance No. 131. London: NICE. http://guidance.nice.org.uk/TA131 (accessed 14 March 2009).

14  Jevon P (2007) Respiratory procedures: use of an inhaler. *Nursing Times* 103(38): 24–25.

15  Asthma UK (2009) Using a spacer. London: Asthma UK,. www.asthma.org.uk/all_about_asthma/medicines_treatments/spacers.html (accessed 14 March 2009).

16  Pearce L (2002) Know how: inhaler devices. *American Journal of Respiratory Critical Care Medicine* 98: 16–21.

17  Newman SP, Pellow PG, Clay MM, Clarke SW (2005) Evaluation of jet nebulisers for use with gentamicin solution. *Chronic Respiratory Disease* 2(1): 35–41.

18  Conway SP (2005) Nebulized antibiotic therapy: the evidence. *Chronic Respiratory Disease* 2(1): 35–41.

19  Rubin BK, Fink JB (2005) Optimizing aerosol delivery by pressurized metered-dose inhalers. *Respiratory Care* 50: 1191–1200.

20  National Formulary British (2008) *British national formulary for children 2008.* London: Pharmaceutical Press. www.bnf.org/bnf/bnf/current/3058.htm?q=%oxygen%#_hit (accessed 14 March 2009).

# Non-invasive respiratory therapy
## B) Oxygen therapy

Marion Aylott

## LEARNING OUTCOMES

*Upon completion of this chapter, the reader should be able to accomplish the following:*

1 Define hypoxia and demonstrate understanding of the indications for oxygen therapy
2 Correctly identify an oxygen cylinder
3 Discuss the health and safety requirements requiring consideration when administering oxygen or handling oxygen equipment
4 Describe safe methods of oxygen administration with reference to flow rate, delivery system, service user monitoring and response
5 Discuss the assembly, care and use of oxygen delivery systems
6 Demonstrate understanding of preparing the child and family for home oxygen therapy

## KEY WORDS

Respiration therapy    Hypoxia    Oxygen
Fire device safety

## CHAPTER OVERVIEW

In contrast to the adult, the paediatric patient presents a spectrum of age-specific physiological differences which are continuously changing during growth and development. Generally, these physiological differences are most striking in the preterm and newborn baby, but also present in infancy, although the situation gradually changes into the adult standard towards the end of puberty. Disease-inflicted changes interfere with this growth and development, thus further modifying structure and function.[1] To add further complexity, there is a changing psychological basis to the nurse–patient interaction throughout childhood[4] and voluntary cooperation and therapeutic techniques will generally not be possible before the end of the pre-school period (4 years of age). It follows that respiratory therapeutic intervention must take a physiological, psychological and developmental approach that differs substantially from the methodology routinely applied in practice.

## Definitions

**Respiration:** the exchange and transport of oxygen and carbon dioxide between cells and the atmosphere

**Oxygenation:** the delivery of oxygen to the body's tissues and cells

**Therapy:** the treatment of disease or of any physical or disorder by physical means

**Hypoxia:** insufficient oxygenation of the tissues

With due consideration to the continuing changes in respiratory structure and function, and the requirement for different applications of oxygen therapy in each age group, this chapter presents a child-friendly approach to the techniques required when administering oxygen therapy.

The air a person normally breathes contains approximately 21 per cent oxygen ($O_2$). An injured or ill child can benefit greatly from receiving air with a higher $O_2$ concentration. Without adequate $O_2$, hypoxia, a condition in which insufficient $O_2$ reaches the cells, will occur. The signs and symptoms of hypoxia include:

- increased breathing and heart rate;
- increased work of breathing;
- changes in level of consciousness;
- restlessness or lethargy;
- cyanosis (bluish lips and nail beds).

Oxygenation of the tissues depends on:

- adequate ventilation of alveolar units;
- diffusion of oxygen across the alveolar–capillary interface;
- appropriate lung perfusion, matched to the area of ventilation.

$O_2$ therapy is prescribed in any acute or chronic condition causing inadequate tissue oxygenation (hypoxaemia). Such conditions most commonly involve the lung, but the $O_2$ cascade can be adversely affected anywhere from the airway to cell oxidative processes. Indeed, in some cases increased metabolic demand for $O_2$ exacerbates the problem. However, giving $O_2$ does not guarantee its arrival at the mitochondria and $O_2$ does not improve ventilation directly.[1] In addition to this, it is important that the nurse remembers at all times that considerable improvement can be obtained by obtaining the child's and parent's confidences as reduced respiratory efforts will lead to improved air entry.

It is important to note that *oxygen has no effect on breathlessness if the oxygen saturation is normal*.[2]

Potential hypoxaemia can occur

- during heavy sedation use with young children, e.g. postoperatively especially after major abdominal or thoracic surgery or if there is evidence of cardiac or respiratory disease;
- following/during use of intravenous anti-convulsants, e.g. lorazepam and diazepam.

---

**KEY POINTS**

- An $SpO_2$ of less than 94 per cent indicates hypoxia
- An $SpO_2$ less than 90 per cent indicates severe hypoxia

---

## OXYGEN THERAPY

Oxygen therapy is the administration of $O_2$ at a concentration greater than ambient air to increase $O_2$ transport by ensuring full saturation of haemoglobin and increasing the level of dissolved $O_2$ in the plasma with the intent of treating or preventing the symptoms and manifestations of hypoxia. The practitioner must bear in mind that $O_2$ is a drug and must be used in accordance with well-recognised pharmacological principles, that is it has certain toxic effects and is not completely harmless (as widely believed) and it should be given only in the lowest dosage or concentration required by the particular child (Box 21.1, page 359). Compared with the adult, the child:[1]

- has less $O_2$ reserve;
- has higher $O_2$ requirement per kg;
- from a small change in supplemental inspired oxygen delivery ($FiO_2$) will show a large change in arterial oxygenation ($PaO_2$);
- with unrestricted $O_2$ therapy will be subject to pulmonary/extrapulmonary hazards;
- with unrestricted $O_2$ therapy will suffer potentially preterm blindness.

However, no specific contraindications exist when hypoxia is judged to be present that is hypoxia. All of the problems listed in Box 21.1 can be reduced by using correct delivery methods and monitoring oxygen saturation levels effectively. Research shows that complications of oxygen therapy in children are most often the result of suboptimal delivery and monitoring techniques.[2]

In 2008, The British Thoracic Society (BTS)[2] published the first national guidance on oxygen use, Although adult focused, this landmark guidance makes important recommendations for principles underpinning safe and effective clinical practice that are equally applicable to the paediatric patient. Nurses have a vital part to play in the use of oxygen, and it is hoped this BTS guidance will help to standardise care in this area (Table 21.3).

**Table 21.3** Practitioners' responsibilities[1]

| Doctors | Nurses and healthcare support workers |
| --- | --- |
| Prescribe $O_2$ | Start $O_2$ and achieve the target immediately |
| Circle the target saturation | Monitor $O_2$ 4-hourly (minimum); record $SpO_2$ and delivery device |
| Sign the drug chart | Titrate and wean off $O_2$ |
| Record the device to be used | Sign the drug chart every drug round |
| Stop $O_2$ when the target $SpO_2$ is achieved on air and the patient is clinically stable | Write and initial codes on the observation chart |

### Box 21.1 $O_2$ therapy: complications/cautions[3,4]

*Pulmonary oxygen toxicity:* excess $O_2$ depletes protective antioxidants. Inflammatory response then occurs

*Central nervous system toxicity:* $O_2$ toxicity is caused by free radicals and may result in seizures when the partial pressure exceeds 200 kPa (1500 mmHg).

*Retinopathy of prematurity:* immature peripheral retina is avascular and sensitive to $O_2$ and constricts if levels are too high. In severe cases, there may be impaired vision and even blindness

*Congenital heart disease:* the administration of supplemental oxygen to patients with certain congenital heart lesions (e.g. hypoplastic left heart, single ventricle) may cause an increase in alveolar oxygen tension and compromise the balance between pulmonary and systemic blood flow

*Tracheobronchitis:* $O_2$-induced inflammation of the trachea

*Discomfort:* prolonged use of dry $O_2$ at high concentrations can lead to drying of mucous membranes

*Absorption atelectasis:* where the absorption of $O_2$ from the alveoli exceeds the replenishment of the alveolar gas

*Fire:* $O_2$ supports combustion[5]

*Respiratory depression with hypoxic drive:* In a small proportion of people with severe chronic pulmonary disease, hyperoxia can depress central respiratory drive, resulting in hypoventilation and hypercapnia. It very rarely occurs in children

*Variable delivery:* oxygen delivery dependent of child's tidal volume as well as delivery method

**KEY POINTS**

- $O_2$ is a life-saving drug;
- Giving too much o $O_2$ is unnecessary as it cannot be stored in the body;
- Too much $O_2$ may be harmful
- Practitioners should give only as much $O_2$ as is needed

**KEY POINTS**

As with all drugs, $O_2$ can cause complications and involves risk. $O_2$ should be regarded as a drug and should be prescribed safely, administered accurately and monitored effectively. All children requiring oxygen therapy will have a prescription for $O_2$ therapy recorded on the patient's drug prescription chart. The only exception is an emergency situation[6]

**VIGNETTE**

**Problem:** It is has been suggested by a member of the medical staff that you administer $O_2$ via a nasopharyngeal catheter (nasogastric tube inserted into the pharynx and connected to $O_2$ tubing).

**Discussion:** A nasogastric tube is not designed or tested for being an $O_2$ delivery device. Furthermore, it is strongly recommended that this method of administering $O_2$ is avoided for a number of reasons as follows:

- improper insertion can cause gagging and nasal or pharyngeal trauma
- improper sizing can lead to nasal obstruction or irritation
- excessive flow can produce pain in the frontal sinuses
- excessive secretions and/or mucosal inflammation can result
- skin irritation can occur
- excessive flow may cause gastric distension.

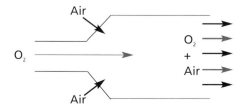

**Figure 21.4** Venturi Bernoulli effect.

Although principally life saving, in certain circumstances it can be lethal if prescribed and/or administered incorrectly. To ensure safe, effective delivery of $O_2$, health professionals dealing with the administration, titration and monitoring of $O_2$ therapy should understand the principles that underpin its use.

## PROCEDURE: General principles

| Procedural steps | Evidence-based rationale |
|---|---|
| **1** Acute care<br>All children and young people requiring $O_2$ therapy should have a prescription for $O_2$ therapy recorded on the drug prescription chart. The only exception is an emergency situation. The prescription should incorporate[2] | $O_2$ should be regarded as a drug and should be prescribed |
| • a target saturation identified by the clinician prescribing the $O_2$ in accordance with the Trust's oxygen guidelines; | Those children at risk of hyperoxaemia require different target ranges for their $O_2$ saturation, particularly the preterm neonate and, rarely, children with chronic respiratory failure |
| • an initial starting dose (i.e. delivery device and flow rate);<br>• in acute circumstances, the drug chart should be signed at every drug round;<br>• but, lack of a prescription should never preclude oxygen being given when it is needed in an emergency situation. A written record must be made of the oxygen therapy given to the patient, as with all emergency treatment[6]<br>• in an emergency $O_2$ can be administered by a registered nurse without a prescription | To provide the nurses with guidance for the appropriate starting point for the $O_2$ delivery system and flow rate<br>To ensure that the patient is receiving oxygen if prescribed and to consider weaning and discontinuation<br>For critically ill patients, high-concentration emergency $O_2$ should be administered immediately to combat actual or potential oxygen deficit without waiting for oxygen saturation (unreliable in these circumstances) and/or blood gas results as this will cause delay during which the child may be exposed to unnecessary hypoxaemia<br>In the first instance $O_2$ should be administered in high concentration via a non-rebreathing mask (with reservoir bag).[6] Flow rate should be at least 10 litres/minute and the child should not be left unattended |
| **2** Long-term $O_2$ therapy (LTOT)<br>LTOT is indicated for chronic hypoxaemia, which may occur as a result of different conditions, e.g. bronchopulmonary dysplasia, cystic fibrosis or for children with nocturnal hypoventilation, which can result from obesity, chest wall disease or obstructive sleep apnoea | $O_2$ should be regarded as a drug and should be prescribed[2] as above and as in Figure 21.3 (page 361). However, due to the geographical displacement at home from specialist care, the prescription must be accompanied by a detailed individual management plan provided by the respiratory consultant, which provides additional information with regards to a sliding scale of parameters of variables with indication of when to seek advice and who to contact for advice, and the necessary information about equipment needs for the $O_2$ supplier and contractor (PCT) |

**Figure 21.3** Medical oxygen prescription.

| DRUG | OXYGEN |
|---|---|
| (Refer to Trust oxygen policy) | |

| Circle target oxygen saturation | STOP DATE |
|---|---|
| 88–92%    94–98%    Other_____ | |

| Starting device/flow rate_____ | |
|---|---|

| PRN/continuous | PHARM |
|---|---|

| Tick if saturation not indicated (Saturation is indicated in almost all cases except for palliative terminal care) | |
|---|---|

| SIGNATURE/PRINT NAME | DATE dd/mm/yy |
|---|---|

## OXYGEN DELIVERY DEVICES

When a child is hypoxic and in respiratory distress, supplemental oxygen, is your first priority. The choice of interface is crucial to the flow rate of $O_2$. In most types of interface, inspired $O_2$ is mixed with entrained air, but the degree of mixing depends on the child's tidal volume and flow rate as well as the type of interface[8] (Tables 21.4 and 21.5). You must endeavour to select a device appropriate to his or her condition and size. Knowing the characteristics of each oxygen delivery device will help you make the right choice. Please note that the bag–valve–mask device with reservoir, used for providing assisted ventilation for the child with absent or ineffective spontaneous breathing,[8] is not included as an $O_2$ delivery device. This device should not be used for 'wafting' $O_2$

delivery, as the flow-back valve may close and result in insignificant levels of $O_2$ delivery.[8]

Please see the website for information on fire safety considerations and $O_2$.

## DELIVERING OXYGEN THERAPY

The need for $O_2$ therapy is determined by measurement of inadequate oxygen tensions and saturations by invasive or non-invasive methods and/or the presence of clinical indicators as previously described. Supplemental $O_2$ flow should be titrated to maintain adequate oxygen saturation as indicated by pulse oximetry $SpO_2$ or appropriate arterial or venous blood gas values.[9] Therapeutic outcome is assessed by determining whether the device selected produces an appropriate increase in $SpO_2$, proves to be appropriate for the child, allows adequate monitoring and facilitates care.

### The procedural goal is to

1 to correct or prevent potentially harmful hypoxaemia;
2 to achieve adequate delivery of oxygen to the tissues without creating oxygen toxicity;
3 to alleviate breathlessness (only if hypoxaemic); remember $O_2$ has no effect on breathlessness if the $O_2$ saturation is normal.

### Equipment

A delivery device: see Tables 21.4 and 21.6 (pages 362–3)
An oxygen supply: piped, cylinder, air compressor
A flow meter: controls the amount of $O_2$ administered in litres per minute (LPM)

**Table 21.4** Variable low-flow $O_2$ delivery devices

| | Simple mask (SM) | Flow-by 'wafting' (W) | Nasal cannulae (NC) | Head box (HB) |
|---|---|---|---|---|
| Description | A plastic cup used to deliver low dose $O_2$. Child must be breathing spontaneously | Method adopted for use with children who require low doses of $O_2$ and do not tolerate SM | A plastic tube which fits behind the ears, and a set of two prongs which are placed in the nostrils. $O_2$ flows from these prongs | Plastic enclosure, typically used for infants, enclose the head and neck in an $O_2$-enriched atmosphere for the infant to breathe in |

| Table 21.4 (continued) | Simple mask (SM) | Flow-by 'wafting' | Nasal cannulae (W) | Head box (NC) (HB) |
|---|---|---|---|---|
| Delivery (%) strengths | 35–50 Cheap | >30 Effective strategy for the delivery of $O_2$ to a child who does not tolerate SM Suitable for an alert child in moderate respiratory distress who requires a low does of $O_2$ | 25–36 Better tolerated in children than in SM system Allows nose to humidify the dry inspired gas Frees mouth for talking/feeding Preferred method for long-term therapy | Up to 40 Suitable for infants: unable to maintain $SpO_2$ >93% with NC or SM this system is advised where thick secretions may preclude NC use or when a child is not tolerating NC or SM use |
| Weaknesses | Effectiveness that is percent oxygen is influenced by: • $O_2$ flow rate (L/min) • leakage between SM and face • child's tidal volume and breathing rate Often poorly tolerated by young children and limits activities, e.g. feeding, talking | Requires constant supervision Highly variable success | Supplies a continuous flow of $O_2$ to the nose, and fills the anterior portion of the nostrils, mixing with inspired air The amount of $O_2$ inspired is limited and difficult to measure Influenced by the child's tidal volume and breathing rate Max. $O_2$ flow: 2 litres/minute in for infants Max. $O_2$ flow for older children: 4 litres/minute | Opening the HB decreases the $O_2$ concentration For infants and children confined to a HB, NC or $WO_2$ may need to be supplied during feeding/nursing care Possibly inhibits infant-to-parent interaction; confining and isolating |
| How to apply | Gently place SM over the child's face, position the strap behind the head or the loops over the ears then carefully pull both ends through the front of the SM until secure | A simple $O_2$ SM placed on the chest can give sufficient $O_2$ therapy | Place the two prongs into the nostrils making sure the prongs face upward and follow the curve of the nostrils. Ensure that the flat tab by the prongs rests above the child's upper lip. Secure tubing behind each ear and adjust it below their chin | Place appropriate sized HB over the head and neck of the infant taking care to ensure box is not trapping fingers or pressing against infant's skin |

| Table 21.4 (continued) | Simple mask (SM) | Flow-by 'wafting' | Nasal cannulae (W) | Head box (NC) (HB) |
|---|---|---|---|---|
| Directions for use | $O_2$ flow *must* be set to a minimum of 5 litres/minute to facilitate clearance of $CO_2$<br>Ventilation holes should never be blocked up as they are there to prevent $CO_2$ build-up | From the top of the SM a flow rate of 8 litres/minute, delivers 30% to an area 35 × 32 cm 10 L/minute, 40% is delivered to an area 16 × 14 cm<br>Note that $O_2$ tubing gives an area too narrow for practicable use | 1 litres/minute gives ~24%<br>2 litres/minute gives ~28%<br>3 litres/minute gives ~32%<br>4 litres/minute gives ~36%<br>Low birth weight/ ex-preterm infants require minute adjustments in flow rate. Low flow meters (0.1–1 litres /minute) and Ultra low flow meters (0.02 and 0.12 litres/minute) are available | Set min. flow rate at 10–15 litres/minute using combination of humidified warm air and oxygen. Flows >7 litres/minute are required to wash out $CO_2$<br>$O_2$ concentrations may vary within the HB: $O_2$ concentrations should be measured by placing a separate $O_2$ analyser as near the nose and mouth as possible<br>Humidify gases to provide a neutral thermal environment |
| Cautions | Not to be used for $CO_2$-retaining children<br>Unheated gas, may induce cold stress in neonates<br>Aspiration of vomit may be more likely when a mask is in place<br>Irritation may result from tight application<br>Rebreathing of $CO_2$ may occur if total $O_2$ flow is inadequate | Stimulation of the superior laryngeal nerve may cause apnoea if the gas flow from the $O_2$ source is cool and is directed at the face of the infant<br>Unheated gas, may induce cold stress in neonates | Skin irritation can result from material used to secure the NC or from local allergic reaction to PVC<br>Improper sizing can lead to nasal obstruction or irritation<br>Displacement can lead to loss of $O_2$ delivery<br>Inadvertent CPAP may be administered depending upon the size of the NC, the gas flow, and the infant's anatomy<br>Irritation can result if flows are excessive<br>Risk of accidental strangulation<br>Use may be limited by the presence of excessive mucus drainage, mucosal oedema, or a deviated septum<br>Contraindicated with nasal obstruction, e.g. nasal polyps, choanal atresia | Monitor temperature within HB closely to reduce the potential for cold stress or apnoea from overheating in neonates<br>High gas flows may produce harmful noise levels<br>Mist may obscure view of infant<br>Use of an improperly sized hood can result in irritation of the infant's skin |

Table 21.5 High (flow) performance devices

|  | Venturi mask (VM) | Non-rebreather mask with reservoir (NRB) |
|---|---|---|
| Description | A modified SM able to deliver precise concentrations of $O_2$ to individuals | A modified face mask used with a reservoir bag in medical emergencies to deliver high concentration $O_2$ |
| Delivery (%) | 24–60 | Up to 98 |
| Strengths | High-performance device designed to deliver a specified and constant mixture of $O_2$ and air at above the maximum inspiratory flow rate<br>Changes in breathing do not affect the $O_2$ concentration delivered | Provides an $O_2$ concentration of 90–95% to the spontaneously breathing child |
| Weaknesses | To change the $O_2$ concentration, you have to change the coloured barrel and flow. | A tight fitting mask is required to deliver higher concentrations of $O_2$<br>Cannot be used with a high degree of humidity |
| How to apply | Gently place VM over the child's face, as for SM (above)<br>Select appropriate Venturi barrel;<br>    Blue = 24%<br>    White = 28%<br>    Yellow = 35%<br>    Red = 40%<br>    Green = 60%<br>Attach barrel firmly into the mask inlet. Set flow rate as indicated on Barrel. This does not affect the concentration of $O_2$ but allows the gas flow rate to match the child's breathing pattern<br>$O_2$ is forced through a short constriction. This has the effect of increasing gas flow; the Bernoulli effect (see Figure 21.4, page 359)<br>After gas is forced through the Venturi valve, the pressure drops suddenly due to the increase in area. The velocity or flow of the gas increases as a result, and air is entrained from either side of the valve | Once the NRB is attached and $O_2$ is flowing through it, ensure that the reservoir bag is inflated; place a gloved finger over the inlet valve of the NRB until the reservoir bag inflates. Then fit by gently placing the mask over the child's face, as for SM above<br>$O_2$ flows directly into the mask during inspiration and into the reservoir bag during exhalation. All exhaled air is vented through a port in the mask and a one-way valve between the bag and mask, which prevents rebreathing<br>$O_2$ is stored in the reservoir bag during exhalation by means of a one-way valve thus achieving high concentration $O_2$<br>Rebreathing of $CO_2$ may occur if total $O_2$ flow is inadequate |
| Directions for use | Ventilation holes should NEVER be blocked up as they are there to prevent $CO_2$ build-up | $O_2$ flow MUST be set to a minimum of 5litres/m to facilitate clearance of $CO_2$ |
| Cautions | Not appropriate for the neonatal population | *Not* to be used for $CO_2$ – retaining patients, except in life-threatening emergencies, or neonate<br>Aspiration of vomit may be more likely when a mask is in place.<br>Irritation may result from tight application |

**Table 21.6** Modes of O₂ delivery and specific considerations

| Mode | O₂ cylinder | O₂ concentrator | Piped O₂ |
|---|---|---|---|
| General description | Black with white collar gas cylinder requires a pressure (psi) valve that indicates how full cylinder is and a flow meter to be fitted[7]<br><br>O₂ temperature in cylinder is 15°C[7]<br><br>Pressure in cylinder is 137 bar[7] | An electrically operated machine which draws in room air, separates the O₂ from the other gases in the air and delivers O₂ at max 4–9 litres/ /minute of 90– 92% O₂ . Concentrator usually limited to 4 litres/minute as higher flows lose O₂ concentration<br><br>The flow regulator on the machine can give 1– 4 litres/minute but flow rates of 0.06 – 0.8 litres /minute can be given using an additional low flow meter<br><br>Most cost-effective and practical devices used to provide home O₂ | Liquid O₂ is stored in a container called a vacuum insulated evaporator (VIE). This allows the liquid O₂ inside to remain very cold at 170°C. Gaseous O₂ above the liquid is passed through a super-heater to raise the temperature to outside ambient levels. It then flows into the hospital pipeline system giving a continuous supply of piped O2 to outlets on wards and units.<br><br>O₂ temperature at outlet 16–18°C<br><br>Pressure at outlet: 10.5 bar<br><br>Cheapest mode. Most convenient in acute care setting |

---

## PROCEDURE:  Delivery oxygen therapy

| Procedural steps | Evidence-based rationale |
|---|---|
| 1 Assess the child's need for O₂ therapy in non-emergency situation aided by SpO₂ | Safe drug administration. Early recognition of the need for oxygen can be difficult as clinical features are often non-specific, including altered mental state, dyspnoea, pallor and central cyanosis, tachypnoea, increased work of breathing arrhythmias and altered mental status |
| 2 Determine the most appropriate method of O₂ administration and gather together equipment | It is the nurse's role to assess the child and select an appropriate system to deliver the O₂ as prescribed and to provide safe and effective delivery |
| 3 Explain the procedure to the child in a manner appropriate for the child's age and understanding, and parents as required. Include the following information: | Enable child and family self-regulatory behaviour and obtain informed consent through partnership with child and family<br>To provide reassurance and psychological support and |

## PROCEDURE: Delivery oxygen therapy (continued)

| | |
|---|---|
| • need for $O_2$ therapy<br>• rationale, explanation and choice (as appropriate) in method of delivery<br>• positive/expected benefits of treatment<br>• possible side-effects of treatment<br>• minimum duration of treatment<br>• inform child and carers as appropriate about the combustibility of $O_2$ | ensure maximum benefit is obtained from treatment Any subsequent changes in the child's status are more likely to be noticed at the earliest opportunity by the child/parent<br>Maintain health and safety; $O_2$ supports combustion. There is always a danger of fire when $O_2$ is being used[10] |
| **4** Allow child to position themselves as comfortably as possible; enlist parental help with young children | Young children in respiratory distress may become frightened or agitated when $O_2$ is administered, causing their clinical conditions to deteriorate. Therefore, they should remain in a position of comfort whenever possible |
| **5** In a non-emergency situation, administer $O_2$ to treat hypoxaemia as prescribed | $O_2$ is a treatment for hypoxaemia. $O_2$ will not have any effect on breathlessness in non-hypoxaemic child. $O_2$ is classed as a drug and the law requires that planned delivery of $O_2$ therapy is prescribed by a doctor |
| **6** In an emergency situation, administer high-concentration emergency $O_2$ immediately via a non-rebreathe mask with reservoir (NRB) with a flow rate of 10–15 litres/min<br><br>Prior to and during delivery, ensure patency of the airway | $O_2$ is used a first response measure to maintain adequate tissue oxygenation. An injured or ill child can benefit greatly from receiving air with a higher oxygen concentration. In an emergency, $O_2$ may be administered by registered nurses without a prescription.[2] Emergency $O_2$ administration is recorded in child's records once the child is stabilised.<br>Effective $O_2$ delivery relies on maintaining a clear and open airway |
| **7** Check that the system of $O_2$ delivery has the capacity to deliver the $O_2$ required for use | Make sure that you always maintain a safe residual for an $O_2$ cylinder. Safe residual for an $O_2$ cylinder is a minimum of 200 psi. Below this point, there is not enough $O_2$ for proper delivery. Before pressure reaches 200 psi, switch to a fresh cylinder<br>A concentrator is able to deliver oxygen at a maximum 5–8 litres/min of 90–92 per cent $O_2$ and requires an electricity supply |
| **8** Before use, ensure that the delivery system's sterile packaging for the tubing, mask and nasal cannulae are not damaged and 'in-date'<br>Set up administration device and supply set-up as per prescription[2] and manufacturer's instructions,[10] e.g. cylinder name, colour code and service history label | To maintain safety |
| **9** Attach the delivery device to the $O_2$ supply using appropriate $O_2$ tubing of sufficient length | Tubing should be of sufficient length to cover all situations but not long enough to kink or touch the floor in hospital (infection control) |
| **10** If portable $O_2$ cylinders being used these should enable adequate oxygen provision<br>Litres in cylinder/litres needed per minute = no. of minutes $O_2$ is available | The number needed to, for example, complete a journey, must be carefully calculated prior to embarking. A nomogram may help you to predict this (Table 21.7, page 000) |
| **11** Administer humidification as required[11]<br>The simplest way of overcoming this with low to | Medical $O_2$ is a cold dry gas, which requires humidification by the upper respiratory tract to bring |

## PROCEDURE: Delivery oxygen therapy (continued)

| | |
|---|---|
| moderate flow $O_2$ is the use of a cold water bubble-through humidifier. These are driven by oxygen and entrain air at the humidifying device according to the $O_2$ percentage setting<br>Please see the website for illustration of a cold water bubble-through system | it to 100 per cent humidity at 37°C.1 At 1–4 litres/min the upper airway usually provides adequate humidification. However, infants receiving flows of greater than 1 litres/min can be uncomfortable causing nasal dryness, irritation or concreted nasal secretions[11]<br>When moderate flow $O_2$ is administered for longer than 24 hours the inspired $O_2$ should be humidified by passing it through fan-driven humidifier<br>Note that fluid hydration is a significant factor in maintaining sufficient humidification |
| 12 Before placing the $O_2$ delivery device in situ as advised by manufacturer, always make sure that $O_2$ is flowing through the device | To maintain safety; check the device is functioning correctly |
| 13 Ensure device is fitted comfortably; the tubing for kinking; is in place and that any required monitoring is correctly attached to the child; commence clinical recordings as required | To maintain comfort, security and safety<br>The effectiveness of oxygen delivery should be monitored with pulse oximetry[2] |
| 14 Observe and record the child's $SpO_2$ for at least 5 minutes after starting oxygen therapy. Adjust delivery devices and flow rates to keep the $SpO_2$ within the target range | To identify if oxygen therapy is maintaining the target $SpO_2$ or if an increase or decrease in $O_2$ therapy is required. Note that there is little value in 'spot check' $SpO_2$ levels to assess ongoing $O_2$ need in any situation that is emergency, acute or chronic illness.[12] A period of monitoring which includes periods of sleep and wakefulness (and at least one feed/meal time) is essential for clinically useful information to be gained) |
| 15 Interpret $SpO_2$ alongside the child's clinical status incorporating respiratory rate, work of breathing, heart rate, temperature, and if necessary, blood pressure | The $O_2$ delivery device and $O_2$ flow rate/inspired $O_2$ concentration should be recorded on the observation chart with the $SpO_2$ reading. To identify early signs of clinical deterioration, e.g. elevated respiratory rate (see Chapter 9) |
| 16 Adjust the flow rate as necessary by turning the finger valve to obtain the desired flow rate. The centre of the ball (float) shows the correct flow rate (Figure 21.5, page 000) | To accurately deliver the prescribed $O_2$ sufficient to achieve and maintain target $SpO_2$ |
| 17 If the child's $SpO_2$ falls outside of the target saturation range, adjust the $O_2$ flow rate accordingly. Monitor $SpO_2$ continuously for at least 5 minutes after any increase or decrease in $O_2$ dose | To ensure that the child achieves the desired saturation range and is maintained within the desired range.<br>The recommended target $SpO_2$ range for the acutely ill child as 94–98 per cent and 88–92 per cent for the child at risk of hypercapnic respiratory failure[2] |
| 18 Repeat vital signs, record per cent/litre flow of $O_2$, $SpO_2$ and delivery system (integrity) observations at intervals determined by the child's clinical situation and documented appropriately,[2] e.g.<br>• emergency situation: every 15 minutes<br>• acute situation: hourly<br>• chronic situation: 4–8 hourly<br>If a child is stable and receiving intermittent therapy, 8-hourly monitoring is recommended[13] | Frequent assessment and observations are an integral part of care, enabling the detection of changes in the child's condition and assessment of therapy effectiveness. To maintain child's clinical safety, all care should be delivered on an individual basis and checked at appropriate intervals to reduce clinical risk e.g. young children appear to be remarkably successful at dislodging nasal cannulae |

## PROCEDURE: Delivery oxygen therapy (continued)

| | |
|---|---|
| 19 If the child's $SpO_2$ is lower than the target specified<br>• check all elements of delivery system for faults or errors<br>• step up $O_2$ therapy as per prescription/emergency protocol<br>• any sudden fall in $SpO_2$ should lead to clinical evaluation and in most cases measurement of blood gases[9] | In most instances a fall in $SpO_2$ is due to deterioration of the child; however, equipment faults should be checked for<br>To assess the child's response to $O_2$ increase, and ensure that $PaCO_2$ has not risen to an unacceptable level, or pH dropped to an unacceptable level and to screen for the cause of deteriorating $O_2$ level, e.g. chest infection[2] |
| 20 If $SpO_2$ is higher than target specified or >98 per cent for an extended period of time,[2] step down $O_2$ flow rate as per prescription and/or consider discontinuation of therapy | $O_2$ is delivered at the lowest concentration possible and for the shortest possible time |
| 21 While $Sp O_2$ is within the target specified,[2] continue with $O_2$ therapy, and monitor child to identify appropriate time for stepping down therapy, once clinical condition allows | $O_2$ is administered in the lowest possible concentration to produce the most acceptable oxygenation without causing toxicity |
| 22 A change in delivery device (without an increase in $O_2$ therapy) does not require review by a doctor[2] | The change may be made in the stable child as regards preference, activity or comfort |
| 23 Check the child's mouth and nose and behind the ears; observe the skin where the cannula tube or mask strap rests against the skin for signs of inflammation according to skin integrity status, e.g. 1–2 hourly for infants<br>Check mask and cannula device at least 2 hourly for cleanliness/blockage. Use a water-soluble lubricating jelly, such as K-Y Jelly on lips and nose. Do not get the lubricating jelly in the cannula or mask | To identify signs of infection and pressure sores as soon as possible and intervene as appropriate, e.g. it is recommended that a hydrocolloid dressing is often used below nasal cannulae tubing to protect the cheeks of infants from pressure sores<br>Epistaxsis and crustation are common problems associated with long-term use of oxygen through nasal prongs in children suffering from chronic lung disease. The nasal prong can cause direct trauma to the septal mucosa.[14] Also dried secretions can obstruct small airways. Petroleum-based products are contraindicated as they constitute a fire hazard |
| 24 Check $O_2$ tubing daily for any obvious signs of damage such as kinking, flattening or splitting. If you notice any damage, replace the tubing immediately. Keep spare masks and cannulae to hand at all times | To maintain patency of delivery system. Take care that tubing does not become trapped, e.g. in furniture, doors, infants' cots, infants' high chairs as this will restrict, or even stop, the flow of $O_2$ |
| 25 In the absence of definitive studies to support change-out intervals, institution-specific and patient-specific surveillance measures should dictate the frequency with which such equipment is replaced. It is generally recommended that $O_2$ masks are washed daily using hot water and detergent and air dried thoroughly. Do not wash and re-use nasal cannulae as they cannot be dried thoroughly; replace these with new at least once a week | Infection control: $O_2$ devices should be kept as clean as possible.<br>Under normal circumstances, low-flow reservoir and head box systems do not present a clinically important risk of infection and do not require routine replacement on the same child. However, high-flow systems should be changed every 24 hours when applied to a child with an artificial airway |
| 26 Following use, ensure that flow valves (and cylinder/concentrator valves) are closed properly and equipment is stored correctly | For fire safety (please see the website for information on fire safety) |

**Table 21.7** Nomogram: $O_2$ cylinder capacity[15]

| Flow rate at litres/minute | D (340 litres) | E (680 litres) | F (1,360 litres) | PD (300 litres) |
|---|---|---|---|---|
| 0.1 | 56 h | 113 h | 226 h | 50 h |
| 0.2 | 28 h | 56 h | 113 h | 25 h |
| 0.3 | 18 h | 37 h | 75 h | 16 h |
| 0.4 | 14 h | 28 h | 56 h | 12 h |
| 0.5 | 11 h | 22 h | 45 h | 10 h |
| 0.6 | 9 h | 18 h | 37 h | 8 h |
| 0.7 | 8 h | 16 h | 32 h | 7 h |
| 0.8 | 7 h | 14 h | 28 h | 6 h |
| 0.9 | 6 h | 12 h | 25 h | 5 h |
| 1.0 | 5 h | 11 h | 22 h | 5 h |

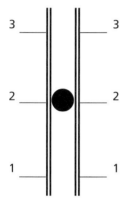

**Figure 21.5** Correct setting for 2 litres/min oxygen.

## DISCHARGE PLANNING FOR HOME OXYGEN THERAPY

The clinical decision that a child will receive home $O_2$ is made by the consultant in charge of the child's care in conjunction with the parents. Parents should understand the need for home $O_2$ therapy, be aware of the risks involved and willing and competent to look after the child at home. This includes being able to assess their child's respiratory pattern, recognise respiratory distress and be able to take relevant, timely and appropriate action. Discharge planning should begin on admission in line with the British Thoracic Society Guidelines.[2] The child's community team should be contacted as soon as discharge planning is started to facilitate a plan in a consistent, systematic process, and conducted in a collaborative manner. Communication of information between professionals and families is vital in order to ensure best follow-up care.[16] To ensure smooth transition of care from hospital to home, a child's management plan should include the following:

- $O_2$ prescription;
- amount of $O_2$ required;
- sliding scale of parameters with indications of when to seek advice and from whom;
- mode of delivery;
- delivery system required;
- all relevant equipment for home $O_2$ therapy;
- health and safety information.

Medical decisions required regarding the use of a pulse oximeter and/or apnoea alarm is appropriate for the home environment.[2] Limited evidence that the use of $O_2$ saturation monitors improves a patient's care at home shows that they can result in carers increasing the flow of $O_2$.[17] An adequate respiratory assessment should be used and reliance should not be placed on the $O_2$ saturation monitor,[18] although some support the use of oximeters in the home because they feel it reduces the providence of hospital admissions.[19]

## CONCLUSION

The objective of $O_2$ therapy is to give the child as much $O_2$ as is required to return their $O_2$ saturation to what is normal for the particular child. There is nothing to be gained by giving too much, and a huge amount to be lost by not giving enough.

Go to the website to find the PowerPoint presentation for this chapter and MCQs to test your knowledge. **www.hodderplus.com/childnursingskills**

## REFERENCES

1 Chamley CA, Carson P, Randall D, Sandwell M (2005) *Developmental anatomy and physiology of children: a practical approach*. Edinburgh: Elsevier & Churchill Livingstone.

2 O'Driscoll BR, L S Howard LS, Davison AG (2008) BTS guideline for emergency oxygen use in adult Patients. *Thorax* 63 (Suppl VI): vi1–vi68. www.brit-thoracic.org.uk/ClinicalInformation/EmergencyOxygen/tabid/219/Default.aspx (accessed 10 February 2009).

3 Firestone K, Adams, H (2007) Evidence-based oxygen therapy for very low birth weight infants, *Journal of Pediatric Nursing* 22(2): 145–180.

4 Primhak R (2007) Home oxygen therapy in children. *Paediatrics and Child Health*, 15(5): 202–205.

5 Ward L, Monaghan M, Flowers D, *et al.* (2008) *Teaching aids for nurses*. London: BTS. www.brit-thoracic.org.uk (accessed 10–02–09).

6 British Medical Association/Royal Pharmaceutical Society of Great Britain (2007) *British National Formulary 54*. London: BMA/RPSGB. www.bnf.org/bnf (accessed 12 February 2009).

7 Bailey P, Torrey SB, Wiley JF (2008) Oxygen delivery systems for infants and children. *UpToDate* 16(3): 11–16 http://www.uptodate.com/patients/content/topic.do?topicKey=~_Nu.n1gTObgzu (accessed 12 February 2009).

8 Davies P, Cheng D, Fox A, Lee L (2002) The efficacy of noncontact oxygen delivery methods *Pediatrics*, 110: 964–967.

9 Leach RM, Treacher DF (2006) The pulmonary physician in critical care. 2: oxygen delivery and consumption in the critically ill. *Thorax* 57(2): 170–177.

10 MHRA (2008) *Oxygen cylinders and their regulators: top tips on care and handling: advice for healthcare professionals*. London, DH. www.mhra.gov.uk/Publications/Postersandleaflets/CON01486 (accessed 11 February 2009).

11 Chandler T (2001) Oxygen administration. *Paediatric Nursing* 13(8): 37–42.

12 Pilkington F (2004) Humidification for oxygen in non-ventilated patients. *British Journal of Nursing* 13(2): 111–115.

13 Balfour-Lynn IM, Primhak RA, Shaw BNJ (2005) Clinical component for the domiciliary oxygen service for children in England and Wales. www.library.nhs.uk/respiratory/ViewResource.aspx?resID=111558 (accessed 21 February 2009).

14 McCoskey, L (2008) Nursing care guidelines for prevention of nasal breakdown in neonates receiving nasal CPAP. *Advances in Neonatal Care* 8(2): 116–124.

15 Lutman D, Petros AJ (2006) How many oxygen cylinders do you need to take on transport? A nomogram for cylinder size and duration. *Emergency Medicine Journal* 23: 703–704.

16 Primhak R (2001) Oxygen saturation and retinopathy of prematurity. *Archives of Disease in Childhood: Fetal & Neonatal Edition* 85(1): F75.

17 American Thoracic Society (2003) *Respiratory function in infants: measurement conditions*. www.thoracic.org/sections/publications/statements/pages/respiratory-disease-pediatric/402.html (accessed 12 February 2009).

18 American Thoracic Society (2003) Care of the child with chronic lung disease of infancy and childhood. www.thoracic.org/sections/publications/statements/pages/respiratory-disease-pediatric/childcare.html (accessed 12 February 2009).

19 Zhu Z, Barnette R, Fussell K, *et al.* (2005) Continuous oxygen monitoring- better way to prescribe long-term oxygen therapy. *Respiratory Medicine* 99: 1386–1392.

# Tracheostomy care

## Marion Aylott

### LEARNING OUTCOMES

*Upon completion of this chapter, the reader should be able to accomplish the following:*

1 Define tracheostomy and list two indications for it use in children
2 Identify three types of tracheostomy tube
3 List the emergency equipment and checks that should be performed at the beginning of a shift when looking after a child with a tracheostomy
4 Describe the potential complications a child with a tracheostomy might experience
5 Discuss the nursing care of a child with a tracheostomy including management of tracheostomy tube obstruction
6 Illustrate the importance of humidification
7 Discuss with rationale the recommended suction pressure, types, sizes and effects of suction catheters
8 Discuss with rationale the recommended techniques for delivering artificial breaths during basic life support

## CHAPTER OVERVIEW

Nurses often care for infants, children and young people with tracheostomy tubes. Within the first year of life, we can expect 3000 infants to undergo a tracheostomy.[1] Eighty-five per cent of these children requiring tracheostomies are less than 1 year old. The need for a tracheostomy may extend to several months or even years and some may require a permanent tracheostomy. The focus of this chapter is on clinical tracheostomy care skills; long-term care will be discussed in Chapter 23.

Tracheostomy care is a complex nursing activity and has many potential complications. Aspects of tracheostomy care are often carried out without much uniformity and with some confusion about correct techniques, especially outside the ear, nose and throat and intensive care environments. Some aspects of literature appear contradictory, leaving nurses to make sometimes ill-informed judgements about procedures. It is the nurse who is accountable for the care given; therefore, with the wealth of knowledge available, it is important that the nurse is adequately informed. The majority of tracheostomy-related complications are preventable or may be minimised by evidence-based care.

### KEY WORDS

| | | |
|---|---|---|
| Tracheostomy | Obstruction | Suction |
| Skin integrity | Dislodgement | |

### Indications for tracheostomy[6]

- To provide of an artificial airway
- To protect of airway
- To facilitate weaning from mechanical ventilation
- To provide of long-term ventilation.

## Definitions

A 'tracheostomy' (also called a 'stoma') refers to a surgically created passage from the skin to the trachea in the anterior neck into which a tube is placed to provide an artificial patent (open) airway.

Typically, the opening is created below the level of the vocal cords between the second and third tracheal rings.[5]

# PHYSIOLOGICAL CHANGES WITH A TRACHEOSTOMY

To maintain cellular respiration the upper and lower airways must be free of obstruction. In normal respiration, the upper airway plays an essential role in the conduction of air from the nose and mouth down to the thoracic inlet: its influence is due to its anatomical structure and the functional properties of the mucosa, cartilages and neural and lymphatic tissues present. The main functions of the nose are

- to regulate of air-stream
- to pre-warm and moisten the inhaled air
- to clean the inhaled air.

The nose is able to pre-warm air to 32–34°C and humidify air irrespective of ambient conditions. Inspired air reaches 37°C and 100 per cent relative humidity just below the carina.[2] The nasal mucociliary system can usually hold up to 70 per cent of passing dust particles, which are moved towards the nasopharynx by ciliary activity. However, a tracheostomy bypasses the nose and upper airway so that cold, dry and particulate air is delivered to the lungs. Cold, dry air and cold gases have been shown to damage the mucociliary system which lines the bronchial tree thus leading to impaired sputum clearance, making the child at risk for pneumonia.[3]

The lower part of the larynx consists of a circular piece of cartilage called the cricoid cartilage. In adults this is cylindrical and the narrowest part of the airway is at the vocal cord. But in the child before puberty, the airway is narrowest at the cricoid area and is cone shaped,[4] providing a natural cuff and thus an uncuffed tracheal tube is used.

# THE TRACHEOSTOMY TUBE

## Term

A tracheostomy may be formed selectively or as an emergency procedure and may be temporary or long term.

# Components

Tracheostomy tubes (TTs) are available in different designs and come with different features depending on their intended use. Uncuffed single-lumen tubes are preferred in children (Figure 22.1) under most circumstances because of the natural cuff provided by the trachea at the cricoid level.[4] TTs consist of three component parts (Figure 22.2).

Older children, post puberty, might require a cuffed tube (Figure 22.3).

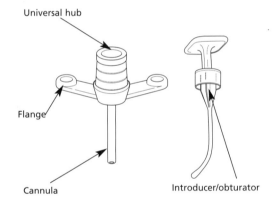

**Figure 22.1** Uncuffed Shiley.

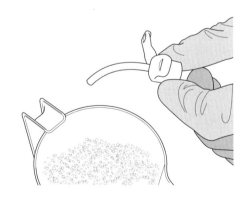

**Figure 22.2** Single lumen tube component parts.

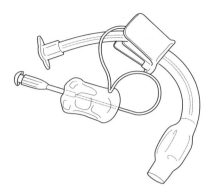

**Figure 22.3** Cuffed Shiley.

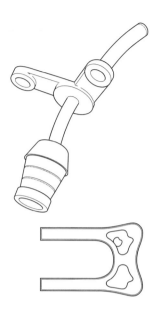

**Figure 22.4** Bivona tube and disconnect wedge.

## Composition

Synthetic TTs are mostly made of polyvinyl chloride, e.g. Shiley. However, when more flexibility is required, silicone tubes, for example Bivona or Arcadia, may be preferred (Figure 22.4). The Bivona has a wire-reinforced silicone shaft, which reduces the risk of kinking due to its length. These are particularly useful with young infants who naturally have short thick necks and need to spend time playing in the prone position. These tubes are not magnetic resonance imaging (MRI) compatible because of the wire reinforcement. A 'disconnect wedge' must be used when removing connections from the tracheal tube (Figure 22.4).

The use of metal TTs (Figure 22.5) is limited to special circumstances, e.g. allergy or after tracheal reconstruction. They consist of a double cannula: outer cannula remains in situ, through which a smaller inner cannula is inserted.

A fenestrated TT, which has holes (fenestration(s) in the middle of the upper aspect of an inner tube, is very rarely used in paediatrics. This allows the passage of air and secretions into the mouth and nose, thus facilitating speech and better clearance of secretions[6] by allowing better translaryngeal air flow.

## Size

Tracheostomy tubes have three dimensions:

- inner diameter (ID) (mm)
- outer diameter (OD)
- length.

The size is marked on the packaging and on the flange of each tracheostomy tube. In practice the ID is used for reference. All TTs have a standard 15-mm opening so that they can be attached to respiratory equipment. The choice and size of TT is made by the ear, nose and throat (ENT) consultant driven by clinical requirements.

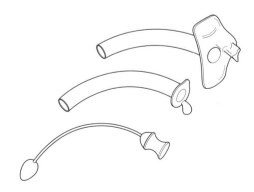

**Figure 22.5** Metal tracheostomy tube.

# COMPLICATIONS

The single most important risk and the greatest cause of morbidity and mortality is accidental obstruction due to mucous plugging or dislodgement of the tube.[14] Therefore, there should always be ready access to emergency equipment, and supplies should be readily available at the bedside. It is the nurse's responsibility to ensure that all emergency equipment is present and fully functioning. It is good clinical risk management to check all equipment at the beginning of each shift yourself. Other common complications include:

- haemorrhage
- inadvertent false passage during tube change
- subcutaneous emphysema
- tracheitis
- granuloma formation.

# EMERGENCY BEDSIDE TRACHEOSTOMY EQUIPMENT

It is recommended[6] that every person with a tracheostomy tube must have the following equipment available at the bedside:

- spare tracheostomy tube (same size and brand as one in situ);
- tracheostomy tube one size smaller than one currently in situ;
- appropriate tracheostomy ties;
- blunt-ended (bandage) scissors;
- self-inflating ventilation bag;
- suction equipment (assembled and working);
- suction tubing (change daily);
- suction catheters (correct size) with distal and lateral holes;
- humidification;
- non-sterile gloves, disposable aprons, goggles;
- clinical waste bag.

# HUMIDIFICATION

Air-conditioning mechanisms are bypassed when a tracheostomy tube is in situ; therefore, alternative methods of conditioning inspired air must be used. Failure to provide adequate humidity in inspired air may lead to damage to the airway mucosa. There are two approaches to humidification, selection depends on context and individual circumstances. In the initial postoperative period, heated humidification is advocated[7] and is mandatory when a TT is present. Later, children who do not require or those who are managed off mechanical ventilation for periods of time may use a heat–moisture exchanger (HME) (see Chapter 23).

## Equipment

Heating unit
1-litre bag of sterile water for irrigation
Appropriate giving set for disposable chamber unit and circuit

## The procedural goal is to

- achieve the desired humidity and temperature of 32–34°C at the carina
- prevent tube obstruction/viscous secretions.

## Rationale

Maximum mucosal function occurs in a relatively narrow range of warmth and humidity above and below the optimum physiological humidity. Large positive or negative deviations may cause deterioration in mucosal function to the point that cell damage occurs with resulting atelectasis.

## PROCEDURE:  Using a heated humidifier

| Procedural steps | Evidence-based rationale |
|---|---|
| **1** Set up as per operators manual | To promote safety[8] |
| **2** Prior to use and during start of shift: check and inspect the child-ventilator system and the humidification device visually. Ensure that heated-wire circuits are not covered and that circuits and humidifiers are compatible | Hazards and complications associated with the use of heated humidification devices include: potential for electrical shock, burns to patient and staff, tubing melt-down[9] |
| **3** If necessary remove condensate from the patient circuit as necessary. NEVER drain condensate back into the humidifier reservoir. If condensation collects in tubing; drain tubing onto paper towels and dispose of in clinical waste receptacle | Inadvertent tracheal lavage from pooled condensate in patient circuit[9]. Condensate is infectious waste |
| **4** Monitor the temperature of inspired gases. Set humidifier to deliver an inspired gas temperature of 38°C which should provide a minimum of 30 mg/litre of water vapour | This setting allows for the fall in temperature and humidity level between circuit temperature probe and patient so that inspiratory gas should not exceed 37°C |
| **5** The temperature probe should be located outside of the incubator or away from the direct heat of the radiant warmer | To reduce the risk of thermal injury and unintentional tracheal lavage from condensation ('rain-out') |
| **6** Set high temperature alarm to no higher than 39°C, and the low temperature alarm no lower than 34°C | To reduce the risk of thermal injury to the child[9] |
| **7** Check water level is at level as advised by manufacturer and automatic feed system is functioning correctly (if applicable). | Inadvertent over-filling can lead to unintentional tracheal lavage[9] |
| **8** Use a clean non-touch technique when manually filling the water reservoir. Use sterile water | To reduce the risk of cross infection |
| **9** Replace circuits weekly | To reduce the risk of cross infection |
| **10** Reusable heated humidifier devices should be disinfected between patients | To reduce the risk of cross infection |

## SKIN CARE AND TRACHEOSTOMY TIE CHANGE

The dressing should be intact for 24 hours if possible as the tracheostomy is a fresh wound, and during the first week it should be cleansed using an aseptic technique.[10] Dressings are not used once the wound has healed (after 7–10 days). Once the surgical wound has healed the stoma site is cleansed using a clean technique twice a day, usually morning and evening. The skin may need to be cleaned more often if it becomes dirty, moist, red or infected. It is often useful to plan to change the tracheostomy ties at the same time. The securing of the tie is as important as the type in children. There are two common types of material used for tracheostomy ties in the short-term period:

- twill tape
- Velcro ties.

Soiled ties contain mucus and micro-organisms. They should be changed as needed to maintain clean and dry skin. Moreover, ties, particularly twill tape, once soiled with saliva and allowed to dry, become like sharp blades which can cut into the child's skin. Also, try to avoid the routine use of ointment and dressings that trap moisture.

*Do not* perform procedure within 2 hours of feeding to minimise risk of vomiting and aspiration.

### The procedural goal is to

- maintain wound/skin hygiene, skin integrity and safety
- reduce the risk or accidental tube misplacement/displacement

### Equipment

Tracheostomy dressing (e.g. Trachi Dress, Trach Sponge, Lyofoam)
Sterile scissors
Sterile gloves
Minor dressing pack
Cleaned and disinfected dressing trolley/surface
Sterile normal saline
Sterile gauze swabs
Sterile pink mouth cleansing sponges (not cotton-tipped Q-tips)
Non-sterile gloves
Alcohol hand rub
Disposable apron × 2
Goggles
Clinical waste bag
Clean tracheostomy ties
Blunt-ended scissors

## PROCEDURE: Tracheostomy tie change

| Procedural steps | Evidence-based rationale |
| --- | --- |
| 1 Two people are required to perform this procedure one of whom should be experienced in tracheostomy care | Removing the tapes increases the risk of accidental tube dislodgement. The second person or assistant is required to hold the tube in place at all times[11] |
| 2 Select appropriate tie method. Is the child at risk of dislodging the tube? (age, agitation, neurological status)<br>Do not use Velcro ties if the child:<br>• is known to pick at tapes<br>• is not cognitively aware of importance and role of tube (usually under 5 years old)<br>• is confused or agitated<br>Is the surrounding skin intact and able to withstand the pressure/abrasion from a tape? | Secure the tube safely |
| 3 Explain procedure to the child and parents as appropriate | Informing the child and encouraging their participation has been identified as a strategy to reduce stress and anxiety |
| 4 Assemble equipment and supplies, including emergency equipment and place near to hand on an appropriate surface. | Maintain a safe environment. Emergency equipment may be needed in the event of accidental decannulation. *This equipment is required at the bedside with the child at all times.* |
| 5 If appropriate prepare dressing trolley/surface, including opening outside wrapping of dressing pack, opening sterile gloves and laying them on the top of the unopened inner wrap of the dressing pack | Easily accessible equipment reduces the risk of infection |
| 6 Screen the bed or cubicle | To ensure privacy |
| 7 Position child as appropriate;<br>• semi-recumbent position<br>• supine with a small rolled towel or blanket under the shoulder<br>• swaddle infants | To promote ease of change and child comfort. A Semi-Fowler's position decreases abdominal pressure on the diaphragm, which in-turn promotes lung expansion. Shoulder roll extends the child's neck slightly to allow easy access to the stoma |

## PROCEDURE:  Tracheostomy tie change (continued)

| | |
|---|---|
| 8  Prior to main procedure, suction tracheostomy/ or ask the child to cough[18] | To reduce the need for suctioning during the procedure |
| 9  Both must wash their hands and put on non-sterile gloves, apron and goggles[11] | To prevent cross-infection from splash back, spills and aerosol sprays from coughs.[11] To comply with standard precautions |
| 10  Person (a) holds the TT in place. They should hold the tube so that their hand is gently resting on the child's chest. This must be maintained throughout the whole procedure whilst observing and supporting the child. This is their only responsibility. Person (b) performs the procedure | To avoid potential dislodgement of the tube as this procedure may cause the child to cough. Holding the tube with the hand gently resting on the child's chest allows secure positioning should the child suddenly move and promotes access to the tube for person (b) (performing the procedure) |
| 11  Ask your assistant to hold the tracheostomy in place whilst you carefully remove the old dressing. Inspect the dressing for colour consistency and odour of wound leakage. Discard the dressing within gloves into the clinical waste bag | Stabilise the TT and reduce risks of dislodgement Early detection of infection facilitates early intervention |
| 12  Observe the stoma site for signs of infection or excessive inflammation, excessive redness and/or swelling, purulent discharge. Take a wound swab if any sign of infection is apparent. Assess these observations in conjunction with general signs and symptoms of infection: pyrexia; malaise | Tracheostomy stoma sites require daily inspection for signs of infection, inflammation, skin breakdown and granuloma formation To facilitate early treatment of infection |
| 13  Person (b): re-wash hands/clean hands with alcohol hand rub and put on sterile gloves | To reduce risk of infection |
| 14  Open inner dressing pack and ask an assistant to open and pour with a non-touch technique the normal saline into the small plastic container (within your dressing pack). Ask them to open gauze swabs, wound swab, tracheostomy dressing and scissors (if needed) using a non-touch technique and drop carefully onto the sterile field | Easily accessible equipment reduces the risk of infection |
| 15  Dip gauze swab, enough to dampen, into the normal saline. Dampen cotton/sponge tipped swab | Gauze swab and/or cotton-tipped swab should be moist enough only to clean without the risk of dripping solution into the tracheostomy |
| 16  Ask your assistant to hold TT in place during the procedure.  At the same time, support the child by explaining what is happening and offering reassurance and praise. Ask your assistant to notify you immediately of any significant changes in the child's condition | Stabilising the tracheostomy tube promotes comfort as children are extremely sensitive to tube movement causing them to cough and this risks dislodgement of the tube. Informing the child and encouraging their participation has been identified as a strategy to reduce stress and anxiety You may be focused on the procedure and not note efficiently changes in the child's condition |
| 17  Visually divide the stoma into four quadrants (like a cake). Clean each quadrant of the stoma inside to out using one single stroke with each swab. Use a clean piece of gauze each time. Repeat in each quadrant until the area around the stoma is clean | Using a single sweep, moving from stoma and outwards with each swab or cotton tipped swab reduces the risk of moving bacteria towards the wound |

## PROCEDURE: Tracheostomy tie change (continued)

| | |
|---|---|
| 18 Use extra swabs to pat dry with clean dry gauze | Excess moisture can predispose the peristomal area to skin breakdown |
| 19 Assess the need for application of a barrier film, e.g. Cavilon barrier film (*not* spray!) if the skin around the stoma (peristomal) is red and inflamed | Reduce the risk of skin excoriation and promote skin integrity |
| 20 If there is cellulitis at the stoma site; inform medical staff who may consider a course of antibiotics | To reduce the risk of infection |
| 21 Change the tracheostomy ties if they are soiled. Untie one side of the old tie and remove that side from the flange. Do not completely remove the old ties until the new one is in place and is securely fastened | Removing old ties before the new ties are put on puts the child at risk for accidental dislodgement of the tracheostomy tube and decannulation<br>If using twill ties: measure and cut a piece of tie long enough to go around the child's neck twice. Cut the tie at an angle so that it is easier to insert the tie into the flange |
| 22 Thread the new ties through the flange tie holes and around the back of the child's neck | |
| 23 Secure the ties. If using twill ties; secure with three reef knots. Pull the tie snug but ensure that you can fit one finger between the tie and the child's neck *Never* use a bow tie | Ensure tracheostomy ties are secure enough to ensure that the tracheostomy tube will not dislodge or cannot be accidentally untied by investigative little fingers. NEVER use a bow tie.[30] A reef knot is unlikely to come undone and lies reasonably flat<br>Promotes comfort, prevents skin damage and reduces risk of reduced blood flow by carotid pressure |
| 24 Carefully identify the old tie clearly and check with assistant. Cut off old tie using blunt ended scissors and discard it. If the child has a cuffed tube, be careful not to cut the cuff balloon when removing the old tie | Identify 'old' tie and check with assistant to reduce risk of inadvertent removal of new tie.<br>Cut, remove and discard the old tie. |
| 25 Apply specifically designed tracheostomy dressing, e. g. Trachi-dress, until wound has healed over. Place the dressing with the smooth shiny side in contact with the child's skin; slide in from bottom of TT | The surrounding skin is at risk of breakdown due to the presence of chest secretions leaking from the stoma site. The purpose of the dressing is to absorb wound exudate and remove from the skin surface and to provide comfort by minimising pressure, shearing and friction from the TT on the healing wound site. Plain gauze pads and other like materials should not be used, as fibres that become loose may be aspirated into the airway. Use a pre-cut tracheostomy dressing to reduce the risk of loose fibres becoming dislodged from the dressing and tracking into the trachea. |
| 26 Assess child for:<br>• Comfort<br>• Respiratory ease<br>• SpO$_2$<br>• Vital signs as necessary to determine distress | To maintain child's safety |
| 27 Dispose of equipment and wash hands | To prevent cross infection |
| 28 Document care given including assessment of secretions, dressing and stoma, as well as the child's tolerance of the procedure | To facilitate on-going evaluation |

**Problem:** You have noted that the lower rim of the tracheostomy flange is eroding the infant's chest over their manubrium (top portion of sternal bone).

**Discussion:** This is not uncommon in young infants. Further skin trauma can be prevented by sticking a small piece of Duoderm in between on the child's chest.

# SUCTIONING

Research has demonstrated that tracheal suction is traumatic and hazardous. There is the potential for mucosal damage, hypoxia, infection and airway collapse by poor technique and inappropriate equipment.[7] Therefore, suction should not be performed on a routine basis, but only as needed.

Optimal humidification is preferable to frequent suction and high suction pressures.[7] There are a number of terms regarding suctioning (Table 22.1).

## Equipment

Suction catheters of the correct size with finger tip control and ideally marked longitudinally for easy control of insertion depth

## The procedural goal is to

- safely and effectively clear secretions from tube thus maintaining a patent airway and allowing adequate respiratory function;
- maintain a aseptic/modified/clean technique as appropriate;
- detect partially obstructed tubes via tactile feedback (Figure 22.6).

**Table 22.1** Suctioning terms, their definitions and their use

| Term | Definitions | Use |
| --- | --- | --- |
| Sterile technique | Use of sterile catheter with freshly washed hands/alcohol hand rub and sterile gloves | In situations where the sterile catheter has to be manipulated by a sterile hand, usually in intensive care[7] |
| Modified sterile technique | Use of sterile catheter with freshly washed hands/alcohol hand rub and non-sterile, gloved hands | Recommended technique for healthcare professionals; standard precautions |
| Clean technique | Use of sterile catheter with freshly washed hands/alcohol hand rub and a non-touch technique: care is taken not to touch the portion of the suction catheter to be inserted | Recommended technique for parents/child as there is theoretically less risk of cross-infection and this simplifies a more child-friendly technique[7] |
| Shallow suctioning | Insertion of a catheter just into the hub of the tube | Removal of secretions the child has coughed into the opening of the tracheostomy |
| Pre-measured suctioning | Use of a catheter with side-holes close to the end of the catheter ($\leq 0.5$ cm), inserted to a pre-measured distance where the most distal side holes just exit the tip of the tube | Avoids epithelial damage due to suctioning too deeply and encrustation of secretions at tracheostomy tip due to suctioning being too shallow |
| Deep suctioning | Insertion of the catheter until resistance is met | For use by experienced intensive care personnel only in order to instigate an artificial cough |
| Routine suctioning | Suctioning according to a pre-set schedule, e.g. twice a day | *Not* recommended. Tube patency is evaluated by respiratory assessment[11] |
| As required suctioning | Based upon assessment of the child | Suctioning should be performed only based on respiratory assessment of the child |

**Table 22.1** Continued

| Size of suction catheter | Use a catheter with an outer diameter of approximately 50% of the tube's lumen for rapid removal of secretions and to prevent loss of lung volume.[7] A suction catheter of greater diameter will lead to obstruction of air flow around the catheter during the procedure and thus hypoxia | To select the size required: double the internal diameter of the tracheostomy tube (mm) size to give you the suction catheter size in Fg. If an odd number size is not available, e.g. 7 Fg, select an 8 Fg |
|---|---|---|
| Negative suction pressure | Use lowest possible vacuum pressure necessary. Increasing negative pressure to >150 mmHg does *not* improve aspiration efficiency; it simply collapses the catheter | 70–100 mmHg/10–15 kPa children[7] <150 mmHg/20kPa adults[11] |
| Bag ventilation | Provides: hyperoxygenation, hyperinflation and hyperventilation | Often done in intensive care units in young people post puberty. It is of no benefit to infants and young children |
| Normal saline instillation | May stimulate a cough but may cause oxygen desaturation and contamination | *Not* recommended as saline does not mix with mucous unless nebulised[10] |

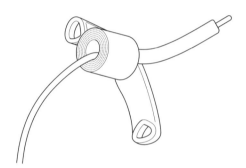

**Figure 22.7** Measuring suction catheter length. A length of catheter is inserted to a depth where the side holes of the catheter reach the tip of a spare tube (a). Alternatively, measure the length of the introducer/obturator.

**VIGNETTE**

**Problem:** You notice that a colleague is reinserting the same catheter during suctioning procedure.

**Discussion:** Policies and procedures do vary between institutions. However, the principles of tracheostomy suctioning are constant. Deviations from standard practice, such as reinserting suction catheters, may represent a serious health risk to the child and should be addressed in consultation with a charge nurse/team leader.

## PROCEDURE: Suctioning

| Procedural steps | Evidence-based rationale |
|---|---|
| 1 Perform suction only on an 'as required basis'.[7] Identify indications for suctioning. Indications that suctioning is required:<br>• child is unable to clear secretions by coughing<br>• sound of mucus bubbling in tracheostomy tube<br>• gurgles heard on auscultation/ felt on palpation of thorax<br>• difficulty breathing<br>• restless<br>• low $SpO_2$<br>• central cyanosis<br>• increased ventilator inspiratory pressure (if relevant)<br>• stridor or changes in breathing sounds\<br>• non-vocal child suddenly vocalises | Research has demonstrated that suctioning has inherent risks.[11] Therefore, suction should not be given on a routine basis, but only performed as needed. Applying suction to remove secretions may cause hypoxaemia, bronchospasm, arrhythmias, bleeding, infection or trauma, pain, anxiety<br>Frequency usually is influenced by<br>• the child's ability to generate an effective cough<br>• the viscosity and amount of secretions<br>Always encourage the child to cough independently to limit the frequency and degree of suctioning[7] |
| 2 Explain the procedure to the child and/or parent | Help decrease anxiety and fears. This procedure is unpleasant and can be frightening |
| 3 Screen bed | To povide privacy |
| 4 Ensure bed is at a safe working level[12] | To maintain a safe working environment |
| 5 Wash hands/apply alcohol hand rub, put on gloves, apron and goggles (standard precautions) | Prevent cross-infection from splash back, spills and aerosol sprays from coughs |
| 6 Identify the correct suction catheter and suction depth as above<br>If appropriate ensure that non-fenestrated inner cannula is in situ[11] | See Table 22.1<br><br>To reduce risk of tracheal damage[7] |
| 7 Set the suction pressures at between 50 and 100 mmHg (6–12 kPa) on full occlusion for a child[7] and does not exceed 150 mmHg on full occlusion for an adolescent or adult[11] | Too high a suction pressure can cause lung collapse and/or damage tracheal tissue; too little will be ineffective |
| 8 Hyperoxygenate, if necessary pre-suctioning | Suctioning is a hypoxic event and some children, particularly infants may require pre-oxygenation to reduce the effects of the inherent hypoxic insult[7] |
| 9 Open end of suction catheter package, leaving catheter inside package. Attach catheter to suction tubing (catheter remains in package) | To maintain sterility of equipment<br>The addition of the suction catheter generates greater pressure at its tip as compared to the suction tubing because it is narrower it will generate a much higher pressure at its tip |
| 10 Check working pressure by occluding tip of the suction catheter immediately before use | Do not test suction pressure setting by occluding suction tubing; suction catheter should be attached for check as narrow catheter significantly increases pressure |
| 11 Open sterile packaging and hold suction catheter in dominant hand taking care to hold it at a point below that which is going into the tracheostomy. Loop it in your hand or wrap it around your fingers so that you are holding it at the suction port | The suction procedure is a potential risk for contamination and infection. Adhere to aseptic/non-touch technique to maintain sterility of equipment |

## PROCEDURE: Suctioning (continued)

| | | |
|---|---|---|
| 12 | Disconnect ventilator tubing/HME device/speaking valve with the non-dominant hand or ask an assistant to do so. Note that with Bivona tubes, the connection can become 'stuck'. Do not use force to disconnect, always use the wedge provided | Use Bivona wedge provided to prevent causing damage to the tube or distressing the child |
| 13 | Encourage the child to take a deep breath while stabilising the tube and immediately prior to inserting the suction catheter in step [14] | This will act as a distraction, prepare them and stimulate a cough as you pass the catheter, thereby increasing the efficiency of the suctioning episode |
| 14 | Stabilise tube with non-dominant hand while inserting catheter into tracheostomy quickly but gently; using non-dominant hand insert catheter up to pre-measured depth | Deep suction causes mucosal damage and irritation; too shallow causes secretions to encrust the tube |
| 15 | Do not apply suction while inserting the catheter! | Decrease the volume of air removed from the lungs and decrease hypoxic effect and trauma to the delicate airway mucosa[7] |
| 16 | Apply negative pressure, using finger tip control as you withdraw the catheter gently straight back over 2–4 seconds. Observe the child throughout the procedure to ensure their general condition is not affected | Reduces the risk of atelectasis, hypoxia and bradycardia. Rolling of the catheter is not necessary as suction catheters now have circumferential holes and exacerbates atelectasis<br>Tracheal suction may cause vagal stimulation leading to bradycardia, especially in neonates |
| 17 | As soon as the catheter is withdrawn, re-connect to ventilator or oxygen supply source if required | Resume ventilator or oxygen delivery as soon as possible to re-ventilate and/or re-oxygenate the child |
| 18 | Reassess child's respiratory status for expected and unexpected outcomes:<br>• self-reported improvement<br>• comfort/decreased anxiety<br>• thorough respiratory assessment:<br>• respiratory ease/non-laboured respiration<br>• $SpO_2$<br>• behaviour<br>• lung sounds/palpation<br>• vital signs as necessary to determine distress;<br>• heart rate, blood pressure and $SpO_2$ (if used continuously) return to baseline parameters | Allows child to recover following each suctioning. Child should have oxygen saturations above 92%, be free of respiratory distress and be calm and comfortable. In contrast, restlessness, agitation, confusion, tachycardia, bradycardia and oxygen saturations below 92% indicate hypoxia and/or hypercapnia and appropriate therapeutic intervention is required immediately[17] |
| 19 | After suctioning the tracheostomy, you may suction the nose and mouth if needed | Children have uncuffed tubes and therefore accumulation of secretions may still accumulate in the upper airway of the child with a reduced ability to cough or swallow secretions |
| 20 | Disconnect catheter from suction tubing. Coil catheter inside gloved hand and remove glove by inverting it over the used catheter | To reduce the risk of cross-infection |
| 21 | Dispose of catheter in glove into clinical waste bag | To reduce the risk of cross-infection |
| 22 | If necessary, repeat suctioning procedure as detailed above | To perform suction only on an 'as required basis'[7] |
| 23 | Clear the suction tubing with water and turn off suction. In practice areas, a child usually has their own bottle of water allocated for this purpose only, changed daily | To maintain a comfortable and dignifies environment for the child |

## PROCEDURE: Suctioning (continued)

| **24** Remove apron and goggles and wash your hands | To reduce the risk of cross-infection |
|---|---|
| **25** Document time of suctioning and consistency, colour, quantity and any odour of secretions. Assess these observations in the light of general observations made: pyrexia, malaise | Early identification of signs and symptoms of respiratory infection or respiratory insufficiency secondary to secretions and/or inflammation Facilitates ongoing evaluation |

## TRACHEOSTOMY TUBE CHANGE

### Acute tracheostomy obstruction/dislodgement

A child with a tracheostomy tube with respiratory distress is considered to have a cannula obstruction or dislodgement until proven otherwise.[14] Maintain a high index of suspicion and suspect obstruction if the child exhibits little chest rise during spontaneous respiration or is unable to breathe alone after assisted ventilation. Airway patency and assessment of adequacy of breathing should be assessed through the usual physical assessment and monitoring means. The following findings may indicate a tracheostomy obstruction:

- signs of respiratory distress or failure with or without abnormal breath sounds;
- increased work of breathing;
- altered mental status with agitation;
- diminished breath sounds bilaterally despite significant work of breathing;
- inadequate chest rise during assisted ventilation;
- tachycardia;
- late findings: cyanosis, bradycardia and unresponsiveness.

*For the first 5–7 days the tracheocutaneous tract is not mature and replacement of the tracheostomy tube may be difficult.*[15] Therefore, stay sutures are used to help replace tube without delay and trauma to stoma.

### Elective Tracheostomy Tube Change

After the first week (tube change) unless otherwise indicated elective tube changes are then carried out by nursing staff until the parents and child, if appropriate, are trained and feel competent and confident to do so. Tube manufacturers generally recommend a tube change every 28 days. There is no consensus regarding the frequency of changing.[7]

To some extent, the frequency of tube change depends on the material of the tube and the presence of infection and/or secretions. All are subject to deterioration from regular use. Polyvinylchloride tubes become more rigid and develop cracks/splits as the plasticiser that provides flexibility leaches out with use after 3–4 months.

**KEY POINTS**

It was once thought that instilling 1–2 mL of normal saline into the bronchial tree via the tracheostomy tube would liquefy secretions prior to suctioning them out. However, research indicates that the instillation of liquid into the lungs is not effective in liquefying secretions.[7] The only consistent benefit in instilling seems to be in causing the child to cough strongly and subsequently loosen secretions. For this reason and the risk of 'drowning' the child, bacterial spread downward into the bronchial tree and formation of a mucus plug, its practice is to be questioned. Viscosity and expectoration of lung secretions are best managed by:[13]
- systemic hydration
- humidity
- suctioning, coughs and assisted coughs
- mobility/turning/change of position
- chest physiotherapy.

**KEY POINTS**

A TT change should be performed by two people, one of whom must be trained and assessed to be competent in tracheostomy changes, decannulations and airway management.

Silicone tubes do not stiffen despite repeated use and cleaning but occasionally develop cracks or tears. Metal TTs may be used indefinitely, although they can develop cracks at the soldered joints. The corrosion is due either to exposure to body fluids over a long period or to the malpractice of using hypochlorite solutions for cleaning and disinfection.[11] Therefore, all TTs must be inspected before each use. Damaged tubes or tubes that are becoming rigid should be discarded and replaced.

### Equipment

Emergency equipment as recommended earlier
Two pairs of non-sterile gloves
Apron
Goggles
New tracheostomy tube (same size)
Spare tracheostomy tube (one size smaller)
Sachet sterile water-soluble lubricant
Alcohol hand cleansing agent
Clinical waste bag/receptacle
Blunt-ended scissors
Ties as appropriate
10 mL syringe (if cuffed tube)

### *The procedural goal is to*

- safely and effectively replace the tube and establish a patent tube;
- rid the tracheostomy of bacteria that may be harmful to the child;
- maintain a clean technique.

## PROCEDURE: Tracheostomy tube change

| Procedural steps | Evidence-based rationale |
|---|---|
| 1 Two people are required to carry out this procedure one of whom is trained and experienced in tracheostomy changes, decannulations and airway management<br>In the acute unplanned situation: call for help | This is a potentially hazardous procedure and the person carrying out the procedure will need an assistant. The following procedures are best accomplished by two people: one to hold the tube in place and observe the child's condition throughout the procedure and the other person to perform the procedure. During the first week, a third person may be required to pull gently on the 'stay sutures' |
| 2 Cleanse hands with alcohol hand rub and put on non-sterile gloves, disposable apron and goggles | To prevent cross-infection including recognition of risk to carer from splash back, spills and aerosol sprays from coughs |
| 3 Taking an appropriate amount of time, explain the procedure to the child and/or parent. Children often fear that they will not be able to breathe while the tube is out and many nurses believe that the stoma will close as soon as the tube is removed. In reality, the stoma will not close, and the child will continue to breathe freely while the tube is out | Informing the child and encouraging their participation has been identified as a strategy to reduce stress and anxiety. Take care to explain this to the child clearly to alleviate any undue anxiety Child gives their consent |
| 4 Screen the bed | To provide privacy |
| 5 Ensure that the bed is at a safe working level[12] | To maintain a safe working environment |
| 6 Position the child as appropriate:<br>• supine will a small rolled towel or blanket under the shoulder<br>• swaddle infants<br>• semi-recumbent position<br>• older children may prefer to be sitting up | Shoulder roll extends the child's neck slightly to allow easy access to the stoma. A semi-recumbent position decreases abdominal pressure on the diaphragm, which in turn promotes lung expansion. Support behind the child helps to guard against sudden movement backwards<br>It is important to give the child choice as appropriate as this promotes feelings of control and autonomy |

## PROCEDURE:  Tracheostomy tube change (continued)

| | |
|---|---|
| **7** Suction the tube or ask the child to cough<br>If necessary administer oxygen or assisted<br>ventilation via the TT before and after suctioning<br>If the child has a double lumen cannula, in the first<br>instance, remove the inner cannula and replace it | Reduce the need for suctioning during an elective<br>procedure<br>Children who breathe through a tracheostomy should<br>receive assisted ventilation through the<br>tracheostomy.[19] Besides improving oxygenation, this<br>manoeuvre will help you to determine whether the TT<br>is open in the case of a sudden acute deterioration;<br>difficulty delivering assisted ventilation and poor chest<br>rise indicate a potential obstruction; proceed to<br>change the cannula: step 9 |
| **8** If <7 days (before first tube change) an ENT<br>anaesthetist must be called and follow local protocol | This is an emergency situation and the child may<br>require resuscitation expertise |
| **9** Open new TT pack and prepare the new tube<br>• Hold the top end of the tube taking care<br>  not to touch the<br>  cannula part of the tracheostomy set<br><br>• If reusing a tube it is essential to inspect the tube<br>  for possible damage and for reduced flexibility<br>  with time and repeated use<br><br>• Place introducer into the tube and check that<br>  it slides in and out easily<br>• If using a cuffed tube; test the cuff for leakage<br>  and ensure that air is out of cuff prior to insertion<br>• For Bivona, check that 15-mm swivel connector<br>  is attached correctly | TTs are packed sterile; prevent cross-contamination by<br>using a non-touch technique<br>• Ensure that all parts fit together correctly before<br>  insertion into the trachea and are ready for<br>  immediate insertion:<br>• Ensures that the tube has not been damaged by<br>  being used too many times<br>• TTs are packed sterile. To prevent cross<br>  contamination by using a non-touch technique<br>• Ensures that all parts fit together correctly before<br>  insertion into the trachea<br>• Partly inflated cuff will make insertion difficult and<br>  potentially cause trauma<br>• The 15-mm swivel connector is removed for cleaning<br>  and must be securely reconnected before use |
| **10** Secure the trach-hold ties to one side of flange | Ready for securing as soon as tube confirmed as<br>properly placed |
| **11** In the rare circumstance that the stoma site<br>appears dry, place a small blob of sterile water<br>soluble lubricant onto a sterile gauze swab and<br>apply a thin film to the tube and protruding<br>portion of the obturator | It is unusual to require lubrication to facilitate tube<br>insertion |
| **12** Prepare child for the next part of the procedure<br>and inform them what is expected of them | Encourages the child's active participation as a<br>strategy to reduce stress and anxiety |
| **13** Person (a): hold the TT in place with hand resting<br>gently onto the child's chest. This must be<br>maintained throughout the whole procedure<br>while observing and supporting the child. This is<br>their only responsibility. Person (b) performs the<br>procedure | Avoid potential dislodgement of the tube as this<br>procedure may cause the child to cough<br>Holding the tube with the hand gently resting on the<br>child's chest allows secure positioning should the child<br>suddenly move, and promotes access to the tube for<br>person (b) (performing the procedure) |
| **14** Person (b): cut off the ties with round-ended scissors | To release the tube ready for removal |
| **15** Person (b): Take hold of the 'new' tracheostomy<br>with introducer inserted at the top end of the<br>tube taking care not to touch the cannula part<br>of the tracheostomy set | To reduce time delay between removal of the 'old'<br>tube and insertion of the 'new' |

## PROCEDURE: Tracheostomy tube change (continued)

| | |
|---|---|
| **16** Ask the child to take a big breath in | Conscious inspiration distracts the child while reducing the risk of coughing. Coughing can result in unwanted spasm (closure) of the stoma |
| **17** If <7 days the tracheocutaneous tract is not mature and replacement of the tracheostomy tube may be difficult. Ask a third assistant to pull gently on 'stay sutures' to establish a patent stoma[15] If >7 days the stoma should usually remain patent | Displacement of the tracheostomy tube is a potentially fatal complication. 'Stay sutures' are put in place by the surgeon help to facilitate emergency tube replacement in the first week postoperatively |
| **18** Person (b): remove the old tube with your non-dominant hand using a curved downward movement as the child is asked to breathe out | Conscious expiration relaxes the child and reduces the risk of coughing. Coughing can result in unwanted spasm (closure) of the stoma |
| **19** Person (b): upon removal of 'old' tube, immediately attempt to replace with 'new' tube by placing the tube through the stoma and into the trachea using gentle pressure and an arc-like motion, pushing the cannula posteriorly and downward until the flange is flush against the neck[16] | To prevent trauma to trachea and surrounding tissue by directing the tube along the contour of the trachea |
| **20** Remove the introducer immediately | The child cannot breathe with the introducer in place: allow air entry to airway |
| **21** If *successful*, confirm proper positioning of the tube by assessment of bilateral chest movement and clinical improvement. Secure with tracheostomy ties. If cuffed, inflate cuff with 10 mL syringe to achieve a cuff pressure of 15–20 mmHg with the aide of a manometer[11] | Follow principles of basic life support: effective chest movement confirms achievement of patent airway by establishment of respiration.[16] Misplacement of the tracheostomy tube into the dreaded false passage, usually in the pretracheal space, should be suspected in the presence of difficult ventilation |
| **22** If *unsuccessful*, remain calm since an outward appearance of panic may cause the child and/or parents to panic and lose confidence. Remove the introducer from the 'new' tube and thread it over an appropriate sized suction catheter Insert the suction catheter into the stoma, and using it as a guiding wire, pass the TT over the suction catheter[17] Once in place remove the suction catheter | In the event that stomal constriction prevents insertion of the replacement TT:<br>• use a guiding wire technique to pass the same size TT<br>• use a guiding wire technique to pass a tube one size smaller<br>Research comparing different strategies recommend a guiding wire/railroad approach as the best technique used to optimise the safeguarding of the airway during a TT change[17]<br>*Note that tracheal dilators are no longer advocated as their use results in substantial tracheal trauma*[16] |
| **23** If successful, replace humidification/oxygen/ventilator tubing as appropriate If a cuffed tube inserted, use a 10-mL syringe to inflate the cuff of the tube until the air seal is achieved/15–20 mmHg with manometer[11] Fasten the ties with Velcro or three reef knots. Leave enough slack to be able to insert one finger between the ties and the child's neck. Trim excess length off | To maintain oxygenation and moisten airway To protect and maintain airway but prevent trauma to the trachea. A cuff pressure above 20 mmHg may cause damage to the tracheal mucosa.[11] A cuff pressure < 15 mmHg may lead to aspiration[11] To secure the tube and promote comfort. Ensure that the ties are not too loose as the tube may become dislodged while at the same time ensuring that they are not too tight as pressure sores may occur |
| **24** If unsuccessful repeat the procedure above and attempt to pass the TT one size smaller over a suction catheter as above[17] | Establishment of a smaller airway is preferable to no airway |

## PROCEDURE:  Tracheostomy tube change (continued)

| | |
|---|---|
| 25 If unsuccessful support the child as appropriate following the principles of basic life support and call for emergency help appropriate to context[16] | See basic life support concerns below<br>Obtain specialist emergency assistance as appropriate to context |
| 26 Once the child is stabilised, reposition and make sure that they are comfortable | To ensure safety and comfort |
| 27 Dispose of equipment and clinical waste as appropriate | To reduce the risk of cross-infection |
| 28 Remove gloves, apron and goggles and wash your hands | To reduce the risk of cross-infection |
| 29 Document the procedure and any observations made, actions taken and report concerns immediately to the appropriate person, e.g. senior nurse, medical staff | Legal requirement for safety and facilitate future reference and evaluation |

# BASIC LIFE SUPPORT CONCERNS: TRACHEOSTOMY

Any child with airway obstruction can deteriorate quickly, particularly small infants. Metabolic rate and oxygen consumption are higher, functional residual capacity is smaller and the diaphragm has fewer fatigue-resistant fibres.[17] Overall, respiratory reserve is small and fatigue occurs sooner. Therefore, careful ongoing and regular assessment of the child is paramount. The approach to basic life support when a child has a tracheostomy follows the same approach as for other children as advocated by the UK Resuscitation Council.[16] However, there are some adjustments. A safe approach is advocated and this usually entails the use of a face-shield for basic life support, but these are not easy to use over a tracheostomy tube or stoma. Therefore, use a face mask connector (filter) and appropriate size mask. Note that a neonatal face mask fits snugly directly over a stoma if necessary.

**VIGNETTE**

**Problem:** An infant you are nursing keeps occluding their tracheostomy with their chubby chin.

**Discussion:** This is a common problem with infants who have a large heavy head in comparison to a short neck. Protector caps are available with side ventilation holes to prevent complete obstruction if this should occur.[18]

**KEY POINTS**

- Always follow ABC (airway, breathing, circulation)
- A blocked tube is invariably the problem
- Remove tube if rapid suctioning fails or is even slightly delayed
- Direct ventilation over stoma is usually the most effective

## PROCEDURE: Basic life support

| Procedural steps | Evidence-based rationale |
|---|---|
| **1** Is the child breathing?<br>• Make sure that the tracheostomy tube is properly positioned and that the introducer has been removed (decannulation plug removed if fenestrated)<br>• Slightly extend the chin of sleeping infants<br>• Check that nothing is inadvertently covering the tracheostomy tube<br>• Remove inner cannula<br>• Increase oxygen therapy via face mask and tracheostomy<br>• Monitor SaO$_2$<br>• Check position of tracheostomy tube<br>• Perform tracheal suction immediately<br><br>Is the child breathing effectively?<br><br>**Yes?**<br>• Maintain high flow oxygen<br>• Ensure adequate humidification<br><br>• Reposition patient to facilitate effective breathing pattern<br>**No?**<br>• Seek urgent medical assistance | Infants with chubby chins can occasionally obstruct the tracheostomy opening<br>Suctioning of the tracheostomy tube will help to evaluate the patency of the tube and clearance of secretions may be helpful in alleviating symptoms. But do not be falsely reassured by a tube entering into the stoma site as it may actually descend into the soft tissues of the neck rather than into the trachea, especially if a prior TT change was attempted and unknowingly resulted in a false passage |
| **2** Lay the child supine with a small rolled towel or blanket under the shoulder to expose the neck<br>*Unable to pass suction catheter?*<br>Call for help<br>*Is the child breathing effectively?*<br>**Yes?**<br>See steps above | Shoulder roll extends the child's neck slightly to open airway and allows easy access to the stoma<br>As there is ineffective breathing and you are unable to pass a suction catheter, an emergency tube change is required[17]<br>A tube change is best accomplished by two people: one to secure the child, deflate the cuff (if present), and remove the old tube and the other person to replace the new tube and assess it for proper positioning<br>Change TT (see p. 384) |
| **No?**<br>**3** Look, listen and feel for breathing (ear to tube, chest wall movement, auscultation)<br>Is the chest moving up and down?<br>Can you feel air coming out of the tracheostomy tube?<br>Can you hear any noise? | Assess for breathing. Take less than 10 seconds to do this |
| **4** Noisy, small inadequate breaths or minimal breath sound where is *no* visible chest rise and fall?<br>Call for trained emergency help appropriate to context | Ineffective breathing is pre-terminal; trained resuscitation help is required |
| **5** Administer five rescue breaths via the tracheostomy tube[16]<br>Administer rescue breaths by mouth-to-tracheostomy tube or mouth-to-stoma or as required | Children who breathe through a tracheostomy should receive assisted ventilation through the tracheostomy[16]<br>Besides improving oxygenation, this manoeuvre will help you to determine whether the tracheostomy tube |

## PROCEDURE:  Using a slide sheet (continued)

| | |
|---|---|
| If trained to do so, administer rescue breaths use manual ventilation bag connected to 15 litres/minute of oxygen<br>If adequate chest movement is not achieved with bag-valve-tracheostomy tube; remove tube immediately and deliver artificial breaths via stoma either by mouth-to-stoma using infection control protector and neonatal face mask or via bag-valve-mask via stoma if trained to do so and available | is open. Difficulty delivering assisted ventilation and poor chest rise indicate a potential obstruction; proceed to change the cannula if not done already<br><br>Deliver breaths slowly and gently over 1–1.5 seconds until you see the chest rise; this tells you that the lungs are inflating[16] |
| 6 If mask-to-stoma ventilation does not result in visible chest rise, deliver artificial ventilation to the child's nose and mouth while occluding the stoma with a gloved hand[20]<br>Or if trained to do so and available, apply bag-mask-ventilation to the child's nose and mouth while occluding the stoma with a gloved hand | Offers an alternative approach if above is unsuccessful[20] |
| 7 After five rescue breaths, check the circulation as described in Chapter 9 | Now continue as usual with basic life support guidelines using the airway and breathing methods described above[16] |

## CONCLUSION

Tracheostomies in children are increasingly performed for chronic medical conditions. Airway assessment is one of the primary responsibilities of nurses caring for children with tracheostomies. This requires the nurse to have a fundamental understanding of the indications, applications and complications of tracheostomy for each individual child. The purpose of this chapter has been to provide evidence-based practical guidance regarding care for the child who has a TT. Chapter 22 examines long-term aspects of caring for a child with a tracheostomy such as cleaning of tubes, use of speaker valves and passive humidification as well as parent/child education and transfer home with a TT.

 Go to the website to find the PowerPoint presentation for this chapter and MCQs to test your knowledge. **www.hodderplus.com/childnursingskills**

# REFERENCES

1 Butnaru CS, Colreavy MP, Ayari S, *et al.* (2006) The changing indications for pediatric tracheostomy. *International Journal of Pediatric Otorhinolaryngologyy* **70**: 115–119.

2 Tortora GJ, Derrickson B (2006) *Principles of anatomy and physiology*, 11th edition. Danvers: Wiley.

3 McChance KL, Huether SE (2006) *Pathophysiology: the biologic basis for disease in adults and children,* 5th edition. St Louis: Elsevier.

4 Chamley CA, Carson P, Randall R (2005) *Developmental anatomy and physiology of children: a practical approach.* Edinburgh, Elsevier & Churchill Livingstone.

5 Daudia A, Gibbin KP (2006) Management of tracheostomy. *Current Paediatrics* **16**: 225–229.

6 Kremer B Botos-Kremer AI, Eckel HE *et al.* (2002) Indications, complications and surgical techniques for pediatric tracheostomies: an update. *Journal of Pediatric Surgery,* **37**: 1556–1562.

7 Quality Improvement Scotland: NHS (2008) *Caring for the child/young person with a tracheostomy.* Edinburgh: NHS QIS www.nhshealthquality.org (Accessed 24 March 2009).

8 Department of Health (2001) *Building a safer NHS for patients.* London: HMSO.

9 DHSS (1987) *Evaluation of heated humidifiers.* Health Equipment Information, 177. London: DHSS.

10 Barnett M (2004) Tracheostomy management and care. *Journal of Community Nursing,* **19**(1).

11 Quality Improvement Scotland: NHS (2007) *Caring for the patient with a tracheostomy.* Edinburgh: NHS QIS www.nhshealthquality.org (accessed 24 March 2009).

12 Smith J (2005) *The guide to the handling of people,* 5th edition. Teddington: ARJO.

13 Barnett M (2005) Tracheostomy management and care. *Journal of Community Nursing* **19**(1): 4–8.

14 Posner JC, Ward RJ, Cheney FW, *et al.* (2006) Emergency care of the technology-assisted child. *Clinical pediatric emergency medicine* **7**: 38–51.

15 Craig MF, Bajaj Y, Hartley BE, *et al.* (2005) Maturation sutures for the paediatric tracheostomy: an extra safety measure. *The Journal of Laryngology and Otology.* **119**: 985–987.

16 Resuscitation Council UK (2005). *Guidelines for paediatric basic life support.* London: Resuscitation Council UK.

17 Mirza S, Cameron DS (2001) The tracheostomy tube change: a review of techniques. *Hospital Medicine* **62**(3): 158–163.

18 Oberwaldner B, Eber E (2006) Tracheostomy care in the home. *Paediatric Respiratory Review* **7**: 185–195.

19 Spaulding LL (2006) Preventing the spread of infection from medical devices. ECPN: *Extended Care Professional News* **110**(5): 34–39.

20 Great Ormond Street Hospital for Children NHS Trust (2006) *Basic life support of babies and children with a tracheostomy: information for families.* GOSH Trust, London www.goshfamilies.nhs.uk (Accessed 24 March 2009).

## CHAPTER 23

# Caring for a child requiring long-term ventilation

Naomi Campbell

## LEARNING OUTCOMES

*Upon completion of this chapter, the reader should be able to accomplish the following:*

1 Define long-term ventilation (LTV)
2 Understand common reasons for LTV
3 Describe common modes of ventilation used with LTV
4 Discuss advantages and disadvantages of invasive versus non-invasive ventilation
5 Develop insight into the general nursing skills required to care for a child on LTV
6 Explore the role of humidification and HME filters (wet and dry circuits)
7 Appraise the use of speaking valves
8 Gain insight into the teaching of parents and children including the discharge process
9 Describe the considerations of LTV at home including psychosocial implications

## CHAPTER OVERVIEW

Over the last decade, there has been a significant increase in the number of ventilator-dependent children. In 1990 there were 24 LTV children in the UK, 38 per cent of whom were managed at home.[1] These figures have increased significantly over the years to 141 children in 1999.[2] Of these, 68 per cent were cared for at home. The most common underlying conditions requiring LTV are as follows:

- neuromuscular disease;
- congenital central hypoventilation syndrome (CCHS);
- spinal injury;
- bronchopulmonary dysplasia (BPD);
- tracheal–bronchial malacia (floppy airways).

The exponential growth in the number of LTV children managed in the community has been partly driven by advances in technology, changes in attitude and perception of long-term disability, in addition to the increasing numbers of children now surviving resuscitation yet not making a full recovery.[3,4] Home ventilation is advocated as practical and advantageous,[5] with its aim to prolong life, relieve discomfort and improve a child's outcome in an environment that will best enhance developmental potential.[6]

The number of hours a child requires ventilation varies depending on the underlying condition. For example, children with CCHS require nocturnal support only when sleeping, whereas those with BPD may require ventilation 24 hours a day.

Despite evidence promoting home ventilation, children remain in hospital for prolonged periods.[6]

## KEY WORDS

| | |
|---|---|
| Long-term ventilation | Invasive ventilation |
| Non-invasive ventilation | Tracheostomy |

In the case of an LTV patient, their respiratory system cannot be maintained without support. In spite of this, these children are considered to be medically stable. It has long been recognised that in order to relieve expensive resources, interventions are required to facilitate discharge of these children into a thriving, nurturing home environment, giving the child a sense of normalisation as soon as possible.[7,8]

Planning the discharge home is complex. The handing over of care responsibilities, and the importance of an interprofessional approach calls for meticulous preparation. This preparation often appears to focus mainly on technological competencies and practical issues, with little psychosocial preparation and support being given. Although this chapter will address the technical competence and practical skills, it also seeks to re-address this balance and give the reader insight into what it is like to be a parent or a child about to go home ventilator dependent.

In order for children to go home, family members must be available every hour of the day and trained in all aspects of care, such as how the ventilator works, suctioning, tracheostomy tube changes and cardiopulmonary resuscitation. Many stress that the child needs to be observed 24 hours a day as, for example, ventilator disconnection or a blockage of a tracheostomy tube could be fatal.[9] Such responsibility can have a major effect on parents, leaving them anxious and apprehensive. An insight, therefore, into the experience of children and parents living the phenomenon is arguably valuable and may potentially make a great contribution to the preparation for discharge and care at home for LTV children and their families.

# VENTILATION

Ventilators are used to mechanically assist breathing by delivering oxygen ($O_2$) to the lungs and removing carbon dioxide ($CO_2$). Indications for ventilation include apnoea and respiratory distress causing acidosis with a high $CO_2$ and poor oxygenation.[10] There are a number of modes of ventilation as discussed in Chapter 25. However, there are two distinct classifications of modes used in LTV; continuous positive airway pressure (CPAP) and pressure support used for an intact respiratory drive, and pressure control for those without (see Table 23.1). These modes can be delivered invasively and by non-invasive means. These are discussed in Table 23.2 (page 393).

**Table 23.1** Ventilation modes used in long-term ventilation

**Intact respiratory drive**

CPAP (continuous positive airway pressure)

- No back-up rate, therefore risk of apnoea
- Patient generates respiratory rate, inspiratory time, tidal volume and peak inspiratory pressure
- Maintains positive end expiratory pressure (PEEP) at all times, reducing work of breathing.

Pressure support sometimes referred to as BiPAP

- IPAP (inspiratory positive airway pressure) and EPAP (expiratory positive airway pressure) are set (bi-level)
- Ventilator supports each spontaneous breath taken by patient
- If the patient's rate falls, a timed breath (Ti back-up) is initiated at the back up rate. Simply put, modifying CPAP to also provide IPAP to assist inspiration
- Commonly used with neuromuscular disease

**Absent respiratory drive**

Pressure control

- IPAP, EPAP, Ti (inspiratory time) and respiratory rate are all set on the ventilator
- Used on children with no respiratory drive, e.g. congenital central hypoventilation syndrome, spinal injury/paralysis

**Table 23.2** Invasive versus non-invasive ventilation

| Invasive ventilation: administered via a tracheostomy | Non-invasive ventilation (NIV): administered via a facemask covering just the nose, or nose and mouth |
|---|---|
| **Advantages** | **Advantages** |
| Enables child to feed and play as normal, therefore suitable for the child requiring ventilation >12–16 hours a day | No real altered body image/scars |
| | Child can cough, swallow and speak freely |
| Maintains difficult airways via tracheostomy | Less specialist skills required to care for child |
| **Disadvantages**[11] | **Disadvantages**[5,12,13] |
| Altered body image | Not usually tolerated by young children, or children with severe learning disabilities |
| Dysphasia: poor speech and language development. Alteration in communication due to position of tracheostomy bypassing vocal folds | Not suitable for children with bulbar impairment and swallowing difficulties, severe laryngomalacia, tracheomalacia and deformities of upper airway |
| Dysphagia: difficulty swallowing, may lead to feeding difficulties | Claustrophobic |
| Impairs cough: patient reliant on suctioning to maintain a clear airway | Risk of pressure sores/skin ulceration |
| Behavioural issues due to communication barrier | Midfacial deformity: distortion to the normal growth and structure of midfacial bones and maxillary dentition |
| Poor socialisation and habituation | Easy for circuit leaks: can be difficult to get a good seal. Relies on patient keeping mouth shut with nasal masks |
| Diverse skills required to care for tracheostomy. Child must be supervised by skilled parents/carers 24 hours a day | Poor mask fit: air leaks into the eyes can cause conjunctivitis |
| | Abdominal distension due to unintentional swallowing of air |
| | Risk of aspiration |
| | Not suitable for >16 hours/day ventilation as the presence of the mask can limit the use of hands, facial expressions and interpersonal contact, especially with young children and infants |

**Definitions**

**Long-term ventilator dependent:** 'Any child who, when medically stable, continues to require a mechanical aid for breathing, after an acknowledged failure to wean, or a slow wean, three months after institution of ventilation.'[3,p.762]

**Ventilation:** process of moving air in and out of the lungs.

**Respiration:** process during which the exchange of oxygen and carbon dioxide occurs in the alveoli of the lungs.

# NURSING SKILLS FOR A CHILD REQUIRING LTV

Chapter 22 discusses specific nursing skills to care for a tracheostomy. Competence in these skills is essential in the care of a child requiring invasive LTV. This chapter will now identify further skills required to care for the child with a long-term tracheostomy outwith the hospital environment.

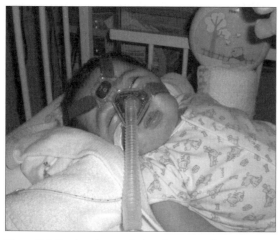

**Figure 23.1** Non-invasive ventilation via nose mask.

## Equipment

Non-sterile gloves
Gauze sponges
Basin/container with water and mild-detergent
Clinical waste bag/receptacle
Sterile normal saline or cooled boiled water (at home)

### The procedural goal is to

- rid the tracheostomy tube of bacteria that may be harmful to the child;
- maintain the useful life of the equipment.

## Non-invasive ventilation

As demonstrated in Table 23.2 non-invasive ventilation (NIV) is an increasingly practical alternative to ventilation via a tracheostomy.[13] As the number of LTV children increases in the UK, when their condition allows, NIV will be commenced rather than tracheostomy ventilation. Although there are disadvantages to both forms of ventilation delivery, when used appropriately, and with efficient nursing care (Table 23.3), the introduction or transfer to NIV can alleviate the disadvantages of tracheostomy and improve the child's freedom and quality of life.

## PROCEDURE: Cleaning of tracheostomy tubes

| Procedural steps | Evidence-based rationale |
|---|---|
| **1** Wash hands put on non-sterile gloves | To prevent cross-infection |
| **2** Place cannula directly into a container of hot soapy detergent and water | A short-term soak (5–10 minutes) in hot water with mild detergent helps to loosen the crusts and mucus from the tube |
| **3** Clean the tracheostomy tube gently with cotton-tipped swabs. If the cannula is occluded with secretions and impossible to clean, dispose of and do not attempt to clean | Before equipment is to be disinfected or sterilised, it should be thoroughly cleaned to remove visible dirt and secretions, as dirt causes disinfectant to lose activity. Do not use a brush (unless supplied by the manufacturer of the tracheostomy tube) as these are abrasive and will damage the tube and increase the risk of bacterial growth[14] |
| **4** After cleansing thoroughly, hold the tube at the top end with dominant hand (to maintain a clean no-touch technique) and rinse the tube with sterile normal saline or freshly cooled boiled water (at home). Leave to air dry | Alcohol and hypochlorite disinfectants are not recommended as they cause tube hardening, brittleness and can cause loosening of the connection between fixation flange and shaft |
| | Thermal methods are not recommended as they are likely to cause material damage |
| **5** Once dry, store in a clean closed container in a cool place until required | To prevent soiling and contamination[15] |

**Table 23.3** Non-invasive ventilation (NIV) nursing considerations

| NIV issue | Nursing consideration |
|---|---|
| **Masks**<br>• Made from soft material such as silicone, rubber or gel | • Frequent inspection of pressure areas, especially the bridge of nose and forehead to ensure skin integrity is maintained |
| • Held in place with headgear using Velcro to fasten. This allows for best fit and positioning to ensure comfort, as well as quick removal if needed | • Ensure the mask fits accurately to achieve best possible results and tolerance, reducing risk of air leaks, leading to conjunctivitis. |
| • Skin injury was observed in up to 48 per cent of children in the PICU setting.[16]<br>**Observation of child** | • Mask should not be fitted tightly, but secured using the Velcro headgear that should maintain an equal gentle pressure around the mask.[5] |
| • O$_2$ saturations (SaO$_2$), respiratory rate, and work of breathing | • Observation will indicate how the child is tolerating and responding to the ventilation. As child's condition improves, respiratory rate and accessory muscle use should ease[12] |
|  | • In the home environment once NIV is well established, formal monitoring may not always be indicated.[13] However, it is important to use nursing assessment skills without the use of monitoring equipment, by having an awareness of the child's normal work of breathing and where condition changes which may require intervention or medical advice |
| • Monitor abdominal distension | • In rare cases, children may require aspiration of air from a gastrostomy, or nasogastric tube if insitu to alleviate abdominal distension and prevent excess pressure on diaphragm |
| • Psychological support | • Children and families will require a high level of psychological preparation and support[12] |
|  | • Thorough explanation of equipment used, and understanding of how equipment works, the importance of it, and how it will help the child's condition |

## Nippy Junior ventilator

LTV ventilators are very different to those seen in the acute setting. The Nippy Junior ventilator by B&D Electromedics[17] is especially designed for the use of LTV in paediatric patients. It is portable, and provides the modes of positive pressure ventilation described in Table 23.1. The Nippy Junior works by compressing ambient air and delivers it to the patient via invasive and non-invasive means. The ventilation mode, set pressure, inspiratory time, rate and estimated tidal volume are all displayed on the main colour screen, making it easy to assess accurate ventilation delivery. Please see the website

for illustration of the Nippy Junior ventilator. The Nippy Junior is easy to use, and has a number of useful hints when troubleshooting various alarms. An in-depth instruction manual can be found at http://www.nippyventilator.com; however, anyone using this piece of equipment must have formal training to ensure the safety of the patient at all times. Ventilator settings must be prescribed by the child's consultant, and should not be altered without formal instruction. All LTV patients will have at least two portable ventilators, so there is a spare if there are any faults.

### Batteries and power supply

The Nippy Junior runs off the mains power supply. However, if the power fails, the ventilator will switch off, putting the child at risk. To avoid this problem, the mains supply can be backed up with external batteries. When stationary, a fully charged battery should be connected into the back of the ventilator; therefore, if the mains power fails, the ventilator will automatically switch to battery power and continue to work. Back-up batteries can last between 4 and 8 hours, but are very heavy and large. To fulfil day-to-day activities, it is not always possible to be connected to a power supply. To make the child more mobile, smaller 2-hour batteries are available for short trips.

All batteries have their own chargers. When caring for patients it is important that these batteries are fully charged when not in use, and recharged as soon as possible after discharge. Although they have recommended running times, as the batteries get older, running time should not be relied on. Battery life will also depend on the mode and level of ventilation set; therefore, the higher the pressures required, the shorter the battery will last. Trips out must be planned with these time scales in mind, and reasonable precautions taken, including plugging the ventilator into the mains supply at any possible opportunity.

For safety and convenience, the new Nippy Junior+ has been installed with an internal battery, providing back-up for up to 6 hours. In addition, it has one portable battery that can provide an additional 6 hours. The ventilator recharges both the internal and external battery when plugged into mains supply and therefore does not require separate battery chargers. Be sure to identify which type of ventilator the patient is using, and ensure competency to use the different batteries and chargers.

**KEY POINTS**

1 Ensure all batteries are charging when not in use
2 Charge batteries as soon as possible after discharge
3 Alternate batteries used to prolong life
4 Test battery running time monthly
5 Report any faults immediately
6 Always carry double the amount of battery back-up time required to ensure ventilator does not fail
7 Alternate the two ventilators used at least monthly to prolong life and ensure correct working order
8 Take mains supply cable on all outings and connect to power supply wherever possible

Battery running time should be tested monthly. Run the spare ventilator on battery power until the low battery warning alarms and record running time. Table 23.4 shows recommendations by the manufacturer for efficient and safe running of the ventilator.

### Air inlet filter

The air input filter is located on the rear of the Nippy Junior. This is where ambient air is drawn into the ventilator to provide positive pressure to the patient. This filter is important as it prevents small particles from the air being drawn into the ventilator and causing a fault. This filter should be inspected weekly. The filter can be washed in warm, soapy water and left to air dry. Ensure the filter is dry before replacement. This should be done only when the ventilator is switched off and disconnected from the mains supply.

**Table 23.4** Nippy Junior user maintenance: recommendations by B&D[17]

|  | Before Use | Daily | Weekly | Monthly |
|---|---|---|---|---|
| Alarms | Test | Test |  |  |
| Batteries | Ensure fully charged | Ensure fully charged | Ensure fully charged | Test |
| Breathing circuits | Inspect | Inspect | Replace |  |
| Inlet filter |  |  | Inspect/replace |  |
| Power cord | Inspect |  |  |  |

# HUMIDIFICATION: USING A HEAT–MOISTURE EXCHANGER DEVICE

The upper airway serves as an anatomical heat-and-moisture exchanger (HME), helping to

- filter
- warm
- humidify inspired air/gas.[18]

Under normal conditions, the upper airway efficiently adds heat and moisture and produces a temperature gradient, starting with ambient at the nose to body temperature in the lungs. The insertion of a tracheostomy causes the normal processes of warming, humidification and filtering of the inspired air to be bypassed, producing an unwanted humidity deficit. The small airways and low body weights of infants and children make them much more susceptible to minor changes in systemic fluid balance, increasing the risk of airway/secretion drying. In view of this, it is recommended that supplemental heat and moisture should be maintained for the child with a long-term tracheostomy, especially when the child is artificially ventilated.[19]

The introduction of wet, heated humidification in the ventilator circuit causes restrictions to the child, as it is not portable (Figure 23.2). The child must also not be positioned lower than the humidifier because of the risk of aspiration of condensed water. Therefore, children are weaned off a 'wet' circuit on to a dry circuit during the day, allowing them freedom and flexibility to move around. Commonly the wet circuit is used at night while the child is stationary.

Children whose condition allows them to come off their ventilator for periods during the day use an HME that can be placed on the end of the tracheostomy tube to provide humidification. This

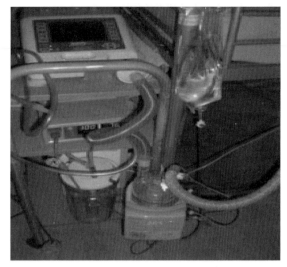

**Figure 23.2** A heated humidifier.

is commonly described as a Swedish nose. The HME capitalises on the body's counter-current mechanism of heat and moisture exchange in the airways, with nasal cooling on inspiration and warming on exhalation. Research indicates that passive airway humidification with an HME device is quickly effective;[20] however, there is no research at present to determine how long they are effective for.

## Equipment

Non-sterile gloves
HME device
Oxygen tubing to fit filter if required

## The procedural goal is to

- partly restore the important respiratory functions of the nose;
- prevent drying of pulmonary secretions;
- preserve mucociliary function;
- bacterial filtration.

## PROCEDURE: Correct use of HME on a tracheostomy

| Procedural steps | Evidence-based rationale |
| --- | --- |
| 1 Review child suitability for HME device. Child must be adequately hydrated and mobile[20] | HME is not suitable for children who are not adequately hydrated, immobile, experiencing tenacious secretions[20] |

## PROCEDURE: Correct use of HME on a tracheostomy (continued)

| | |
|---|---|
| **2** Select appropriate HME device for self-ventilating child | Please see the website for illustration of two different sizes of HME: the smaller HME is recommended for neonates and young infants; the larger HME can be used for children and adults |
| **3** Wash hands and put on non-sterile gloves before handling, connecting or disconnecting HME device | Standard precautions |
| **4** Regularly (hourly to 4 hourly) monitor the child's work of breathing and viscosity of secretions, which may indicate inadequate humidity | Each child will have an optimal level of humidification, and as the condition of the child changes so may their humidity requirements. Decreased humidity can negatively affect lung mechanics. Adverse effects of low humidity are proportional to exposure. Viscosity is resistance to flow; therefore lowering viscosity of mucus improves clearance |
| **5** Check the filter for clogging by secretions; replace if this occurs | The filter should be clean and dry. A build-up of secretions can block the filter causing obstruction and significantly increases resistance to airflow and therefore, increases breathing effort[20] |
| **6** Replace HME at least every 24 hours | HME device should be changed regularly as, over time, bacterial growth will accumulate in the filter |
| **7** HME devices can be easily 'coughed off'; replace with a new HME device if this occurs | To reduce the risk of cross-infection |
| **8** Wear non-sterile gloves to remove and discard soiled HME devices in clinical waste receptacle. Remove gloves and wash hands | To reduce the risk of cross-infection |
| **9** Monitor the number of HME devices used per day[20] | To facilitate ongoing evaluation |

### Nippy Junior breathing circuits

As many children require ventilatory support all day, it is not feasible to have them on a wet circuit continuously as it is not easily portable. For these children, there are dry circuits available that have an inbuilt HME, therefore allowing mobility. Please  see the website for illustration of dry circuit.

Dry circuits should be used with caution as they are not as effective as a heated humidifier; therefore, tolerance can vary from child to child. Careful monitoring and continuous assessment of tolerance should be maintained. For some children, saline nebulisers may be considered to loosen secretions while on dry circuits. If tolerance is low, indicated by increased work of breathing, low oxygen saturation levels, increased respiratory rate and heart rate, the child should be put straight back on their wet circuit if possible, and dry circuit use should be limited to outings.

## SPEAKING VALVES

For patients with a tracheostomy, the natural inspiration and expiration flow of air from the nose and oropharynx is interrupted because of the placement of the tube below the level of the vocal folds. Air flows to the path of least resistance, the artificial opening of the tracheostomy tube, resulting in minimal airflow across the vocal folds, causing aphonia (the inability to create a voice).[11,21] As a result of this, it is well recognised that speech and language development can be delayed since aphonia causes the child to miss out on many critical steps towards speech development, including early forms of communication such as cooing, babbling and crying.[21] If small children are unable to communicate in these ways, it has been noted that care givers will talk to them less frequently, and the child can become frustrated as

VIGNETTE

**Problem:** Manufacturer guidelines state that HME shown on the child in Figure 23.3 should be used only on neonates and infants.

**Discussion:** The child in Figure 23.3 has been established on the smaller HME and is using it every day. Although they are recommended for smaller children, he is clearly a very happy, healthy child and not showing any signs of respiratory distress. An HME that is too small may cause $CO_2$ retention due to inefficient tidal volumes and insufficient humidification. However, this child has a significant leak around his tracheostomy, allowing him to breath around it; therefore, this particular HME meets his individual need. It is important to be aware that those children with a more 'snug' fitting tracheostomy and no leak may not be able to tolerate a smaller HME. Observation and assessment of the child's clinical condition is essential.

**KEY POINTS**

Effective humidification is sometimes difficult to achieve in children when normal mechanisms are bypassed by a tracheostomy in situ. No standards exist for humidification of spontaneously breathing tracheostomy patients. The effective humidification options available in the paediatric population are HMEs and heated humidifiers, both of which are reviewed and discussed. In some circumstances the humidification achieved with HMEs is inadequate.

| Over-humidification | Under-humidification |
| --- | --- |
| Poor gas exchange | Heat loss |
| Increased secretions due to decreased evaporation | Dehydration of respiratory tract |
| Degeneration and adhesion of cilia | Epithelial damage |
| Condensation of water droplets causing atelectasis | Impaired function of mucociliary elevator |
| Mucosal cooling/burning | Sputum retention |
| | Atelectasis |
| | Bronchospasm from dry gases/cold water |

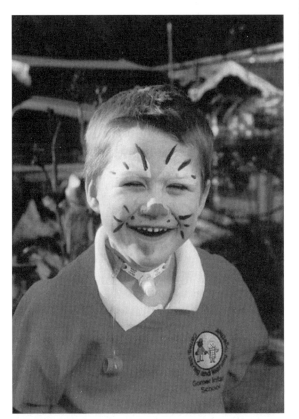

**Figure 23.3** A child with a small heat-and-moisture exchanger on his tracheostomy.

his/her needs and wants cannot be easily understood. In addition to speech and language difficulties, the lack of airflow through the upper airway can reduce vital senses such as smell and taste, which may then contribute to feeding difficulties.

To overcome these difficulties, the patented Passy–Muir speaking valve (PMV) was invented by David Muir in 1985, a 23-year-old quadriplegic patient suffering from muscular dystrophy.[22] David Muir, having a tracheostomy himself, invented the PMV to assist with his own communication needs after becoming very frustrated with people struggling to understand him.

The speaking valve is placed onto the tracheostomy in the same way as a Swedish nose and allows the patient to produce a voice by using a one-way valve. On inspiration, the valve opens allowing inspired air into the tracheostomy tube. During exhalation, the valve closes and airflow will again follow the path of least resistance, but as the valve is one way, airflow will travel around the tracheostomy tube, through the larynx, vocal folds, nasal passages and oral cavity (Figure 23.4). This airflow past the vocal folds allows restoration of spontaneous communication with a natural voice.[22] The use of speaking valves allows patients to develop speech and language skills, essential for socialisation with family members and care providers.

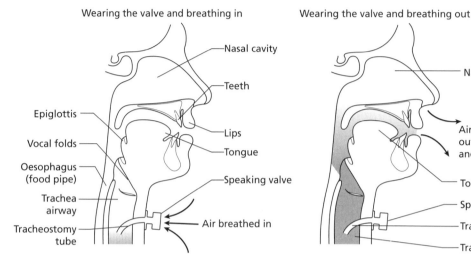
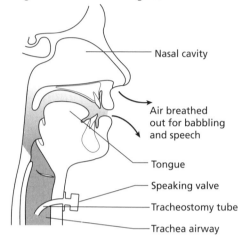

Wearing the valve and breathing in

Wearing the valve and breathing out

**Figure 23.4** Air flow with use of speaking valve.

In addition to the restoration of communication, speaking valves have been shown to provide several other physiological benefits, such as (a) improved secretion management, (b) decreased chest infections as the valve filters and cleans air, (c) improved swallow, reducing the risk of aspiration, (d) improved sense of smell and taste, and (e) in some cases expedited weaning of ventilation and decannulation as the child can get used to normal airflow patterns in oral and nasal passages.[21,22]

There are a number of studies identifying the benefits of speaking valves, but very limited research into the disadvantages of them. Current practice has identified that speaking valves are not suitable for all children with a tracheostomy, as their clinical condition cannot always tolerate the different path of airflow. Children must have a patent upper airway and be medically stable before a speaking valve should be considered. Trials should start over a short period of time, and ideally lead to extended use of the speaking valve for up to several hours each day with a diminishing need for direct supervision.[21]

### Equipment

Non-sterile gloves
Speaking valve
SaO$_2$ monitor

### The procedural goal is to

- restore the child's ability to vocalise;
- facilitate communication to enhance socialisation and bonding with family and care givers;
- ensure child's safety at all times.

## PROCEDURE: Nursing considerations for using a speaking valve

| Procedural steps | Evidence-based rationale[21] |
|---|---|
| 1 Review child suitability for speaking valve. The child must be medically stable; awake and alert; supervised and have a patent upper airway | Unsuitable children are those clinically unwell; with tracheal or laryngeal stenosis; have excessive secretions; are asleep; are unsupervised |
| 2 Suction the tracheostomy | To remove excess secretions<br>To ensure a patent airway |
| 3 Assess heart rate, respiratory rate and effort, SaO$_2$ | Baseline set of observations to look back to, if there is a question of intolerance |
| 4 Apply non-sterile gloves, remove Swedish nose and attach speaking valve directly to tracheostomy tube | Standard precautions<br>*Ensure speaking valve is clean and patent prior to use* |
| 5 Continually assess physiological parameters: heart rate, respiratory rate and effort, SaO$_2$, effectiveness of cough and ability to clear secretions | Compare with baseline observations to ensure the child's condition and safety remains stable<br>*Discontinue* immediately if there are significant changes to observations with sign of intolerance to speaking valve |
| 6 Remove speaking valve and replace Swedish nose. Wash with water and mild soap, leave to air dry | Standard precautions<br>Speaking valves are reusable. Discard if valve becomes sticky, noisy or vibrates |

## TEACHING FAMILIES TO PROVIDE CARE AT HOME

In order for the LTV child to be able to be discharged, in-depth training of family members must be undertaken. Parents are seen as the primary care givers and therefore must be competent in providing all aspects of their child's care. LTV children and their families will be supported by nurses and carers in the community providing respite, especially at night. A child dependent on LTV cannot be left unattended at any time because of the risks involved. It is exceptionally rare for community support to be funded for a 24-hour period. Therefore, there will be periods when the parents are left alone to care for their child, highlighting the importance of competency.

### Specific knowledge and skills required of parents of a child with a tracheostomy[24]

- Knowledge and understanding of their child's underlying condition, and the reason for the need of LTV.
- Understanding airway anatomy, tracheostomy tube location and challenges: tracheostomy changes (emergency and routine), cleaning and care of the stoma
- Recognition of signs and symptoms of respiratory distress, and how to respond accordingly.
- Clinical assessment techniques: not just relying on monitoring, but visual assessment of child.
- Suctioning concepts and techniques.
- Knowledge and understanding of ventilator and accompanying equipment, such as batteries: how they work, care of equipment and trouble-shooting.
- Knowledge and understanding of how to respond in an emergency situation: basic life support and cardiopulmonary resuscitation training, what to do if unable to reinsert a dislodged tracheostomy.
- Standard precautions: hand hygiene, the importance of a clean, smoke-free environment.

This complex teaching involves very close communication and teamwork with the multidisciplinary team, ensuring all aspects are covered in significant detail. Documentation of education is important. Education should be started from an early stage, teaching basic care concepts, and then cascading when appropriate to critical thinking and decision-making skills. Teaching with resources such as tracheostomy dolls and resuscitation dummies are very effective, as well as providing mock scenarios requiring parents to practise problem-solving and practical skills. Comprehensive teaching plans will enable effective and timely education, ensuring all aspects of care are covered. Please see the website for examples of competency documents.

These provide an area to document initial teaching and subsequent supervised practical skills, until the parent is deemed competent. It is important not to forget teaching the child to live and care for their tracheostomy, dependent on their age and understanding. If the child is too young to understand about their tracheostomy, teaching should be facilitated in their everyday development.

## OUTINGS AWAY FROM HOME

LTV children are highly dependent on a vast amount of equipment to ensure their safety. Therefore, before going anywhere, safety checks must be completed to ensure all their equipment is available and in working order (Table 23.5). If the child requires ventilatory support only for certain periods of the day, all equipment must still be taken in the event of deterioration.

**Table 23.5** Equipment and safety checks to be made prior to outings

| Equipment | Checks/considerations |
| --- | --- |
| Emergency tracheostomy kit | Contains everything required for an routine or emergency trachy change and care on the go |
| • Spare tracheostomy of same size | Clean, ready to use in case of dislodgement/blockage |
| • Spare tracheostomy one size smaller | In case stoma closes/unable to pass current size tracheostomy |
| • Tapes to secure tracheostomy | Ensure cotton tapes are cut to size, ready to use and attached through one side of trachy flange |
| • Scissors | To cut tapes quickly |
| • Gauze and saline | To clean site |
| • Tracheostomy dressing | To protect stoma area |
| • Lubricating gel | To ease insertion |
| • Bagging circuit and appropriate size face mask | In case of need to hand ventilate child, &/or unable to pass tracheostomy |
| Ventilators (usually × 2) and mains lead | Check settings and alarms correct with care plan |
| Dry breathing circuit | Check intact, no cracks |
| Batteries | Fully charged, adequate running time for outing Consider taking chargers for longer trips |
| Portable suction machine and mains lead | Check suction pressure Fully charged Empty collection bowel |
| Suction catheters | Appropriate size and quantity |
| Oxygen cylinder | > ¼ full (even if no current oxygen requirement) Adequate amount for trip? |
| Oxygen supply connecter (for Swedish nose and/or breathing circuit) | Tubing intact Adequate length |
| Saturation monitor and mains lead and/or batteries | Check alarm limits appropriate to child's care plan |
| Spare saturation probe | Replacement if current probe gets damaged |
| Swedish noses | Adequate number for trip (should replace daily and if soiled) |
| Gloves (non-sterile) | Standard precautions |
| Mobile phone fully charged | Contact help if required |

# THE DISCHARGE PROCESS: FROM HOSPITAL TO HOME

The handing over of care and responsibility for LTV children transferred home from the hospital is a complex process involving a vast number of different healthcare agencies and joint planning. It has been well recognised from the Platt report[7] to the NSF for children that the best place for a child to be cared for is in the familiar surroundings of their own home and family. Sadly the reality is that stable, LTV children are still spending inappropriately long periods of time in acute hospital settings awaiting provision of a 'package of care' that will provide care and support for them to be discharged and remain at home.[8] Such care packages include the financing, contracting and supply of both human and equipment resources required for the individual child and each must be tailor-made as these children often require complex and complicated care from technological, practical, social and psycho-emotional perspectives. Consequently, approximately 15 per cent of paediatric intensive care unit (PICU) and paediatric high-dependency unit (PHDU) beds are occupied by medically fit, LTV children. Owing to the acuteness of these areas the child's emotional, social and psychological needs are often not met adequately, and in many cases are made worse because of their experiences.[8] In order to mitigate this problem, transitional care units are beginning to open to care especially for LTV children,

providing a more developmentally and emotionally favourable environment.

The discharge process comprises a complex multiagency assessment, planning and management process involving representatives from the hospital and community teams as well as the child and family. It is recommended that a key worker acts as the child's discharge coordinator who is involved in the assessment and development of the care package.[25] Nurses providing the day-to-day care of the child while in hospital need not be involved in all elements; however, it is paramount that they remain informed of progress with clear lines of communication agreed with the key worker. Effective communication between all involved is crucial. Regular discharge meetings should take place, providing a forum for discussion of progress to date. The family of the child should be informed of progress as it happens, giving them insight into the planning of their child's discharge. In addition to this, the entire process must be documented well, ensuring availability to all the agencies involved.

For detailed advice regarding the discharge process and a recommended care pathway please go to www.longtermventilation.nhs.uk, where you will find a number of clinical guidelines that have been developed to help you.

Please see below the key steps required for a successful transfer home. When following this process please remember, as it takes some time, the next process can be commenced prior to the previous step being fully completed.

## PROCEDURE: A step-by-step guide to the discharge process[25]

| Procedural steps | Evidence-based rationale |
|---|---|
| 1 Establish a named consultant and designated team of named nurses who will develop a care plan and closely follow the discharge-planning progress | To ensure all key stages are acted on without repetition<br>Designated key workers to avoid any communication barriers<br>These people to liaise with outside agencies and be responsible for discharge plan |
| 2 Inform community nurses of child as soon as it is established that the child will require LTV | Discharge planning can commence straight away<br>Key worker within the community to be identified and coordinate the child's discharge plan. This key worker to be responsible to meet with all involved in child's care |

## PROCEDURE: A step-by-step guide to the discharge process (continued)

| | |
|---|---|
| 3 Contact relevant primary care trust (PCT) and local authority commissioners directly to make child known to them so PCT planning can commence | To be followed up by multiagency care package proposal following first MDT meeting and formal assessment. To include care requirements and estimated costs involved<br>Funding to be agreed in principle |
| 4 Refer family to hospital and local social services team with their permission to discuss services available | Hospital social services team should automatically see patient after being an inpatient for 90 days |
| 5 Begin parental involvement in every aspect of child's care | Competency training to be documented and follow a written plan |
| 6 Establish equipment that will be required by the child and is suitable to the home environment. Order this equipment and begin to use. Develop a disposables list to make available for when provision is handed over to PCT | Ensure family is familiar with use of equipment.<br>To include<br>2 × Nippy Junior Ventilators (£4800 each) and batteries<br>1 Humidifier unit (£1.600)<br>2 Suction machines (£600 each)<br>1 Nebuliser (£600)<br>Oxygen saturation monitor (£1000)<br>Portable saturation monitor<br>Disposable equipment (gloves, trachy ties, suction catheters, ventilator circuits, etc.)<br>Pushchair: suitable to carry the weight of all equipment needed to make the child mobile |
| 7 First multidisciplinary/multiagency meeting. Attendees to include specialist consultant, key nurses in hospital, key worker for community nurses/care provider, representative from PCT, family's assigned social worker, physiotherapist, occupational therapist, dietician, general practitioner, paediatrician and nurse representative from local hospital, child and parents | Confirm child's physical needs, and identify additional support that will be required specific to individual family circumstances<br>Identify an housing adaptations that may be required to accommodate child's care needs<br>Chance for all of MDT to meet key worker and discuss any issues to date. Communication methods agreed between parties<br>Key worker to be a link between family and multiagencies |
| 8 Formal assessment using the Framework of Assessment of Children in Need and their families as a guide with health professionals adding on assessments specific to technological needs of child | Key worker to coordinate<br>Needs assessment of child and family members, housing assessment, risk assessment<br>Proposal for preliminary funding agreement can be submitted following assessment |
| 9 Formal funding agreed by relevant local authority | Carers can now be recruited by care provider and trained in the care of the child |
| 10 Agreement of care | To be agreed between community care provider and family. Establish working partnerships between family and carers clarifying roles and responsibilities |
| 11 Begin day trips out of the hospital with child and family<br>Incorporate home visits | Full risk assessment must be taken before each outing<br>Initially to be accompanied by nursing staff to ensure child's safety<br>Following competency training, allow times away with just parents (ensure there is always two tracheostomy trained people with the child at all times) |

## PROCEDURE:  A step-by-step guide to the discharge process (continued)

| | |
|---|---|
| **12** Following any adaptations required ensure home is set up to accommodate child and equipment. | Contact utility providers so they are aware of child's requirements and ensure they will be priority should a power failure occur<br>Equipment and disposables required to be handed over from hospital funding to PCT budget<br>Contact insurance companies for home and car, making them aware of carrying oxygen<br>Contact local emergency service to inform them of child's condition should a 999 call be made from that household |
| **13** Final discharge meeting | Once everything is in place regarding funding, equipment, housing alterations, and carers are fully trained and competent, hold a last meeting to ensure all parties are happy with the plan of care<br>Ensure guidelines regarding criteria for readmission are agreed<br>Agree final discharge date and time |
| **14** Trial night at home with carers | This to take place prior to official discharge date. Hospital bed to be kept open for child in case of any teething problems |
| **15** Patient is discharged home | Care is fully transferred from hospital to the community. Detailed transfer letters should be sent from the hospital to community care providers, GP and emergency services<br>Child will have 'open access' to the hospital should problems occur and their safety be compromised at any time |

## Barriers to discharge

Unfortunately there is no central agreement for the funding of LTV packages at present. Children are dealt with individually by their local PCT, contributing to long delays in the discharge process. Additionally, the need to re-house a family, recruit and train a team of staff, and the purchasing of equipment, can also delay this process.

Although we, as healthcare professionals, cannot directly improve the funding issues, and the process of re-housing and employing carers, we can foster sound communication and documentation directly, which acts to facilitate the process.

## SUPPORTING CHILDREN AND FAMILIES

LTV children can be cared for at home only if parents are provided with support to enable them to meet their child's needs. Support can include practical assistance, advice and information; however, it is important not to overlook psycho-emotional support. There is much emphasis on the physical and technological support that LTV children and families will require; however, psycho-emotional aspects can be overlooked, perhaps because of the huge element of the unknown as all families respond differently. It is suggested that care needs to be taken to prevent an unequal balance between the technical, and psychosocial aspects of care.[26]

Without insight into what it is like to be a child or family member of a child requiring LTV, it is difficult to imagine the psychsocial and psycho-emotional implications that impinge on everyday life. However, as healthcare professionals caring for these families, we must consider all aspects of support in order to improve the welfare of these children and their parents, which should be paramount to family-centred care.[27]

Feelings of frustration, isolation, lack of control over daily living, and the feeling of being watched continuously are commonly emphasised by parents and children. The major issue highlighted by most families is that their family life can no longer be kept private due to the large number of carers working in the family home. Some parents have referred to these carers as an intrusion, as they feel they are being watched and judgments being made on their lifestyles and parenting approaches.[28] These feelings will have an effect on the natural running on the family. The ideal working relationship between the family and carers will vary for each individual family; therefore, assumptions cannot be made regarding the correct approach. To avoid conflict and provide high-quality support individual to family need, negotiation between the family and carers is vital. Negotiation regarding roles and responsibilities from a medical and, perhaps more importantly, from a non-medical point of view must be made: for example, negotiating family preferences in relation to routines, discipline and general child-rearing expectations. Additionally, major consideration needs to take place regarding relationships between the family and staff, and how the family home will be used by staff.

Home-based support can be very satisfying, but, as identified, can produce many challenges to the family and carers. Unfortunately, because of the dependency of LTV on medical supervision, the intrusion made by staff on family life cannot be completely removed. Preparation is needed for the feelings that children and parents may encounter, giving opportunity to think and reflect on coping mechanisms they might adopt prior to discharge. With understanding and respect for individual personal lives and space, it is anticipated that a good working relationship can be developed and adapted, allowing for all the needs of the child, family and carer be met.

## CONCLUSION

This chapter has given a brief overview of the skills needed to care for children and families affected by LTV. With the increase in LTV children in the UK and continuing improvements in technology and treatments, the future impact of LTV on paediatric nursing will be great. For hospitals where transitional care units have not yet been built, the future of the nursing care of LTV children will move towards a general ward area, so as not to adversely impact valuable resources within intensive and high care settings. Therefore, it is important to have an understanding and knowledge of the implications of LTV, with the associated nursing skills required to care for these children and their families. Although these children are seen as medically stable, they have an extremely high life dependence on technology, thus competence in the specific nursing skills are essential to ensure the child's safety at all times.

 Go to the website to find the PowerPoint presentation for this chapter and MCQs to test your knowledge. **www.hodderplus.com/childnursingskills**

## REFERENCES

1  Robinson RO (1990) Ventilator dependence in the United Kingdom. *Archives of Disease in Childhood* **65**: 1235–1236.

2  Jardine E, O'Toole M, Wallis C (1999). Current status of long term ventilation of children in the United Kingdom: questionnaire survey. *British Medical Journal* **318**: 295–299.

3  Jardine E, Wallis C (1998) Core guidelines for the discharge home of the child on long term assisted

ventilation in the United Kingdom. *Thorax* **53**: 762–767.

4  Amin RS, Fitton CM (2003) Tracheostomy and home ventilation in children. *Seminars in Neonatology* **8**: 127–135.

5  Wallis C (2000) Non-invasive home ventilation. *Paediatric Respiratory Reviews* **1**: 165–171.

6  Boosfeld B, O'Toole M (2000) Technology dependent children: Transition from hospital to

home. *Paediatric Nursing* **12**(6): 20–22.

7  Department of Health (1997) *Paediatric intensive care 'A Framework for the Future'*. London: DH.

7a Ministry of Health (1959) *The welfare of children in hospital. 'The Platt Report'*. London: HMSO.

8  Murphy J (2008) Medically stable children in PICU: better at home. *Paediatric Nursing* **20**(1): 14–16.

9  Haffner JC, Schurman SJ (2001) The technology dependent child. *Pediatric Clinics of North America* **48**(3): 751–764.

10 Davies JH, Hassell LL (2007) *Children in intensive care: a survival guide*, 2nd edn. London: Churchill Livingstone.

11 Torres LY, Sirbegovic DJ (2004) Problems caused by tracheostomy tube placement. *Neonatal Intensive Care* **16**(1): 52–54.

12 Preston R (2001) Introducing non-invasive positive pressure ventilation. *Nursing Standard* **15**(26): 42–45.

13 Samuels M, Boit P (2007) Non-invasive ventilation in children. *Paediatrics & Child Health* **17**(5): 167–173.

14 Medical Devices Agency (2000) *Single use medical devices: implications and consequences of re-use*, DB 2000 (04). London: MDA.

15 Quality Improvement Scotland – NHS (2007) *Caring for the patient with a tracheostomy*. Edinburgh: NHS QIS: www.nhshealthquality.org

16 Fauroux B, Lavis JF, Nicot F, *et al.* (2005) Facial side effects during non-invasive positive pressure ventilation in children. *Intensive Care Medicine* **31**(7): 965–969.

17 B&D Electromedical (2007) *Instruction manual for the Nippy Junior + positive pressure ventilator*. Stratford-Upon-Avon: B&D Electromedical www.nippyventilator.com.

18 Lewarski JS (2005) Long-term care of the patent with a tracheostomy. *Respiratory Care* **50**: 534–538.

19 Gracey K, Fiske E (2004) Tracheostomy home care guide. *Advanced Neonatal Care* **4**: 54–55.

20 Rozsasi A, Leiacher R, Fischer Y, Kack T (2006) Influence of passive humidification on respiratory heat loss in tracheotomised patients. *Head & Neck* **28**(7): 609–613.

21 Hull EM, Dumas HM, Crowley RA, Kharasch VS (2005) Tracheostomy speaking valves for children: tolerance and clinical benefits. *Pediatric Rehabilitation* **8**(3): 214–219.

22 Torres LY, Sirbegovic DJ (2004) Clinical benefits of the Passy-Muir tracheostomy and ventilator speaking valves in the NICU. *Neonatal Intensive Care* **17**(4): 20–23.

23 GOSH NHS Trust. Great Ormand Street Hospital for children NHS Trust: *Information for Families, Speaking Valves 08F0532*. London, 2008.

24 Fiske E (2004). Effective strategies to prepare infants and families for home tracheostomy care. *Advances in Neonatal Care* **4**(1): 42–53.

25 Noyes J, Lewis M (2004) *From hospital to home, guidance on discharge management and community support for children using long-term ventilation*. Ilford, Essex: Barnardos.

26 Hewitt-Taylor J (2004) Children who require long-term ventilation: staff education and training. *Intensive and Critical Care Nursing* **20**: 93–102.

27 Department of Health (2003) *Getting the right start: NSF for children*. London: DH.

28 Hewitt-Taylor J (2007) Providing support at home for families whose children have complex needs. *Journal of Children & Young Peoples Nursing* **1**(4): 195–200.

# Invasive monitoring

Jane Shelswell

## LEARNING OUTCOMES

*Upon completion of this chapter, the reader should be able to accomplish the following:*

1 Define invasive monitoring and list two indications for its use in children
2 Identify three types of invasive monitoring
3 List the equipment and checks that should be performed at the beginning of a shift when looking after a child with invasive monitoring
4 Describe the potential complications a child with invasive monitoring might experience
5 Discuss the nursing care of a child with invasive monitoring including management of common problems
6 Discuss with rationale for the recommended 'normal' values
7 Discuss with rationale the usual 'abnormal' readings, what they tell you and your nursing action

## CHAPTER OVERVIEW

There are many types of invasive monitoring equipment available and in common use in high dependency and intensive care environments. They offer an aid when managing seriously ill or compromised children. An understanding of the individual roles of invasive equipment and the data transmitted on to a screen can enhance the nurse's ability to assess the child's changing condition. This can aid appropriate adjustments in the

management of the child in order to provide optimum care.

This chapter presents practical evidence-based guidance on the use of arterial blood sampling that shows an acid–base balance, which will assist a practitioner in making changes to the ventilation or medication of a child within the medical prescription. The analysis of blood gases can appear daunting but this chapter will present a 'need to know' guide for nursing interpretation of acid–base balance and an excellent website for reference and self-testing.

In addition, this chapter discusses the use of an arterial cannula and central venous catheter (CVC) to give continuous blood pressure and central venous pressure data, which is essential for monitoring haemodynamic changes; it can provide immediate information about the treatment given such as drug therapy as well as data that need to be reported to medical staff immediately for their due attention. These tools are not without risks and these are discussed under each subject heading.

Owing to the complexity of monitoring cerebral (brain) perfusion, a brief overview of the anatomy and physiology is covered to help the reader understand how intracerebral pressure monitoring can give important information. The possibility of false readings due to equipment failure or inappropriate set-up will be highlighted. Examples will be given of such events and how to deal with them. The use of an extra ventricular drain is also covered within this chapter, highlighting how intracerebral pressure monitoring and subsequent drainage of cerebral spinal fluid (CSF) can be life saving.

It is hoped that this chapter will teach nurses that monitoring is a part of the overall care of a child. It is important to note that equipment can go wrong and sole reliance on machinery is not advocated. It teaches the nurse to be aware of the quality checks needed of any monitoring including the signs of failing or unreliable monitoring and what to do. Monitoring is a useful sequential tool to observation and recording.

### KEY WORDS

Arterial venous pressure monitoring
Invasive monitoring    Blood gas analysis
External ventricular drain (EVD)
Intracranial pressure (ICP)    Central venous catheter

## ARTERIAL PRESSURE MONITORING

The first recorded arterial blood pressure was done by Reverend Stephen Hales in 1733.[1,2] He inserted a brass pipe into an artery of a horse and connected it to a glass tube to demonstrate a rise in pressure. We have come a long way since then and it is now common practice for a doctor to cannulate an artery of a child. An appropriately sized cannula is inserted into an artery. Data are transmitted via a transducer and digitalised for on-screen monitoring. Access can be gained from the cannula to aspirate blood for gas analysis as regularly as required.

### Indications for arterial pressure monitoring

Any child who is compromised or likely to become compromised through their illness, such as:

- a respiratory illness such as pneumonia;
- severe sepsis such as meningococcal disease;
- circulatory or cardiac conditions;
- receiving drug therapy, e.g. inotropic support;
- neurological injury.

## PHYSIOLOGY OF HAEMODYNAMIC MONITORING

Blood vessels that carry blood away from the heart are anatomically known as arteries. Inserting a cannula into an artery enables serial blood gas sampling and analysis, continuous blood pressure monitoring and the added ability to calculate intracranial pressure when an intracranial measuring device is in situ.

The left ventricle expels blood into the aorta during contraction or systole, the blood stretches the elastic walls of the aorta and aortic pressure reaches its peak. This is the systolic pressure. The elastic recoil of the arteries provides the force for the blood to continue to flow passively to the arterioles. The aortic valve closes as the pressure in the aorta exceeds that in the ventricle, preventing blood flowing back into the heart. When the aortic valve has closed, the pressure in the aorta and larger arteries falls as the blood flows downstream along the large arteries to the arterioles and capillaries. This pressure recorded before the next beat is called diastolic pressure.

Aortic pressure changes with every heart beat and therefore it is important to consider the mean arterial pressure (MAP) as this is the driving force through the vascular system to the tissues. Diastole lasts longer than systole, so the mean pressure is approximately equal to the diastolic pressure plus one third of the pulse pressure (difference between diastolic and systolic pressures).

### Definitions

**Arterial pressure monitoring:** The use of a cannula inserted directly into an artery. A transducer within the system directly measures pressure which is the amount of force exerted by circulating blood against the arterial wall. This is represented by a waveform displayed on a monitor (see Figure 24.1)

This type of invasive monitoring enables accurate assessment of blood pressure status; allows for serial blood samples to analyse acid base and oxygenation status[3,4]

Common arterial sites used are
- radial
- ulna
- brachial (see Figure 24.2)
- axillary
- dorsalis pedis
- femoral

Please see the website for illustration of a dorsalis pedis and a femoral arterial line.

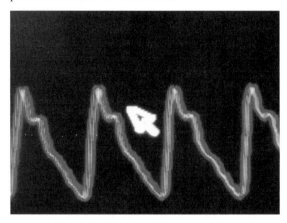

**Figure 24.1** Arterial waveform illustrating the dicrotic notch, shown by the arrow.

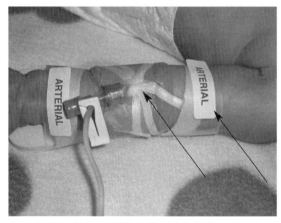

**Figure 24.2** Brachial arterial line, clearly labelled and clear dressing to observe the site.

Doctors generally prefer to use the radial artery due to its proximity to the surface and collateral circulation. Also, they prefer not to locate a cannula near a large vein or nerve as there may be a risk of puncturing these sites.[5] The superficial temporal artery can be used in infants while in the newborn the umbilical artery can be accessed for sampling, although it can close within 48 hours if not catheterised.[6] It is of note that early removal of a catheter may prevent the risk of infection and necrotising enterocolitis.[2]

By monitoring a child's condition before and after treatments the nursing and medical staff can alter the care accordingly in a more precise way.[6] It enables prescribed drug treatments to be evaluated and titrated more accurately than in non-invasive monitoring. It primarily serves to enable early recognition of haemodynamic changes, which are changes to blood pressure, pulse rate and rhythm, and enables regular blood gas analysis without frequent puncturing of the skin.

## THE ARTERIAL LINE

Arterial blood pressures are significantly higher in distally located arterial sites therefore the pedal pressure will be higher than the brachial as it is more distally located (Figure 24.2).[2] The more peripheral the higher the systolic pressure and lower the diastolic.[7]

### The procedural goal is to

- cannulate an artery using an aseptic technique, to secure and label the site clearly;
- enable continuous invasive monitoring and blood gas sampling to enhance optimal care.

### Equipment

Arterial cannula appropriate for size of child
Dressing pack/sterile paper towel
Sterile gloves × 1/non-sterile gloves × 1, apron and eye protection as per infection control policy
Chloraprep® one-step or skin preparation solution as per local policy
T-piece connector
Sterile sodium chloride 0.9 per cent
10 mL syringe
Needle
Tape for securing/Steri-strips or as per local policy
Clear bio-occlusive dressing
Pressure bag/or 50-mL luer lock syringe with infusion line (if using for neonates and small infants but dependent on local policy)
Syringe driver
Transducer set (single or triple line set dependent on monitoring required, i.e. single for arterial only)
500 mL of IV (intravenous) heparinised saline to flush system, usually 1 IU/ml (can be 0.9 per cent saline dependent on local policy)

## PROCEDURE:  The nurse's role in setting up an arterial line using a vamp system

| Procedural steps | Evidence-based rationale |
|---|---|
| 1 Set up transducer as per operators manual or if not available then ensure the following | To promote safety[10] |
| • Use flushing solution as per local policy: some areas use 0.9 per cent saline and others use heparinised saline[8,9] | To prevent clotting in the line<br>In the case of a neonate a 50-mL syringe may be used to infuse flushing solution when fluid accuracy is paramount Use a syringe driver to deliver the solution via a luer lock line connected to transducer |
| • Hang the prescribed fluid inside the pressure bag and ensure all roller clamps are turned off, spike bag of fluid with the transducer set | |
| • Inflate the pressure between 150–300 mmHg (20–40 kPa), local policy dictates pressure to be used. This allows 1.5–3 mL/hour of flush | To prevent backflow of arterial blood into transducer tubing |
| • Prime transducer set by opening each line singly. | Prevents air bubbles if you do this slowly |
| • Ensure the vamp section is withdrawn. Pull on the quick flush tag to allow flow of fluid through the system | Withdrawing the vamp allows fluid to fill the chamber on priming |
| • When the solution gets to the vamp section turn the vamp plunger downwards and withdraw slowly to prime the vamp while still pulling on the flush. When filled, plunge the chamber to expel fluid and air to end of the arterial line | It is a frequent problem that air can get into this part of the system, air rises and can easily be purged from the system |
| • Ensure all connectors are tight and secure[3] | To prevent haemorrhage, air embolism, backflow of fluid, clotting and subsequent dampening of arterial waveform |
| 2 Explain procedure to child if awake and parents Local anaesthetic may be required in an awake child, but the doctor will assess situation at the time | Informed consent allays fears and maintains communication |
| 3 Wash hands as per infection control policy, don gloves, apron and protective eye wear<br>Ensure doctor uses aseptic technique and dons protective clothing as per policy | To minimise infection. Minimal contact with bodily fluid maintained |
| 4 Ensure a sterile field is available on which to empty packs, also ensure a sterile paper towel available for use under the chosen arterial site | To prevent contamination from non-sterile objects |
| 5 Open packs but do not touch the contents: drop on to sterile field | Prevents contamination from nurse's non-sterile gloves |
| 6 Allow the doctor to draw up 10 mL of saline into the syringe using a needle and without touching the outside of the container. The doctor will prime the T-piece connector. Discard all sharps into appropriate container | Aseptic preparation excludes risk of infection T-piece allows transducer set to be changed every 72 hours or as per policy, without disconnecting and exposing to air. This reduces the risk of infection |
| 7 Once the artery is cannulated, connect the primed T-piece. Ensure the site is secured with steri-strips (dependent on your local unit policy), tape and cotton padding under the hub if necessary to prevent pressure on skin surface. Ensure site is *highly visible, labelled* and the *procedure documented*[11,12] as per visual phlebitis signs (VIPS); see *Figure 24.2 to demonstrate clear labelling* | Some areas suture arterial lines but always ensure security to prevent dislodgement, visibility to prevent haemorrhage going unnoticed, labelling ensures all medical and nursing staff are aware this is an arterial line and for monitoring and blood sampling. Drugs are never administered via this route – it could cause necrosis, death of tissue and occlusion of the artery |

## PROCEDURE: The nurse's role in setting up an arterial line (continued)

| | |
|---|---|
| 8 Ensure the transducer is connected to the monitor by means of non-disposable cable. Turn the monitor parameters on, ready to display a waveform. Zero the transducer as per manufacturer's instructions. Connect the primed line to the T-piece | The transducer detects pressure changes within the artery and converts mechanical pressure into electrical energy and displays it on a monitor[6,13,14] (see below 'How to re-zero transducer to monitor waveform' for further help) |

## PROCEDURE: How to re-zero the transducer to monitor a waveform

| Procedural steps | Evidence-based rationale |
|---|---|
| 1 Silence the alarm. The transducer will be turned off to the patient, therefore there will be no waveform to the monitor, it will alarm! Do not walk away at this point, in case your patient becomes unwell during the alarm silence. Ensure your child is positioned as described in the Key Points (page 413).[13,14] All pressure monitoring devices are zeroed to ambient atmospheric pressure[2] | Be safe and be aware of the use of alarms in arterial monitoring. They are set for a reason To ensure calibration is set from a universal landmark The external level of the heart is known as the phlebostatic axis |
| 2 Turn the arterial lever on the transducer plate off to the patient, therefore lever upwards, but check individual devices – they may differ | The flow of flushing solution is now stemmed by the position of the on/off valve. This prevents air going to the patient when the valve is opened to air |
| 3 Open the valve that has a manufacturer's bung. This is an open valve for priming the lines. This is now open to the atmosphere and off to the patient You will notice the trace is flat on your monitor | There is no air entry or flushing solution to the patient if you follow this instruction No information to the monitor as lever is closed to the patient |
| 4 If you have more than one invasive pressure, do them separately until you are proficient with the procedure Go to the arterial monitoring area of your screen and press 'zero' (the transducer port must be open to air at this stage or else it will not be able to calibrate). The display for Art BP will show '0' in the window. Replace the manufacturer's bung with an airtight bung | Sometimes there is more than one invasive pressure and they all need zeroing to the atmosphere but until you are proficient it is safer to do them individually Once '0' is seen the transducer is calibrated The one in place when the set is opened is for priming the set initially |
| 5 Turn the lever on to the patient allowing the line to remain patent and flushed when in operation (neutral position). Check the waveform is transmitted to the screen. Ensure blood pressure values appear and all alarm limits are set according to age of the child | If there is no waveform then check all connections are tight and lever turned on to allow flushing fluid to flow. Check to see if BP corresponds to previous trends. Check cables are connected properly. Varying age groups have different acceptable limits due to their physiological state |

# Arterial line waveform[7]
## Characteristics of a waveform (Figure 24.1)

A – An initial sharp rise: rapid upstroke, the anacrotic rise and it occurs during early systole with the opening of the aortic valve. Reflects the pressure pulse by left ventricular contraction[2]

B – Peaked top: represents left ventricular systole or filling of the aorta with blood

C – Dicrotic notch represents aortic valve closure and occurs on the way down the waveform. Shown by the arrow in Figure 24.1

D – Tapering off from the dicrotic notch represents ventricular diastole and coronary perfusion

### Anacrotic notch

As the ventricles enter the systole phase there is an increase in pressure. This rise is called the anacrotic notch and occurs just before the opening of the aortic valve.

### Peak systolic pressure

The peak systolic pressure reflects the maximum ejection force of the left ventricle. As the aortic valve opens a sharp uprise is seen in the tracing that is reflective of the outflow of blood from the ventricle into the arterial system.

### The dicrotic notch

As the pressure falls in the left ventricle, the aortic valve closes and the aorta subsequently relaxes. The closure and relaxation of the aorta is seen on the arterial tracing as the dicrotic notch. Please see the website for illustration of a femoral arterial line. This marks the end of systole and the onset of diastole. The location of the dicrotic notch varies according to the timing of aortic closure in the cardiac cycle. It is delayed in patients with hypovolaemia; this would be illustrated by seeing the dicrotic notch further down the dicrotic limb. It is further away again in patients who have a more peripherally located arterial line.[2]

### Diastolic pressure

This represents the amount of vasoconstriction in the arterial system. During diastole, blood moves in the arterial system and onward into the smaller arteriole branches. There must be enough time for this to occur; therefore if the heart rate is faster and the diastolic time is shortened, there is less time for movement of blood into the smaller branches, the result of this is higher diastolic pressure.

### Problems associated with waveforms[2]

*Flattening of the curve* or loss of the characteristics indicates loss of vibration sensed by the transducer. Causes include obstruction of the cannula due to clot formation: cannula pushed against arterial wall, bubbles in tubing or kinked tubing. Air transmits impulses differently from fluid; air bubbles in the tubing are one of the most frequent and important source of error. They can dampen the mechanical signal and cause erroneous measurements. *This is why it is so important when priming the line to ensure no air bubbles are present. For this reason, it is generally recommended that line extensions and/or the addition of stopcocks is avoided.*

*Dampened waveforms* lose their characteristic landmarks and appear rounded and smooth in appearance. There is a less noticeable dicrotic notch or it may be completely absent. The results can give a falsely low systolic and a falsely high diastolic pressure reading. In an under-dampened trace, there is often a tall, narrow waveform and an artificially high systolic blood pressure. This pattern could be due to small air bubbles or long tubing. In an over-dampened trace there is a low return to base line after flushing, the waveform more rounded and a slow upstroke, a poorly defined dicrotic notch and a narrow pulse pressure. This could be caused by large air bubbles or a blood clot in the system. This can result in an artificially low systolic blood pressure and a raised diastolic pressure. In both instances the mean pressure remains relatively unaffected.

In each case you should *check that the pressure bag is inflated and fluid not empty.* (This should be checked at the beginning of every shift.) Ensure the arterial site is appropriately positioned. Use the quick flush tag to flush the line, review to see if the waveform has returned. Aspirate back using the vamp system and monitor for clots. *If clots are seen in the arterial line, DO NOT flush them back into the system.*

Inform the doctor who may have to disconnect the system aseptically and remove the clots by aspirating the line (see Figure 24.3) The doctor has removed the dressing and in this case, removed the arterial line tubing in an attempt to assess viability. The cannula is being aspirated to see if clots are present that may have occluded the line. There are no clots so he is seen gently flushing the cannula, which clearly blanches and is unusable.

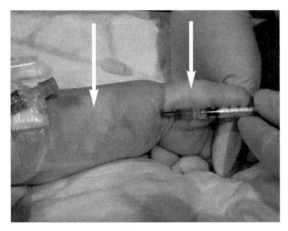

**Figure 24.3** Blanching arterial line. The areas indicated by arrows illustrate blanching.

## Complications of an arterial line[2]

### Bleeding from the site or from disconnection of the cannula

Check site regularly and ensure connections tightened prior to set up and continuously throughout duration of cannula.

### Thrombosis

Causes of thrombosis include:

- lack of flushing solution either by the bag deflating or fluid run out;
- debris can be flushed into an artery from the catheter device accidentally;
- multiple cannulation attempt;
- thrombogenic disorders, length of time cannula in situ;
- size of the cannula in relation to the diameter of the artery.

There can be a problem with the femoral site if venous and arterial lines are in same leg.

### Haematoma

This can be caused by clotting disorders, oozing around site or not enough pressure applied when cannula is removed (5 minutes or more recommended if clotting derangement evident).

### Infection

Ensure pressure bag is always inflated to prevent backflow and consequent stasis of blood in line; ensure adequate fluid in pressure bag and remove the cannula as soon as it is no longer required. Use aseptic technique when changing dressings or dealing with line. Record date and time of insertion and record VIPS score at every shift change. Change giving sets as per local policy.

### Vascular compromise and occlusion

This is particularly of note in children who are having vasoconstrictive drugs, e.g. adrenaline (epinephrine) and children with vascular compromise, e.g. cardiac disease and severe sepsis when peripheral circulation may be diminished.

### Nerve damage

This is especially of note with axillary lines; there is a risk of brachial plexus damage.

### Accidental injection of air or drugs

This can be caused by human error, not having the site labelled clearly, port left open when transducing, causing air to be drawn into circuit, or cannula becoming detached.

### Digital necrosis

This can be a result of inadequate blood flow. Lack of regular observation to limbs distal to arterial catheter could result in missing this complication. This can also be caused by possible drug administration inserted into an arterial line, thus causing death of tissues.

In Figure 24.3 the dressing has been removed after waiting a short period to see if the artery recovers from possible spasm. Vasospasm and thrombosis are the principle causes of arterial cannula failure.[2] Further assessment is made of the site. You can clearly see the blanched areas on flushing. This is no longer a viable line and should be removed.

The consequence of leaving a line in when it has extravasated can be seen in Figure 24.4. On removal the nurse should press on the site for 5 minutes to exclude a possible haematoma or bruising. Pulses should be checked, capillary refill noted and the arm monitored frequently to ensure adequate perfusion still persists. Inform the doctor if any further circulatory concerns are evident.

**Problem:** You are asked to assist with taking a blood sample for blood gas analysis. Your colleague is finding it hard to withdraw blood using the vamp system. The hand and arm become blanched on flushin. What should you do?

**Discussion:** The artery can go into spasm; mostly this is a sign that the line is no longer viable. Blanching often denotes that the flushing solution is being forced into the surrounding tissues under pressure or restricted blood flow due to pressure being exerted within the area. Therefore, notify the doctor and leave the cannula alone to see if the artery recovers from spasm or the line needs removing (see Figure 24.3).

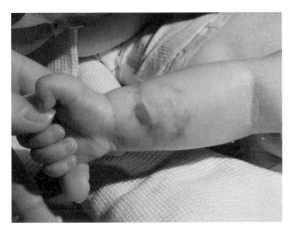

Figure 24.4 A badly extravasated site and pressure point noted.

# ARTERIAL BLOOD GASES

## Acid–base balance: understanding blood gas analysis

Table 24.1 Normal blood gas values16

| Infant/child | Neonate |
| --- | --- |
| pH 7.35–7.45 | 7.3–7.4 |
| PCO$_2$ (kPa) 4.5–6.0 (35–45 mmHg) | 4.6–6.0 |
| PO$_2$ (kPa) 10 –13 (75–100 mmHg) | 7.3 –12 (55–90 mmHg) |
| Bicarbonate (mmol/litre) 22–26 | 18–25 |
| Base (mmol/litre) –2 to +2 | –4 to +4 |

Arterial blood is superior to peripheral venous blood in both acid-base and oxygenation assessment because it reflects overall blood or body conditions. Arterial blood is uniform regardless of which artery it is drawn from.[1]

Ensure after *any* change in the child's position that the transducer level is checked. It should be level with the midaxillary line, the 4th intercostal space which is level with the right atrium.[13,14] Measure from the black dot/marker on the transducer to the landmarks described. In some areas a spirit level can be used for greater accuracy. Re-zero the transducer, as described in 'How to re-zero a transducer to monitor a waveform' (page 410). You should check the transducer at the beginning of your shift and regularly thereafter if there is any doubt about accurate measurements. Be aware of your patient's haemodynamic status, e.g. fluid balance or sepsis, that may affect the readings significantly.

Convenient ways to calculate mean arterial blood pressure (MABP)[1,15] are:

MABP = (systolic pressure) + (2 × diastolic pressure)/3, e.g.

80 + 35 × 2 = 150 ÷ 3 = 50 mmHg = 80/35 (50)

MABP = 1 ÷ 3 systolic pressure + 2 ÷ 3 diastolic pressure, e.g.

80 ÷ 3 = 27 + 35 ÷ 3 × 2 = 23 = 50 mmHg

MABP = diastolic pressure + (pulse pressure ÷ 3), e.g. 90/50 calculates into:

50 + (40 ÷ 3) = 63 mmHg

If the transducer is lower than the landmarks, then you will get a falsely high reading. Likewise, higher positions give pressure falsely lower readings.[2] Check a non-invasive cuff pressure if you are unsure of the measurement to see how they correspond.

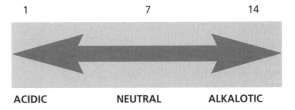

## Related physiology

The pH scale is a scale upon which hydrogen ions are measured. At one end of the scale, 1 is the most acidotic and 14 the most alkalotic. The normal values are between 7.35 and 7.45 for normal metabolism to take place. Hydrogen ions (H+) are inversely related, therefore *the more H+ in the blood the lower (more acidic) and the lower H+ ions the higher the pH (more alkalotic).*

If the pH is more acidotic, it can diminish cardiac contractions, decrease the normal vascular response to catecholamines and reduce the effects of some drugs.

If the pH is more alkalotic, it can interfere with tissue oxygenation, neurological and muscular function. A pH of about 7.8 and below 6.8 will interfere with cellular function and lead to death if left uncorrected.

The body self-regulates its acid–base balance to maintain the pH within the normal range. How does it do this? Buffers are substances with the ability to bind and release H+ thus maintaining a constant pH. Three main buffers are bicarbonate, haemoglobin and phosphate. The buffer system converts strong acid to weak acid or strong base to weak base.

There are buffer mechanisms between the respiratory and renal systems.

*Respiratory buffer response:* the by-product of respiration is $CO_2$. This is excreted in the lungs. Excess $CO_2$ combines with $H_2O$ to form carbonic acid, $H_2CO_3$. The blood pH changes according to the amount of carbonic acid present. Once there is an imbalance the lungs are activated to increase respirations to blow off excess or decrease respirations to hold on to $CO_2$. This is done by increasing or decreasing rate and depth of breathing. This occurs relatively quickly in response to the imbalance (1–3 minutes).

*Renal buffer response:* the kidneys excrete or retain $HCO_3$ in response to a change in pH (remember how the lungs react in the same way but with $CO_2$). As the pH decreases (becomes more acidic) the kidneys compensate by retaining bicarbonate. As the pH increases (becomes more alkalotic) the kidneys excrete bicarbonate through the urine. This is by no means a quick process; it can take from hours to days to correct an imbalance.

### Things to note when looking at blood gases[17]

$O_2$: A patient with low oxygen $O_2$ is not respiring properly and is hypoxic but be aware of the child's underlying condition, e.g. hyperplastic left heart syndrome prior to surgery, and may have a very low oxygen figure due to the anatomical differences associated with the disease.

$PCO_2$: The carbon dioxide and partial pressure indicate respiratory related problems; the $PCO_2$ is determined entirely by ventilation. A high $PCO_2$ (respiratory acidosis) indicates under ventilation, because you are not 'blowing off' $CO_2$. A low $PCO_2$ (respiratory alkalosis) indicates over ventilation. Again, be aware of individual lung pathology as this may mean the child has a permitted higher value.

$HCO_3$: The $HCO_3^-$ ions indicate whether a metabolic problem is present (e.g. ketoacidosis). A low $HCO_3^-$ indicates metabolic acidosis; a high $HCO_3^-$ indicates metabolic alkalosis. Note the $HCO_3^-$ values move the same way as the pH scale

**Base excess:** this indicates whether the patient is acidotic or alkalotic. An exceeded negative base excess indicates the patient is acidotic; therefore, a positive exceeded base excess means they are alkalotic.

| KEY POINTS[18] | The only two ways an acidotic state can exist is from either too much $PCO_2$ or too little $HCO_3$: high $PCo_2$ and low pH value and low $HCO_3$ = acidosis<br>The only two ways an alkalotic state can exist is from either too little $PCO_2$ or too much $HCO_3$: low $PCO_2$ and high pH value and high $HCO_3$ = alkalosis)<br>An excellent self-learning package on arterial blood gases[18] can be found at www.orlandohealth.com/pdf%20folder/SLP/2007ABG_rev.pdf |
| --- | --- |

Please note that for areas of practice that do not have heparinised syringes use a 2-mL syringe and draw up 1 mL of 1:1000 heparin. Plunge the syringe back and forth to coat the inside of the barrel. Expel heparin and dispose of the needle in sharps container. The minimal amount of heparin left in the hub of the syringe does not alter blood gas results. It is not advisable to use higher concentrations of anticoagulant as this may alter pH and ionised calcium[6]

## PROCEDURE:  Taking an arterial blood sample from the arterial line using a closed vamp system

| Procedural steps | Evidence-based rationale |
|---|---|
| 1 Ensure use of universal precautions: gloves, apron and protective eye wear<br>Have alcohol wipe, heparinised syringe and necessary equipment to hand in suitable container | To reduce risk of accidental contamination and transmission of blood borne viruses<br>To prevent entry of micro-organisms into system<br>The risk of line disruption and clotting could ensue if left for a long period of time. |
| 2 Silence alarm on monitor if safe to do so. Make patient aware of possible alarm if appropriate; reassure parents in case alarm is activated | Withdrawing blood into the vamp system will cause the monitor to alarm due to disruption of arterial waveform |
| 3 Withdraw blood into the vamp system at a steady rate but not too fast. The vamp withdraws approximately 2–4 mL when it has reached the hilt<br>Turn the tap *off* to the patient.<br><br>Swab the top with appropriate cleansing pad as per local policy and leave to dry | This allows the heparinised blood to be withdrawn and therefore not contaminate the result<br><br>This prevents heparinised blood being withdrawn back from the vamp system when the sample is taken<br>Prevents micro-organisms entering the port and causing infection in the line and systemically |
| 4 Attach heparinised syringe to the needle less connector and push securely onto the bung on the arterial line<br>*Do not push connector onto bung without syringe* | This will enable blood to be aspirated from the arterial blood vessel<br><br>*This will open the pathway for arterial blood to come out and the patient will lose unnecessary blood* |
| 5 Holding the *syringe and connector securely* together withdraw 0.5 mL of blood for a blood gas or more if blood samples are required<br>Be aware of the age group when you are sampling and note possible small circulating volumes. Note condition of patient for example do they have a low haemoglobin and is the sample necessary?<br>Record on fluid balance chart | The two can come apart and cause blood loss If not held together<br><br>Minimal amounts taken for sampling allows patient not to be depleted of vital circulating blood volume. This is especially important in low birth weight or young babies due to minimal circulating volume, e.g. an infant has a circulating volume of 70-80 mL/kg[19] therefore a 10-kg infant has 700–800 mL of blood circulating |
| 6 When appropriate amount is withdrawn remove the syringe and connector together (0.5 mL)<br>Put airtight cap on the gas syringe<br>If wishing to obtain further samples use a separate syringe of appropriate size and a new connector and repeat process of applying them together (non-heparinised syringes for other blood tests) | This prevents blood loss if removed together, if the syringe is accidentally removed before the connector it will squirt blood due to the pressure from the artery, If this happens, remove the connector as soon as possible to prevent further blood loss. Blood is a living cell therefore it will continue to metabolise if not sealed with a cap, allowing further diffusion of gases[20] |
| 7 Sometimes blood has oozed from the bung when removal takes place, swab with appropriate wipe and leave to dry.<br>Turn the tap *on* to the patient, but *off* to flush. Push the vamp down to allow the heparinised blood to return to the patient. Observe the site for blanching as you do so and ensure the line is patent. Turn the tap *on* to the patient and flushing solution, *off* to sampling port.<br>Use the fast flush tag to flush the line | To prevent infection<br>To prevent the blood going back up the line towards the flushing solution<br><br><br>This allows heparinised saline/ saline to flush the line and prevent clotting and line failure |
| 8 Ensure trace returns to monitor | Check tap position, patient position, non-disposable cables, pressure and fluid bag |

# CENTRAL VENOUS CATHETER (CVC)

## Indications[22]

- Any large fluid bolus or blood products
- Total parenteral nutrition
- Cytotoxic drug therapy
- Inotropic drugs which are better administered through a large vein to minimise damage to the vessels; likewise, some none inotropic drugs such as erythromycin, which can be an irritant.
- Measurement of central venous pressure (CVP)
- postoperative measurement of haemodynamic status whereby the child may be haemodynamically compromised
- Route may be used for insertion of pacing line
- Blood sampling if arterial line not sited, or simultaneously for venous sampling or blood tests. Mixed venous samples enable trends in cardiac output when other cardiac output devices are not available[2]
- Administration of resuscitation drugs

## Common puncture sites[23]

- *Internal jugular vein (IJV):* in the neck, carries blood from the head to the heart.
- *Subclavian vein (SV):* under the collar bone, carrying blood from the arm to the heart (Figure 24.5).
- *Femoral vein (FV):* the main vein in the leg, and the upper limbs used for insertion of peripherally inserted central catheters (PICCs).

## Complications of CVC lines[24]

- *Pneumothorax:* this can occur during the insertion of the CVC. A chest X-ray should always be requested post procedure to validate the position of the line.

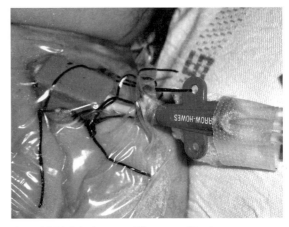

**Figure 24.5** Subclavian central line sutured in place; a transparent dressing is in situ for high visibility.

- *Cardiac arrhythmia:* if the catheter is over-advanced then cardiac arrhythmias can occur, so cardiac monitoring should always be in place when the procedure is being carried out.
- *Air embolism:* this is another potential complication from central line insertion. All connections should be checked and left visible. Care should be taken to ensure no damage occurs to the line while it is being sutured in place. Be careful if scissors are used for removing dressings, they may cause accidental damage to line.
- *Infection:* this is the most common complication. This is a serious potential risk especially if the femoral vein is used because of the proximity to the genitalia. Strict aseptic technique should be adhered to throughout insertion of the CVC and when dealing with the site thereafter. Dressing changes should be every 7 days unless otherwise indicated by moisture-related problems. Large-

bore and multilumen catheters are associated with higher risks of infection; therefore, remove as soon as possible: line-related infections can be associated with the length of time the line is left in situ unnecessarily. Ensure the line is observed at each shift handover to check for patency and signs of infection (Figure 24.6).

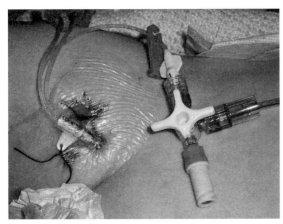

**Figure 24.6** Femoral central line with transparent dressing.

- *Exsanguination:* ensure all ports are secure at time of insertion. At the beginning and throughout the nursing shift ensure all lumens have an end bung to prevent accidental blood loss. Ensure the site is visible at all times.
- *Occlusion:* a continuous infusion can prevent this from occurring. Dependent on how many ports are available, all ports should be flushed before and after drug administration and local policy will dictate how often a free port should be flushed and the solution to be used.
- *Thrombosis:* if resistance is felt during injection, force should not be exerted as this may cause further damage to occur or flush a clot into the system. Use of a pressurised infusion via the CVP port; will help to maintain patency.

- *Catheter fracture:* this can occur externally or internally. Beware of using scissors to prevent external fracture occurring; frequent clamping of a line may weaken it. Internal fracture is another complication that requires discontinuation of the line until reviewed by a doctor. The fracture is denoted by swelling around the site and fluid leakage. It can be a serious condition, dependent on the degree of disruption within the internal part of the catheter. Seek medical assistance as soon as possible.

### The procedural goal is to

- cannulate a large vein using aseptic technique;
- enable continuous monitoring to guide therapy and enhance optimal care.

### Equipment

Central venous catheters appropriate to size of child
Dressing pack and sterile drapes
Sterile gloves × 1 and gown/non-sterile gloves × 1, apron and eye protection as per infection control policy
Chloraprep® one-prep or skin preparation solution as per local policy
Three-way taps for as many lumens you require
Sterile sodium chloride 20 mL
20-mL syringe and blue needle
Transparent bio-occlusive dressing
Suture material preferably with a curved needle
Pressure bag or 50-mL luer lock syringe with infusion line (if using for neonates and small infants, but dependent on local policy)
Syringe driver
500 mL of 0.9 per cent saline solution or pre-heparinised solution, as per local policy
Transducer set (note, if arterial monitoring in progress there may be a double lumen measuring device already in situ – if not, follow guidelines to prime the line as for arterial line)

## PROCEDURE: The nurse's role in setting up a central line

| Procedural steps | Evidence-based rationale |
|---|---|
| **1** Set up transducer as per operators manual or if not available then ensure the following:<br>Use flushing solution as per local policy: some areas use 0.9% saline and others use Heparinised saline[8,9]<br>Hang the prescribed fluid inside the pressure bag and ensure all roller clamps are turned off, spike bag of fluid with the transducer set<br>Inflate the pressure between 150 and 300 mmHg tubing (20–40 kPa), local policy dictates pressure to be used<br>This allows 1.5–3 mL/hour of flush<br>Prime transducer set by opening each line singly<br>Pull on the quick flush tag to allow flow of fluid through the system | To promote safety[10]<br><br>To prevent clotting in the line.<br>In the case of a neonate a 50-ml syringe may be used to infuse flushing solution when fluid accuracy is paramount. Use a syringe driver to deliver the solution via a luer lock line connected to transducer<br><br>To prevent backflow of arterial blood into transducer<br><br><br>Prevents air bubbles if you do this slowly. |
| **2** Wash hands as per infection control policy, don gloves, apron and protective eye wear<br>Ensure doctor uses aseptic technique and dons protective sterile clothing as per policy | To minimise infection. Minimal contact with bodily fluid maintained |
| **3** Ensure a sterile field is available on which to empty packs, also ensure a sterile drape is available for the doctor to use over the chosen central venous access site | Strict asepsis to be maintained throughout procedure to minimise risk of infection |
| **4** Open packs but do not touch the contents: drop onto sterile field | |
| **5** The site and insertion are decided by the doctor carrying out the procedure. It is recommended by NICE[24] that real-time ultrasound guidance should be carried out in the non-emergency situation | This provides the operator with visualisation of the exact vein to be cannulated and the surrounding anatomical structures |
| **6** Allow the doctor to draw up 20 mL of saline into the syringe using a needle and without touching the outside of the container<br>The doctor will aspirate the central line when it is positioned<br>There are stoppers on the end of lines when the pack is opened. These are usually changed for bungs and three-way taps to allow for greater access (as per your local unit policy). Discard all sharps into appropriate container | For priming lines to prevent clotting after insertion<br><br><br>This excludes the risk of air in the line, i.e. blood is drawn back and then flushed with saline<br>Applying bungs means the line is free from contamination when three-way taps changed for example, they maintain a closed system<br>The person inserting the line is responsible for disposing of their sharps to prevent accidental needlestick injury |

## PROCEDURE: The nurse's role in setting up a central line (continued)

| | |
|---|---|
| **7** Once the vein is cannulated, connect to the dislodgement, primed central line tubing. CVP monitoring can take place. An X-ray is done to check placement. The site is secured with sutures, cotton padding under the hub (if necessary) to prevent pressure on skin surface. Ensure site is highly visible, labelled and procedure documented[11,12] (see Figures 24.5 and 24.6, pages 418, 419). | *Always* ensure security of site to prevent visibility to prevent haemorrhage going unnoticed; labelling ensures all medical and nursing staff are aware this is a central line and for monitoring and blood sampling if an arterial line not present or for mixed venous saturation reference |
| **8** Ensure the transducer is connected to the monitor by means of a non-disposable cable. Ensure transducer plate is *secure* to minimise artefact. Please see the website for an illustration of a transducer. Turn the monitor parameters on, ready to display a waveform. Zero the transducer as per manufacturer's instructions (see instructions above for zeroing arterial line, same procedure) | The transducer detects pressure changes and converts mechanical pressure into electrical energy and displays it on a monitor[6,13,14] |

### Definitions

An **intracranial pressure device** is a pressure-sensitive device which is inserted inside the head. The most common methods of monitoring are with intraventricular and intraparenchymal catheters.[25]

The device is connected to a transducer which converts the pressure into a continuous waveform. It is used to guide early intervention and treatment. The aim of monitoring and managing elevated intracranial

pressure (ICP) is the prevention of cerebral ischaemia.

Raised ICP may be the first sign of worsening intracranial pathology.

The National Institute of Clinical Excellence (NICE) considers ICP monitoring a standard clinical practice with risks and benefits that are sufficiently well known.[26]

## INTRACRANIAL PRESSURE MONITORING

### Indications[27,28]

- Severe head injury denoted by CT scan and referral to neurosurgeon[29]
- Intracerebral and subarachnoid haemorrhage: localised mass lesions
- Hydrocephalus
- Brain oedema or swelling: encephalitis, meningitis
- Hypoxic brain injury
- Central nervous system infections
- Focal oedema secondary to trauma, infarction and tumour

### Monro–Kellie hypothesis[30]

In 1783, Scottish physician Alexander Monro (1733–1817) deduced that the cranium was 'a rigid box' of unchanging size containing three things: brain, blood and cerebrospinal fluid. He therefore proposed that any addition to the intracranial compartment must push something else out or increase intracranial pressure. This hypothesis was later supported by experiments by George Kellie (1758–1829).

What is now referred to as the Monro–Kellie doctrine, or hypothesis, is that the sum of volumes of brain (80 per cent), cerebral spinal fluid (CSF) (10 per cent) and intracranial blood (10 per cent) is constant. An increase in one should cause a decrease in one or both of the remaining two. The

Monro–Kellie hypothesis provides the physiological basis for the management and treatment of raised ICP. These include opening the skull, using diuretics such as mannitol to remove water; careful and minimal handling of the patient, and in those with refractory ICP, imposing hyperventilation to reduce blood carbon dioxide and constrict blood vessels.

### Causes of raised ICP

- *Mass effect:* brain tumour, infarction with oedema, contusions, subdural or epidural haematoma, or abscess.
- *Generalised brain swelling:* trauma, ischaemic–anoxia states, acute liver failure, encephalopathy, Reye's syndrome
- *Increased venous pressure:* thrombosis, heart failure, or obstruction of superior mediastinal or jugular veins
- *Obstruction to CSF flow and or absorption:* hydrocephalus (blockage of ventricles or subarachnoid space at base of brain) extensive meningeal disease

ICP is measured in millimetres of mercury (mmHg). In the vertical position it becomes negative (–10 mmHg (–1.3 kPa)).[31] ICP is normally 0–10 mmHg (0–1.3 kPa). In term infants 1.5–6 mmHg (0.2–0.8 kPa) is considered normal, whereas in children values have been suggested as 3 and 7 mmHg (0.4 and 0.9 kPa). It fluctuates dependent on the child's activity such as coughing, exercising and the respiratory cycle.[32]

Depending on the reason for ICP elevation, e.g. hydrocephalus, this can determine a lower ICP acceptance value.[27] At 20–25 mmHg (2.7–3.3 kPa), the upper limit of normal, treatment to reduce ICP is always required.[33]

### How does the brain compensate?

The circulating blood volume provides a constant supply of oxygen and glucose to the tissues. The components, that are brain, blood and CSF, may alter a small degree in relation to one another but in healthy people homeostatic mechanisms maintain a constant ICP. Therefore, small increases in brain volume do not lead to an immediate increase in ICP. However, if the brain suffers an insult, for example swelling from trauma, a decrease in blood volume and CSF volume occur, and in accordance with the Monro–Kellie hypothesis, the pressure (ICP) inside the cranium will rise. Once the ICP reaches 25 mmHg (3.3 kPa), small increases in brain volume can lead to comparatively greater elevations in ICP as there is less room for compensation.

## What is cerebral perfusion pressure?[32]

Cerebral perfusion pressure (CPP) is the pressure that facilitates blood flow to the brain, which remains fairly constant due to autoregulation. It is calculated by subtracting the ICP from the mean arterial pressure (MAP). In intensive care situations, where invasive monitoring is commonplace, a patient who is in need of ICP monitoring will have arterial pressure monitoring in progress simultaneously. CPP = MAP – ICP.

When the ICP increases it can cause a decrease in CPP. The optimum pressure at which the brain is perfused is >60 mmHg (8 kPa) to maintain the brain's supply of oxygen and glucose. A raised ICP will produce signs and symptoms but does not cause neuronal damage; however, a CPP of <40 mmHg (5.3 kPa) will cause neuronal damage and ischaemia.[34]

When the ICP reaches the MAP, cerebral blood flow ceases. The body's response to a decreased CPP is to raise blood pressure and dilate blood vessels in the brain. This in turn increases blood volume, which increases ICP, thus lowering CPP further. There are many interventions to reduce and prevent this phenomenon. This is a basis guide and further reading in the care of neurological patients is advised.

### Pressure waveforms

Normal individual ICP pulse waveforms generally have three characteristic peaks of decreasing height that correlate with the arterial pulse waveform and are referred to as P1 (percussion wave), P2 (tidal wave), and P3 (dicrotic wave). P1 generally has a sharp peak and fairly constant amplitude. P2 is more variable and ends on the dicrotic notch. P3 follows the dicrotic notch. There may be additional smaller peaks following the three main peaks, but these vary by individual and may not always be present.

### Waveform analysis

P1 – represents arterial pulsations
P2 – represents intracranial compliance (when brain compliance reduces P2 exceeds P1)
P3 – represents venous pulsations (Figure 24.7)

The waveforms follow the pulse wave: increasing size of the wave corresponds to increasing ICP. Plateau waves show evidence of ischaemia and brain damage, but can follow respiratory patterns. Interference with the waveforms can occur due to poor calibration, kinks or air in the line and repositioning the patient.

There are three distinct waveforms: Lundberg's pressure waves.

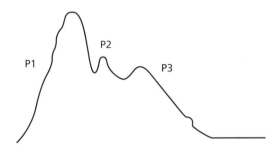

**Figure 24.7** Waveform.

- A waves: plateau wave. Sharp increase in ICP to 30–70 mmHg (4–9.3 kPa); they remain high for 2–20 minutes; they cause reduced cerebral perfusion which in turn caused ischaemia.
- B waves: sharp sawtooth with ICP 5–70 mmHg (0.7–9.3 kPa) occurring every 30 seconds to 2 minutes. This reflects the fluctuation in blood pressure.
- C waves: small rhythmical waves occurring every

4–8 minutes. They are related to normal fluctuation in respiratory pattern.

A and B waves need acting upon. ICP waveforms give information on autoregulation and cerebrospinal compliance.

## THE NURSE'S ROLE: CHILD WITH ICP MONITORING DEVICE

The neurosurgeon or trained technician will insert an ICP bolt into the parenchymal area of the brain when the condition of the patient warrants invasive pressure monitoring. A small hole is drilled in the skull through which a strain gauge is passed and sited into the parenchyma. This is then transduced to give an estimate of the ICP, which in turn is used to guide therapy.

The nurse must assist in setting up the equipment and help to maintain an aseptic technique.

### The procedural goal is to

- ensure asepsis maintained and assist medical practitioner;
- enable continuous invasive monitoring throughout procedure and maintain patient safety.

### Equipment

Surgical gown
Appropriate insertion pack
Dressing pack/sterile drape if not included
Razor to shave site
Sterile gloves ×1/non-sterile gloves ×1, apron and eye protection as per infection control policy
Chloraprep® one-step or skin preparation solution as per local policy
Sterile sodium chloride 0.9 per cent
5-mL syringe
Needle
Local anaesthetic: lignocaine 1 per cent
Betadine for soaking gauze to be placed around bolt entrance (as per local policy as a means of prevention of infection at entry site)
Steri-strips
Monitor for ICP transducing

---

**KEY POINTS**[15]

Neonates and infants respond differently to the effects of raised ICP because their cranial sutures have not yet fused, thus allowing the fontanelle to bulge under pressure. This mechanism gives practitioners a limited opportunity over time to identify raised ICP before serious neurological symptoms occur.

For example, an infant who has sustained a head injury has been admitted to your ward for observation. You observe that the fontanelle is raised; it is your duty to ensure that the doctor is alerted of this finding *immediately*.
Fontanelle assessment is a basic nursing assessment tool that can be life saving!

## PROCEDURE: Setting up an ICP monitoring device

| Procedural steps | Evidence-based rationale |
|---|---|
| **1** Open packs onto a sterile working area using an aseptic technique | To maintain asepsis |
| **2** Assist the surgeon in donning sterile gown and gloves | To prevent the gown becoming contaminated |
| **3** Pass the required equipment in accordance with the principles of asepsis, i.e. not touching the equipment inside the packs but opening and dropping onto the sterile field | To prevent contamination |
| **4** *Local anaesthetic should be checked by a trained nurse and the doctor who will be using it.* Snapping the ampoule and allowing the doctor to draw the solution into the syringe with a sterile blue needle attached <br><br> Ensure the administration is documented in the patients notes | To ensure the correct drug is used and prevent a drug error occurring. Follow hospital protocol for checking subcutaneous drug administration <br><br> To ensure legal documentation of administration of a drug via any means |
| **5** The cleansing solution checked for strength and appropriate usage <br> Ensure the patient is not allergic to any product by asking a family member if possible <br> Explain to parents or legal guardian what the procedure involves | To maintain safety when using cleaning products on the skin site <br> To prevent an allergic skin reaction to products. Iodine solutions can sometimes cause skin irritation, so be aware this may become evident <br> The area is shaved and the skin may be discoloured with the cleaning solution, depended on what is used to prepare the skin site. Prior knowledge may allay subsequent fears for parents |
| **6** The procedure is carried out under aseptic conditions at all times | *There is a risk of infection to the brain, therefore use aseptic conditions throughout* |
| **7** The catheter is inserted through a burr hole made in the skull. The connector is zeroed, by the surgeon; the fine gauge catheter is then connected. An opening pressure should be seen on the monitor <br> If no numeric values are shown on the monitor, then check all connections and see if the monitor is plugged in and turned on <br> Dependent on local preference, some equipment set up may be different, for example the Codman System requires zeroing the connector in water prior to insertion. See the manufacturer's instructions | This ensures asepsis: all equipment for procedure is sterile <br> The opening pressure can act as an immediate guide for treatment and act as a baseline of the immediate condition within the skull <br> There may be loose connectors causing inability to transduce. Ensure the monitor is turned on remembering the ICP is zeroed from the box connected to the patient; therefore there is no worry with the height of the transducer. Please see the website for an illustration of a zeroed box |
| **8** There is a depth indicator on the inserted catheter; this is situated between the armoured casing and is often taped either side to ensure it is easily recognisable and lies between both borders This must remain within the areas taped. | This denotes the depth of insertion. If it moves from within the taped markings the nurse should inform the doctor immediately. This may alter ICP readings as the catheter tip will have been dislodged |
| **9** The waveform should be seen along with numeric representation of ICP and CPP pressures | Note that if an arterial blood gas is being taken, the blood pressure reading will not be seen on the screen as the waveform is interrupted. The CPP pressure will not be accurate as there is no MAP to initiate the calculation (remember CPP = MAP – ICP) |

## PROCEDURE:  Setting up an ICP monitoring device (continued)

| | |
|---|---|
| **10** The surgeon may place Betadine-soaked gauze around the bolt entrance site. Please see the website for illustration of Betadine-soaked gauze. This is left in situ for 5 days unless otherwise instructed | As per local policy, used in some centres as a means to help prevent infection. If this becomes dislodged, then ensure area covered or reapply as instructed. Care for the entry site as per unit policy |

## Nursing recommendations following insertion of an ICP device

- Ensure the depth indicator stays within the marked area; report immediately if it is not.
- The device is calibrated at the box as described but daily zeroing of the main monitor is advised.
- Ensure alarms and settings are set appropriately.
- Ensure the cable connector is secured to the bed and not dragging on the ICP catheter in any way.
- Detach connector when moving a stable child to limit drag effect and possible dislodgement. When disconnecting, you will not need to recalibrate. Ensure a waveform returns to monitor when you reconnect.
- Ensure iodine dressing remains around ICP bolt at insertion point. This remains in situ for 5 days unless otherwise instructed; it can be changed after this time or of the ICP device can be removed by the surgeon. Pay attention to wound site and any possible signs of infection.
- If the ICP bolt is removed the site will be sutured to prevent entry of micro-organisms. The suture(s) remains in situ for 5 days unless otherwise instructed.

## EXTRAVENTRICULAR DRAIN

### Indications

Acute hydrocephalus

**VIGNETTE**

**Problem:** You are turning a child who has an ICP monitoring device in situ. You are using the log roll technique. You carry out the cares and notice that when you return your child to their previous position the ICP is 28. You initiate methods to reduce the pressure as per your unit protocols. You wait a few minutes and it seems unchanged.

You note the coloured area inside the armoured casing has moved. What should you do?

**Discussion:** Remember to disconnect the transducer box prior to moving to reduce drag effect. This is an acceptable practice in a stable patient. Check the depth gauge prior to moving. A dislodged ICP catheter requires referral to a doctor immediately as there is no longer a reliable measurement.

Head injury with reduced Glasgow coma score (GCS <8)
Purulent meningitis: infected CSF drains and allows direct administration of antibiotics into CSF
Posterior fossa tumours
Subarachnoid haemorrhages
Infected shunt replaced with EVD temporarily

Ventricular cannulation was originally a method assessed by Lindberg in 1960, and is thought to provide the most accurate measurements[25,36] and is classed as the 'gold standard'. There may be

## Definitions[29,35]

| | |
|---|---|
| **Extraventricular drain (EVD):** a *temporary* device used to drain CSF from the ventricles and relieve pressure in the skull. It is used when production, drainage or absorption of CSF is abnormal. It is a hollow flexible silicone tube that is inserted via a burr hole. It is placed in either the right or left lateral ventricle. It is either sutured at the insertion point or tunnelled for 4–5 cm and exits at a separate scalp site. It is then | connected to a drainage system. Note that the EVD is used to drain fluid but it can have a transducer attached to measure ICP. An intraventricular catheter connected to a pressure transducer is considered to be the most accurate and reliable method.[25] This is done under aseptic conditions should it be required or at time of insertion. The drain must be closed to measure ICP intermittently or a dual-lumen catheter used. |

difficulty placing the catheter in some instances as the ventricles can change shape under increased pressure and are often quite small if the brain is swollen from injury. The catheter is inserted under general anaesthetic via a burr hole into the frontal horn of the lateral ventricle. *The child will return to the care area after the procedure and the nurse has responsibilities associated specifically to the care of the EVD.*

## Risks associated with insertion of an EVD device

- Infection: particularly after 5 days
- Bleeding: particularly on insertion, in 0.5–2 per cent of cases
- Damage to brain tissue with continued neurological effects
- Risks from general anaesthesia
- Inability to find ventricle and accurately place catheter

## The nursing recommendations following the insertion of an EVD device[37]

- Drainage depends on gravity; this means the amount of CSF draining depends on the position of the chamber beneath the ventricles. The 'zero reference point' is located at the foramen of Munro or level with the external auditory meatus (top of the child's ear).
- The set drainage pressure is advised by the neurosurgeon. It is usually 10 cm $H_2O$ from the zero reference. This means that when the pressure inside the head reaches >10 cm $H_2O$ the system will drain.
- Hourly observation includes EVD integrity, levelling of the drainage system to reference points as described. Volume of drainage ± ICP and CPP pressure if transducer in situ.
- The system suspends on a corded attachment next to the patient, *visible at all times.*
- Dressings remain in situ at all times. If the dressing gets wet, then aseptic technique must be used to replace the dressing.
- Check all connections and equipment every shift to ensure safety and patency of tubing.
- The drain should *never be clamped* unless specified by a doctor
- Following any movement of the child, the zero

reference must be maintained, i.e. the 0-cm mark must be in line as described above. Care must be taken when the child is likely to be higher or lower than the zero mark, this effects the drainage of CSF. See the complications associated with EVDs. Record neurological observations and report changes.

> **KEY POINTS**
>
> Measurements are in cm $H_2O$ so do not confuse with mmHg, which is also a scale on the device and very different. Ensure attached drainage bag is set to the zero reference point. Ensure the slide chamber is at the correct height. This allows the brain fluid to stay at the correct pressure but allows fluid to drain should the pressure be exerted above the prescribed pressure level set by the surgeon.

## Complications of an EVD

Inadequate drainage of CSF may occur if:

- the system is placed too high;
- the tubing is kinked;
- the three-way tap is off to drainage
- the drainage bag is full: empty when three-quarters full under aseptic conditions;
- thick CSF is blocking the system.

Excessive drainage of CSF may occur if the system is placed too low which may cause collapsed ventricles. This could cause the brain tissue to pull away from the dura, initiating tearing of blood vessels and a subdural or subarachnoid haemorrhage.

Tentorial herniation from either too much or too little drainage. Symptoms to be aware of are as follows:

- severe headache
- lethargy
- drowsiness
- irritability
- apnoea
- sluggish pupil response
- abnormal reflexes
- changes in heart rate and blood pressure.

*Infection*

- This is a major complication and can lead to ventriculitis.
- Samples of CSF fluid for laboratory review

should be taken under strict aseptic technique.

- Dressings should be changed when soiled; monitor for signs of CSF leak and report. Re-dress using aseptic technique.
- Observe for signs of infection.
- Report any changes to ensure treatment instigated.

*Accidental disconnection*

- In this situation, clamp the catheter to prevent complications of excessive CSF drainage.
- Maintain asepsis to prevent infection.
- Observe for signs of raised ICP in case there is inadequate absorption of CSF. Contact the surgeon, who may need to change the system if

contamination has occurred.

## Removal of the EVD

This is done by the neurosurgeon under aseptic conditions. They will have specific requests regarding raising or clamping the drain prior to removal.

- Monitor for signs of raised intracranial pressure after removal in the unsedated child.
- Ensure sutured area is inspected for signs of infection over the next few days, i.e. redness, swelling, oozing around wound site or tension on the sutures. Take a wound swab as per unit policy as needed.
- Remove sutures after 5–7 days or as instructed.

Go to the website to find the PowerPoint presentation for this chapter and MCQs to test your knowledge. **www.hodderplus.com/childnursingskills**

## REFERENCES

1  Bass Johnson R, Noble A, Thomas A (2005) Arterial blood pressure. In: Noble A (ed.) *The cardiovascular system, basic science and clinical conditions.* Edinburgh: Churchill Livingstone, Chapter 10.

2  Halley GC, Tibby S (2009) *Hemodynamic monitoring.* In: Nichols G (ed.) *Roger's textbook of pediatric intensive care,* 4th edition. Philadelphia: Lippincott Williams & Wilkins, Chapter 65.

3  McGhee BH, Bridges MEJ (2002) Monitoring arterial blood pressure: what you may not know. *Critical Care Nursing* **22**(2): 60–79.

4  Watson D (2007) Understanding invasive monitoring 1: indications. *Nursing Times.* **103**(49) www.nursingtimes.net (accessed January 2009).

5  Woodrow P (2001) *Intensive care nursing: a framework for practice.* London: Routledge.

6  Malley WJ (2005) *Clinical blood gases: assessment and intervention,* 2nd edition. Philadelphia: Elsevier Saunders.

7  Haemodynamic Monitoring Arterial Pressure Monitoring http://rnbob.tripod.com/artmon.htm (Accessed September 2008).

8  Clark SL (1999) Arterial lines: an analysis of good practice. *Journal of Child Health Care* **3**(1): 23–27.

9  Kaye J, Heald GR, Morton J, Weaver T (2001) Patency of radial arterial catheters. *American Journal of American Critical Care.* **10**(2): 104–111.

10  DH (2001) *Building a safer NHS for patients.* London: HMSO.

11  Nursing Midwifery Council (2004) *Guidelines for records and record keeping.* London: NMC.

12  Royal College of Nursing (2003) *Standards for infusion therapy.* London: RCN.

13  Smith SF, Duell DJ, Martin BC (2004) *Clinical nursing skills basic to advanced,* 6th edition. New Jersey: Pearson Prentice Hall.

14  Imperial-Perez F, McRae M (2002) Arterial pressure monitoring. *Critical Care Nurse* **19**(2): 105–107.

15  Professional Development Unit 15 (1995) Blood pressure week 1: knowledge for practice. *Nursing Times* **91**(14).

16  Davies JH, Hassell LL (2007) *Children in intensive care. A survival guide,* 2nd edition. Edinburgh: Churchill Livingstone.

17  Arterial blood gases: http://en.wikipedia.org/wiki/Arterial_blood_gas (accessed January 2009).

18  Orlando Regional Health Care Education and Development (2007). Interpretation of arterial blood gas. Self-learning package www.orlandohealth.com/pdf%20folder/SLP/2007ABG_rev.pdf (accessed January 2009).

19  Advanced Life Support Group (2005) *Advanced paediatric life support: the practical approach,* 4th edition. London: BMJ Books.

20  Woodrow P (2004) Arterial blood gas analysis. *Nursing Standard* **18**(21): 45–52.

21  Mooney G, Comerford DF (2003) What you need to know about central venous lines. *Nursing Times*; **99**(10): 28–29.

22  Dougherty L (2000) Central venous access devices. *Nursing Standard* **14**(43): 45–49.

23  Smith M (2007) A care bundle for management of central venous catheters. *Paediatric Nursing* **19**(4): 41–45.

24  National Institute for Clinical Excellence (2005) Guidance on the use of ultrasound locating devices for placing central venous catheters. Technology appraisal Guidance No 49. www.nice.org.uk (accessed January 2009).

25  Neuro monitoring for traumatic brain Injury. www.trauma.org/archive/neuro/neuromonitor.html (accessed January 2009).

26  National Institute for Health and Clinical Excellence www.nice.org.uk (accessed January 2009).

27  Mazzola CA, Adelson PD (2002) Critical care management of head trauma in children. *Critical Care Medicine* **30**: S393–401.

28  Rising Intracranial Pressure. www.patient.co.uk/showdoc/40001329/ (accessed January 2009) Intracranial pressure. http://Wikipedia.org/wiki/intracranial_pressure (Accessed November 2008).

29  National Institute for Health and Clinical Excellence (2007) *Triage, assessment, investigation and early management of head injury in infants, children and adults.* NICE Clinical Guideline www.nice.org.uk/guidance/CG56 (accessed January 2009).

30  Mokri B (2001) The Monro-Kellie hypothesis: applications in CSF volume depletion. *Neurology* **56**: 1746–1748.

31  Steiner LA, Andrews PJ (2006) Monitoring the injured brain: ICP and CBF. *British Journal of Anaesthesia* **97**(1): 26–38.

32  Intracranial Pressure http://Wikipedia.org/wiki/intracranial_pressure (accessed January 2009).

33  Gharjar J (2000) Traumatic brain injury. *Lancet* **356**: 923–929.

34  North B, Reilly P (1990) *Raised intracranial pressure: a clinical guide.* Oxford: Heinemann Medical Books.

35  External Ventricular Drains (EVD) and Externalized shunts. www.cw.bc.ca/library/pamphlets/ search_view.asp?keyword=372 (accessed January 2009).

36  Goldstein B, Aboy M, Graham A (2009). *Neurological monitoring.* In: Nichols G. (ed.) *Roger's handbook of pediatric intensive care*, 4th edition. Philadelphia: Lippincott Williams & Wilkin, Chapter 33.

37  Woodward S, Addison C, Shah S, *et al.* (2002) Benchmarking best practice for external ventricular drainage. *British Journal of Nursing* **11**: 4753.

# Invasive respiratory therapy

Sue Robson

## LEARNING OUTCOMES

*Upon completion of this chapter, the reader should be able to accomplish the following:*

1 Identify the reasons a child will require respiratory support provided by mechanical ventilation
2 Understand the principles of mechanical ventilation and the associated complications
3 Identify the differences between the most commonly used modes of ventilation
4 List the equipment needed and the procedure to follow when assisting with the intubation of a child
5 Discuss the importance of effective humidification
6 Discuss with rationale the recommended techniques for undertaking endotracheal suctioning
7 Discuss the nursing priorities when caring for a child who is mechanically ventilated

## CHAPTER OVERVIEW

Infants and children have less respiratory reserve than adults, leading to a relatively high incidence of respiratory failure during severe illness. The PICANet (Paediatric Intensive Care Audit Network) National Report for May 2008[1] recorded that children requiring invasive ventilation procedures accounted for 67 per cent of paediatric intensive care admissions. Invasive respiratory support includes the provision of a secure upper airway and effective ventilatory support. One of the functions of an intensive care unit is to provide advanced respiratory support; therefore, an understanding of the indications and types of mechanical ventilation together with knowledge of the fundamental physiological mechanisms of ventilation is necessary for anyone working within this environment.

The aim of artificial/mechanical ventilation is to improve gas exchange, to reduce the work of breathing and to avoid complications while maintaining optimal conditions for recovery. Whatever the indication for respiratory support, the underlying condition of the child must be reversible, otherwise subsequent weaning may not be possible.

Ventilation allows the manipulation of both oxygenation and carbon dioxide removal and may be necessary for treatment of conditions other than primary respiratory disease:

- to support the cardiovascular system (following cardiac surgery);
- to allow wound healing following tracheal or laryngeal surgery;
- to manipulate $PaCO_2$ when intracranial pressure is raised;
- to maintain respiratory function when pharmacological therapy interferes with effective respiration, for example in the management of status epilepticus;

- to maintain airway patency where obstruction may be anticipated, following smoke inhalation injury.

Respiratory failure, however, does remain the primary indication for respiratory support. It occurs when the child's respiratory system is unable to meet the metabolic demand of removing carbon dioxide and delivering adequate oxygen. The criteria for intubation and ventilation will vary with each child and is based on a clinical assessment. Indicators include:

- altered or decreasing conscious level;
- inability to protect the airway;
- exhaustion with a laboured pattern of breathing;
- significant chest trauma;
- hypoxia: central cyanosis (decreasing oxygen saturations with increasing oxygen demand).

## CAUSES OF RESPIRATORY FAILURE

- Inadequate gas exchange
  - pneumonia, pulmonary oedema, acute respiratory distress syndrome (ARDS)
- Inadequate breathing
  - chest wall problems, e.g. fractured ribs, flail chest
  - pleural wall problems, e.g. pneumothorax, haemothorax
  - respiratory muscle failure, e.g. Guillain–Barré syndrome
  - central nervous system depression, e.g. drugs, brain stem compression
- Obstructed breathing
  - upper airway obstruction, e.g. epiglottitis, croup, oedema, tumour
  - lower airway obstruction, e.g. bronchospasm, bronchiolitis

## PRINCIPLES OF VENTILATION

The primary function of the respiratory system is to deliver oxygen to the body and to remove carbon dioxide. The process of gas movement in and out of the lung is defined as ventilation. The respiratory cycle consists of inspiration and expiration, which both have 'flow' and 'pause' phases. Normal mechanisms of ventilation are dependent on pressure gradients within the respiratory system. The conductive airway begins at the mouth and

nose and ends at the small airways near the alveoli. When the pressure in the mouth and alveoli are equal, as occurs at the end of inspiration or the end of expiration, no gas flow occurs. This is because the pressure throughout the conductive airway is equal, therefore no pressure gradient exists.

During inspiration, the diaphragm muscle contracts causing it to move down towards the abdomen, the chest wall expands, and because the pleural surface of the lungs is kept in contact with the pleura on the chest wall by surface tension the lungs are made to expand. This increases the volume of the air spaces inside the lungs and consequently the air pressure inside the alveoli drops from atmospheric, 100 kPa (760 mmHg) to about 99.74 kPa (758 mmHg). This causes a reduction in intrathoracic pressure. On condition that there is no obstruction in the ventilation pathway, air is sucked into the lung. Oxygen-rich air passes across the alveolar–capillary interface and gas exchange takes place. Oxygen diffuses into the blood and carbon dioxide diffuses out.

During expiration the diaphragm and the chest wall relax, the lung tissue springs back to its non-stretched state and the chest wall and diaphragm move back to their original positions. The thoracic volume decreases, alveoli air pressure increases to about 100.39 kPa (763 mmHg) and carbon dioxide-loaded air is squeezed out of the lungs into the atmosphere.

## PRINCIPLES OF MECHANICAL VENTILATION

Positive pressure ventilation is the usual method of providing mechanical ventilatory support in the paediatric intensive care unit (PICU). In order to do this, pressure is generated by the ventilator at a higher pressure outside the child, causing the gas to be literally blown into the child's lungs, which have a lower pressure. Positive pressure ventilation is the opposite of the physiologically normal negative pressure ventilation.

Important factors to consider affecting positive pressure ventilation are *compliance* and *resistance*.

*Compliance* is a measure of the expandability or elasticity of the lungs – how easily the lung tissue stretches and returns to its non-stretched state. Healthy, compliant lungs will inflate with very low pressures. This is an important point to remember when delivering mechanical ventilation because compliance reflects the amount of pressure required to deliver a given volume of air into the lungs. Increased compliance requires less pressure to distend the lungs with a given volume. Decreased compliance requires more pressure to deliver the same volume of air. Children are not always mechanically ventilated because of problems with their respiratory systems; for example a child with a head injury may require mechanical ventilation for manipulation of carbon dioxide levels to reduce cerebral oedema but would be expected to have healthy, compliant lungs.

*Resistance* is the result of friction between moving parts. The size of the airways is very important in determining how easily air flows into and out of the lungs. The wider the airways, the easier it is for air to flow. Resistance is directly related to the length of the airway, flow rate of the gas and viscosity of the gas. High resistance increases the work of breathing. Careful attention must be paid to maintaining a patent airway as the diameter of the airway lumen and the flow of air into the lungs can decrease as a result of increased resistance caused by bronchospasm, increased secretions, mucosal oedema, tracheal or bronchomalacia or kinks in the endotracheal tube (ETT) or tracheostomy tube.

To force gas into the lungs, pressure is needed to overcome the resistance and elasticity of the respiratory system. The higher the resistance and the reduction in compliance, the greater the pressure required to move a given volume of gas.

To generate the necessary pressure required for mechanical ventilation, access to the child's airway is required. This is normally obtained using an ETT or tracheostomy tube or, if non-invasive ventilation is appropriate, by a tight, well-sealed mask. The important principle here is the tight seal, either by

inflation of the cuff found on an older child's ETT, or inflatable seals on facemasks. Without this tight seal the necessary pressures would not be able to be generated. The narrowest part of a child's airway is at the level of the cricoid cartilage, whereas in adults it is near the glottis. For this reason, children are easily ventilated using uncuffed ETTs with minimal air leak.

A mechanical ventilator is a machine that generates a controlled flow of gas into a child's airways. Oxygen and air are received from cylinders or wall outlets, the gas is pressure reduced and blended according to the prescribed inspired oxygen tension ($FiO_2$), accumulated in a receptacle within the machine, and delivered to the patient using one of many available modes of ventilation.

As previously mentioned, the central premise of positive pressure ventilation is that gas flows along a pressure gradient between the upper airway and the alveoli. Initial settings determine the magnitude, rate and duration of flow. Flow is either volume targeted and pressure variable, or pressure limited and volume variable. Modern ventilators allow different modes of ventilation and the medical and nursing staff must select the safest and most appropriate mode of ventilation for the patient. Mechanical ventilation is designed to maintain lung ventilation in the *absence* of spontaneous breathing effort as well as in the *support* of the patient's existing spontaneous breathing effort.

There are two phases in the respiratory cycle, high lung volume (inspiration) and lower lung volume (expiration). Gas exchange occurs in both phases and the inspiration–expiration (I/E) time ratio can be manipulated with a mechanical ventilator. Inspiration is active and serves to replenish alveolar gas; therefore, prolonging the duration of the higher volume cycle increases

## Definitions

**Positive end-expiratory pressure (PEEP):** PEEP reopens or recruits collapsed alveoli by redistributing fluid in the intra-alveolar space to the interstitial space. The application of PEEP improves a child's oxygenation by increasing the functional residual capacity (FRC) and increasing mean airway pressure.

**Functional residual capacity (FRC):** FRC is the volume of air present in the lungs at the end of expiration.

**Tidal volume (TV):** This is the volume of gas required for one breath (5–7 mL per kg for children[2]).

**Minute volume (MV):** This is the quantity of gas expired by the lungs in 1 minute.
MV = TV 5 respiratory rate.

oxygen uptake. Expiration is passive and thus requires more time to allow alveolar units to empty. If the ventilator is set for the child to receive 20 breaths per minute, then the duration of each cycle is 3 seconds. A conventional I:E ratio is 1:2, so 1 second is set aside for inspiration and 2 for expiration. This mimics normal physiology. A severely hypoxic child, e.g. one with acute respiratory distress syndrome (ARDS), may need a prolonged inspiratory time to improve oxygenation. With inverse-ratio ventilation the I:E is greater than 1:1, often 2:1 or more. Patients do not tolerate inverse-ratio ventilation and may require heavy sedation and paralysis.

## TYPES OF VENTILATION

*Control*: How the ventilator knows how much flow to deliver.

*Volume control*: Ventilation occurs when the ventilator delivers a preset tidal volume regardless of the pressures generated. The lung compliance determines the airway pressure generated, so if the lungs are stiff this pressure may be high with the resultant risk of barotrauma.

*Pressure control*: Ventilation occurs when the ventilator delivers a preset target pressure to the airway during inspiration. The lung compliance and the airway resistance therefore determine resulting tidal volume delivered.

## MODES OF VENTILATION

The term 'mode' describes a breath type and the timing of breath delivery. In general, mechanical ventilation is initiated to accomplish one of two things for the patient: either to control their ventilation and oxygenation when they are unable to do so, or to support them as they recover and wean them from ventilatory support (Figure 25.1).

## Complications of mechanical ventilation

- *Oxygen toxicity*: Patients receiving >50 per cent $FiO_2$ for prolonged periods of time may develop parenchymal changes from oxygen exposure. The lowest $FiO_2$ possible should be used to achieve the level of oxygenation required.
- *Acute lung injury*: A consequence of high airway pressures may be overdistension and rupture of the alveoli leading to injury of the lung tissue (barotrauma) and potentially pneumothorax.
- *Decreased cardiac output*: Flow is always from zones of high pressure to those of low pressure, and the negative intrathoracic pressure associated with normal physiological inspiration will enhance this effect; however, increased intrathoracic pressure as a result of positive pressure ventilation will reduce the pressure gradient along which blood returns to the heart, and decrease venous return. This reduces right ventricular preload, right ventricular output and ultimately cardiac output. This may lead to a reduction in blood pressure and pooling of blood in the abdomen and peripheries.
- *Reduction in urine output*: The reduction in cardiac output may result in neural and hormonal mechanisms (i.e. antidiuretic hormone (ADH) secretion and activation of the renin–

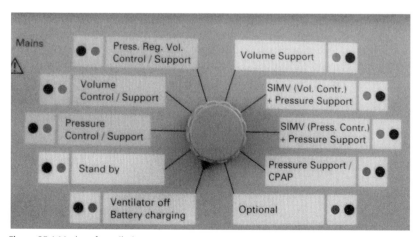

**Figure 25.1** Modes of ventilation.

**Controlled mechanical ventilation (CMV)**

- All breaths determined by machine
- Can be volume or pressure targeted
- Requires child to be sedated and paralysed
- No synchronisation of child's breathing

**Volume control (VC)**

- Preset rate.
- Preset tidal volume (5–7 mL/kg)
- Pressure is not set but depends on lung compliance and resistance

**Pressure control (PC)**

- Preset pressure for each breath
- Tidal volume is not set but depends on lung compliance and resistance

**Supported mechanical ventilation (SMV)**

- Works with child's own respiratory effort
- Senses inspiratory effort and triggers the ventilator to give the breath a 'boost'
- Can give pressure or volume support

**Volume support (VS)**

- Preset minute volume
- Delivers the lowest respiratory support to achieve the preset minute volume
- Patient initiates all breaths

**Pressure support (PS)**

- Patient generates rate and volume
- Supports each spontaneous breath
- Gives a little push to help the breath in
- Helps to overcome resistance of breathing through an ETT

**Pressure-regulated volume control (PRVC)**

- Combines advantages of VC and PC
- Preset tidal and minute volume
- Preset upper pressure limit

**Synchronised intermittent mandatory ventilation (SIMV)**

- Partly controlled and partly supported
- Determines both when a patient gets a breath and what kind of breath they receive
- Patient can initiate breaths but still receives mandatory (preset) breaths

**Combined modes**

- SIMV with VC and PS
- SIMV with PC and PS

**Expiratory support to ventilation**

- PEEP is used with all forms of positive pressure ventilation
- When PEEP is applied in a spontaneously breathing patient it is called continuous positive airway pressure (CPAP)

angiotensin–aldosterone system). These acute compensatory mechanisms aim to increase cardiac output and mean arterial pressure by increasing intravascular blood volume and increasing renal perfusion; however, fluid retention may lead to pulmonary oedema, pleural effusions and ascites.

- *Gastrointestinal disturbances*: A reduction in splanchnic blood flow may be secondary to decreased cardiac output and cause reduced functioning of the gastrointestinal tract. Reduced gut motility may be caused by use of sedative and narcotic drugs and lead to abdominal distension, large gastric aspirates and reduced frequency of bowel movements. A distended abdomen may cause splinting of the diaphragm. Stress ulceration may cause gastrointestinal haemorrhage

- *Nutrition*: The capacity for oral intake is limited due to the presence of an ETT and the child's level of sedation; however, an increased basal metabolic demand due to critical illness is likely. This may lead to malnutrition or metabolic disorders.

- *Infections*: Ventilator-associated pneumonia (VAP) is the second most common hospital acquired infection in PICU patients.[3] VAP is a pneumonia that develops in mechanically ventilated patients who are intubated for more than 48 hours without the presence or likelihood of pneumonia at the time of intubation.[4] Ventilated children have an increased risk of developing nosocomial infections as a result of suppressed immune function, invasive procedures and the presence of artificial tubes

(ETT, urinary catheter, central venous catheters).

- *Immobility*: Sedated and ventilated patients require regular turning to prevent pressure sores and maintain skin integrity.

## ASSISTING WITH TRACHEAL TUBE INTUBATION

Whenever possible, intubation should be undertaken on an elective basis and as a result of clinical indications. Intubation involves insertion of a tube into the trachea through the mouth or nose to establish a patent airway. In emergency situations the oral cavity is used as the route of insertion because orotracheal intubation is easier and faster. However, it is difficult to secure the tube and maintain exact tube placement, and it is also uncomfortable for conscious patients because it stimulates salivation, coughing and retching.

In nasal intubation, the nasal cavity is used as the route of insertion. Nasal intubation is preferred for elective insertion and is more comfortable and secure for the child. However, it is more difficult to perform because the tube passes blindly through the nasal cavity and can potentially cause more tissue damage and increase the risk of infection by introducing nasal bacteria into the trachea. Nasal intubation is contraindicated in patients with facial or basilar skull fractures or a blood clotting abnormality.

## Complications of intubation

- Laryngospasm/bronchospasm
- Hypoxaemia/hypercapnia during intubation
- Laryngeal oedema resulting in stridor when extubated
- Trauma/bleeding to nasal, oral, oesophageal, tracheal or laryngeal sites
- Broken teeth
- Nosocomial infection (pneumonia, sinusitis, abscess)
- Displacement of tube (right mainstem bronchus, gastric intubation)
- Aspiration of oral or gastric contents
- Tracheal stenosis/tracheomalacia
- Laryngeal damage, paralysis and necrosis
- Dysrhythmias, hypertension, hypotension

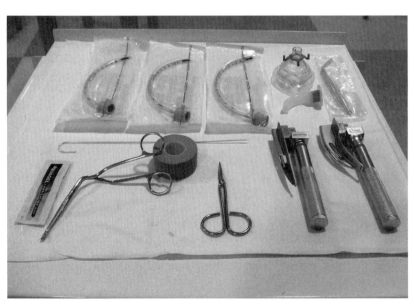

**Figure 25.2** Equipment required for an intubation.

## PROCEDURE:  Intubation of infant/child (Figure 25.2)

| Equipment required for intubation of infant/child | Evidence-based rationale |
|---|---|
| **1** Laryngoscope blade and handle: check bulb is secure and bright | Infant: straight blade to elevate the epiglottis and visualise the vocal cords<br>Child: curved blade to elevate supraglottic structures<br>The anatomical transition from infant to child/adult conformation has significantly progressed by toddler age (18 months to 3years) |
| **2** Tracheal tube of estimated size plus one 0.5 mm smaller and one 0.5 mm larger | Term infant requires an estimated 3.5-mm tube<br>1-year-old an estimated 4.0 mm tube<br>Above 2 years age calculate size using formula as age $\div$ 4 + 4<br>Uncuffed tubes tend to be used in children <8 years so as not to cause oedema at the cricoid ring[5] |
| **3** Stylet | The stylet should be inserted only up to the final 1 cm of the ETT then the proximal end bent over the blue universal adaptor of the tube to prevent the stylet advancing beyond the end of the tube |
| **4** Reliable suction source plus wide bore rigid suction catheter (Yankauer) and soft suction catheters | Size of soft suction catheters calculated by multiplying tracheal tube width by 2 |
| **5** Bag–valve–mask device with $0_2$ | When choosing a mask ensure it fits snugly over both mouth and nose but does not cause pressure on the eyes nor create an air leak by overriding the chin |
| **6** Oropharyngeal and nasopharyngeal airways | Nasal airway is less likely to cause gagging, vomiting and laryngospasm and therefore can be used in a semi-conscious child |
| **7** Magills forceps | For nasal intubation |
| **8** Stethoscope | Auscultate the chest for air entry |
| **9** Nasogastric/orogastric tube | To decompress the stomach |
| **10** Pre-cut tape to secure tube | Regardless of the method of strapping used it is important that tube displacement is prevented |
| **11** End tidal carbon dioxide monitoring equipment | The presence of an exhaled $CO_2$ waveform confirms correct tube position but readings must be combined with other clinical data |
| **12** Ventilator with circuit and humidifier | |

## PROCEDURE: Assisting with tracheal intubation (Figure 25.3, page 438)

| Procedural steps | Evidence-based rationale |
|---|---|
| 1 Advise necessary staff that an intubation is about to take place. At least two experienced practitioners are required to perform this procedure<br>Explain and acknowledge the difficulty of the procedure to the child's parents and the child (if conscious). Ensure that the relative has a choice of remaining with their child or leaving without invoking any feelings of guilt whatever their decision. If they choose to stay it will require another member of staff to remain with them and support them during the procedure | Whatever the indication, tracheal tube intubation should be carried out in a safe, systematic and controlled fashion. A doctor/anaesthetist is required to prescribe the drugs selected for induction and to insert the tracheal tube. An experienced nurse is required for support and assistance. A third person may be required<br>A child that requires intubation will be critically ill and the situation can create significant emotional stress and anxiety for the child's family. Giving clear and concise information has been identified as a strategy to reduce stress and anxiety<br>Current evidence suggests that parents, although distressed during critical incidents, often choose to witness the event and remain with their child[6] |
| 2 Screen the bed or cubicle | To ensure privacy |
| 3 Have appropriate tracheal intubation-sized equipment checked and ready on an appropriate surface near to hand<br>Have emergency drugs to hand<br>Ensure the patient has a minimum of one, patent intravenous cannula. Ensure sedation, paralysing agent and a saline flush have been prescribed, checked, drawn up, labelled accordingly and are ready to use<br>Ensure the environment is clear and the end of the child's bed/cot has been removed and that the bed/cot is flat. Ensure oxygen and suction are within reach and working<br>Ensure that a checked ventilator and circuit with humidification are available together with $CO_2$ monitoring | To maintain a safe environment. Every effort should be made to maximise the likelihood of intubation at the first attempt. Emergency equipment and drugs may be needed in the event of inability to intubate at the first attempt |
| 4 Ensure appropriate monitoring is attached to the child. Heart rate, blood pressure and oxygen saturations are required | The process of intubation can induce bradycardia, and hypoxia<br>The induction of anaesthesia can cause vasodilation |
| 5 Ensure the bed is at a safe working level | To maintain a safe working environment |
| 6 Wash hands/apply alcohol hand rub, put on gloves, apron and goggles (standard precautions) | Prevention of cross-infection can be improved with good hand hygiene and use of gloves[7] |
| 7 Pre-oxygenate the child for a minimum of 15 seconds with 100% oxygen<br>If possible the patient should be pre-oxygenated for a full 3 minutes, to wash all of the nitrogen out of the lungs and create a reservoir of $O_2$ | All children with breathing difficulties should receive high-flow oxygen through a face mask with oxygen as soon as the airway has been demonstrated to be adequate.[1] A self-inflating bag with a reservoir attachment enables high oxygen concentrations to be delivered. Without a reservoir bag, it is difficult to supply more than 50 per cent oxygen to the child whatever the gas flow, whereas with one, an inspired oxygen concentration of 98 per cent can be achieved |

## PROCEDURE: Assisting with tracheal intubation (continued)

| | |
|---|---|
| 8  Ideally an infant/child should be nil by mouth prior to intubation. A nasogastric/orogastric tube should be placed in the stomach and the contents aspirated and discarded prior to intubation | Nil by mouth status or aspiration of gastric contents decrease the risk of emesis and aspiration. An NG/OG tube is also useful to prevent insufflation of the stomach with air during bag–valve–mask procedure. Cricoid pressure may be required to prevent passive regurgitation of gastric contents |
| 9  Position the child as appropriate. In a child of >2 years, place the head on a pillow. This will slightly flex the neck: 'sniffing the morning air position'. In infants and children <2 years the head should be placed on a flat surface in a neutral position[5] | Turn the child on his/her back and position the head to open the airway<br>Appropriate placement of the head allows for easier visualization of the epiglottis and vocal cords. Head elevation and neck flexion are simple manoeuvres to perform that can improve the laryngeal view and assist in successful intubation |
| 10  Reassess the airway<br>Listen to the breathing<br>Reassess the heart rate, blood pressure and oxygen saturations<br>Give the sedation and paralysing agent as prescribed | If the airway sounds 'bubbly' the patient has secretions that will need clearing. The doctor will need a clear view to visualise vocal cords before passing an oral ETT. A wide bore rigid (Yankauer) catheter can provide rapid suction of large volumes of fluid from the mouth and pharynx (see Suctioning, page 441)<br>Suctioning is a hypoxic event<br>Ensure the patient has recovered from the effects of the hypoxic insult before continuing |
| 11  Once the clinician has inserted the tracheal tube confirm correct placement. If a cuffed tube is used inflate the cuff with air<br>Connect to a self-inflating bag and ventilate<br>Look for bilateral and symmetrical chest movement<br>Auscultate the chest over the axilla for breath sounds and listen over the stomach<br>Check end-tidal $CO_2$ | The black markings at the end of the ETT should sit at the level of the vocal cords or, if a cuffed tube is used, the cuff should sit just below the vocal cords. If breath sounds are heard in the stomach this can indicate an incorrect oesophageal intubation<br>The measurement of exhaled $CO_2$ (termed capnography) provides direct evidence of ventilatory function |
| 12  Record the tracheal tube length at the lips | This provides a record for future tracheal tube intubation and detection of tube dislodgement/migration |
| 13  Secure the tube as per local protocol, continue ventilation and continually reassess tube position | Decrease the risk of tube displacement. Excessive head movement can displace the tube: the tube can be displaced further into and out of the airway by head flexion and head extension respectively |
| 14  Connect the tube to a ventilator and ensure the child continues to ventilate effectively | |
| 15  Obtain a chest X-ray | Formal and accurate confirmation of tracheal tube placement |

## Cricoid pressure

The cricoid cartilage is the ring felt below the larynx. If this is displaced posteriorly, because it is circular shaped and solid, it compresses and closes the oesophagus (which lies behind it). This prevents passive regurgitation and aspiration of gastric contents. The pressure should only be released when a tracheal tube protects the airway or unless the patient actually vomits. Cricoid pressure is contraindicated in patients with suspected cricotracheal injury, active vomiting or unstable cervical spine injuries. Too much pressure may compress and obstruct the trachea and could distort the upper airway anatomy making tracheal intubation difficult.[8]

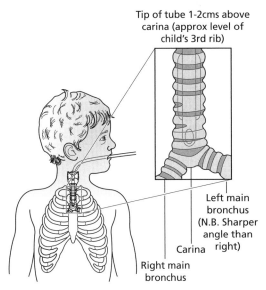

Tip of tube 1-2cms above carina (approx level of child's 3rd rib)

Left main bronchus (N.B. Sharper angle than right)

Carina

Right main bronchus

**Figure 25.3** Correct placement of an endotracheal tube.

## Reasons for ineffective ventilation following tracheal intubation

Ventilation may not be established effectively after intubation or it may become ineffective after a variable period. The main causes of this can be described by the acronym DOPE:

- Displaced tube: into either pharynx/oesophagus, or right/left main bronchus
- Obstructed tube: vomit, blood, secretions or kinked tube
- Pneumothorax
- Equipment failure.

These problems should be recognised and diagnosed by the checks that routinely follow intubation

## HUMIDIFICATION

Normal spontaneous breathing provides 100 per cent relative humidity at 37°C and contains 44 mg/L of water (absolute humidity).[9] Endotracheal intubation results in a bypass of the patient's natural gas humidifier, the nose and upper airway. Medical gases are cold and dry and, therefore, the inspired gas must be warmed and humidified (conditioned) before it is delivered to the patient. This means adding an artificial humidifier to the ventilator circuit. Artificial humidification of medicinal gases can be active or passive. In active humidifiers, known as heated humidifiers (HHs), the inspired gas passes across or over a heated water bath. Passive humidifiers, known as artificial noses or heat and moisture exchangers (HMEs), trap heat and humidity from the patient's exhaled gas and return some to the patient on the subsequent inhalation.

Failure to provide adequate humidity in inspired air may lead to damage to the mucociliary transport system in the airways.[10] Inadequate humidification of the inspired air may lead to increased volume and viscosity of secretions. This leads to increased risk of blocked artificial and anatomical airways. In addition, increased volume and viscosity of secretions will increase the need for suctioning and increase the risk of potential complications from mechanical damage to the tracheal mucosa or a fall in oxygenation and functional residual capacity.

The resistance to gas flow will rise in the presence of secretions. If this results in an increase in peak inspiratory pressure the patient's risk of pneumothorax will increase.

## Equipment

Heating unit
1-litre bag of sterile water for irrigation
Appropriate giving set for disposable chamber unit and circuit

## The procedural goal is to

- achieve the physiologic optimal humidity for invasive ventilation of 37°C, 44 mg/litre $H_2O$ and temperature of 32–34°C at the carina;
- prevent tube obstruction/viscous secretions;
- decrease the risk of infection.

## Rationale

Maximum mucosal function occurs in a relatively narrow range of warmth and humidity above and below the optimum physiologic humidity. Williams et al.[10] and Irlbeck[11] suggested that the mucociliary transport is the most sensitive indicator of appropriate humidity and therefore is optimised when inspired air reaches 37°C and 100 per cent relative humidity. Large positive or negative deviations may cause deterioration in mucosal function to the point that cell damage occurs with resulting atelectasis.

Whenever the temperature in the patient circuit is less than the temperature of the gas leaving the humidifier, condensation will accumulate in the circuit (rain-out). If the temperature of the gas in the patient circuit is higher than the humidifier, the *relative humidity* in the circuit decreases.

## PROCEDURE: Humidification

| Procedural steps | Evidence-based rationale |
|---|---|
| 1 Set up as per operator's manual | To promote safety |
| 2 Prior to use and during start of shift, the humidification device is inspected. Ensure that heated-wire circuits are not covered and that circuits and humidifiers are compatible | Hazards and complications associated with the use of heated humidification devices include: potential for electrical shock, burns to patient and staff, tubing melt-down |
| 3 If necessary, remove condensation from the patient circuit. Never drain condensation back into the humidifier reservoir. If it collects in tubing, drain tubing onto paper towels and dispose of in clinical waste receptacle | Inadvertent tracheal lavage from pooled condensate in patient circuit. Condensate is infectious waste |
| 4 Monitor the temperature of inspired gases. Set humidifier to deliver an inspired gas temperature of 39°C minus 2°C, which should provide a minimum of 30 mg/litre of water vapour | This setting allows for the fall in temperature and humidity level between circuit temperature probe and patient so that inspiratory gas should not exceed 37°C at the airway threshold |
| 5 The temperature probe should be located outside of the incubator or away from the direct heat of the radiant warmer | To reduce the risk of thermal injury and unintentional tracheal lavage from condensation ('rain-out') |
| 6 Set high temperature alarm to no higher than 39°C, and the low temperature alarm no lower than 34°C | To reduce the risk of thermal injury to the child[12] |
| 7 Check water level is at level as advised by manufacturer and function of automatic system is functioning correctly (if applicable) | Inadvertent overfilling can lead to unintentional feed tracheal lavage |
| 8 Use a clean non-touch technique when manually filling the water reservoir. Use sterile water | To reduce the risk of cross-infection |
| 9 Replace circuits weekly[13] | To reduce the risk of cross-infection[14] |
| 10 Reusable heated humidifier devices should be subjected to disinfection between patients | To reduce the risk of cross-infection[14] |

**Problem:** A child is due to be turned and repositioned for postural drainage and water is seen collected in the ventilator tubing.

**Discussion:** Condensate in the ventilator tubing can potentially be a source of accidental lavage when the patient is turned. Prior to turning, the tubing should be emptied or the water directed away from the patient and must never be allowed to enter the patient's airway.

Ensure the water trap in the ventilator tubing is emptied regularly and securely reattached

Condensate within the ventilator tubing may reduce the internal diameter of the circuit and subsequently cause an increase in the resistance to air flow. This will cause a reduction of the inspired oxygen concentration, the inspired ventilatory pressure, or the volume of gas delivered to the patient.

## NURSING CARE OF THE CHILD REQUIRING MECHANICAL VENTILATION

Despite advances in technology, mechanical ventilation is still associated with high morbidity and mortality. The role of the intensive care nurse in caring for a mechanically ventilated child is to continuously monitor patients, observing for changes in their condition to detect early signs of potential problems and prevent acute deterioration. Mechanical ventilation affects many body systems causing physiological changes; therefore an understanding of its principles and adverse effects are required.

### Safety

At the beginning of each shift, the nurse is responsible for conducting safety checks on the equipment in the bed space, alarm limits on monitoring equipment and alarm limits set on the ventilator.

### Emergency bedside airway equipment

- Age-appropriate bag–valve–mask device. The facemask should provide an airtight seal on the face and extend from the bridge of the nose to the cleft of the chin avoiding compression of the eyes.
- Oxygen supply
- An oropharyngeal or Guedel airway may be used in an unconscious child but may stimulate vomiting in a conscious child. A correctly sized airway when placed with its flange at the centre of the incisors, then curved around the face will reach the angle of the mandible.

- Suction catheters should have an external diameter less than half the internal diameter of the ETT.
- Rigid suction catheter (Yankauer sucker) to clear the mouth of thick or particulate matter.

### Assess the security of the ETT and prevent accidental extubation

- Ensure the ETT is securely taped at the correct documented length.
- Ensure there is no kinking or pulling on the ETT or ventilator tubing.
- Support the weight of the tubing.
- Ensure the child's hands cannot interfere with the ETT or ventilator tubing.
- Assess the patency of the ETT and the possible need for suctioning.

### Physical assessment of the child during mechanical ventilation

Physical assessment provides invaluable information concerning the child's interaction with the ventilator. Is the ventilatory support adequate? Is the child under- or over-ventilated depending on their needs? This nursing assessment is particularly important during initiation of mechanical ventilation and following any change in ventilatory parameters. No aspect of airway management is routine.

- Assess and observe the child's colour, breathing pattern, evidence of bilateral air entry and equal chest movement. Is the child's chest moving in synchrony with the ventilator?
- Ensure the adequacy of delivered ventilatory support. Are the minute and tidal volumes, peak inspiratory and end expiratory pressures appropriate for the child's weight and condition?
- Assess the heart rate: extreme tachycardia or bradycardia may be a sign of hypoxia.

- Assess the blood pressure: hypertension may indicate pain.
- Arterial blood gases should be examined in relation to the ventilator settings and previous blood gases with the goal of achieving normal blood gas values.
- Oxygen saturations should be monitored continuously.[2]
- End-tidal CO2 should be used.
- If a child's condition suddenly deteriorates, the child should be disconnected from the ventilator and manually ventilated while the ventilator is checked for malfunction, and the nurse should assess breath sounds to ensure ETT patency.
- If chest expansion is poor and the child continues to deteriorate, suction the ETT.
- If this fails to oxygenate the child, *this is a medical emergency*; call for help.
- If a blockage is suspected and cannot be removed it may be necessary to remove the ETT and hand ventilate the patient via an oropharyngeal airway and facemask until reintubation is performed.

## SUCTIONING

Research has demonstrated that tracheal suction is traumatic and hazardous.[15] There is the potential for mucosal damage, hypoxia, infection and airway collapse by poor technique and inappropriate equipment. Both single-use open and multi-use closed system (in-line) suction are used in PICU. Closed-circuit systems maintain ventilation and PEEP during suctioning and reduce the risk of infection to healthcare workers and patients. Suction may be performed as a single procedure or incorporated into a respiratory physiotherapy regimen. Suctioning is not a benign procedure and adverse physiological effects can be immediate and long term. It is important, therefore, that those undertaking the procedure are aware of the potential risks and practise in a manner that ensures effectiveness and patient safety. Resuscitation equipment should be available to facilitate rapid clinical emergency interventions if necessary.

## Equipment

Suction catheters, of the correct size with finger tip control and ideally marked longitudinally for easy control of insertion depth.

### The procedural goal is to

- safely and effectively clear secretions from tube thus maintaining a patent airway and improving ventilation and oxygenation;
- maintain a sterile technique;
- detect partially obstructed tubes via tactile feedback.

## PROCEDURE: Suctioning

| Procedural steps | Evidence-based rationale |
|---|---|
| 1 The frequency of suction is determined by the child's clinical condition and not predetermined time intervals. Indications that suctioning is required:<br>• presence of an artificial airway<br>• neurological disorder that inhibits/depresses normal cough reflex<br>• sound of mucus bubbling in ETT<br>• gurgles heard on auscultation/ felt on palpation of thorax<br>• difficulty in breathing<br>• restlessness<br>• low SpO$_2$<br>• central cyanosis<br>• increased ventilator inspiratory pressure | Research has demonstrated that suctioning has inherent risks.[15] Therefore, suction should not be given on a routine basis, but only performed as needed by an experienced practitioner. Deleterious effects of suctioning include hypoxia, bronchospasm, tracheobronchial trauma, arrhythmias, decreased cardiac output, raised intracranial pressure, pneumothorax, bacterial infection, pain and anxiety. Frequency usually is influenced by the viscosity and amount of secretions |
| 2 Explain the procedure to the child and/or parent even if the child is apparently unconscious | To help decrease anxiety and fears. This procedure is unpleasant and can be frightening. Reassure them of the benefits of the procedure |

## PROCEDURE: Suctioning (continued)

| | |
|---|---|
| 3 Screen bed | To provide privacy |
| 4 Ensure bed is at a safe working level | To maintain a safe working environment |
| 5 Wash hands/ apply alcohol hand rub, put on gloves, apron and goggles (standard precautions) | To prevent cross-infection from splash back, spills and aerosol sprays from coughs |
| 6 Identify the correct suction catheter. Multiply the size of the child's ETT by 2 | To reduce risk of tracheal damage |
| 7 Identify the distance the suction catheter will be inserted into the ETT<br>Measure the length of the ETT plus connections | To ensure secretions are removed from the child's entire airway<br>To minimise risk of damage to the carina |
| 8 The negative pressure of the suction unit must be checked prior to attaching the catheter to the suction tubing. This is done by turning on the unit, placing a finger over the end of the suction tubing and then noting the suction manometer reading. Set the suction pressures at 60–80 mmHg (8–10 kPa) for neonates or up to 120 mmHg (<16 kPa) for older children | Too high a suction pressure can cause lung collapse and/or damage tracheal tissue; too little will be ineffective |
| 9 Pre-oxygenate if necessary pre-suctioning.<br>A child receiving >40 per cent inspired oxygen will require pre-oxygenation<br>If physiotherapy treatment is required ensure the child has adequate sedation and analgesia | Suctioning is a hypoxic event and the maximum duration of each suction attempt should be determined by the individual child's clinical response, but should be limited to no more than 10–15 seconds<br>To be successful, ET suctioning must remove tracheal secretions; rapid ineffective suctioning is a waste of time |
| 10 Hyperinflation may be required for ventilated children who have reduced lung compliance<br>Only an experienced nurse or physiotherapist should perform hyperinflation | To maintain distension of the terminal alveoli, minimise the development of atelectasis and enhance oxygenation during the procedure<br>The potential haemodynamic stress of this procedure predisposes a high risk of causing cardiac dysrhythmias and reduced cardiac output[15] |
| 11 For open suctioning: open the end of suction catheter package, leaving catheter inside package and attach to suction tubing | Maintain sterility of equipment. The addition of a narrow suction catheter in relation to larger bore suction tubing generates an increased pressure at its tip |
| 12 Check working pressure by occluding the proximal thumb valve of the suction catheter immediately before use. The distal (patient) end remains covered inside the package | Do not test suction pressure setting by occluding suction tubing; the suction catheter should be attached for check as narrow catheter significantly increases pressure |
| 13 Open sterile glove packaging and put a sterile glove onto your dominant hand. Your non-dominant hand remains unsterile and is used to hold the suction catheter in its package so that the catheter can be removed with the dominant sterile hand. Use your non-dominant hand to control the thumb valve while your dominant sterile hand controls the position of the catheter, taking care to hold it at a point below that which is going into the ETT | The suction procedure is a potential risk for contamination and infection. Adhere to aseptic technique to maintain sterility of equipment. There should be no contact between the suction catheter and anything other than the sterile glove and the ETT |

## PROCEDURE: Suctioning (continued)

| | |
|---|---|
| **14** Disconnect ventilator tubing with the non-dominant hand or ask an assistant to do so. For in-line suction attach suction tubing and open the thumb lock. Depress to achieve suction | Maintain sterility of equipment |
| **15** Stabilise tube with non-dominant hand while inserting catheter into ETT quickly but gently with the dominant hand<br>The distance a catheter is inserted into the airway is determined by measuring the length of the child's ETT plus connections (0.5 cm)<br>An in-line catheter has a prerecorded depth marking to limit the distance of catheter advance | Deep suction causes mucosal damage and irritation; too shallow causes secretions to encrust the tube |
| **16** Do *not* apply suction while inserting the catheter! | To decrease the volume of air removed from the lungs and decrease hypoxic effect and trauma to the delicate airway mucosa |
| **17** Apply negative pressure, using fingertip control as you withdraw the catheter gently straight out of the ETT over 2–4 seconds. Observe the child throughout the procedure to ensure their general condition is not affected | Reduces the risk of atelectasis, hypoxia and bradycardia. Rolling of the catheter is not necessary as suction catheters now have circumferential holes<br>Endotracheal suction may cause vagal stimulation leading to bradycardia, especially in neonates<br>If the child's condition deteriorates, appropriate resuscitation procedures must be initiated immediately |
| **18** As soon as the catheter is withdrawn, reconnect to ventilator or continue manual hyperinflations if required | Resume ventilator or oxygen delivery as soon as possible to reventilate and/or reoxygenate the child |
| **19** Reassess child's respiratory status for expected and unexpected outcomes:<br>• thorough respiratory assessment<br>• respiratory rate and quality<br>• colour<br>• SpO$_2$<br>• lung sounds/bilateral air entry<br>• vital signs as necessary to determine distress<br>• heart rate<br>• blood pressure | Allows child to recover following each suctioning. Child should have oxygen saturations above 92 per cent, be free of respiratory distress and be calm and comfortable. In contrast, restlessness, agitation, confusion, tachycardia, bradycardia and oxygen saturations below 92 per cent indicate hypoxia and/or hypercapnia and appropriate therapeutic intervention is required immediately |
| **20** After suctioning the ETT you may suction the nose and mouth if needed<br>Catheters must be changed between suction of an artificial airway and mouth/nostrils | Children below age 8 years have uncuffed tubes and therefore secretions may still accumulate in the upper airway of the child with a reduced ability to cough or swallow secretions<br>To reduce the risk of cross-infection |
| **21** Disconnect catheter from suction tubing. Coil catheter inside gloved hand and remove glove by inverting it over the used catheter | To reduce the risk of cross-infection |
| **22** Dispose of catheter in glove into clinical waste bag | To reduce the risk of cross-infection |
| **23** If necessary, repeat suctioning procedure as detailed above<br>If a child has viscous secretions that are not effectively cleared by suctioning the use of an | Suction should never be 'routine', but performed when indicated<br>Optimal humidification and adequate patient hydration maintain secretion clearance |

## PROCEDURE: Suctioning (continued)

| | |
|---|---|
| irrigant (0.9 per cent sodium chloride) may be considered; however, research indicates that the instillation of fluid into the lungs does not liquefy secretions[4] | |
| 24 Clear the suction tubing with water and turn off suction | To reduce the risk of cross-infection |
| 25 Remove apron and goggles and wash your hands | To reduce the risk of cross-infection |
| 26 Document time of suctioning and consistency, colour, quantity and any odour of secretions | Allows early identification of signs and symptoms of respiratory infection or respiratory insufficiency secondary to secretions and/or inflammation Facilitates ongoing evaluation |

## Positioning

All patients are at an increased risk of gastric reflux and aspiration of gastric contents when laid supine and the considered optimum position for adults is head up 45°. A semi-recumbent position decreases the risk of both aspiration of gastric contents and VAP.[17] The efficacy of semi-recumbent positioning has not yet been established in children but elevating the head of the bed may be instrumental in limiting the risk factors associated with VAP. Regular turning helps in the mobilisation of chest secretions and enables assessment and care of pressure areas.

## Sedation

Ensure the child has adequate sedation, analgesia and muscle relaxants if necessary to enable ventilatory therapy to achieve satisfactory gas exchange. Dysynchrony – where the child 'fights against the ventilator' – leads to increased oxygen consumption and an increased risk of complications, such as accidental extubation and laryngeal damage.

## Oral care

Oral hygiene should include tooth brushing, mouth rinsing, oral suctioning and appropriate storage, rinsing and replacement of suction devices. A reduction in the number of micro-organisms in the mouth through oral care will decrease the risk of translocation and colonisation in the lungs and, therefore, reduce the risk of VAP.[17]

## Eye care

The use of sedation can impair the blink reflex putting the cornea at risk of drying and infection therefore regular eye assessment is necessary. Regular eye care and the application of an ocular lubricant or gel film can prevent a corneal abrasion.

## Care required for systemic effects caused by positive pressure ventilation

*Cardiovascular:* Perfusion is reduced to all systems because of reduced systemic venous return and low cardiac output, causing systemic hypotension. Therefore, appropriate fluid loading or inotropic support may be necessary.

*Renal/endocrine effects:* Owing to the secretion of ADH, water retention and low urine output may occur. Administration of prescribed diuretics, restriction of fluids and maintaining electrolyte balance will help to prevent oedema formation.

*Gastrointestinal effects:* Critical illness causes a compromise in nutritional status. Nutritional support must be administered to prevent wastage of muscles, in particular, respiratory muscles, which may lead to a longer period of ventilation. Additionally, milk feeds will help in the prevention of stress ulcers. Feed absorption must be closely monitored as the use of sedatives may reduce gut motility, requiring administration of prescribed prokinetic agents.

A daily feed break from continuous enteral feeding is necessary to allow the gastric pH to recover to a sufficiently acid level to prevent translocation of bacteria from the gut to the trachea and prevent VAP.[17]

## Communication and psychological support

The child's inability to speak due to intubation through their vocal cords should be explained together with the need for mechanical ventilation. If the child is capable of writing a sign board or pen and paper can be provided. The child and family may require repeated explanations of treatment and procedures and constant reassurance. Intensive care nurses work in close proximity to patients and relatives, and are therefore in an ideal position to offer support and build a trusting relationship.

## Weaning

Weaning from mechanical ventilation can be considered when the underlying illness is treated and an improvement in gas exchange is noted. Prior to weaning, there should be no residual neuromuscular blockade and sedation should be minimised, so that the child is awake. It may be difficult to achieve a balance between weaning sedation, to allow a child to breath spontaneously, and having a distressed child who is endangering the safety of his airway. The child should be observed for early indications of fatigue or failure to wean.

 Go to the website to find the PowerPoint presentation for this chapter and MCQs to test your knowledge. **www.hodderplus.com/childnursingskills**

## REFERENCES

1 Paediatric Intensive Care Audit Network (2008) *National Report of the Paediatric Intensive Care Audit Network: January 2005 to December 2007*. Leeds: Universities of Leeds & Leicester.

2 Cheifetz IM (2003) Invasive and noninvasive pediatric mechanical ventilation. *Respiratory Care* **48**: 442–453.

3 Foglia E, Meier M D, Elward A (2007) Ventilator-associated pneumonia in neonatal and pediatric intensive care unit patients. *Clinical Microbiology Reviews* **20**: 409–425.

4 Raymond SJ (1995) Normal saline instillation before suctioning: helpful or harmful? A review of the literature. *American Journal of Critical Care* **4**(4): 267–271.

5 Jevon P (2004) *Paediatric advanced life support: a practical guide*. Oxford: Butterworth Heinemann.

6 Resuscitation Council UK (1996) *Should relatives witness resuscitation?* London: Resuscitation Council UK.

7 Sacar S, Turrgout H, Kaleli I, *et al.* (2006) Poor hospital infection control practice in hand hygiene, glove utilisation, and usage of tourniquet. *American Journal of Infection Control* **34**: 606–609.

8 Hartsilver EL, Vanner RG (2000) Airway obstruction with cricoid pressure. *Anaesthesia*, **55**(3): 208–211.

9 Pilbeam SP(2006) Final considerations in ventilator set-up: humidification. In: Pilbeam SP and Cairo JM (eds) *Mechanical ventilation: physiological and clinical applications*. St Louis: Mosby Elsevier, Missouri, p. 129.

10 Williams R, Rankin N, Smith T, *et al* (1996) Relationship between the humidity and temperature of inspired gas and the function of the airway mucosa. *Critical Care Medicine* **24**: 1920–1929.

11 Irlbeck D (1998) Normal mechanisms of heat and moisture exchange in the respiratory tract. *Respiratory Care Clinics of North America* **4**: 189–198.

12 DH (2001) *Building a safer NHS for patients*. London: HMSO.

13 Martin C, Perrin G, Gevaudan MJ, *et al.* (1990) Heat and moisture exchangers and vaporizing humidifiers in the intensive care unit. *Chest* **97**: 144–149.

14 Craven DE, Steger KA (1989) Pathogenesis and prevention of nosocomial pneumonia in the mechanically ventilated patient. *Respiratory Care* **34**: 85–97.

15 Walsh J M, Vanderwarf C, Hoscheit D (1989) Unsuspected hemodynamic alterations during endotracheal suctioning *Chest*, 95, 162–165.

16 Ruffell A, Adamcova L (2008) Ventilator-associated pneumonia: prevention is better than cure. *Nursing in Critical Care* **13**(1): 44–53

17 Munro C, Grap M (2004) Oral health and care in intensive care unit: state of the science. *American Journal of Critical Care* **13**: 25–33

# FURTHER READING

Advanced Life Support Group (2005) The child with breathing difficulties. In: *Advanced paediatric life support: the practical approach*, 4th edition. BMJ Books: London, Chapter 8.

Hatherill M, Murdoch I A, Marsh M. (1996) Paediatric ventilation. *Current Anaesthesia and Critical Care* 7: 248–253.

HSE (1992) *Manual handling: manual handling operations regulations 1992*. London: HSE.

DHS (1987) *Evaluation of heated humidifiers. Health Equipment Information*. p 177.

MacLeod P, Bucknall R (2006) Mechanical ventilation with heated humidifiers or with heat and moisture exchangers. *Evidence Based Nursing* 9: 82.

Shelly MP, Lloyd GM, Park GR (1988) A review of the mechanisms and methods of humidification of inspired gas. *Intensive Care Medicine* 14: 1–9.

## LEARNING OUTCOMES

*Upon completion of this chapter, the reader should be able to accomplish the following:*

1 Define invasive cardiovascular support, and list different methods of providing this support
2 List the emergency equipment and checks that should be performed at the beginning of a shift when looking after a child with invasive cardiovascular support
3 Describe types of pacemaker and methods of pacing
4 Describe the modes of pacing
5 Describe the parameters that can be set with external pacing
6 Describe the potential complications associated with external pacing
7 Discuss the nursing care of a child with a pacemaker
8 Describe the procedure for removal of temporary pacing wires
9 Describe the action of inotropes
10 Describe four commonly used inotropic agents and when they may be used
11 Describe the nursing care required for a child receiving inotropic support
12 List the indications for a chest drain, and types of chest drain
13 Describe the risks associated with chest drains
14 Describe the nursing care of a child with a chest drain

## CHAPTER OVERVIEW

Children may require cardiovascular support after cardiac surgery, or for a variety of conditions that affect the circulatory or respiratory systems. This chapter provides an overview of the following types of support: pacing, inotropic support and chest drains. Although the application of these aspects of care will be most common on intensive care units or cardiothoracic wards, children with cardiac conditions may be admitted to general paediatric wards, and nurses working in these areas could find themselves caring for these children. A basic understanding of the principles of care is therefore essential for all nurses caring for children in the acute care setting.

## PACING

Contraction of cardiac muscle occurs when an electrical-type impulse passes through the myocardium. In some conditions, the impulse may not occur, may occur irregularly or follow an abnormal (accessory) pathway. If this causes haemodynamic instability, an impulse may be generated artificially to mimic the heart's own intrinsic impulse. This is the role of the pacemaker.

### KEY WORDS

Pacemaker   Transvenous pacing   Epicardial pacing
Endocardial pacing   Internal cardioverter
Defibrillator mode

## Normal conduction physiology

In order to understand pacing, it is important to have a basic understanding of normal conduction. Please see the website for a summary of normal conduction.

## Physiology of pacing

Pacing occurs when a small electrical charge is delivered to the cardiac muscle (myocardium). This small charge initiates an impulse through the heart muscle, causing contraction of the cardiac muscle. If the impulse begins in the atria, it may be picked up by the AV node, and pass through the normal pathway to the ventricles. If it does not, a charge will be delivered to the ventricles, and will pass through the ventricular muscle, causing contraction of the ventricles. The impulse will not follow the 'normal' conduction route. Please see the website for further details. The charge can be delivered to the atria and ventricles (dual chamber), or one of these (single chamber). The wires that provide the impulse may pass through the vascular system to the myocardium (transvenous/endocardial pacing) or may be attached directly to the epicardium on the outside of the heart (epicardial pacing).

## Indications for pacing

- Following cardiac surgery
  - Suppression/treatment of arrhythmias
    Following cardiac surgery, arrhythmias are relatively common. The reported incidence varies from 15 per cent[1] to 28 per cent.[2] Complete atrioventricular block after some types of surgery has an incidence of 1–3 per cent. This is often transient, typically resolving within 10 days of surgery,[3] but may sometimes require permanent pacemaker insertion.

Owing to the risk of postoperative arrhythmia, it is common practice for pacing wires to be inserted during surgery. Heart blocks leading to bradycardias may require pacing to ensure a heart rate that provides an adequate cardiac output.
- To augment cardiac output
After surgery, the contractility of the myocardium may be temporarily reduced, causing a corresponding reduction in stroke volume. In this case, maintaining a satisfactory blood pressure (BP) may require pacing at a higher heart rate than 'normal' for the age of the child.
  - In tachyarrhythmias, cardiac output may be compromised because of reduced filling time. In this situation, cardiac resynchronisation therapy (CRT) ('overdrive pacing' or 'anti-tachycardia pacing', ATP) may be useful. The pacemaker is set to a rate above the patient's intrinsic rate, and the rate is then gradually reduced. If treatment is successful, the heart rate will drop, increasing cardiac output. This allows longer filling times and longer diastole, during which the cardiac muscle is perfused.
- *Arrhythmias*
  - Heart block
    Heart block occurs when the impulse cannot follow the usual path. It may be partial, such as right bundle branch block, or complete heart block, where the impulse from the P wave does not reach the ventricles, and they are activated by an escape rhythm, starting within the muscle of the ventricles. The associated bradycardia may require pacing to ensure an adequate cardiac output.
  - Long Q–T syndrome
    Long Q–T syndrome is a congenital condition

with a risk of life-threatening arrhythmias. Owing to the risk of sudden cardiac death associated with this condition, an internal cardioversion defibrillator (ICD) may be inserted.

- Bradycardias

  Sinus bradycardias rarely require pacing, but this may be necessary if drug therapy is not effective.

## Methods of pacing

Methods of pacing can be categorised in various ways:

- endocardial versus epicardial pacing;
- temporary versus permanent;
- single chamber versus dual chamber.

### Endocardial pacing

The pacing wires are attached to the endocardium (inside the heart). They are usually inserted via the venous system, and this method is therefore often referred to as *transvenous pacing*. This may be permanent or temporary.

Temporary endocaridal pacing is most commonly used in acute settings, where quick access is required. It is usually performed in a cardiac catheter laboratory. The pacing wires are passed through the venous system into the heart where they are inserted into the myocardium of the right atrium and ventricle. They attach to the muscle by a variety of methods, such as coils and hooks. The distal ends of the wires are attached to an external pacing box and the mode, rate, and other settings may be set and changed easily.

### Epicardial pacing

In this method of pacing, the wires attach to the epicardium (outer surface of the heart). This type of pacing may be temporary or permanent. Epicardial pacing has historically been the method of choice for permanent pacing, but is now less common. Insertion of the pacemaker is a surgical procedure, and is performed under general anaesthetic. Fibrosis of the cardiac muscle is a common complication, leading to an increased pacing threshold requiring increased voltage and as a consequence shortens the pacemaker's life. Recent advances in lead technology have produced a steroid-eluting lead that reduces inflammation, thereby reducing the pacing threshold and

lengthening the life of the pacemaker. [6]

Temporary epicardial pacing is common after cardiac surgery. Wires are placed into the myocardium during the surgical procedure. The wires exit the skin on the upper abdomen. There are usually four wires: two atrial and two ventricular. The wires attach to the pacing box in the same way as in transvenous pacing (above).

Higher pacing thresholds are usually required for epicardial pacing than for endocardial pacing.[4] Epicardial leads are more prone to failure than endocardial leads, although steroid eluting leads have a similar failure rate to endocardial leads.[5]

### Permanent pacemakers

If pacing is required long term, e.g. for chronic rhythm problems such as sick sinus syndrome, heart block or long Q–T interval,[7] a permanent pacemaker may be inserted. The pacemaker device is situated under the skin, usually on the chest wall or in the abdomen. It contains electrical circuitry, a small radio transceiver and a battery. Permanent pacemakers may be single chamber or dual chamber. These terms specify whether both the atrium and the ventricle are paced (dual chamber), or only one is paced (single chamber). In permanent pacemakers, the controls are not accessible, and the mode and other settings must be changed using a radio device. Devices can be interrogated through a programmer header which allows access to the device history (Figure 26.1).

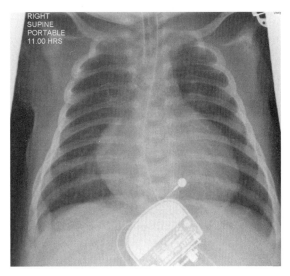

**Figure 26:1** Chest X-ray: permanent epicardial pacemaker (single chamber).

## Temporary pacemakers

A temporary pacing system is a pulse generator that can both sense the heart's intrinsic electrical activity and deliver an electrical impulse to initiate depolarisation of the myocardium. The pacing wires of temporary pacemakers exit from the patient, either from a vein (endocardial pacing) or through the abdominal wall (epicardial pacing). The mode, rate and voltage of sensing and pacing can be altered easily with the control unit, which usually contains a display (Figures 26.2–26.4).

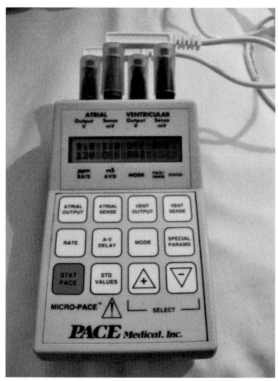

**Figure 26.2** Temporary pacing box.

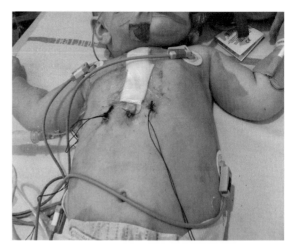

**Figure 26.3** Epicardial pacing wires exiting the skin.

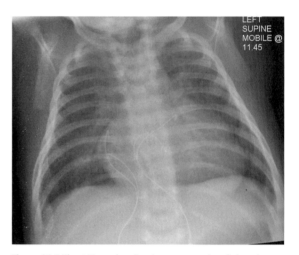

**Figure 26.4** Chest X-ray showing temporary epicardial pacing wires.

## Transcutaneous pacing

This method of pacing is used temporarily in an emergency if no pacing wires are in situ. It provides an impulse through the skin via hands-free defibrillation pads. This method is extremely uncomfortable and should only be used in an emergency with adequate sedation and analgesia until a more appropriate method can be initiated.

## Percussion pacing

This may be used in an emergency, but its success rate is poor and it is not advocated in children who have undergone cardiac surgery. Short, sharp 'thumps' to the chest over the heart stimulate an impulse. It is only appropriate for a very short time, until a more appropriate method can be initiated.

## Implantable cardioverter defibrillators

Some conditions pose a high risk of ventricular fibrillation (VF) or ventricular tachycardia (VT) with significant haemodynamic instability. For children with a high risk of sudden cardiac death due to these rhythms, an implantable cardioverter defibrillators (ICD) may be inserted to monitor the cardiac rhythm and automatically defibrillate if VF or VT is detected.

Children with these devices in situ are at significant risk of emotional disturbances and depression, and psychological support is required. There is a small risk of inappropriate activation of the device, which causes increased anxiety in the children concerned.[8]

## Pacing modes

The pacemaker can *sense* intrinsic impulses of the heart, and can *pace* by sending an impulse to the muscle to stimulate muscular contraction. Each chamber may be sensed and/or paced independently. A generic code system for pacing modes has been developed by the North American Society of Pacing and Electrophysiology and the British Pacing and Electrophysiology Group. Permanent pacemakers have five letters, as shown in Table 26.1. Temporary pacemakers use only the first three letters (Table 26.2).

As well as the mode, other settings include:

- voltage (measured in millivolts) of the sensing and the pacing: atrial pacing uses lower voltage

than ventricular; the lowest voltage that 'captures' (causes an impulse to be initiated in the cardiac muscle) should be used;
- rate;
- AV delay. This is the time between pacing of the atria and pacing of the ventricles.

## Safety and risk management

Please refer to Table 26.3 for safety and risk management.

## Nursing care of the child with a temporary pacemaker

### Safety

Emergency life support equipment should be available and the defibrillator should be capable of pacing via hands-free pads in case the pacemaker fails.

The doses of emergency drugs (adrenaline [epinephrine]; atropine) should be known and these drugs should be easily available in case of failure of pacing and life-threatening arrhythmias.

**Table 26.1** Permanent pacemaker modes

| Chamber paced | Chamber sensed | Mode of response | Programmable functions | Antitachycardia functions |
|---|---|---|---|---|
| O – None | O – None | O –None | O – None | O –None |
| A – Atrium | A – Atrium | T – Triggered | P – Simple programmable | P – Pacing |
| V – Ventricle | V – Ventricle | I – Inhibited | M – Multi-programmable | S – Shock |
| D – Dual (A and V) | D – Dual (A and V) | D –Dual | R – Rate modulation | D –Dual (P and S) |

**Table 26.2** Temporary pacemaker modes

| | Atrial sensing | Atrial pacing | Ventricular sensing | Ventricular pacing | Response |
|---|---|---|---|---|---|
| DDD | ✓ | ✓ | ✓ | ✓ | Both chambers are sensed and paced |
| AAI | ✓ | ✓ | ✗ | ✗ | Inhibits when intrinsic atrial rate is above the rate |
| VVI | ✗ | ✗ | ✓ | ✓ | Inhibits when intrinsic ventricular rate is above the set rate |
| DVI | ✗ | ✓ | ✓ | ✓ | If AV conduction is successful, ventricular output of pacemaker is inhibited; otherwise, ventricles are paced after a set AV delay |
| AOO | ✗ | ✓ | ✗ | ✗ | Atria are paced, despite any intrinsic activity (rarely used) |

**Table 26.3** Safety and risk management

| Risk | Signs | Action |
|---|---|---|
| Failure to pace: <br><br> Lead dislodgement at myocardium <br><br> Lead disconnection at pacing box <br><br> Fracture or damage to wire <br><br> Failure of capture; fibrosis at lead site | Non-paced rhythm seen on cardiac monitor, with heart rate lower than set rate | Check that pacing wires are attached to box <br><br> Call for help <br><br> Swap polarity of leads <br><br> Medical staff will check pacing threshold and may increase or change mode <br><br> If these actions are not successful, emergency measures may be required, e.g. transcutaneous pacing or reinsertion of pacing wires by reopening the chest |
| Bleeding (rare, but possible after lead removal) | External: visible blood from wire insertion site <br><br> Internal (rare): signs of hypovolaemia <br><br> Possible signs of tamponade: tachycardia, hypotension, increasing central venous pressure, signs of reduced cardiac output | Apply pressure to site <br><br> Check clotting <br><br> Observe closely for signs of tamponade <br><br> Echocardiogram may be required to show extent of bleeding <br><br> A needle cardiocentesis may be required, or drain insertion |
| Infection <br><br> Incidence reported as 0.5–2% Most common microbe: *Staphylococcus*[9] | Pyrexia <br><br> Tachycardia <br><br> Increased WCC; increased CRP; <br><br> Possible vegetation seen on echocardiogram | Take blood cultures <br><br> Administer antibiotic therapy: usually 6 weeks' duration <br><br> Remove pacing wires <br><br> Consider epicardial pacing until infection resolved |
| Inappropriate muscle stimulation: diaphragmatic stimulation via phrenic nerve | | Less common in bipolar stimulation with lower output. Consider changing to this |

Pacing wires are thin and easily fracture; they can become dislodged or disconnected. It is therefore vital that the pacing box is placed in a position where it will not fall, and that the leads are kept neat and not caught around other items or lines. Although they are held in place with a suture, they can be pulled out inadvertently, especially by an awake toddler. Extra taping of wires, with loops to allow for some accidental pulling, is a sensible precaution.

A spare pacing box should always be kept to hand, with the settings preconfigured, in case the main pacing box fails.

### General checks

Most pacing boxes have a locking mechanism so that they cannot be inadvertently changed or switched off.

The battery life should be checked regularly. Most boxes have two batteries, which may be changed independently without a break in the pacing. However, for safety, a second pacing box should be available with the same settings as the box in use.

The attachment of the wires to the box should be secure. Adaptors should not be used: the wires should be directly compatible with the box.

If the wires are not in use, they should be coiled and secured with easy access to the ends in case pacing is required quickly. The wires should not be bent and inserted into tubing as the risk of fracture is increased.

### Monitoring

All children with temporary pacemakers should have continuous ECG monitoring to allow problems with the pacing to be quickly identified. The alarms of the ECG monitor should be set to just above and below the set rate, so that failure to pace can be quickly identified.

A cardiac monitor will pick up the pacing 'spike', which will be visible on the display. Most monitors allow the user to select 'paced', which helps the monitor software to interpret the paced rhythm.

A 12-lead ECG should be taken at the beginning of each shift, and any changes reported.

### Documentation

All the pacemaker settings should be recorded at the beginning of each shift, and again if any changes are made.

The rhythm should be observed on the cardiac monitor, and recorded with the observations e.g. paced, sinus rhythm, etc.

## Procedures

### Removal of pacing wires

There is variation in the timing of pacing wire removal, within and between institutions. Local policy will guide the timing. Jowett et al.[2] found that, of the children who required pacing after cardiac surgery, all developed arrhythmias within 24 hours of surgery. They argue that if there have been no arrhythmias during this time, the wires may be safely removed after 24 hours. However, a timing of 5 days post operatively is more common in most institutions.

Please see the website for the procedure for removing pacing wires.

## INOTROPIC THERAPY

### What are inotropes?

The term 'inotrope' refers to a group of drugs that increase the force of contraction of the heart. However, inotropic drugs may also have other

---

**VIGNETTE**

**Problem**: A 2-year-old child with Down's syndrome has returned from theatre after repair of an AVSD (atrioventricular septal defect). The child had an arrhythmia when coming off bypass. The pacing wires are attached to the pacing box, but it is not switched on. The plan is to warm the child, then wake and extubate.

**Discussion**: The precaution of attaching the wires to the pacing box in case it is needed can be justified. However, the risk of the wires becoming dislodged or damaged as the child wakes probably outweighs the benefits. This risk is higher in a child with developmental delay, who may be unable to follow instructions; also in a child with Down's syndrome, who may be difficult to sedate. If the pacing wires are not being used and the child is in sinus rhythm with an adequate rate and cardiac output, the box should be disconnected and the wires coiled and stuck to the skin, allowing quick access if required, but preventing accidental pulling or damaging.

---

**KEY POINTS**

Pacemakers are life-saving devices, but their correct use is vitally important to prevent life-threatening complications. Safety issues are paramount, and a good working knowledge of the modes, and trouble-shooting, is vital for the nurse caring for a child with a temporary pacemaker.

---

**KEY WORDS**

Cardiac output   Inotrope   Chronotrope
Contractility   Vasopressor

---

effects that affect cardiac output, such as peripheral vasoconstriction, vasodilation or an increase in heart rate. A more accurate term would be catecholamine: a substance which acts on the adrenergic receptors in the heart and blood vessels. However, the term inotrope is more often used in clinical practice.

Inotropic support is directed at establishing or maintaining a reasonable arterial pressure and ensuring adequate tissue perfusion by improving cardiac output (CO). In order to understand how these drugs work, it is important to understand the concept of cardiac output. Please see the website for a summary.

| **Definitions** | |
|---|---|
| **Cardiac output (CO):** the amount of blood ejected from the heart per minute (stroke volume × heart rate). | **Chronotrope:** a drug that increases the heart rate. |
| **Stroke volume (SV):** the amount of blood ejected by the heart with each beat. | **Vasodilator:** a drug which causes dilation of blood vessels by relaxing the smooth muscle of the vessel wall. |
| **Contractility:** the ability of the cardiac muscle fibres to contract. | **Vasopressor:** a drug which causes constriction of blood vessels by causing contraction of the smooth muscle of the vessel wall. |
| **Catecholamine:** a substance containing catechol and amine groups, which acts at adrenergic receptors. | **Preload:** the amount of blood entering the heart. |
| **Inotrope:** a drug that increases the force of cardiac muscular contraction. | **Afterload:** the effort required to push blood out of the heart. |

## How do inotropes work?

Inotropes act on the α, β1 and β2 receptors within the heart and blood vessels. Different drugs act on different receptors, and therefore have different effects. Please see Table 26.4 for a summary of this.

## When are inotropes used?

### Following cardiac surgery

Inotropes are commonly used after cardiac surgery. Cardiopulmonary bypass, aortic cross-clamping and hypothermia-induced cardiac arrest can precipitate a complex systemic inflammatory response, which affects multiple organs, and can cause severe haemodynamic instability; inotropic therapy may be required to support cardiac function until the inflammatory response resolves.[10]

### Shock

In states of shock, there is a hypoperfusion of vital organs, usually with low CO and low BP. Inotropic support is directed at establishing or maintaining a reasonable BP and ensuring adequate tissue perfusion by improving CO.

In septic shock, massive vasodilation produces a fall in systemic vascular resistance (SVR) and BP. If fluid resuscitation is ineffective, the BP may be improved pharmacologically, with inotropic drugs. Noradrenaline (norepinephrine) is often the drug of choice as its predominant action is vasoconstriction. Noradrenaline (norepinephrine) may be used in conjunction with other inotropes to improve both BP and cardiac output.

In cardiogenic shock, e.g. following myocardial infarction or cardiac surgery, CO and BP are lowered, but SVR is raised. The goal in this situation is to increase contractility, coronary blood flow and CO. Dobutamine or dopamine may be used here. If the right ventricle is affected, milrinone may also be used.

### Preterm neonatal hypotension

Preterm neonates may present with hypotension unrelated to hypovolaemia. It is thought that adrenal insufficiency may account for some cases. If the hypotension does not respond to one cautious fluid bolus and there are no signs of hypovolaemia, inotropic therapy may be initiated.[11] The inotrope of choice is dopamine, with dobutamine added if the maximum dose of dopamine is not effective.

### To maintain clinical state until further treatment is possible, or in life-limiting conditions

Milrinone may be used in children for extended periods while awaiting further treatment for severe cardiac conditions, e.g. transplantation for cardiomyopathy.[12] Milrinone has also been used to prolong life in children with cardiomyopathy relating to Duchenne's muscular dystrophy, where transplantation is inappropriate or impossible.[13]

## Commonly used inotropic drugs

For commonly used inotropic drugs, please refer to Table 26.4 (page 455).

## Care of the child receiving inotropic agents

The biological half-life of inotropic agents is 1–2 minutes, because of re-uptake into tissues and breakdown within the body. They therefore have an extremely fast action and a very short half-life,

Table 26.4 Commonly used inotropic drugs

| Drug | Receptor | Effect on contractility | Effect on heart rate | Effect on BP | Clinical use | Dose/administration | Adverse effects |
|---|---|---|---|---|---|---|---|
| **Dopamine** A naturally occurring substance, the precursor of noradrenaline (norepinephrine) | Dopamine +++ α+++ β1 ++ β2 +++ | + | + | Vasodilation Dose-dependent vasoconstriction (minimal action) | After surgery, to improve BP by increasing cardiac output. Hypotension of unknown cause with hypovolaemia ruled out, in preterm neonates | Dose dependent: 2–5 µg/kg/min: vasodilation of renal arteries, increasing urine output. 5–10 µg/kg/min: increased heart rate and BP. 10–20 µg/kg/min: increased vasoconstriction, increasing BP | Tachycardia; angina; arrhythmias; headache; hypertension; vasoconstriction; nausea and vomiting |
| **Milrinone** Does not act in same way as other inotropes | Does not act on adrenergic receptors. Inhibitors of phosphodiesterase (enzyme which breaks down cAMP) | +++ Improves ventricular function | Minimal effect | Reduces BP (vasodilation) | After surgery, especially affecting right ventricle or septum. Long-term use in conditions that reduce cardiac output | May require initial bolus over 10 minutes, then rate of 0.2–0.75 µg/kg/minute | Supraventricular and ventricular arrhythmias, hypotension, fluid retention, hypokalaemia, tremor, diarrhoea, thrombocytopaenia |
| **Adrenaline** A naturally occurring hormone and neurotransmitter (use in cardiac arrest is not discussed here) | β1 +++ β2 ++ α+++ | +++ | ++ Increases | Increases BP | Emergency use in cardiac arrest – increases cardiac responsiveness to cardioversion. Used to increase cardiac output in low output states. Use is limited in this setting, because it increases myocardial oxygen requirements and can lead to ischaemia | Starting dose 0.05 mcg/kg/min. May increase as required. Administer centrally, as in infusion in low cardiac output state | Cardiac ischaemia; tremor; headache; peripheral ischaemia; nausea and vomiting; cerebral haemorrhage; pulmonary oedema; sweating; weakness; dizziness; hyperglycaemia |
| **Noradrenaline** (norepinephrine) A naturally occurring neurotransmitter | α+++ β1+ | + | ++ Increases heart rate | Increases BP ++ Vasoconstriction | Used mainly in treatment of hypotension in shock, e.g. septic shock | Starting dose: 0.05 mcg/kg/min. May increase as required. Administer centrally as infusion; NO BOLUS | Hypertension; headache; bradycardia; arrhythmias; peripheral ischaemia |
| **Dobutamine** A synthetic drug, not produced by the body | β1 +++ β2 ++ | +++ | + Increases heart rate at higher doses | Minimal effect on BP, possible reduction | Rarely used in children because of increased cardiac oxygen demand | Dose: 2.5–10 µg/kg/min | Tachycardia, arrhythmias, angina, nausea, tremor, anxiety, hypokalaemia |

meaning changes in the rate of infusion may have profound effects on the cardiovascular status of the child. For this reason, most inotropic agents are administered only in critical care areas or under the guidance and supervision of medical or outreach teams. Owing to their slightly longer half-life, dopamine, dobutamine and milrinone may be used on specialist cardiac wards with appropriate monitoring, staff training and medical cover. These drugs are sometimes administered long term to patients awaiting transplant or patients with cardiomyopathy on specialist cardiac wards with appropriate staff training and medical cover.[14]

Cardiac monitoring is essential, and invasive BP monitoring should be available. If it is not, a non-invasive BP reading should be taken at least every 5 minutes until invasive BP monitoring can be initiated. Among the drugs discussed in this chapter, the exception to this rule is milrinone, which has a longer action time and half-life and is therefore safer to use in the ward setting[15] with appropriate patient monitoring and staff training.

### Administration

Owing to the fast action, inotropes must be administered as a continuous infusion, preferably into a large central vein. Steady state is achieved within 5–10 minutes after the start of an infusion. The rate of delivery of each inotrope is titrated against specified end-points, e.g. BP, CO, SVR. Prolonged use may lead to loss of efficacy due to the downregulation of β receptors.

No other drugs may be infused with inotropes, because of the risks of the child receiving a bolus of the drug as rates are changed. Inotropes may be administered together, however, via a single lumen of a central venous catheter.

Each organisation will have a standard method for dilution. Rates of administration are discussed in terms of μg/kg/minute. This allows universal understanding of the amount that the child is receiving, whatever the weight of the child or the dilution of the drug. In order to work this out use the formula in Table 26.5 (page 457).

## Safety and risk management

Owing to the quick action and short half-life of these drugs, any reduction in the flow of the inotrope or small bolus can cause significant and potentially life-threatening changes in BP.

Note that the use of needleless devices within inotrope giving sets and systems is not advised because of some reported problems with initiation of new therapy and higher infusion pressures, leading to a reduction in the amount of the drug received, followed by a surge of drug when the connector is tightened.

## PROCEDURE: Changing inotrope syringes

| Procedural steps | Evidence-based rationale |
| --- | --- |
| **1** Prepare the new infusion, using the same concentration as the old infusion | In order to be ready to change syringe with no delay or pause in therapy |
| **2** Prime the giving set | To avoid air embolus |
| **3** Place infusion in new syringe driver, and start infusion at same rate as current infusion (without connecting to the patient) | To allow pump to build up to infusion pressure (not required in some modern pumps) |
| **4** Watch for drug infusing from end of giving set | To ensure no reduction in administration during change-over |
| **5** Using a three-way tap, attach giving set of new infusion and immediately turn tap on to new infusion and off to old infusion | To allow for quick change from one syringe to the other without 'double-pumping' or risk of reduction in therapy |
| **6** Place old infusion on 'hold' | So that old infusion may be restarted in case of problems with new infusion |
| **7** When cardiovascular stability is ensured, turn off the old infusion and remove | To ensure cardiovascular stability |

**Table 26.5** Calculating inotrope rates

| Formula | Example: 20-kg child, 4 mg of noradrenaline (norepinephrine) in 50 mL of saline, running at 2 mL/h |
| --- | --- |
| Amount of drug in syringe (mg) | 4 |
| ÷ volume in syringe = mg/mL | ÷ 50 (mL) = 0.08 mg/mL |
| × 1000 = µg/mL | × 1000 = 80 µg/mL |
| × rate of infusion = µg/hour | × 2 = 160 µg/hour |
| ÷ weight of child (kg) = µg/kg/hour | ÷ 20 = 8 µg/kg/hour |
| ÷ 60 = µg/kg/minute | ÷ 60 = 0.13 µg/kg/minute |

### Changing the rate of infusion

Only those familiar with the effects of inotropic therapy should change the rate, within previously agreed parameters and under medical guidance. The rate may be titrated to BP or other parameters by senior nursing staff in some areas.

> **KEY POINTS**
>
> Inotropic drugs *must* not be suddenly stopped or bolused, except in cardiac arrest situations, as this may cause severe and life-threatening changes in BP and cardiac output

The changes in BP will be transitory, and should return to 'normal' within a few minutes. However, severe consequences can occur during this short time. Medical help must be summoned, and an experienced nurse may reduce the rate of infusion until the BP begins to come down, at which point the infusion is returned to the original rate. This should be done only if the BP is at a life-threatening level, and only by nurses who are experienced in titrating inotropes, and with a doctor on hand.

Many other types of drugs provide cardiovascular support, and may be used in cardiac surgical or cardiology settings. Examples of these include:

- drugs which alter the heart rate (e.g. beta-blockers);
- drugs which alter the BP (e.g. ACE [angiotensin-converting enzyme] inhibitors);
- drugs to correct arrhythmias (e.g. amiodarone, digoxin);
- drugs which alter fluid balance (e.g. diuretics);
- drugs to correct electrolyte imbalances.

These drugs are not discussed in detail here, but a knowledge of them is vital for nurses working in these settings.

> **VIGNETTE**
>
> **Problem**: A 5-year-old child has septic shock and has a noradrenaline (norepinephrine) infusion running through an internal jugular central line, which becomes kinked when the child moves. The child's BP drops to 60/30. The child's neck is straightened and the line becomes patent again, allowing the noradrenaline to flow. The build up of pressure in the line causes a bolus of noradrenaline (norepinephrine) to be infused and the BP rises sharply to 180/100.
>
> **Discussion**: The risk of swings in BP due to access problems is high, especially with central lines in the internal jugular or femoral vein, due to the risk of them becoming occluded or kinked when moving. Ensure the line is taped securely, and in such a way that kinking is minimised.

## CHEST DRAIN MANAGEMENT

> **KEY WORDS**
>
> Chest drain   Pneumothorax   Haemothorax
> Pleural effusion   Chylothorax   Underwater seal

### Reasons for drain insertion

Please refer to Table 26.6 (page 458) for reasons for drain insertion.

### Position of drain

An apical pleural drain is inserted to resolve a pneumothorax, or to assist with the reinflation of a lung or prevent a pneumothorax after surgery

## Definitions

**Chest drain:** a tube inserted between the visceral and parietal pleura or into the mediastinal space to remove or prevent build up of air or fluid in the pleural space or mediastinasstrium.

**Apical:** towards the apex of the lung.

**Basal:** towards the base of the lung.

**Pneumothorax:** air within the pleural cavity, outside the lung.

**Haemothorax:** blood within the pleural cavity, outside the lung.

**Chylothorax:** chyle (lymph) within the pleural cavity, outside the lung.

**Tamponade:** pressure on the heart, usually caused by blood around the heart, reducing the heart's ability to pump effectively. A potentially life-threatening situation that requires emergency treatment.

**Tension pneumothorax:** a pneumothorax in which the pressure builds up in the affected side of the chest and moves the mediastinum towards the other side. A potentially life-threatening situation that requires emergency treatment.

**Table 26.6** Reasons for drain insertion

| | |
|---|---|
| Pneumothorax | To remove air from the pleural space after surgery with lung deflation, or after spontaneous or traumatic pneumothorax |
| Haemothorax | To remove or prevent a build-up of blood in the pleural space after surgery or trauma |
| Pleural effusion | To remove serous fluid from the pleural space caused by fluid shifts and pressure changes in the pulmonary circulation |
| Chylothorax | To remove chyle from the pleural space, if the thymus gland or lymph vessels have been damaged during surgery |
| Empyema | To remove pus from the pleural space caused by infection within the pleura |
| Post surgery | Mediastinal: to prevent a build-up of blood or serous fluid in mediastinal space<br>Pleural: to encourage reinflation of the lung after surgery |

within the thoracic cavity, e.g. thoracic, cardiac or spinal surgery.

A basal pleural drain is inserted to drain fluid from the pleural cavity. The fluid may be blood (haemothorax), serous fluid (pleural effusion), pus (empyema) or chyle (chylothorax).

A mediastinal drain is inserted during surgery to prevent a collection of blood or serous fluid around the heart after cardiac surgery.

## Types of drainage system

### Underwater seal systems

These rely on the end of the drainage tube being under water. This allows the escape of air or fluid, but prevents air going up the tubing and entering the pleural space. The drainage bottle must be kept below the level of the chest to prevent syphoning of the fluid back into the chest. The bottle must be kept upright, to maintain the underwater seal and to prevent air entering the end of the tubing. Some modern drainage systems involve a closed system,

where there is no visible tube entering the water. However, they still require water to be placed in the bottle in order to prevent backflow.

### One-way valve systems

These are portable bags that contain a one-way valve allowing air or fluid to enter the bag, but preventing any ingress back into the tube. They may be lifted above the level of the chest for short periods without risk of air or fluid entering the pleural space. However, they will not drain unless below the level of the insertion point.

## Drain insertion

This may be done in theatre, or on the ward or intensive care unit. The location of the procedure will depend on the availability of appropriately trained staff, the age and developmental stage of the child, and psychological factors. Sedation or general anaesthetic will be required, and the child may be transferred to theatre, intensive care or a specialist treatment area within the ward for closer monitoring following the insertion. However, older children may not require anaesthetic, and the procedure can be done on the ward.

As well as the equipment required for inserting the drain, the following must be available during the procedure:

- suction;
- oxygen, with a method of giving it, e.g. bag–valve–mask if the child is to be sedated, non-rebreathe mask for high concentration $O_2$ in a self-ventilating child.

Analgesia must be considered. Older children may find Entonox useful, but the reason for drain insertion must be considered, as Entonox is contraindicated with pneumothorax. Local anaesthetic is used at the insertion site, but insertion is still painful and an opiate may be required.

The child must be closely monitored during drain insertion, with at least monitoring of oxygen saturation and respiratory rate and effort, and preferably with ECG monitoring and regular BP recordings.

Unless drains are being inserted under direct vision during thoracic or cardiac surgery, a chest X-ray should be obtained after insertion to identify the correct position of the drain.

Please see the website for the requirements for assisting with drain insertion.

## Care of the child with a chest drain

### Pain

Chest drains are painful. The wound site, sutures and the presence of the drain in the pleural space will cause pain. Any pulling or movement of the drain can cause pain. Adequate analgesia must be provided, weighing up the risks of respiratory depression with opiate analgesics against guarded, shallow breaths caused by pain. Distraction techniques and reassurance can help to overcome fear and psychological problems caused by the drain. Children often tolerate drains very well with minimal analgesia, once they have become accustomed to them. Each child must be individually assessed and managed accordingly.

### Positioning

An underwater seal drainage system must remain below the level of the chest to prevent water syphoning back into the chest.

Movement and positioning of the child must be undertaken with care to ensure that drains are not pulled. The tubing should not be attached to bedding as it may be pulled when the child moves

### Keeping the drains patent

The drains must be kept patent, and this can be achieved by several methods:

- gently tapping the drain;
- applying low vacuum suction (3–5 kPa [23–38 mmHg]) to the drain.

The drain tubing should *not* be 'milked' using roller clamps or other devices. The pressure changes this creates within the chest can dislodge clots forming within the wound or heart and cause increased bleeding.

### Education

The child and parents must be educated about the reasons for the drain, the risks and care of the drain.

### When to clamp the drain

Drains should not be clamped routinely. The drain should be clamped only if it becomes disconnected, either accidentally or for a procedure such as changing the bottle. It should not be clamped for moving the patient or as a 'trial' to assess readiness for drain removal.

The only indications for clamping a drain are:

- if the drain becomes disconnected it should be clamped until a new drainage system can be attached;
- after instillation of drugs, e.g. urokinase; antibiotics; drugs for pleuradhesis;
- when changing the drainage system.

If the drain is clamped for any of these reasons, the child must be closely observed for signs of tension pneumothorax or fluid build-up.

Drain clamps must be kept with the patient at all times, in case of unexpected disconnection. In the short term, the drain may be kinked by the nurse while help is summoned. A drainage system must then be reattached under sterile conditions.

### Instillation of drugs via chest drain

Some drugs may be given into the pleural cavity, e.g. antibiotics, drugs for pleuradhesis in recurrent pneumothoraces; chemotherapy drugs. This is done under sterile conditions and only by medical staff or specialist nurses.

### Taping the drain

The connections between the drain and the tubing should not be taped as disconnection of the drain from the tubing cannot be seen if the join is obscured by tape.

### Safety and risk management

The most serious risk associated with chest drains is *tension pneumothorax* if the drain becomes blocked. This is a life-threatening complication and the nurse caring for a child with a chest drain must be aware of the causes, signs and emergency action to take if a tension pneumothorax is suspected.

Other risks include drain displacement, kinking, bleeding and infection (Table 26.7)

### Equipment

Emergency equipment must be available at the bedspace of a child with a chest drain. This must include:

- clamps
- oxygen
- suction.

**Table 26.7** Identifying adverse events

| Risk | Signs | Action |
|---|---|---|
| Tension pneumothorax | Increased work of breathing Increased respiratory rate Pain Tracheal shift towards side of pneumothorax Circulatory compromise or collapse | Emergency needle thoracocentesis. See Advanced Paediatric Life Support guidelines[16] for detailed procedure |
| Drain displacement | Leaking around site Observed change in length of tube, or position of stay suture Observed drainage holes in tube outside skin | If drainage holes can be seen outside the skin, they should be immediately covered with an occlusive dressing to prevent air from entering the pleural space and possibly causing tension pneumothorax. The drain must then be replaced. |
| Kinking or blocking of drain | Drain stops draining or bubbling; Signs of worsening pneumothorax or increasing fluid in pleural space despite drain in place | Having the drain on a low level of suction (2–5 kPa [15–38 mmHg]) can prevent blocking. The drain should not be actively 'milked' as the changes in pressure can damage the pleural or mediastinal tissues or dislodge clots which are forming around wounds. Gentle tapping of the tubing can ensure continued drainage |
| Bleeding | Bleeding around site | Apply pressure Check clotting If bleeding is seen around the site, consider a suture around the site |
| Infection | Redness around site Pyrexia Raised white cell count; Raised C-reactive protein (a non-specific inflammatory marker) | The most important activity for infection control is prevention. Strict aseptic technique in all aspects of care, and basic preventative actions such as hand washing, are essential If infection is suspected: Swab the drain site Sample drainage fluid Administer antibiotics if they are clinically indicated |

Please see the website for the procedure for changing the chest drain bottle.

## Removal of the chest drain

The chest drain should be removed on medical advice, when drainage has reduced or a pneumothorax has resolved. The presence of a drain will cause some serous fluid to be produced by the pleura, as the presence of a foreign object in the pleural space will cause irritation and mild inflammation. It is therefore unrealistic to expect drainage to stop completely.

Please see the website for information for removing the chest drain.

Different types of drains are being developed that could replace traditional chest drains after surgery, such as Blake drains[17–19] and bulb-suction drains.[20]

## OTHER TYPES OF INVASIVE CARDIOVASCULAR SUPPORT

Other types of invasive cardiovascular support include intra-aortic balloon pumping, and extracorporeal membrane oxygenation, both of

**VIGNETTE**

**Problem:** You are caring for a child with two chest drains after cardiac surgery. The drains are both on suction, and have drained minimal amounts over the past 3 hours. The child has begun to show signs of respiratory distress, including tachypnoea, sternal and intercostal muscle recession, and dropping oxygen saturations.

**Action:** The child must be fully assessed to determine if the cause of the respiratory distress is a tension pneumothorax, caused by the drain tubing becoming blocked. Tension pneumothorax is an emergency and requires immediate action. The chest should be observed for symmetry of movement, and tracheal deviation looked and felt for (this is not always apparent). Medical assistance must be called for if tension pneumothorax is suspected, and needle thoracocentesis performed. If the deterioration is slow, a chest X-ray may be obtained, but this should not delay treatment for suspected tension pneumothorax.

which are outside the scope of this book. Some pictures of these types of support are available on the website, but a specialist paediatric intensive care text should be used for more detail on these types of therapies.

## ACKNOWLEDGEMENTS

Thanks to Patrick Phillips, Peter Wilson and Caroline Cole for their expert help and guidance. Also to the staff of PICU for their helpful comments, and to Markus and Lesley for their patience.

**KEY POINTS**

Chest drains have the potential to cause significant harm if not cared for appropriately, or if signs of problems are ignored. Nurses caring for children with chest drains must be appropriately trained and competent to care for them, and must identify and deal with any complications that arise.

Go to the website to find the PowerPoint presentation for this chapter and MCQs to test your knowledge. **www.hodderplus.com/childnursingskills**

# REFERENCES

1 Delaney JW, Moltedo JM, Dziura JD, *et al.* (2006) Early postoperative arrhythmias after pediatric cardiac surgery. *Journal of Thoracic and Cardiovascular Surgery* **131**: 1296–1300.

2 Jowett V, Hayes N, Sridharan S, *et al.* (2007) Timing of removal of pacing wires following paediatric cardiac surgery. *Cardiology in the Young* **17**: 512–516.

3 Gross GJ, Chiu CC, Hamilton RM, *et al.* (2006) Natural history of postoperative heart block in congenital heart disease: Implications for pacing intervention. *Heart Rhythm* **3**: 601–604.

4 Silvetti MS, Drago F, De Santis A, *et al.* (2007) Single-centre experience on endocardial and epicardial pacemaker system function in neonates and infants. *Europace* **9**: 426–431.

5 Silvetti MS, Drago F, Grutte G (2006) Twenty years of paediatric cardiac pacing: 515 pacemakers and 480 leads implanted in 292 patients. *Europace* **8**: 530–536.

6 Brzezinska-Paszke M (2006) Steroid-eluting epicardial pacing in Children. *Via Medica* **13**: 312–318.

7 Bar-Cohen Y, Silka MJ (2006) Congenital long QT syndrome: Diagnosis and management in pediatric patients. *Current Treatment Options in Cardiovascular Medicine* **8**: 387–395.

8 Eiken A, Kolb C, Lange S, *et al.* (2006) Implantable cardioverter defibrillator in children. *International Journal of Cardiology* **107**(1): 30–35.

9 Massoure PL, Reuter S, Lafitte S, *et al.* (2007) Pacemaker endocarditis: features and management. *PACE* **30**: 12–19

10 Roth SJ Adatia I, Pearson GD, *et al.* (2006) Summary proceedings from the cardiology group on postoperative cardiac dysfunction. *Pediatrics* **117**(3): S39–46

11 Soni NB, Barr S (2006) Evidence based guideline in management of hypotension in neonates. *Welsh Paediatric Journal* **24**: 31–33

12 McMahon CJ, Murchan H, Prendiville T, Burch M (2007) Long-term support with milrinone prior to cardiac transplantation in a neonate with left ventricular noncompaction. *Cardiomyopathy* **28**: 317–318.

13 Cripe LH, Barber BJ, Spicer RL, *et al.* (2006) Outpatient continuous inotrope infusion as an adjunct to heart failure therapy in Duchenne muscular dystrophy. *Neuromuscular disorders* **16**: 745–748.

14 Allan S, Houston A, Richens T (2005) The safety profile of IV inotropes in the ward setting. *Archives of Disease in Childhood* **90** (Suppl.): A67.

15 Bailey JM, Miller B E, Lu W, *et al.* (1999) The pharmacokinetics of milrinone in pediatric patients after cardiac surgery. *Anesthesiology* **90**: 1012–1018.

16 Advanced Life Support Group (2005) Advanced paediatric life support: the practical approach, 4th edition. Oxford: Blackwell Publishing.

17 Sakopoulos AG, Gundry S, Razzou AJ, *et al.* (2005) Efficacy of Blake drains for mediastinal and pleural drainage following cardiac operations. *Journal of Cardiac Surgery* **20**: 574–577.

18 Kejriwal N, Kejriwal K, Newman MAJ (2005) Use of a single silastic drain following thoracotomy: initial evaluation. *ANZ Journal of Surgery* **75**: 710–712.

19 Ishikura H, Kimura S (2006) The use of flexible silastic drains after chest surgery: novel thoracic drainage. *Annals of Thoracic Surgery* **81**: 331–333.

20 Valusec PA, Tsao K, St Peter SD, et al. (2006) A comparison of chest tubes versus bulb-suction drains in pediatric thoracic surgery. *Journal of Pediatric Surgery* **42**(5): 812–814.

## CHAPTER 27

# Caring for children suffering from burn injuries

## Maureen Betts and Shirin Pomeroy

## LEARNING OUTCOMES

*Upon completion of this chapter, the reader should be able to accomplish the following:*

1. Gain an insight into the care of a child/family with a burn injury
2. Identify when fluid resuscitation is required and know how to calculate fluid requirements
3. Understand when and why referral to a specialist burns service is necessary
4. Gain an overview of the multidisciplinary nature of burn care
5. Provide rationales for the care of the burn wound and choice of dressings used
6. Understand the complications associated with burn injury and how they might be prevented

## CHAPTER OVERVIEW

Burn care is a complex subspecialty within plastic surgery that is not just skin deep. Around 50 000 children annually under the age of 15 suffer from a burn injury in the UK,[1] and although the majority of these are relatively minor injuries, the impact on the child and family cannot be quantified. As well as physical, there are also emotional, psychological, social and spiritual components to a burn injury. All of these can potentially have long-term effects on the child and family, irrespective of the size of the initial burn. This can sometimes go unnoticed, as often problems arise after the child has been discharged from hospital. It is an important nursing skill to be able to provide and facilitate holistic care for the burn-injured child and their family, ensuring that all their needs are being met.

The most common thermal injuries in children are scalds from hot fluid (e.g. cups of tea), and this is predominantly seen in those under 3 years old.[2] The second most common injury in children is contact burns. The injury sustained is generally on the palms of hands, and the cause of the injury can be from ceramic hobs, ovens, heaters/radiators or even hair straighteners. However, severe burn injuries in children are still most frequently caused by hot bath water, whereby the child is either left unattended in the bathroom and turns on the hot tap, or the bath is only filled with hot water and the child either climbs or falls in.

In essence, burn care can be subdivided into seven different phases: rescue, resuscitate, retrieve, resurface, rehabilitate, reconstruct and review.[3] With this is mind, the full range of healthcare professionals can play a part in ensuring the best possible outcome for the child. In severe cases this input may be necessary until the child reaches adulthood and beyond. The purpose of this chapter is to assist nurses in having a better understanding of burn care and to know how best to manage a child who presents with a burn injury.

## Definitions

**Bronchoconstriction:** constriction of the airways in the lungs due to the tightening of surrounding smooth muscle

**Carboxyhaemoglobin:** resultant of carbon monoxide binding with haemoglobin in the blood, usually as a result of inhalation injury

**Circumferential:** burn injury that goes all the way around a limb or the body

**Compartment syndrome:** a complication that can result when a burn injury causes pressure which affects the blood supply beneath it. Loss of limbs/organ damage can result if the pressure is not released

**Contracture:** a permanent tightening of muscle or tendon

**Cyanosis:** this can occur when tissues in the body are lacking in oxygen supply

**Debridement:** the removal of dead, damaged or infected tissue to promote healing

**De-roof:** the process of cutting away the dead tissue part of a blister

**Dyspnoea:** difficulty in breathing

**Epithelialise:** the process of regrowth of the epithelium layer of skin

**Eschar:** the dead skin that results from burn injury

**Escharotomy:** Surgical knife or electrocautery incisions of the burn eschar (damaged skin surface) to allow for better peripheral perfusion and if performed on the chest, better ventilation.[9] This does not affect the underlying fascia.

**Exudate:** a fluid that filters from the capillary system to the wound surface. It contains a mixture of water, plasma solutes, white blood cells and platelets

**Fasciotomy:** A deep surgical incision (usually of limbs) right into the fascia to relieve tension or pressure that had caused circulatory compromise to an area of tissue or muscle.[10]Glasgow Coma Score (GCS): a neurological scale that determines a person's level of consciousness

**Hypoglycaemia:** low blood sugar

**Hypoperfusion:** low oxygen and nutrient supply to the tissues/organs

**Hypotension:** low blood pressure

**Hypothermia:** low temperature (<36°C)

**Hypovolaemia:** low blood volume and in particular low plasma volume in the blood

**Hypoxia:** a shortage of oxygen in the body

**Oedema:** abnormal accumulation of fluid in the body causing swelling. Results from injury or disease

**Split skin graft:** a slicing of epidermis and dermis skin that is used to replace skin loss in another area of the body. It can be different thicknesses

**Stridor:** noisy breathing. It can be inspiratory or expiratory depending on the cause

**Tachypnoea:** fast breathing

**Vasoconstriction:** a narrowing of the blood vessels as a result of muscle tightening in order to restrict or slow down the flow of blood. Blood pressure increases

**Vasodilation:** a widening of the blood vessels as a result of muscle relaxation in order to increase the flow of blood. Blood pressure drops

# PATHOPHYSIOLOGY OF A BURN INJURY

Knowledge of the pathophysiology of a burn wound provides the rationale for why certain treatment modalities are necessary. Reading Chapter 19 on the anatomy and physiology of skin and wound healing is a good starting point.

Thermal injury initiates both a local and a systemic response, and the main difference between a burn wound and any other wound is its dynamic nature. The local response to the body can best be described by the three zones of a burn wound as presented by Jackson.[4] This classification can enable better understanding of why particular interventions are necessary (Table 27.1, page 466).

> **KEY POINTS**
>
> These three zones described by Jackson are three dimensional: they apply to the surface of the skin (as in the area that is visible), but also below the skin surface (what is not visible). Any loss of tissue in the zone of stasis may make the wound deepen as well as widen.

The systemic response to burn injury is much more complex and to a greater extent applies to larger burns. There are four main systemic changes and these are cardiovascular, respiratory, metabolic and immunological in nature (Table 27.2, page 466).

## FIRST AID

The aim of first aid after burn injury is to stop the burning process by cooling the burn, to remove (if possible) the causative agent, and to provide pain relief.[6] Correct first aid can have an effect on the level of injury sustained, so it is important to get it right. As with any basic life support and first aid training it is important to start with the SAFE approach[1] (Table 27.3, page 466), and then proceed to managing the burn injury (Table 27.4, page 467).

> **KEY POINTS**
>
> - Do not use ice to cool the burn, as this causes vasoconstriction and may increase tissue injury.
> - Do not apply any creams or ointments to the burn.
> - Do not intentionally burst any blisters.
> - Do not remove clothing or substances that are stuck to the burn.
> - Do not 'wrap' the Clingfilm around the wound: apply it in layers, to prevent constrictions.

## ASSESSMENT

The assessment of a burn must always be considered as a structured approach as per the *Advanced Paediatric Life Support* guidelines of airway, breathing, circulation, etc.[1] It is important not to be distracted from this sequential assessment as this may precipitate the exclusion of other major trauma that is more serious than the burn. The diagram in Figure 27.1 (page 466) has been designed to help in this sequential assessment.

> **KEY POINTS**
>
> Always be vigilant to the signs and symptoms of inhalation injury such as:
> - history of flame burns or burns in enclosed space
> - full thickness or deep dermal burns to face, neck and upper torso
> - singed nasal hair
> - carbonaceous sputum or carbon particles in the oropharynx.
>
> Have a low threshold for intubation if the following signs are evident:
> - erythema or swelling of the oropharynx on direct visualisation
> - change in voice with hoarseness or harsh cough
> - stridor, tachypnoea or dyspnoea.

**Table 27.1** Jackson's classification of burn injury[4]

| Zone of coagulation or necrosis | The central, most severely damaged part of the injury. Irreversible tissue loss because the cells are coagulated or necrotic. Tissue in this area will require debridement. The necrotic area affected can be wide, i.e. cover a large area of the body, but it can also be deep, i.e.: affect both epidermal and dermal layers of skin |
|---|---|
| Zone of stasis | This area surrounds the central area of coagulation. It is an area of decreased tissue perfusion (vasoconstriction). Cells in this area are injured but recoverable. The main aim of burns resuscitation is to increase tissue perfusion in this area and thus prevent the worsening progression of the injury. Other insults such as prolonged hypotension, infection or oedema can convert this zone of stasis to a zone of coagulation from where there is no recovery |
| Zone of hyperaemia | The outermost area of the burn where tissue perfusion is increased. This occurs as part of the inflammatory response to injury and is the body's way of trying to get rid of excess heat. It presents as erythema and should recover unless there is severe sepsis or prolonged hypoperfusion |

**Table 27.2** Systemic response to burn injury

| System affected | Effect after burn injury |
|---|---|
| Cardiovascular | An initial vasoconstriction is soon reversed by inflammatory mediators to vasodilation and an increased capillary permeability (leakage of fluid, intravascular proteins and neutrophils into the tissue spaces)[4] which occurs in both the injured and non-injured areas of the body. Combined with fluid losses from the burn wound this can lead to systemic hypotension and end organ hypoperfusion with a high risk of hypovolaemic shock if treatment is delayed |
| Respiratory | Inflammatory mediators cause bronchoconstriction. With this and oedema, the child's airway can easily be compromised |
| Metabolic | The basal metabolic rate increases significantly, along with an enhanced production of glucose from non-sugar carbon substrates, insulin resistance and increased protein break down. There is also a loss in the thermoregulatory function of the damaged skin and if the child is too hot or too cold, this can have an added effect on the metabolic rate. Body heat can be lost very quickly in the more severe injuries[5] |
| Immune | The exact reasons are unknown, but the immune response is depressed which affects both humeral and cellular lines of defence |

**Table 27.3** The SAFE approach

**S**hout or call for help

**A**ssess the scene for dangers to rescuer or patient

**F**ree the area around the patient from danger

**E**valuate the casualty

**Table 27.4** Managing the burn injury

| Aim | Action |
|---|---|
| To stop the burning process | Remove the heat source: douse flames, remove from hot liquid, disconnect from electricity |
| | Cool the burn: immediately get the wound under tepid, clean, running water (if possible) as this reduces the heat, removes noxious agents and provides pain relief |
| | Continue this cooling process for 20 minutes if tolerated |
| | Always be aware that cooling large areas can cause hypothermia (so continue to observe the child)[6] |
| | Chemical burns require copious water irrigation in order to bring the skin pH back to normal |
| | Remove any jewellery or constrictions around the burn |
| To provide pain relief | Cooling the burn |
| | Covering burn with simple dressing, e.g. Clingfilm |
| | Administer pain relief[7] |
| To prevent shock | After the cooling process keep the patient warm and reassure[7] |

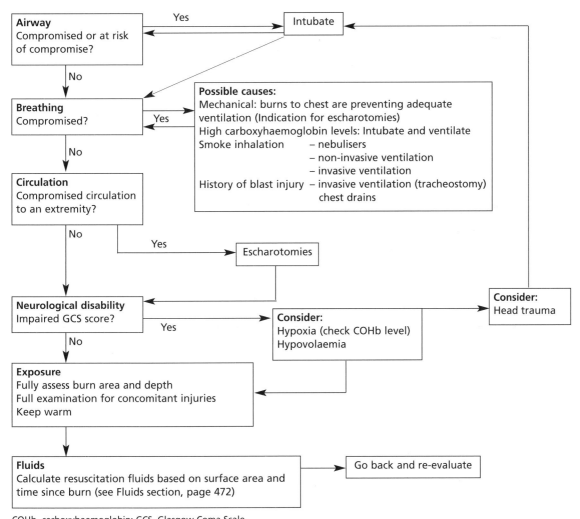

COHb, carboxyhaemoglobin; GCS, Glasgow Coma Scale.

**Figure 27.1** Sequential assessment of a burn

## PROCEDURE: Assessing the child with a burn injury[8]

| Look for | Procedure guidelines | Evidence-based rationale |
|---|---|---|
| **1 Airway**<br>Mouth/nostril burns or sooting<br>Hoarse voice<br><br>Uvula oedema<br>Circumferential burns to neck<br>Risk of cervical injury<br>Risk of inhalation injury | If in doubt enlist senior help and consider endotracheal intubation with an uncut tube<br><br>Protect cervical spine unless confirmed there is no injury<br>Anticipate the burn and surrounding area to become oedematous.<br><br>If facial burns present have a low threshold for intubation | To ensure airway is clear and there is no compromise |
| **2 Breathing**<br>Dyspnoea, stridor<br>Is chest expansion full?<br><br>Is there a history of inhalation injury?<br><br>Is there a history of blast injury?<br>Is there a history of penetrating injury?<br><br>Take note of circumferential chest wounds<br>Lungfield crackles or wheezes<br>Cyanosis or low oxygen saturations<br>High COHb (carboxyhaemoglobin) levels will cause false $SaO_2$ readings | Give 100% oxygen via face mask with reservoir bag<br>Escharotomies may be indicated if there is a mechanical restriction of breathing by the burn injury[7]<br>Inhalation injuries may need a period of ventilation to allow adequate oxygenation and regular lung toileting<br><br>Obtain blood gas | To ensure there is no compromise to breathing<br><br><br><br><br><br>Blood gas will ascertain COHb levels |
| **3 Circulation**<br>Monitor heart rate, blood pressure, capillary refill time and temperature<br>Take note of circumferential wounds to limbs and check peripheral pulses<br>History of electrical injury?<br>Consider haemorrhage<br>Look for hypothermia<br><br>Urine output | Obtain two large peripheral or intra-osseous lines.<br>Take bloods<br><br><br><br>Fluid resuscitation (see fluids section) only if 10% of total body surface area of injury<br>If circumferential wounds are present, neurovascular observations and elevation of limbs are essential<br>Increased burn wound oedema may cause progressive extremity ischaemia or compartment syndrome. In such cases fasciotomies or escharotomies would need to be performed<br>Insert urinary catheter | To ensure there is no circulatory compromise<br>To monitor potential for circulatory compromise<br>To relieve any compromise to peripheral circulation<br>To observe fluid balance |

## PROCEDURE:  Assessing the child with a burn injury[8] (continued)

| | | |
|---|---|---|
| | Hypovolaemia is not a normal initial response to burn injury unless there has been a delayed presentation, cardiogenic dysfunction or a source of blood loss from a differing cause | |
| **4 Disability**<br>Assess Glasgow Coma Scale (GCS)<br>Are the pupils equal and reactive to light?<br>Assess pain levels<br>Is fluorescein eye examination required? | **Record results**<br>A reduced GCS may indicate that endotracheal intubation is required.<br><br>Give pain relief<br><br>Consider trauma series (C-spine, pelvis and chest X-ray)<br><br>Record results of fluorescein test | A reduced GCS might be due to hypoxia, head trauma or hypovolaemia<br><br>An eye examination may be required to assess corneal damage and visual acuity |
| **5 Exposure** with environmental control | Always keep child warm<br><br>Remove jewellery (ensure all clothing goes with the child to the Burn Unit)<br><br>Use Clingfilm only to cover the wounds or sterile plastic bags to limbs<br><br>Assess the whole body noting all injuries, e.g. bruising/fractures, etc.<br><br>Assess the wound percentage and depth using appropriate assessment tools (see Burn assessment section below) | To prevent hypothermia and reduce progression of the burn injury<br><br>Clingfilm is an easy, non-stick, temporary dressing for the wounds until a more definitive wound management plan has been ascertained<br><br>To rule out or confirm non-accidental injury |
| **6 Fluids** | Use the Parkland formula to calculate fluid requirements based on an estimation of the burn size (see fluids section)<br><br>Keep the child nil by mouth (NBM) until a plan has been ascertained | To prevent hypovolaemia and reduce the progression of the burn injury |
| **7 Glucose** | Check blood sugar and act as indicated | To prevent hypoglycaemia |

## ASSESSING THE EXTENT OF THE BURN INJURY

Burn assessment is a two-fold process. It involves assessing the extent of the burn in terms of its percentage and its depth. There are a variety of methods used to assess the percentage.

The Wallace 'rule of nines' is a well known and simple formula, but it is based on an adult head being 9 per cent of the total body area and has to be adapted for children. It also does not account for the differing surface area variations of a child at different ages (Table 27.5, page 469).

**Table 27.5** Extent of burn injury

| Body part | Adult (%) | Child (%) |
| --- | --- | --- |
| Head | 9 | 18 |
| Each arm | 9 | 9 |
| Anterior torso | 18 | 18 |
| Posterior torso | 18 | 18 |
| Each leg | 18 | 14 |
| Genitals/perineum | 1 | Not counted separately |

Another method is called the '1 per cent' rule or 'rule of palms'. This is where the surface area of the child's palm including the fingers is considered to be 1 per cent. Again, a crude method, and there is evidence to suggest that a more accurate figure for a child's palm is in fact 0.5 per cent. The most accurate tool for assessing percentage burn in children is the

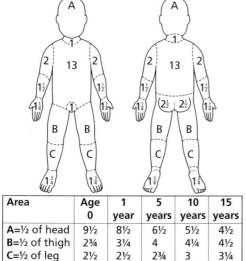

| Area | Age 0 | 1 year | 5 years | 10 years | 15 years |
| --- | --- | --- | --- | --- | --- |
| A=½ of head | 9½ | 8½ | 6½ | 5½ | 4½ |
| B=½ of thigh | 2¾ | 3¼ | 4 | 4¼ | 4½ |
| C=½ of leg | 2½ | 2½ | 2¾ | 3 | 3¼ |

**Figure 27.2** Body surface area chart, adapted from the Lund and Browder model

Lund and Browder chart[7,11] as it takes into account the body surface area changes with age. Figure 27.2 is an adapted version of the chart.

The area of simple erythema (zone of hyperaemia) is not counted in the overall percentage burn and it is a very important skill to be able to distinguish between what is simple erythema and actual burn. Always seek expert advice with burn assessment.

The second part of the assessment process is calculating the burn injury depth. This is a much more difficult process due to the dynamic nature of burn injury. This means that what is assessed on day 1 is not necessarily the same on days 2 or 3. Burns are generally classified into two groups by the amount of skin loss. A partial thickness burn is one where not all layers of skin have been affected whereas a full thickness burn involves all the layers and the subcutaneous tissue.[12] Partial thickness burns can be further divided into superficial, superficial dermal and deep dermal (Table 27.6).

There are a number of ways in which the depth of a burn can be ascertained (Table 27.7, page 471). It can be assumed that by their nature, a flame burn is likely to produce a deeper burn than a scald, and a contact burn might also be deep, depending on the length of time the heat source was in contact with the skin. However, assumptions aside, it is necessary to obtain a full account of the cause and

**Table 27.6** Subdivisions of partial thickness burns

| | |
| --- | --- |
| Superficial | The epidermis is effected but not the dermis. It is often called an epidermal burn. It presents as a reddening of the skin of which sunburn is a good example[13] |
| Superficial dermal | The burn extends through the epidermis into the upper layers of the dermis and is associated with blistering as serous exudate is released from the damaged capillary network |
| Deep dermal | The burn extends through the epidermis into the deeper layers of the dermis but not through the entire dermis |

**Table 27.7** Ascertaining the depth of a burn

|  | Superficial | Superficial dermal | Deep dermal | Full thickness |
|---|---|---|---|---|
| Sensation | Painful | Painful | Dull | None |
| Appearance | Red, glistening | Dry, whiter | Cherry red | Dry, white, leathery |
| Blanching to pressure | Yes, brisk return | Yes, slow return | No | No |

mechanism of injury alongside the wound assessment in order to gather a more accurate picture of the depth of injury.

Most burns, however, are a mixture of depths. Assessment of depth is important for planning appropriate treatment options. More superficial burns tend to heal naturally with appropriate dressings, whereas deeper burns will take a long time to heal and are likely to need surgical intervention. It is always worth seeking advice from your nearest burn unit as to what action to take.

It is also very important to assess the pattern of burn injury. There are specific descriptors for burn injuries that are likely to have been caused by deliberate harm rather than accidental injury. Table 27.8 below gives a summary.

While it is important to be aware of the above, it is also inappropriate to make false judgements. Always seek the advice of more senior personnel if any suspicions are raised.

**KEY POINTS**

Be aware of the indicators that might suggest a non-accidental injury has occurred and activate safe-guarding children procedures where necessary:

- Evasive or changing history
- Delayed presentation
- No explanation or a implausible mechanism given for the burn
- Inconsistency between age of the burn and age given by the history
- History not matching developmental ability of the child
- Inadequate supervision, such as child left in the care of inappropriate person (older sibling)
- Lack of guilt about the incident
- Lack of concern about treatment or prognosis

**Table 27.8** Injury pattern of non-accidental burns

Obvious pattern from cigarettes, lighters, irons

Burns to soles, palms, genitalia, buttocks, perineum

Symmetrical burns of uniform depth

No splash marks in a scald injury. A child falling into a bath will splash; one that is placed may not

Restraint injuries on upper limbs

Is there sparing of flexion creases, i.e. was the child in fetal position (position of protection) when burnt? Does this correlate to a 'tide line' of scald, i.e. if child is put into a fetal position, do the burns line up?

'Doughnut' sign, an area of spared skin surrounded by scald. If a child is forcibly held down in a bath of hot water, the part in contact with the bottom of the bath will not burn, but the tissue around will

Other signs of physical abuse: bruises of varied age, poorly kempt, lack of compliance with healthcare (such as no immunisations)

## HISTORY-TAKING

A full an accurate history of the mechanism of injury is as much the responsibility of the nurse as it is the medical team. It should be obtained as part of the history taking sequence and is especially important when there are concerns with child protection. This includes the history of the presenting illness, the child's past history, social history and family history and then a systems review (see Table 27.9, page 472).

**Table 27.9** History-taking

| Presenting/ principal symptom or complaint | History of complaint | Past history | Social history | Family history | Systems review |
|---|---|---|---|---|---|
| Percentage and depth of burn injury detailing any circumferential wounds | Detailed account of when, where and how the injury occurred | Other medical conditions Other injuries/ complaints | Development/ school details Lifestyle: smoker/alcohol Travel/immunisations Living conditions/ social support | Parents/siblings Foster care/ guardianship | Full examination of all systems |

All healthcare personnel have a responsibility for safeguarding children in their care. Always seek advice from your nearest burn unit if there is a high suspicion of non-accidental injury.

Once the assessment process, immediate treatment required and history has been carried out, it is necessary to then decide where the best place is for the continuing care of the child. Burn care, even for the relatively minor injuries (<5 per cent), can be complex, and decisions around where to continue caring for the child should be made after discussion with the nearest specialist burn unit. The National Burn Care Review committee report[3] has produced indicative criteria for referral to a specialist burn unit. These have been summarised in Table 27.10. There may also be other non-burn skin conditions that also require transfer to a specialist burn service. Examples of such are toxic epidermal necrolysis, staphylococcal scalded skin syndrome or purpura fulminans. Such conditions require the same multidisciplinary management as for a burn injury and the treatment

of these children might require the specialist skills of a burns team.

Once the decision to refer and transfer the child has been made in collaboration with the receiving burn service, it is important to make sure it is carried out safely. Table 27.11, page 473 may help in this.

## PRINCIPLES OF MANAGEMENT

The general care of the minor burn involves pain relief, infection control, wound care and follow-up. Where the burn injury involves special areas such as the face, hands, feet and perineum its management might require a more involved team approach, so it is important to consider discussing even the minor burns with your nearest burn service, to ascertain whether referral is indicated. A minor burn that is also a deep burn should also be considered for referral, as surgical invention is likely to be indicated. Always regard the term 'minor' burn loosely as there may be a lot of factors to consider, even for the smaller burn.

**Table 27.10** Indications for referral

Any burn exceeding 5% of the total body surface area (TBSA)

Any small (<1%), full thickness burns which might benefit from early excision and grafting

Burns or scalds to functionally important areas, such as the face, hands, feet, perineum, joints or flexor surfaces

Children with other medical conditions, such as diabetes or epilepsy

If there is any suspicion that the injury is non-accidental

Burns with associated injuries, such as smoke or gas inhalation or electric shock

Children whose wounds show any sign of infection or is unwell and has a burn wound

Any wound that is circumferential

Any wound that is slow to heal or has got worse

**Table 27.11** Transferring patients

| Issues to consider when transferring patients | Rationale |
|---|---|
| Is the transfer urgent? | Urgent transfers are indicated when immediate specialist treatment is indicated |
| Transportation mode in relation to burn severity and bed dependency level required. | For minor injuries it may be acceptable for child/family to use their own means of transport |
| Child/family travelling in own transport | For timely, urgent transfers always consider all the available transport options |
| Retrieval team | |
| Ambulance, helicopter, or aeroplane | |
| Airway management | If in any doubt about potential airway compromise as a result of oedema, intubate before transfer[10] after discussion with receiving burn service |
| Venous access | For injuries ≥10%, peripheral access should be obtained before transfer. If however, IV access is difficult, discuss this with receiving burn service. Do not delay transfer to achieve central venous access unless discussed with receiving burn unit |
| Urinary catheter | Do not delay transfer to insert a urinary catheter unless discussed with receiving burn service |
| Body temperature | Hypothermia is a particular problem during transportation. Observe temperature and ensure the child is warm (>37°C) |

**KEY POINTS**

The insertion of central venous access (including femoral access) must not be taken lightly at it can cause a significant increase in the risk of septicaemia.

**VIGNETTE**

**Problem:** A child presents with a history of possible inhalation injury but shows no immediate signs of airway compromise. After a few minutes, however, the child shows noticeable dyspnoea.

**Discussion:** This is not uncommon as the inflammatory response can be delayed. Always think and respond to the structured assessment: ABC (airway, breathing, circulation) and keep re-evaluating.

Burn injuries of ≥10 per cent total body surface area (or ≥5 per cent in infants), irrespective of their depth, require formal fluid resuscitation. This is the most important part of the early management of the burn, and should take precedence as soon as possible after the percentage burn has been assessed.

## FLUID MANAGEMENT

Fluid is lost from the wound immediately after injury. The heat damage to the capillaries causes increased permeability, leading to a loss of water, sodium, and, later, plasma proteins (especially albumin) from the intravascular circulation into the interstitial space. Oedema occurs in both burned and non-burned tissue[8] as a combined result of wound-released mediators and hypoproteinaemia, which is why it is so important in facial burns to anticipate potential airway compromise. Children, unlike adults, have, among other things, a large surface area-to-volume ratio and a higher percentage of extracellular fluid,[14] which means they are at increased risk of losing more fluid.

The aim of fluid replacement is to replace deficits, prevent hypovolaemic shock and maintain adequate tissue perfusion; however, there is no single formula that will accurately meet the fluid

**Table 27.12** Parkland formula for fluid resuscitation

| |
|---|
| **Accurate weight of child $\times$ % TBSA burn $\times$ 2 – 4 (factor to be agreed by nearest burns unit) of Hartmann's solution** |
| Half the total to be administered over 8 hours from the time of injury |
| Second half of the total to be administered over the next 16 hours |

volume requirement of the child[9] and each case requires careful management to prevent secondary complications. The most widely accepted formula is the Parkland formula for calculating resuscitation fluids,[9] and although there may be slight modifications of the amount to be given, it is generally accepted that Hartmann's solution is the fluid type used[8] (Table 27.12). It is advisable that early contact with your nearest burns service is made in order to discuss appropriate fluid management of the child prior to transfer. Unfortunately, inaccuracies in burn size estimation and the child's weight can precipitate inaccurate fluid resuscitation and can therefore contribute to further complications.

The resuscitation fluid should be coupled with maintenance fluids using a 0.45 per cent normal saline and 5 per cent glucose fluid mixture in order to help prevent hypoglycaemia[8] and hyponatraemia, although it is worth discussing this first with the burn service as local guidelines may differ slightly.

Throughout fluid resuscitation and for some time after, it is vitally important to maintain an accurate fluid balance. The child's homeostatic balance can be disrupted for a long time afterwards and, in order to prevent any permanent organ failure, close observation of the child's input/output fluid and electrolyte levels[14] (in particular serum sodium) are essential. Invasive monitoring such as central venous pressure and arterial blood pressure monitoring might be indicated to assert accuracy along with regular observation of the child's vital signs.

## THE MULTIFACETED NATURE OF BURN INJURY

The management of a burn injury requires a whole-team approach. Even relatively minor injuries can have an effect on metabolism and movement and so may require dietetic and physiotherapy input. The more severe the injury, the more the body's systems are affected. The children's burns multidisciplinary team comprises surgeons, paediatricians, nurses, pain specialists, dieticians, physiotherapists, occupational therapists, clinical psychologists, play and school teams, anaesthetists and intensivists (if required). Other input from pharmacists and microbiologists are often called upon as and when needed. The child/family will see many professionals when the child is an inpatient and an outpatient, and treatment/care is often coordinated with all the relevant disciplines involved.

Effective pain control is vital for any child with a burn injury. Immediately after the burn injury, the pain experienced is due to the stimulation of skin nociceptors (pain-sensing nerves). In deep burns these might be completely destroyed, but in those that remain intact, pain will be triggered until the wound is healed. Any nerves that are regenerating will also be painful. Chemical mediators released during the inflammatory response to the injury will sensitise active nociceptors. This will make the wound very sensitive to stimuli such as touch, rubbing, debridement as well as antiseptics or other topical agents. The analgesic requirements for the child depends as much on the child as it does on the size of the burn and at what phase the injury is in: emergency phase, acute phase or rehabilitation phase.[10] All types of pain must be considered within each phase of injury, and these include background, procedural and breakthrough.[15] The best way to address pain is through having a care plan that is tailored to the individual and which includes both pharmacologic and non-pharmacologic approaches,[15] and uses appropriate assessment tools such as visual analogue scales.[16]

Background pain is pain at rest: dull, continuous and of a lower intensity. If not treated with regular analgesia it will lead to exacerbated anxiety and pain experienced during procedures. For moderate to large burns, opioid medication as an infusion or patient-controlled analgesia is the most widely recommended. For smaller burns, simple analgesia such as paracetamol and ibuprofen will suffice.

Procedural pain relief must be considered in addition to the resting analgesic requirement. For smaller burns, oral morphine or an equivalent along with a mild sedative such as midazolam are perfectly acceptable alongside oral paracetamol and ibuprofen in order achieve successful dressing changes as well as aid physiotherapy interventions. Non-pharmacological methods of pain management with relaxation techniques and distraction therapy must not be undervalued. The play specialist can have a vital role in procedural pain relief. The involvement of the pain team can also be very useful in considering alternative analgesic options. Also, the psychologist can work with the child/family to help prepare them and find ways of coping with all painful procedures. For older children, nitrous oxide (Entonox) can help to take away the fear and anticipatory pain of dressing changes. For larger burns it may be necessary in the initial phases of recovery to consider a general anaesthetic for dressing changes.

Breakthrough pain is defined as that which increases above baseline level for reasons not related to procedures. This is exacerbated by anxiety and can affect everyday activities such as turning in bed or being able to eat/drink independently for example.

Anxiety, depression and pain are interrelated in patients with burns. It is well known that anxiety increases the pain experience and with lots of painful procedures happening on a daily basis, it is important to acknowledge the extent to which this affects the child/family. The psychologist is a useful resource in this respect and can help the child/family work through their anxieties.

During the wound-healing process, pruritis (itching) can become a major problem due to the regrowth of the nerves. Antihistamine medication such as chlorphenamine can help with this, and if the wound is healed creaming and massaging the new skin with aqueous cream can also lessen the itchy sensation. If the antihistamine alone is ineffective, gabapentin can be prescribed. Given regularly this is an effective treatment for neuropathic pain and itching.[17]

To help ensure a good outcome for the child, enabling the child to return home and to fulfil their full potential, it is important the rehabilitation begins on admission. This means involving the *physiotherapists* and *occupational therapists* at an early stage whereby appropriate positioning, splinting and exercise all contribute to a much better functional outcome. Positioning and splinting protects wounds and joints, reduces oedema, achieves anatomical positioning and can reduce scar contracture. Exercising, both passive and active, increases circulation, reduces oedema and contractures and preserves motor function. It is important that exercising is done regularly, several times a day, as this helps rebuild strength, endurance and prevents/minimises contracture formation. If left, contractures will develop quickly and further surgery will be needed to release them to aid better function.

Early *dietetic* input is vital to support the nutritional needs of the burn-injured child and prevent weight loss. The metabolic rate increases after burn injury, whereby resting energy expenditure and cardiac output is increased in proportion to the size of the injury. This is coupled by an enhanced production of glucose from non-sugar carbon substrates, insulin resistance and increased protein breakdown. In minor injuries this effect is not so apparent and normal dietary intake is all that is required, although observation of intake should take place. In the larger burns where fluid resuscitation is required, this can have major implications for the care of the child and can delay wound healing if not appropriately managed. Investigations into finding a definitive way of reducing or eliminating this hypermetabolic response have been attempted, but more research is needed. In order to reduce the amount of protein breakdown and supplement the calorific requirements that the child needs, nasogastric feeding is essential and may be required even after the wounds have healed. There is a natural tendency for loss of appetite to occur, but if the child can tolerate the high-calorie and high-protein food requirements then this is encouraged. Regular weight and height checks are needed to keep track of any weight loss and the child's body mass index (BMI). There may also be a need to observe and respond to vitamin and mineral deficits, which can have a direct effect on wound healing.[18]

The *psychological* effects of burn injury to child and carer must not be taken lightly. In a society where body image is so important, even what appears as the smallest scar can seem like the biggest disfigurement to a child/family. Child and family need to learn to adapt to the change and to re-establish confidence and independence.[12] Long hospital stays, being isolated in a cubicle and sometimes being miles away from home and from supportive family/friends can all add to the problem. The whole multidisciplinary team needs to be aware of this and help them be more prepared for the losses that will occur along with providing the coping mechanisms for child/family for addressing difficult issues in the future. Many burns services have dedicated clinical psychology input to help the child/family cope both during their hospital stay and beyond. The hospital play/school teams can also be valuable resources in helping children regain some normality in their daily life while in the recovery phase. Children/families must be informed of what help/support is available both while they are in a hospital environment and also when discharged home.

Any child with ongoing needs on discharge must be referred to the relevant community services to ensure continued monitoring, support and care. Some burn services have Outreach teams attached to them and they are best placed to coordinate the care required in the community.

# WOUND CARE: SURGICAL/ NON-SURGICAL

As previously mentioned in the assessment section, treatment options are often decided once assessment of the extent (as a percentage) and the depth of injury has been ascertained. Early surgery for severe injuries to remove the dead eschar and prevent secondary complications is now widely accepted.[19]

A *deep dermal* or *full thickness burn* usually requires early surgical intervention under general anaesthesia. Early surgery to remove the burn eschar (dead tissue) and then cover with a skin graft can happen within the first 2 weeks after injury. This split skin graft is taken from unburned skin and applied to the wound (known as an autograft). The transferred skin is either glued, stapled or sutured in place. Often parents/carers ask if they can donate their own skin instead, but it is not the same, as the child's body would reject it as a 'foreign body'. The newly grafted wound is then covered first with a non-adherent layer such as a silicone mesh dressing, an absorbent gauze layer

and finally secured with childproof bandaging and/or adhesive tape. It may be necessary to keep the child on bed rest or immobilise the grafted area by splinting it at least until the first dressing change in order to allow the new skin the best possible chance of adhering to the wound bed. This first dressing change after grafting can be anything from 3 to 5 days after which the graft is assessed for 'skin take'. Further periodic dressing changes are required to protect the graft from bacterial invasion, friction and interfering fingers until the wound has completely healed.

*Care of the skin graft* continues even after it has healed as the new graft does not produce sufficient natural oil to lubricate the skin. When fully healed, a non-perfumed, non-lanolin-based moisturising cream should be massaged into the graft at least three times a day, as it often gets very dry and can become very itchy for the child. The process of firm, slow massaging not only replaces the skin oils but is therapeutic in encouraging the scar to stretch, stay soft and supple, and helps to control itching. Further scar management treatment may be necessary, such as silicone gel and pressure garments to control the scar tissue during the maturation phase, when there is a tendency for it to become raised and lumpy (hypertrophic scarring). This treatment may need to be continued for some time, as it can take up to 2 years for the burn scar to mature, i.e. become pale in colour, soft and supple. Sun care advice must be given to the child/family to ensure that the immature scar is not permanently damaged. The appropriate advice is to protect the area for at least two summers if not three, with high-factor sun block and/or clothing.

The *donor* wound (where the split skin graft is taken from) is a superficial wound that heals within 10–14 days. The most common choice of donor area is the thigh or buttock, but in the larger burns other sites will also be used. Often the donor site is described as a big 'graze', and can be more painful for the child than the grafted wound so regular analgesia is needed. This donor site wound is dressed in theatre, usually with a calcium alginate dressing and gauze padding. The dressing is left in situ for a minimum of 10 days to allow the wound to fully re-epithelialise. It is therefore essential that the dressing is secured to prevent slipping, especially for thigh dressings. Additional padding can be added to the outer dressing if bleeding occurs, which is common in the first 48 hours. When healed, the donor area will look red initially but should gradually fade over several months, during which time it will require massaging with a moisturising cream in a similar way to the grafted wound.

*Partial thickness burns* should be thoroughly cleaned with warm normal saline or with tap water in the form of a bath/shower in order to remove contaminants and any devitalised tissue, such as loose blistered skin. This helps to avoid prolonging the inflammatory stage of healing and to reduce the risk of wound infection. Cleansing practices and the use of antiseptics have been the subject of study and debate for many years and continues to be so. It is important not to be guided by ritualistic practices, and make rationale-based treatment decisions after accurate assessment of the wound's age and stage of healing.

In some units it is routine to consider a general anaesthetic to facilitate the initial cleansing procedure when the depth of injury can also be more accurately assessed and, if required, surgical debridement of the wound bed can take place. Specialised dressings that promote re-epithelialisation, reduce pain and wound exudates, such as Biobrane, Aquacel or Veloderm, may be applied if the depth of injury is less than full thickness. If a general anaesthetic is not appropriate then adequate pain relief is essential before attempting wound cleansing and debridement.

The treatment of blisters remains a subject for debate and has been for many years. Some evidence suggests that blisters should be completely de-roofed and removed to assist the assessment of burn depth, to prevent the conversion of a superficial wound to a deeper one and to prevent restriction of movement if the burn affects a joint. Other evidence suggests that a blister which is not tense or likely to rupture should be left intact, as it forms a biological dressing that will assist the healing process and even help prevent infection. This is particularly pertinent when treating burns to the palms of hands and plantar aspect of feet. The epithelium to these areas is much thicker than elsewhere and most burns will heal without the need for skin grafting. Advocates of leaving the blisters intact, suggest that only minimum dressings are required in order to allow the child a full range of movement. Applying 'childproof' dressings that allow a full range of movement is difficult, whereas

an intact blister that is unlikely to rupture can be left with minimum protective dressings. Always remember that if the blister has been removed, then it will be much more painful for the child.

An appropriate *dressing* should be applied that provides the ideal wound environment. There are many varied dressings now available and it is often difficult for nurses to make evidence-based choices regarding the right dressing to use. Burn wounds can often be difficult to dress because of their non-uniformity in shape or depth, and children can add another challenging dimension to the procedure. The following factors to consider are

- coping with high levels of wound exudates;
- a tendency for dressings to stick to the wound surface;
- an irregular distribution of epithelial/dermal damage;
- wounds covering a large body surface with high risk of infection;
- pain;
- the need to apply a childproof dressing while allowing a full range of movement to assist physiotherapy;
- multiple separate wound areas and/or areas of the body where dressing choices are challenged, such as the scalp, face, ears, neck and perineum.

A moist wound environment is beneficial to wound healing, but the high levels of exudate produced in the inflammatory phase can cause maceration and 'strike through', increasing the risk of infection. Therefore the dressing must be sufficiently absorbent and changed at least every 48 hours until the level of exudate settles. The periods between dressing changes can then be increased with emphasis on minimum changes so not to disturb re-epithelialisation.

The irregular distribution and size of the wound can also dictate the dressing of choice. A non-adherent wound contact layer that will minimise trauma to the wound or pain on removal, such as a silicone mesh, can be used with layers of absorbent gauze. The thickness of the absorbent layer can be adjusted according to the level of exudate after 4 or 5 days. As discussed previously, the dressing should be secured with bandage or adhesive tape allowing for a full range of movement. A thin hydrocolloid dressing can be used when the exudate level is much less. This dressing is ideal as it can be cut to size, is comfortable to wear, is shower proof and is not restrictive and therefore supports early mobilisation and physiotherapy. It is also recommended for burns to hands and when there are small unevenly distributed wounds left to heal. Table 27.13 will help with deciding on the suitability of dressings.

Burns to *hands/feet* can become very swollen as a direct result of the inflammatory response to thermal injury. For short-term use, sterile polythene bags with an antibacterial cream may be used. The bags keep the wounds moist, allow observation of the swelling and neurovascular observation of the injured limb, and also enable physiotherapy. However, this treatment should be used with caution in young children due to the risk of suffocation. The affected limb must be elevated with either pillows or slings to help reduce swelling.

*Facial* burns can be left exposed and managed by twice daily cleansing with normal saline and application of Vaseline or liquid paraffin several times a day to keep the wound surface moist. As the wounds start to re-epithelialise, Vaseline can be replaced with a moisturising cream. The swelling effect (oedema) of a burn injury is more apparent with facial burns especially around the peri-orbital area, which usually reaches its peak at 48 hours after injury. Sitting more upright against several pillows can help to reduce the oedema to the face. Facial burns can also be managed with dressings and these include Aquacel and Biobrane.

The initial assessment to determine the depth of injury is only a guide, and some wounds will prove with time to be deeper than first thought. A superficial burn will heal within 7–12 days. At 14 days post injury any unhealed areas greater than 2.5 cm$^2$ that have no islands of epithelium will be assessed for skin grafting.

Undertaking *dressing changes* and gaining the cooperation of a fearful child can be difficult. Each dressing change requires careful planning and employs the following measures:

- xareful reassurance and explanation appropriate to the child's age and level of understanding prior to and during the dressing change;
- ensuring adequate, prior pain relief is given for the outpatient as well as the inpatient;
- using play and distraction therapy, helping to make the experience as least stressful as possible for the patient and parent/carer;
- always praising and rewarding at the end of the procedure.

**KEY POINTS**

- All burn and scald injuries will require massaging with a moisturising cream until the affected epithelium ceases to be dry and flaky.
- A deeper burn that has taken longer than 2 weeks to heal may develop areas of hypertrophic scarring. In this case additional scar management therapy is required in the form of silicone products and/or pressure garments.
- All wounds, including donor wounds must be protected from the sun with a high factor sun cream (minimum SPF 30) and clothing for the following 2 or 3 summers. Without protection these areas will burn because of lack of melanocytes within the scar tissue.[13]

**Table 27.13** Types of dressings

| Dressing type | Dressing name | Suitability of use |
|---|---|---|
| Hydrocolloid | Duoderm | Low exudate wounds |
| | | All depths |
| | Aquacel | Low-medium exudate wounds |
| | | Superficial: mid-dermal wounds |
| Calcium alginate | Sorbsan | Medium: High exudate wounds |
| | Kaltostat | Superficial: mid-dermal wounds |
| Silicone mesh | Mepitel | All wounds |
| | Urgotul | All depths |
| Biosynthetic dressings | Biobrane | Superficial: mid dermal wounds |
| Paraffin gauze | Jelonet | All wound types |

## PREVENTION OF INFECTION AND OTHER ASSOCIATED COMPLICATIONS

Timely, appropriate management of the burn-injured child should help to reduce the risks of secondary complications. Such complications include fluid overload, which can then result in pulmonary oedema, right heart failure, abdominal deep muscle compartment syndromes and cerebral oedema.[10] Other complications include hypothermia and sepsis. In order to prevent hypothermia, the burn-injured child should be nursed at higher than 'normal' temperatures in ambient temperatures of 30–33°C. This will help to reduce the child's energy demands and control heat loss.[10] In view of this, for the more severe burns, the child's temperature would sit at between 37 and 38°C and this would still be within an acceptable/normal range. It is suggested that sepsis is caused by a combination of factors: a colonisation of bacteria on the wound bed as well as deep into the underlying tissues, the child's suppressed immunity and the translocation of bacteria and their by-products from the gut.

Normal skin hosts a small selection of bacterial flora of mainly diphtheroids and *Staphylococcus epidermidis*, and occasionally *Staphylococcus aureus*.[10] The burn injury actually sterilises the area affected initially, but is then subsequently dominated by *S. aureus*. The important part of *controlling wound infection* is to try to reduce the build up of bacteria to a point of critical colonisation and eventually infection. Cleansing the wound with topical antimicrobial agents can help to control bacterial growth, along with early wound excision.[10] However, burn injury causes immunosuppression, so children are much more susceptible to developing infections. The subject of prophylactic antibiotics is much debated, and there are both valid arguments for and against. Some reports state that antibiotics can increase bacterial resistance and can actually precipitate fungal infections; however, other work in favour of antibiotics suggests that it can reduce incidences of *toxic shock syndrome (TSS)*.

TSS is an added complication of burn injury that results from toxin-producing (TSST-1) strains of *S. aureus* and is also a subject of much debate in the burn care literature. The reason being is that accurate diagnosis of it is complex and there is no universally agreed management of it. Young children (particularly 6 months to 3 years) are considered to be more susceptible to it as they do not have the levels of antibodies required to fight the toxins until the age of about 10 years. There is a range of symptoms that have been collated as indicative of TSS, and these include a high temperature (>39°C), widespread macular rash, sickness and/or diarrhoea, tachycardia, irritability, confusion and/or lethargy.[20] If any of these symptoms are not noted or acted upon early, the child is at a high risk of organ failure and mortality. A specific management criteria has been suggested:

- resuscitation and stabilisation in a high-dependency area;
- inspection and cleaning of the burn wound;
- treatment with anti-staphylococcal (and streptococcal) antibiotics;
- provision of passive immunity against TSST-1 with fresh frozen plasma or intravenous immunoglobulin.[20]

If a child presents with a burn wound and is unwell, always consider TSS. The wound itself can be small and appear clean (i.e. uninfected). Discussion with your nearest burn service as the most suitable course of management is vital.

## REHABILITATION AND AFTER-BURN CARE

To ensure the best outcome for the child following a burn injury it is vital to begin discharge planning and rehabilitation on admission. The aim of rehabilitation is to enable the child to return to as normal a life as possible and be able to reach their full potential. It is expected that there may be a regression in age-appropriate development in the younger age group, but this can soon be overcome with the right intervention and support. For older children, the challenge is much greater, but once again, with the right support, the child should be able grow to lead a happy and fulfilling life.

Following a burn injury children may be left with permanent scarring, and or suffer from nightmares, sleep problems, behavioural problems and reduced appetite. They may have an altered body image and have problems accepting how they look, which has been described as having a social difficulty. The parents/carers may also be suffering from feelings of guilt and anger for the loss of the child they had before the injury. All these issues, which may be minimal or all-consuming, must be dealt with accordingly. Professional psychological support and counselling may be required and should be sourced at the earliest opportunity. This might be initiated in the burn service, but is likely to need continuation in the community.

Many burn services have burn support groups and clubs that are affiliated to them. It has been recognised that such groups are needed for the continual psychosocial support of the child where perhaps community services are lacking.[3] These groups enable the child/family to build up a network of support with other children/families who also have been affected by a burn injury. Often these group gatherings involve child-friendly activities and camps, where the burn-injured child can be free from ridicule and enjoy outdoor pursuits that challenge their character in a supportive way.

Go to the website to find the PowerPoint presentation for this chapter and MCQs to test your knowledge. **www.hodderplus.com/childnursingskills**

## REFERENCES

1   Advanced Life Support Group (2005) *Advanced paediatric life support: the practical approach*, 4th edition. Oxford: BMJ Books.

2   Taylor K (2001) The management of minor burns and scalds in children. *Nursing Standard.* **16**(11): 45–51.

3   National Burn Care Committee Report (2001) *Standards and strategies for burn care*. London: British Association of Plastic Surgeons.

4   Jackson D (1953) The diagnosis of the depth of burning. *British Journal of Surgery* 40: 588–596.

5   Bosworth Bousfield C (ed) (2002) *Burn trauma management & nursing care*. London: Whurr Publishers.

6   Lawrence JC (1987) British Burn Association recommended first aid for burns and scalds. *Burns* **13**(2): 153.

7   Allison K, Porter K (2004) Consensus on the prehospital approach to burns patient management. *Emergency Medicine Journal* 21: 112–114.

8   Yowler C, Fratianne RB (2000) Current status of burn resuscitation. *Burn Care and Management* 27(1): 1–47.

9   Hettiaratchy S, Papini R (2004) ABC of burns. Initial management of a major burn: II – assessment and resuscitation. *British Medical Journal* 329: 101–103.

10  Herndon.D.N. (2007) *Total burn care*, 3rd edition. Philadelphia: Saunders Elesvier.

11  Lund CC, Browder NC (1944) Estimation of areas of burns. *Surgery, Gynaecology and Obstetrics* **79**: 352–358.

12  Papini R (2004) ABC of burns. Management of burn injuries of various depths. *British Medical Journal* 329: 158–160.

13  Richard R, Johnson RM (2002) Managing superficial burn wounds. *Advances in Skin and Wound Care* 15(5): 246–247.

14  Glasper A, Richardson J (eds) (2006) *A textbook of children's and young people's nursing*. Churchill Livingstone Elsevier: London

15  Faucher L, Furukawa K (2006) Practice guidelines for the management of burn pain. *Journal of Burn Care & Research* 27: 659–668.

16  Raghavan R, Sharma P, Kumar P (1999) Abacus VAS in burn pain assessment. *The Clinical Journal of Pain* 15(3): 238.

17  Mendham J (2004) Gabapentin for the treatment of itching produced by burns and wound healing in children: a pilot study. *Burns* 30: 851–853.

18  Casey G (1998) The importance of nutrition in wound healing. *Nursing Standard* 13(3): 51–56.

19  Xiao-Wu W, Herndon D N, Spies M (2002) Effects of delayed wound excision and grafting in severely burned children. *Archives in Surgery* 137: 1049–1054.

20  Young A, Thornton K (2007) Toxic shock syndrome in burns: diagnosis and management. *British Medical Journal* 92: 97–100.

## CHAPTER 28

# Transporting and transferring sick children and young people

Jill Thistlethwaite

## LEARNING OUTCOMES

*On completion of the chapter the reader should be able to:*

1. Outline the risk management and legal implications of inter-hospital transport
2. Discuss the importance of a structured approach to assessment and stabilisation of a critically sick child
3. Describe the support required by the specialist transport team
4. Explain the care priorities and their general implementation in the emergency transfer of a critically sick child to another hospital
5. State the special considerations required when transporting a sick child to X-ray, computed tomography or magnetic resonance imaging scan

## CHAPTER OVERVIEW

This chapter will address the process of inter- and intra-hospital transfers, focusing predominantly on the care of the critically sick child within the referral hospital. It will demonstrate how a referral team can safely assess, stabilise and refer a critically sick child to a paediatric intensive care unit (PICU) and how they may best support the visiting specialist transport team (STT). The process of conducting an emergency transfer to a receiving unit will also be discussed as a guide for the referring hospital team (RT), who will at times be required to conduct such transfers. Although the chapter focuses on the child requiring transfer to a PICU, the process described can be followed for the care and transfer of the child requiring high dependency care, which at the time of writing within the UK remains the responsibility of the RT.

## INTER-HOSPITAL TRANSFER

### Why we do it?

The vast majority of children requiring paediatric intensive care (PIC) do not present in a hospital that has the facilities or staff to provide this service and therefore require transfer to an institution able to provide the level of care needed.

### Who should do it?

The transportation of critically ill children cannot be achieved without risk to the child and several studies have highlighted the morbidity associated with this activity.[1,2] Studies, of non-specialist transfer teams originating from referring hospitals, identified life-threatening events during the referral and transfer process, such as failure to provide adequate airway support, inadequate monitoring and failure to record vital signs during the transfer, hypoxia, inadequate fluid resuscitation, absence of or insufficient intravenous (IV) access and the use of inappropriate maintenance fluids. Further studies suggest specialist intensive care transport teams prevent avoidable secondary insults to the patient, such as loss of IV access, accidental extubation, failure of equipment and oxygen supply.[1,3] The STT's experience, specialised clinical skill and familiarity with the transport environment including the equipment used, assist their ability to

## Definitions

**Apgar score:** A system used in the assessment of the newborn[15]

**Ayers T piece:** Manual ventilation system used by anaesthetists, which has an open ended bag, allowing varying levels of positive end expiratory pressure to be delivered to the patient.

**Catheter mount:** Corrugated extension piece which can be attached to end tracheal tubes (ETTs) to facilitate safer positioning of the tube

**Cricothyroidotomy:** Incision made in the cricothyroid membrane in the event of complete airway obstruction. It facilitates oxygen delivery to the lungs temporarily whilst preparing to perform a surgical airway procedure such as a tracheostomy

**Definitive care:** Care specific to the patients individual condition or disorder

**End tracheal tube:** Airway catheter which is inserted into the trachea when a patient requires ventilator support. It also allows the removal of secretions by suction[15]

**End tidal carbon dioxide monitoring:** Sensor positioned on the end of the ETT that measures expired carbon dioxide levels. The presence of carbon dioxide determines the correct position of the ETT. If the ETT is displaced into the oesophagus carbon dioxide will not be detected

**Extubation:** Removal of end tracheal tube

**Erythematous:** Red patches on the skin caused by congestion of capillaries in its lower layers[15]

**Gestation:** The period of development of a foetus from fertilisation to birth. Normally 40 weeks.[15]

**Inotropes:** Drugs affecting the force or energy of muscular contractions in the heart muscle

**Intra–osseous needle:** Needle inserted into a bone facilitating drug infusion into the bone marrow. Most common sites for insertion are the tibia and femoral bone

**Intubation:** Insertion of an ETT into the trachea[15]

**Invasive blood pressure monitoring:** Monitoring of B/P via an arterial line in the patient. This line also facilitates frequent blood sampling from the patient eliminating the need for frequent venepuncture

**Laryngoscope:** Instrument used to view airway and facilitate intubation

**Maculopapular:** A rash consisting of maculae (spot or discoloured area) and papules (pimple or small elevation) on the skin[15]

**Magills forceps:** Angled forceps used in intubation

**Muscle relaxant:** Drug given to facilitate neuromuscular blockade which stops the patient moving

**Petechia:** Small spot due to effusion of blood under the skin[15]

**Pulse oximetry:** Sensor attached to a finger or toes which records oxygen saturation levels in the blood

**Purpura:** A condition characterised by extravasations of blood in the skin and mucous membranes, causing purple spots and patches[15]

**Referring Hospital:** This is usually a District General Hospital, or other medical institution.

**Specialist Transfer Team:** PICU Team specifically trained in, and equipped for, transfer process.

**Tertiary care centre:** A hospital where patients are referred for specialist care

**Urticaria:** An eruption of wheals on the skin which cause great irritation[15]

**Ventilation (Mechanical):** Ventilating the lungs using a ventilator in the case of extreme illness where the patient cannot breath by themselves

**Vital signs:** Heart rate, blood pressure, respiratory rate and other parameters necessary to monitor the patient's condition

---

deal with failing equipment when necessary and is a significant factor in improving outcomes.

In 1995 the Paediatric Intensive Care Society (PICS)[4] followed by the Framework for the future document (1997)[5] recommended that all PICUs should provide a consultant-led transfer service,

with each transfer undertaken by a specialised PICU physician and nurse. It is now commonplace within the UK that children requiring PIC will be transferred by a specialist transport service, most of which are based in the receiving PICUs. There remains, however, situations where an STT is unavailable, or the clinical situation warrants an immediate transfer, such as the child with a traumatic brain injury (TBI) requiring urgent surgical intervention. These are known as time-critical transfers and in these cases it is appropriate for the RT to undertake the transfer. This eliminates the outward journey by the STT, reducing the overall transfer time. In these infrequent situations, RTs must be prepared to undertake transport procedures to ensure optimum and timely treatment is delivered to the child. Where this is necessary, advice should always be sought from the STT on how to stabilise and transfer the patient. The practice of 'scoop and run' is no longer acceptable. In the event that the child requires intubation and ventilation, a physician competent in airway management must accompany the patient, together with a senior nurse competent in advanced paediatric life support.

## What mode of transport should be used?

Most transfers will be carried out by road, using a front-line ambulance carrying emergency equipment such as oxygen, suction and a defibrillator. STTs often have their own vehicles modified to carry all transport equipment with designated storage space. RTs normally use a local front-line ambulance and consequently their equipment has to be stored in the space available. Occasionally STTs have to travel by air. These considerations fall outside the remit of this chapter and therefore will not be discussed.

## When should a child not be transferred?

There are situations where intensive care may be inappropriate for a child; for example, where the child has a life-limiting illness. These situations have often been discussed with the family prior to the onset of acute illness. Any decision made regarding the withholding or withdrawal of care in an acute clinical situation requires great sensitivity and will pose a huge challenge to the healthcare team. Decisions of this nature are always made at consultant level. In the event of brainstem death post TBI it is generally inappropriate to transfer a child into a PICU, as it removes the family from their support networks (family and friends) into an unfamiliar environment, solely for the purpose of discontinuing treatment. The one exception to this

is where consent to organ donation has been given. However, with the advent of organ transplant coordinators support is available to both the RT and family to locally facilitate the harvesting (surgical removal of organs) process. It remains undesirable and often unnecessary to transfer these children in these circumstances.

The inter-hospital transportation of critically sick children poses many risks to both staff and patients. It is essential that careful and thorough preparation is made and adherence to hospital policies is imperative to prevent unnecessary harm to either the patient, or staff.

## Legal considerations and transport

The responsibility for patient care during the referral process is shared between the consultant leading the STT, usually the consultant in charge of the receiving PICU, and the consultant responsible for the patient in the referring hospital, usually the consultant paediatrician. Sole responsibility for the patient is transferred to the STT at the time they leave the referring hospital.

### Responsibility of the referring hospital team

It is the responsibility of the RT to assess and stabilise the critically sick child and all personnel are accountable for the care they deliver. It is imperative that protocols based on best practice and national guidelines are in place, and that personnel presented with critically sick children are suitably trained in the skills required. Most UK hospitals will base their protocols on Advanced Paediatric Life Support (APLS) guidelines and will have a number of personnel who hold the APLS certificate.

### Responsibility of the specialist transport team

The personnel on this team (medical and nursing) must hold the appropriate qualifications and have the necessary experience in paediatric critical care. Clearance from the criminal records bureau (CRB) is also a requirement. This team works at all times during the transfer process under the legal framework of their employing hospital and must follow the guidelines set down by that institution, set within the components of clinical governance. They function as agents of their base hospital. In the case of the independent STT, they work within the legal framework of their host NHS trust.

## PROCEDURE: Risk management and transport

| Procedural steps | Evidence-based rationale |
|---|---|
| **1** *Team*<br>Wherever possible use a specifically trained team of an appropriate size (not too large) to ensure that all members achieve a minimum level of activity to maintain their skills | Evidence suggests that patient outcome is improved if a specially trained team undertakes the transport and if available such a team should be used.[3,6] The STTs have expert clinical skills in the field of paediatric critical care and will have sound knowledge of the transport process and equipment used. They are able to anticipate common problems likely to occur during the transport process, having all drugs and equipment readily at hand and are able to deal effectively with malfunctioning equipment |
| **2** *Equipment: characteristics*<br>All equipment should be, lightweight, compact and should be safely secured in the ambulance to avoid injury to staff or patients during the transfer process | Any loose equipment however light becomes a dangerous missile during acceleration or deceleration in a moving vehicle. Equipment must be robust to prevent damage and be regularly checked and maintained by the biomedical department to ensure it is always in good working order[7] |
| **3** *Equipment: energy supply/capacity*<br>All equipment relying on an energy supply must have a fully charged battery back-up prior to the commencement of any journey. To prolong battery life electric power cables should be used whenever possible | |
| **4** *Equipment: safe storage*<br>During transfer to and from the ambulance, equipment on the stretcher should be secured to a fixed point, such as a drip stand | To prevent injury to the patient/staff or equipment itself. In all cases avoid securing or placing any heavy equipment close to the patient's head |
| **5** *Equipment: supply/availability*<br>It is essential that all transport kits are checked before and after transport by trained personnel | To ensure all necessary items are available and, where appropriate, within their expiry date |
| **6** *Communication*<br>All communication between referring and receiving teams must be documented throughout the whole process, beginning with the initial referral | This ensures that all staff have consistent information about the advice given enabling them to develop a clear picture of the clinical issues related to the patient[7] |
| **7** *Protocols*<br>All teams involved in the process of assessment, stabilisation and transfer of critically sick children must follow the protocols set out by their hospital. These protocols must be in place and readily available when required. District general hospitals (DGHs) may choose to adopt the protocols written by their local PICU. It is good practice for these protocols to be placed in a file or laminated and displayed on the wall in the resuscitation room, where they are at hand when needed. It is now possible in some areas for referral teams to access up-to-date protocols by way of web links to the local PICU transport team | To ensure optimum, standardised care is delivered to all patients[7] |

## PROCEDURE:  Risk management and transport (continued)

| | |
|---|---|
| **8** *Patient monitoring* <br> Patients must be continually monitored during the stabilisation and transfer process. <br> End tidal $CO_2$ and invasive blood pressure monitoring would be considered standard in the ventilated child | This will facilitate accurate assessment and timely treatment promoting patient stabilisation and safety[7] |
| **9** *Critical incident reporting* <br> Owing to the nature of the transport environment, critical incidents are not uncommon. Any adverse incident occurring during the transfer process must be reported according to hospital policy | Transport teams work at all times according to the policies of the hospital that employs them. Policy, protocol and procedure may change as a result of critical incident reports, thereby protecting staff and patients from a repetition of adverse events[7] |
| **10** *Critical incident reporting: feedback forms* <br> Some teams use two-way feedback forms, allowing the RT and STT an opportunity to feed back to each other anything about their conduct and action that could have been improved | This promotes examination of local practice and identifies training needs with the aim of promoting optimum patient care[7] |
| **11** *The use of lights and sirens* <br> If a patient has been stabilised appropriately and the traffic is free flowing, then the use of lights and sirens is inappropriate. The use of lights and sirens should be monitored and only used when absolutely necessary, i.e. to make progress through heavy traffic | Travelling above the speed limit and using exemptions to the law, such as driving through red lights, puts ambulance crews and their passengers at 11 times greater risk of injury than is the case when travelling at a normal speed[7] |
| **12** *Checklists* <br> A comprehensive pre-departure checklist should completed prior to transfer (see Table 28.2, page 496) | To ensure nothing is forgotten, that all essential be procedures are completed prior to transfer, with all necessary equipment, documentation and drugs accompanying the patient |
| **13** *Managed clinical networks/outreach education* <br> Some PICUs offer a service of outreach education to those DGHs who use their service | This aims to provide assessment, recognition and stabilisation skills to those medical and nursing personnel who are the first point of contact for most critically sick children, leading to better understanding between teams and improved patient care[7] |

### Insurance

Insurance policies must adequately cover transport team activities,[8] including air medical transfers if appropriate. Personal membership of the Paediatric Intensive Care Society (PICS) gives personnel additional cover during the transport process.

### Consent for transfer

Written consent is not yet required within the UK for critical care transfer, although the parents/guardian of any child must be kept fully informed of all ongoing care and the intention to transfer a child to another institution must be discussed with them. In the case of a terminally ill child who is nearing the end of their life, the family may refuse transfer on the grounds that they consider intensive care to be inappropriate. The physician responsible for the child's long-term care should be involved at this point to ensure that any treatment decision is made in the best interest of the child and family.

### Patient with a 'do not resuscitate' order

These patients are at times successfully resuscitated because a team is not aware of the 'do not resuscitate' DNR order when the child presents in their department. Transfer to a PICU is then required as withdrawal of care after successful

## PROCEDURE: Monitoring the critically ill child

| Procedural steps | Evidence-based rationale |
|---|---|
| 1 *Electrocardiograph (ECG) and blood pressure (BP) monitoring*<br>ECG monitoring should be continuous and the BP can be monitored continuously via an invasive arterial line if available. BP can also be monitored via non-invasive means (cuff), and in the acute stage this should be at least in 5-minute cycles | To ensure that any deterioration in the patient's heart rate, rhythm or cardiac output is detected immediately promoting prompt reassessment and treatment of the cause[1,7,9,10] |
| 2 *Pulse oximetry and blood gas analysis*<br>Pulse oximetry, to monitor oxygen saturations, should be continuous, and blood gas analysis, which can be taken from an artery, vein or capillary sample, should be done at regular intervals, as frequently as every 15–30 minutes in the critically unstable child | To ensure that the patient's ventilation parameters are kept within normal limits, promoting early detection and prompt treatment of abnormalities and reducing patient morbidity[1,7,8] |
| 3 *End tidal carbon dioxide monitoring (capnography)*<br>This is essential in any intubated patient | Capnography is the gold standard to assess that the endotracheal tube is correctly placed in the trachea and not dislodged into the oesophagus.[9] It is also provides a continuous assessment of the patient's ventilation status and so can reduce the frequency of blood gas analysis[7,9,10] |
| 4 *Peripheral skin temperature*<br>Continuous monitoring via temperature probe on an extremity (usually foot) | A low peripheral temperature, in the absence of exposure, indicates a reduction in peripheral perfusion, and may be an indicator of reduced organ perfusion[9] |
| 5 *Urine output*<br>An indwelling urinary catheter should be placed in all haemodynamically unstable children, to allow continuous urine output monitoring | Reduced urine output, <1 mL/kg/h indicates reduced organ perfusion[9] |

resuscitation is often not acceptable to the family. Unless a DNR order has been obtained through the law courts, which is rare, the family can revoke it at any time. In cases where PICU treatment is considered to be inappropriate, further treatment must be discussed with the family and all teams involved in the child's treatment to facilitate an appropriate plan of care.

### If a transport team refuses to collect a patient

In the case of time-critical transfers, as previously discussed, it remains the responsibility of the RT to transfer the child. Facilities to conduct transfers should be in place within all hospitals accepting acute admissions. If an STT refuses to collect a patient on the grounds that there is no available bed, it remains the responsibility of the RT to continue with the resuscitation process until a

suitable bed can be located. The independent STT may resolve this problem by taking responsibility for the transfer of the child whether they can place it within their region or not. Unfortunately, most PICU transfer teams in the UK are based within a working unit and are commissioned only to transfer patients into their own unit.

### When a child dies during the transfer process

In the event that a child dies during transfer to another facility, a regional boundary should not be crossed and the child should remain within that region, to comply with the coroner's jurisdiction. In practice, the transport team would resuscitate the patient until reaching the receiving unit, or in the event that this distance is too great, divert to the nearest accident and emergency department or return to the referring hospital.

## Preparation for inter-hospital transport

### Assessment and stabilisation

Critically sick children will often present in an A&E department or may collapse during a procedure, such as during a computed tomography (CT) or magnetic resonance imaging (MRI) scan, or in interventional radiology or in a cardiac catheter laboratory. In other cases staff on a ward may be alerted to a patient by a high score on a paediatric early-warning score (PEWS). Wherever these children present, it is the responsibility of the team caring for the child to conduct a comprehensive assessment of the patient and to initiate, as far as possible, appropriate treatment to promote stability. Assessment and stabilisation of any critically ill child should be carried out using a systematic approach.[9] Please see the website for further information on patient assessment and stabilisation.

After successful resuscitation the child must be closely monitored (Figure 28.1).

### The referral

The referral of a critically sick child who requires tertiary care in another institution must be done only when the initial assessment and stabilisation process has been completed. The physician leading the care will usually make the referral, and this must be done in a systematic manner to facilitate an accurate assessment of the patient by the STT. This allows the STT to appropriately advise the referrer and assist the patient stabilisation process. Referral forms are often used to ensure that necessary and relevant information is given during the referral (Figure 28.2).

Advice given by the STT should be documented in the patient's notes together with details of all treatment given prior to the team's arrival. The receiving unit may request further investigations such as CT scans or X-rays and the RT must be prepared to transfer the patient to the relevant departments maintaining appropriate patient care and monitoring. Please refer to the section on intra-hospital transfer for further information.

| Name of Patient | DOB |
|---|---|
| Address<br><br>Post Code | GP Name<br>Address |
| Telephone number | Telephone number |
| Past medical history | Known allergies<br><br>Vaccination history |
| Presenting clinical signs | Clinical management |
| **Present status** | |
| **Respiratory** | **Cardiovascular** |
| Intubated? | Heart rate |
| Induction drugs | Blood pressure |
| Endotrachael tube size | Capillary refill time |
| | Fluid given? |
| Ventilation parameters | IV access: |
| Blood gas (inc. lactate if possible) | Inotropes? |
| End tidal $CO_2$ | Urine output mL/kg/h |
| | Maintenance fluid |
| **Misc** | Blood results |
| Temperature | |
| Antibiotics given | |
| Advice given by receiving team | Actions taken post referral |
| Patient transferred     Y or N | Patient destination |

**Figure 28.1** Inter-hospital referral form.

## PROCEDURE: Supporting the specialist transport team

| Procedural steps | Evidence-based rationale |
|---|---|
| **1** *Multidisciplinary handover*<br>On arrival of the STT an accurate handover must take place, allowing appropriate resuscitation to continue and preventing repetition or omission of treatment detrimental to the patient<br>The handover should include:<br>• past medical history, vaccinations given, known allergies<br>• for neonatal patients, delivery details including, gestation, apgar scores, antenatal/postnatal care given<br>• presenting history and symptoms<br>• treatments given together with the patient response<br>• investigations conducted and current results if available (X-rays/blood samples)<br>• present clinical condition, clinical signs and treatment in progress<br>• parents or guardians: where they are and what they have been told | A multidisciplinary approach to the handover, with all relevant personnel, will ensure the patient continues to receive the appropriate care[7] |
| **2** *Documentation*<br>All documentation relevant to the patient admission should be photocopied and given to the transfer team, including:<br>• medical referral letter<br>• medical and nursing notes relating to this admission<br>• patient personal information, home address, GP, parent's contact details<br>• all observation charts: vital signs, fluid balance, blood gas analysis<br>• X-rays, scans, which could be on a computer disk if hard copies are not available.<br>• previous hospital discharge letter (where appropriate) | This will ensure all relevant information travels with the patient, so it is readily available to all concerned at the receiving centre, promoting effective continuity in care and improving the patient journey<br>This is useful where children have a complex medical history, as it provides a concise medical history improving the handover process |
| **3** *Working alongside the transport team*<br>Patient responsibility: patient care is shared between the RT and STT until the patient leaves the referral hospital. The STT will usually take responsibility for the direction of care once the patient handover has been completed<br><br>**4** Working alongside the transport team<br>Assisting the team: Assistance in the preparation of IV infusions required for the journey, the location of disposable equipment required, such as needles, syringes and fluids | It is important that the RT continues to assist the STT, who are working in an unfamiliar environment.<br>In particular the RT can be of great support to the STT by contacting relevant members of the multidisciplinary team (MDT), if further investigations are required, or specialist opinions sought, prior to transfer<br><br>This can help to reduce the time to prepare the patient for transfer, enabling a prompt departure[7] |

## PROCEDURE: Supporting the specialist transport team (continued)

| | |
|---|---|
| **5** *Providing equipment*<br>The referring hospital should provide the STT with all the disposable equipment they require while in their department | This prevents depletion of the transport stock that must be saved for use on the journey[7] |
| **6** *Patient monitoring*<br>Equipment: The STT will carry all the monitoring equipment they require for the journey. STTs will use their own monitoring equipment at the earliest opportunity | This assists the STT in developing a familiar working environment and saves time when 'packaging' a patient ready for transfer[7] |
| **7** *Patient monitoring*<br>Electrical equipment: In the case of electrical equipment mains power will be used wherever possible | To conserve battery life for those parts of the journey where an electrical supply is not available[7] |
| **8** *Patient monitoring*<br>Recording vital signs: Documentation of vital signs, etc., will be commenced by the STT on arrival and continue until the patient is delivered to the receiving unit. Some referral units continue to record vital signs until the patient leaves the hospital. As they continue to share patient responsibility this would seem to be appropriate | Evidence of continual monitoring and treatment given is required by all teams involved in the patient's care[7,8,10] |
| **9** *Communication with the patient's family*<br>Although the STT will speak to the patient's family as soon as possible, the RT can help to keep the family up to date while the STT work. In the event that the STT cannot transport the parents with the patient, the RT can help the family to make travel arrangements to the receiving hospital | Parental anxiety levels are lowered if they are kept well informed of their child's progress, which in turn leads to further cooperation by them, and can reduce future litigation claims[11] |
| **10** *Learning and observation opportunities for the referring team*<br>While supporting the STT the RT should take the opportunity to observe the resuscitation and stabilisation process at first hand | This will improve their knowledge and understanding of the assessment and stabilisation process for future occasions |

## Transfer of the critically sick child by the referring hospital

Transport by STTs is now an integral part of regionalised healthcare delivery, where well equipped, properly trained and appropriately directed teams provide a level of care comparable to that provided by most intensive care units.[10]

This section addresses how the RT should plan, organise and implement an inter-hospital transfer, in those clinical situations it is considered to be the most appropriate course of action in providing timely and suitable care reducing mortality and morbidity.

### Assessment, stabilisation and preparation for transfer

This must be continuous throughout the referral and transfer process to ensure optimum care is provided to the patient at all times. Advice regarding definitive care, post initial assessment and stabilisation, should be sought from the receiving physician and implemented by the RT as far as possible, using available experience and equipment. Full cardiovascular and respiratory stability should be achieved prior to transfer in order to give the patient the optimal chance of arriving safely. Most critically ill children require intubation and ventilation prior to transfer. In those cases where this is not warranted during the stabilisation period, serious consideration must be given to intubate prior to transfer. Intubation can be a difficult procedure, particularly for an anaesthetist less experienced in paediatric airway management. It is far safer if done in a controlled manner with the assistance of familiar staff and equipment, rather than in an emergency situation, in the unfamiliar environment of an ambulance, with minimal space, scarce equipment and scant support. Patient stability and readiness for transfer can be assessed effectively by using a checklist (Table 28.1).

**Table 28.1** Patient assessment checklist

| | |
|---|---|
| Respiratory | Endotracheal tube (ETT): Is it secure?<br>Chest X-ray: to check ETT position and assess lung fields<br>Appropriate ventilation parameters for age and weight<br>Blood gas analysis: to assess ventilation<br>Humidification in situ to prevent ETT blockage with thick secretions<br>Portable suction with appropriate suction catheters and Yankauer<br>Nasogastric tube: to deflate stomach and prevent reflux of gastric contents and added pressure on the lungs<br>Appropriate sedation, analgesic and muscle relaxant, usually given as continuous infusions, to ensure comfort of intubated patient and prevent adverse events such as accidental extubation |
| Cardiovascular | Circulatory status: heart rate, blood pressure (BP) and capillary refill<br>Ensure haemodynamic stability prior to transfer<br>Two good intravenous (IV) lines are minimum requirement for transfer (IV/IO (intraosseus) or central)<br>Fluid boluses prepared for the journey (in syringes)<br>Inotrope infusions prepared/in situ (if required)<br>Continuous invasive BP monitoring via an arterial line is preferable if inotrope therapy is required |
| Neurological | AVPU (alert, voice, pain, unresponsive)<br>Pupil reaction<br>CT scan<br>Neuro protection for raised intracranial pressure<br>C-spine immobilisation in situ for all trauma patients |
| Renal | Bladder catheter if accurate urine output required for fluid balance or cardiovascular assessment<br>Urea and creatinine results to assess renal function |
| Biochemisty | Check electrolytes within normal limits<br>Blood sugar |
| Haematology | Haemoglobin and clotting studies |
| Infection | Temperature<br>White cell count and C-reactive protein (CRP) results<br>Cultures and swabs sent<br>Antibiotics/antivirals given |
| Drugs | Documentation of all drugs and infusions given or in progress |
| Lines and tubes | Documented<br>Security of all lines catheters and drains<br>Adequate/appropriate access. Will need central access for inotropes<br>Accessibility to IV lines during transfer for drug or fluid administration |
| Parents and family | Communication and support<br>Transport arrangements |

## Who should conduct the transfer

This should be done by the most experienced or highly trained individuals available, and it is the responsibility of nursing managers in areas where these patients are likely to present, particularly A&E departments, to ensure that appropriate staff are trained for such an eventuality. The nurse should have up-to-date advanced paediatric resuscitation training and must be familiar with the transport equipment. Any child who is intubated must be accompanied by a physician who can manage and replace the ETT should the need arise. Most intensive care transfers require a senior nurse with a doctor who is proficient in airway management. This is commonly an anaesthetist, but may be a paediatrician with previous intensive care experience.

## Transport equipment

The team transporting the child must ensure that all necessary equipment and drugs are readily available, in full working order and familiar to those using them. It cannot be assumed that ambulances will have equipment, although all frontline ambulances carry oxygen and a defibrillator, but these may not be suitable for children. When you are arranging transport, the equipment required must be discussed with ambulance control.

The procedure below contains a list of essential equipment required when conducting a paediatric intensive care transfer. Figure 28.2 shows a suitable transport kit used by a PICU.

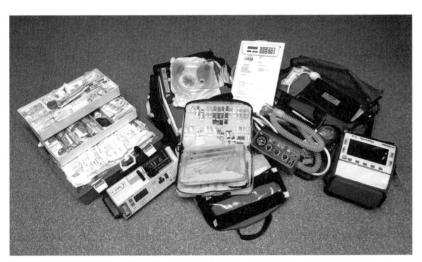

**Figure 28.2** A transport kit used by a paediatric intensive care unit transfer team.

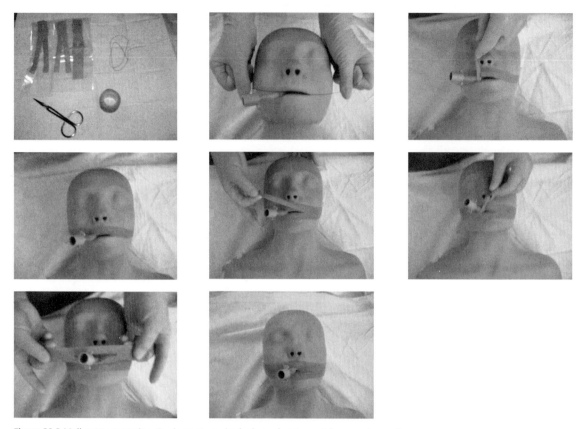

**Figure 28.3** Melbourne strapping. Equipment required: elastoplast tape; string or suture; scissors.

## PROCEDURE: Transport kit

| Procedural steps | Evidence-based rationale |
|---|---|
| **1** *Airway*<br>Oropharyngeal airways sizes 000, 00, 0, 1, 2, 3<br>Tracheal tubes sizes 2.5–7.5 uncuffed, 6.0–8.0 cuffed<br>Laryngoscope handles × 2<br>Selection of straight paediatric blades and curved adult blades<br>Replacement batteries and bulbs<br>Magills forceps<br>Yankauer suckers adult and paediatric<br>Suction catheters size 5–12<br>Humidity moisture exchange unit<br>Needle cricothyroidotomy set | This will allow the transport team to manage the child's airway in both the hospital setting prior to departure and in the event that the patient's airway, mechanical (ETT) or other, becomes unstable or blocked during the journey, the team will have all necessary equipment to intubate or reintubate the patient.[8,14] Figure 28.3 shows how to secure an ETT |

## PROCEDURE: Transport kit (continued)

| | |
|---|---|
| **2** *Breathing*<br>Oxygen mask with reservoir bag attached, adult and paediatric size<br>Self-inflating bags (Ambu) with reservoir attached<br>Infant (240 mL), paediatric (500 mL and 1 litre), adult (2 litre)<br>Face masks: infant 01, 1, 2, child 3, 4, adult 5<br>Catheter mount and connections<br>Ayres T piece: infant (500 mL), child (1 litre), adult (2 litre)<br>Portable ventilator<br>Oxygen cylinders (see below for $O_2$ calculation) | In the event that the patient's breathing becomes compromised, in the self ventilating patient, or the ventilator fails, in the case of the ventilated child, the transport team will be able to deliver oxygen and ventilation using the appropriate sized equipment.[8,14] |
| **3** *Circulation*<br>Vital signs monitor equipped to record ECG invasive and non-invasive BP, respiratory rate saturations and end tidal $CO_2$ Defibrillator with paediatric paddles or pads<br>Intravenous access requirements:<br>Intravenous cannulae: various sizes<br>Intraosseous infusion needles 16–18 g<br>Intravenous giving sets including blood giving set<br>Syringe drive infusion sets<br>Syringes 1–50 mL<br>Needles: various sizes<br>Intravenous syringe pumps (fully charged) with electric cables<br>Cut down set | The team will be able to monitor the patient's respiratory and cardiovascular status throughout the entire transfer process. They will be sufficiently equipped to deliver any drug or fluid therapy required both during the stabilisation process and the journey.[8,9,14] |
| **4** *Fluids*<br>0.9% saline or Hartmann's solution (Ringers lactate)<br>5% and 10% dextrose<br>Gelofusine<br>4.5% human albumin solution | The team will be sufficiently equipped to provide treatment for any haemodynamic instability that occurs to the child both during the stabilisation process and the journey.[8,9,14] |
| **5** *Drugs*<br>Adrenaline (epinephrine) 1:10000 (minijets)<br>Adrenaline 1:1000<br>Atropine (Minijets)<br>Adenosine<br>Sodium bicarbonate 8.4%<br>Dopamine<br>Dobutamine<br>Lidocaine 1%<br>Amiodorone with small bag 5% dextrose for flush<br>Calcium chloride (minijet)<br>Calcium gluconate 10%<br>Furosemide<br>Hydrocortisone<br>Mannitol 20%<br>Strong sodium chloride 30%<br>Noradrenaline (norepinephrine)<br>Midazolam<br>Muscle relaxant, e.g. vecuronium/pancuronium/suxemethonium | The team will have all the emergency drugs necessary to deal with all aspects of cardiovascular instability that can occur to the critically sick child in the transport environment.[8,9,14] |
| **6** *Miscellaneous*<br>Glucose testing strips<br>Spare batteries for syringe drivers | |

### Calculation of oxygen requirement for journey

Always take twice as much oxygen as the estimated journey time requires. E size cylinder contains 680 litres of oxygen when full. Only carry full cylinders.

Number of cylinders = 2 × duration of journey (minutes) × oxygen flow (L/minute)/cylinder capacity in litres

## PROCEDURE:  Conducting the transfer

| Procedural steps | Evidence-based rationale |
|---|---|
| **1** *Monitoring* This must be continuous throughout the transfer process. One member of the transport team must be in a position to constantly view the monitor and have responsibility for recording vital signs, this is usually the nurse. A 15-minute interval for recording of vital signs is considered appropriate | This will ensure prompt treatment of abnormal symptoms, promoting haemodynamic stability and the safe transfer of the patient[7,9,10] |
| **2** *Documentation* All notes, including clinical findings, investigations taken and treatment given, X-rays and consent forms must travel to the receiving hospital with the patient | This enables a thorough handover at the receiving hospital and ensures no treatment is omitted or repeated unnecessarily[7,9,10] |
| **3** *Parents: communication* The physician responsible for the child should keep the parents fully informed of progress and treatment planned, including transportation | |
| **4** *Parents: travel arrangements* If it is not possible for the parents to accompany the child in the ambulance, travel arrangements must be made for them. Full details of the receiving unit, including address, directions and phone number must be given them so they can contact the unit should they themselves experience travel delays. It is a very stressful time for parents and every opportunity to support them must be sought. Where it is practicable at least one parent should travel in the ambulance with the child | Separation from a sick child is a well-recognised cause of extreme stress to the family and should be avoided whenever possible[7] Many transport teams still seem reluctant to allow this giving the reason as possible disruption that can be caused, particularly to the team. Research conducted by teams who offer transport regularly to parents would contradict this belief, demonstrating that it is extremely rare for parents to interfere with the transport process.[12] Some studies have shown that allowing family members to be present during emergency situations including transport may reduce litigation against healthcare institutions.[11] If the ambulance can safely carry one or both of the parents, this is the appropriate course of action, particularly when the child is awake, as this will reduce unnecessary stress to the child that could cause significant clinical deterioration |

## PROCEDURE: Conducting the transfer (continued)

| | |
|---|---|
| 5 *Packaging the patient for transfer*<br>Securing the patient: Once stability is achieved, the referral has been made, the destination confirmed and all documentation prepared, the patient must be packaged securely on the stretcher for transport<br>Children below 5 kg should be transferred in an incubator or similar device. Larger children must be secured appropriately in a well-fitting harness on the ambulance stretcher. Ambulance restraints are generally only suitable for patients above 15 kg, but smaller harnesses are available and should be used<br>Securing the staff: Staff must be seated and wearing seatbelts before the journey commences. In the event that patient deterioration means treatment must be instigated, the ambulance must stop until stability is achieved and staff can return to their seats | All staff and patients travelling within a moving vehicle must be secured at all times to prevent injury[7] |
| 6 *Packaging the patient for transfer*<br>Maintaining body temperature: Blankets must be used and the ambulance heated prior to the transfer<br>Children below 5 kg should be transferred in an incubator or similar device | This will prevent heat loss from the patient and ensure that body heat is maintained during the journey. Hypothermia, particularly within neonatal patients, is associated with increased mortality and morbidity[7] |
| 7 *Packaging the patient for transfer*<br>Securing equipment: all lines must be secure and easily accessible<br>All equipment should be secured to a fixed part of the trolley or ambulance to prevent movement during the journey. All unfixed moveable items must be stored in cupboards if possible, or wedged under the trolley. No equipment, however light, should be left free to move as in the event of sudden acceleration or deceleration as this may lead to injury. When the patient is transferred onto the ambulance trolley or into the incubator, it is safer to move all the equipment first followed by the patient. The equipment is often tangled by this stage, and by sorting and securing it on the trolley first you ensure all lines are long enough and free moving | This will allow the team to deliver drug and fluid therapy during the journey if necessary[7]<br>This reduces the risk of lines and tubes being pulled out, preventing critical incidents leading to patient deterioration and transfer delays[7] |
| 8 *Packaging the patient for transfer*<br>Securing the patient: The patient's head must be positioned appropriately and immobilised using rolled up towels to ensure that the ETT does not kink and that the ventilator tubing is not caught between the patient and ventilator | This will reduce the risk of accidental extubation during the journey[7] |

## PROCEDURE: Conducting the transfer (continued)

| | |
|---|---|
| **9** *Be prepared for all eventualities*<br>All cannulae and tubes must be secured well to prevent misplacement during the journey. The adage is, 'If it can fall out, it will fall out' | This can cause journey delay if the team has to stop and replace the cannulae, increasing the level of risk to the patient[7] |
| **10** *Emergency equipment*<br>Emergency equipment for airway, breathing and circulation should be readily available<br><br>It is commonplace for reintubation equipment, including appropriate laryngoscopes, ETTs (one the patient's size and one the size below), facemask, airway, tape and scissors to resecure the new tube, to be contained in a small bag secured to the end of the stretcher | This will allow the team to reintubate the patient immediately should the ETT become blocked or dislodged during the journey[7] |
| **11** *Ventilator*<br>In the event that the ventilator fails or the patient deteriorates, an alternative manual ventilation device must be available. Most anaesthetists prefer to use an open-ended bag, known as an Ayres T piece; this must be readily available and attached to a spare oxygen supply in the ambulance. In the event of oxygen supply failure, a self-inflating bag, commonly known as an Ambu bag, must also be available and within easy reach | This will allow the team to manage the airway and breathing manually in the event of a ventilator failure[7] |
| **12** *Emergency drugs*<br>An emergency drug bag is also advised containing adrenaline (epinephrine) and atropine minijets, and any other drugs that are likely to be required, including infusions and fluid bolus's drawn up in 50-mL syringes. | This allows the team to manage circulatory instability in a timely manner[7] |
| **13** *Maintenance fluid*<br>When maintenance fluid is in progress, sufficient must be available for the journey. This usually has to be delivered via a syringe pump, as normal fluid delivery pumps are considered too bulky for transport. Additional 50-mL syringes of maintenance fluid may be required depending on the length of the journey and the size of patient. Anticipate the journey to be twice as long as expected and prepare accordingly. The fluid requirement for critically sick children is ongoing and must also be readily available during the journey | Small children will require maintenance fluid during even the shortest journey to prevent a fall in blood sugar, which is associated with increased mortality and morbidity[7] |
| **14** *Blood transfusions*<br>Blood may also be required during the journey and this must be carried in an appropriate container provided by blood bank | Blood should be carried only if likely to be used during the journey. Receiving hospitals are unlikely to use blood not cross-matched by them |
| **15** *Pre-departure checklist*<br>To ensure that the patient is ready for transfer most dedicated teams will use a pre-departure checklist | This serves as a prompt for the team to ensure that all that is required to optimise a safe transfer has been done or is available with the patient (Table 28.2) |

**Table 28.2** Pre-departure checklist

| | Yes | No |
|---|---|---|
| Is the airway protected? | | |
| Is the endotracheal tube (ETT) taped securely? | | |
| Is ventilation satisfactory on the transport ventilator (blood gas analysis and pulse oximetry)? | | |
| Is the neck immobilised properly (if appropriate)? | | |
| Is there sufficient oxygen available for the journey? | | |
| Is intravenous (IV) access sufficient (at least two IV cannulae)? | | |
| Is appropriate monitoring in situ? | | |
| Are drug and airway bags on the stretcher? | | |
| Is the manual ventilation bag attached to oxygen supply? | | |
| Is Ambu bag on the stretcher? | | |
| Is the patient secure in harness or incubator with sufficient blankets? | | |
| Is all equipment and kit stored securely? | | |
| Are the patients notes, X-rays and consent forms, if appropriate, present? | | |
| Has the case been discussed with the receiving unit? | | |
| Have the plans been discussed with the parents/guardians? | | |
| Are the parents'/guardians' contact details available? | | |
| Contact details for the receiving unit? | | |

**VIGNETTE**

**Problem:** The child is likely to require a fluid bolus during the journey but the line cannot be reached without the nurse leaving her seat, which is forbidden in a moving vehicle.

**Discussion:** Fluid should be attached to the patient via a free IV line. In order that it can be given easily a 50-mL syringe of fluid should be attached to a three-way tap and then to along plain IV line. Once this has been attached to the patient the clamp on the cannula should be opened. The three-way tap at the syringe is then closed preventing bleeding back into the IV line, ensuring patency is maintained. When fluid is required the nurse is able to open the three-way tap and administer fluid while seated. When infusion is complete the three-way tap is closed to the patient. Both drugs and fluid can be delivered in this manner.

### Arrival at the receiving hospital

On arrival at the receiving unit a comprehensive handover must be given while the patient remains on the transport trolley. It is advisable that this is multidisciplinary between the RT and all relevant personnel in the receiving team, ensuring the undivided attention of all staff involved. The first transfer of the patient to the bed often leads to divided attention, as staff busy themselves connecting monitors, etc. The RT continue to hold responsibility for the patient until the receiving team has full knowledge of the patient's case. Having received a comprehensive handover the receiving team are fully equipped with the knowledge to safely transfer the patient to a bed and provide appropriate treatment. Once the patient has been transferred safely into the care of the receiving team, the RT must ensure that all transfer notes are fully completed and a copy left with the receiving team. The original copy must return with the RT to be placed in the patient's notes at the referral hospital.

Prior to leaving the receiving unit, the RT must collect all their equipment, as it is a costly exercise to return forgotten items to the referring unit. When the RT returns to their own unit, all equipment must be cleaned, and where necessary recharged. The transport kits must be restocked so they are immediately ready for use. Any equipment failure must be checked and repaired by the biomedical engineering department before it is returned to circulation.

## INTRA-HOSPITAL TRANSFER

This section will deal with the transportation of children between departments within a hospital, including to and from A&E, X-ray, CT or MRI scanning, or admission to an internal PICU.

The principles of intra-hospital transfer are the same as those previously set out regarding inter-hospital transport when transferring a critically sick child to or from any internal department. Stability must be achieved as far as is reasonably possible and the equipment and monitoring must be appropriate to enable the accompanying staff to assess and treat the patient effectively throughout the transfer process. All equipment should be secured to a fixed point on the bed, and cot sides must be in place to ensure patient safety. The intubated, ventilated patient must at all times be accompanied by an appropriately competent physician, with the necessary equipment for reintubation, including oxygen, suction and drugs. Please refer to the section 'Be prepared for all eventualities' (point 9, page 495). All the equipment and monitoring a critically sick child needs when being transferred to a CT scanner is the same as that required for the inter-hospital transfer to a neurosurgical centre should this be an immediate necessity.

When patients collapse on a ward or present in the A&E department of a hospital with a PICU, assessment and resuscitation will immediately be commenced. However, the PICU team should be approached at an early stage to give advice and practical support. Some PICUs provide an outreach service within their hospital; this team is trained and equipped to attend all paediatric intra-hospital collapses. Whether such a team exists or not, it is usually the responsibility of the PICU team to collect patients from other hospital departments when they require PICU admission. This allows the instigation of intensive care treatment within the referral department by qualified staff using appropriate monitoring equipment, optimising a safe transfer into PICU.

The remainder of this section will address the transfer of non-ITU patients requiring intra-hospital transfer.

## PROCEDURE: Transfer to the X-ray department

| Procedural steps | Evidence-based rationale |
|---|---|
| 1 *Inform parent or carer*<br>Although written consent is not required within the UK to conduct many investigative procedures on hospitalised children, the parents must be informed prior to their child's transfer and wherever possible be allowed to accompany the child, even though they may not be able to enter the X-ray or scanning room | In accordance with the principles of family-centred care this reduces both parental and child stress, leading to greater cooperation from both[11] |
| 2 *Escort the child*<br>Where the patient's condition allows, it will be appropriate for the parent to take the child to the relevant department without supervision. In any case where the child requires sedation, more commonly seen in interventional radiology, then a nurse holding a paediatric nursing qualification must be in attendance at all times | This ensures patient safety and timely treatment, if necessary, during the procedure |

## PROCEDURE:  Transfer to the X-ray department (continued)

| | |
|---|---|
| **3** *Equipment*<br>If the patient's clinical condition is such that a nurse escort is not necessary, no equipment will be required. In the event the patient requires sedation, then a nurse together with oxygen, suction, appropriately sized catheters, Yankauer sucker, facemasks, airways, Ambu bag and saturation monitor must accompany the patient | If the patient has an adverse reaction to the sedation, airway and breathing can easily be managed using the simple adjuncts available while awaiting further assistance[9] |
| **4** *Equipment*<br>The monitor: this must be clearly visible at all times to the accompanying nurse, especially in those cases where the nurse cannot be in the same room but needs to be protected by a screen or glass window<br>Security: infusion pumps and any monitoring equipment must be attached to a fixed part of the bed and only equipment currently in use should be taken. Any excess unnecessary equipment previously in use should be removed prior to transfer | The nurse is protected from high levels of radiation while still able to continually monitor the patient's condition.<br><br>This will minimise potential injury to patient or staff and reduce damage to equipment. It will also make the bed/ stretcher easier to move, further reducing staff injury |
| **5** *Mode of transport*<br>This will be determined according to the age and clinical condition of the patient, ranging from the child who can walk or be carried, to those who need to be transferred in a pushchair, wheelchair, trolley or bed | The patient will be transferred using the most appropriate equipment to ensure safety throughout the process |
| **6** *Mode of transport: Safety*<br>A bed or trolley must be fitted with two fully functioning cot sides | This will ensure patient safety is maintained throughout the transfer |
| **7** *Mode of transport: Staff escort*<br>The mode of transport determines how many staff/personnel must accompany the patient. A bed or trolley requires two members of staff, usually one nurse and a porter. Whether the nurse has specialist training will be determined by the patient's condition | This will ensure that the patient is transferred comfortably and that risk to staff and patient is kept to its lowest level |
| **8** *Notes and X-rays*<br>The patient's notes and previous X-rays (if appropriate) together with a request form should accompany the patient, although in many hospitals X-rays are now in computerised format accessible by any department via the computer network, negating the need for hard copies. If the child requires only parental escort, the notes should be placed in a sealed envelope | If all relevant documentation travels with the patient, the investigative and report process will be done more efficiently, improving the patient's journey throughout their hospital stay |

## Transfer to CT or MRI scanner

When a child is transferred for a CT or MRI scan, the same considerations apply as for transfer to the X-ray department. There are, however, several additional factors that must be considered to ensure patient safety, particularly if it is part of an emergency assessment.

### CT scanner

When transferring a child to undergo a planned CT scan the considerations for transfer are no different than transferring to X-ray.

However, in the acutely ill child, particularly the child with a fluctuating conscious level, intubation and ventilation is recommended prior to scanning. The alternative term 'Donut of Death' sometimes used for the CT scanner is not unfounded, as a consequence of the number of inadequately stabilised children who collapse during the procedure.

### MRI scanner

This scanner uses a powerful static magnetic field to produce detailed anatomic or functional images of soft tissue. Any metal objects containing iron, such as scissors, laryngoscopes and IV poles, are magnetised turning them into dangerous missiles.[12] It is the responsibility of the transfer team to ensure that all equipment, for example ventilator and cardiac monitor, that must enter the scanner is MRI compatible. Equipment that is not MRI compatible must be kept outside the magnetic field. Essential drug infusions must be kept to a minimum (i.e. those with a very short half-life, such as inotropes); infusion lines must be extended to allow continuous delivery of the drugs during the scan while ensuring the pump remains outside the magnetic field. A bolus of IV sedation may be used instead of constant infusion, and IV maintenance should be stopped for the duration of the scan. Standard oxygen cylinders must not cross the magnetic field; therefore, oxygen/ventilator tubing must be transferred onto MRI compatible cylinders located within the scanning room. The patient must be inspected prior to transfer and metal objects, such as hairgrips and name bands, removed. Biomedical implants, such as pacemakers and cochlear implants, may not be MRI compatible and advice must be sought before scanning children who have such devices in place. MRI-compatible ECG and pulse oximetry cables must be used to prevent thermal injury caused by wires forming conductive loops within themselves, or parts of the body, because of radiofrequency fields.[13] As the patient is not visible during the scan it is imperative all monitoring equipment is visible to staff observing from the control room. Noise levels within the scanner can be extremely loud and it may be appropriate to use earplugs for some children to reduce distress and optimise sedation therapy.[12] In all cases where an MRI scan is necessary, trained MRI staff should be consulted to ensure safety is maintained throughout the procedure.

 Go to the website to find the PowerPoint presentation for this chapter and MCQs to test your knowledge. **www.hodderplus.com/childnursingskills**

## REFERENCES

1 Barry PW, Ralston C (1994) Adverse events occurring during interhospital transfer of the critically ill. *Archives of Disease in Childhood* **71**: 8–11.

2 Sharples A, O'Neill M, Dearlove O (1996) Children are still transferred by non specialist teams (Letter) *British Medical Journal* **312** (7032): 120.

3 Edge WE, Kanter RK, Weigle CGM, Walsh RF (1994) Reduction in morbidity in interhospital transport by specialized paediatric staff. *Critical Care Medicine* **22**: 1186–1189.

4 Paediatric Intensive Care Society (1995) *Standards for paediatric intensive care*. London: PICS.

5 Department of Health (1997) Paediatric intensive care. *A framework for the future*. London: Department of Health.

6 Britto J, Nadel S, et al. (1995) Morbidity and severity of illness during interhospital transfer: impact of a specialist retrieval team. *British Medical Journal* **311**: 836–839.

7   Byron YA, McCloskey K (1992) *Evaluation, stabilization and transport of the critically ill child.* London: Mosby Year Book.

8   Advanced Life Support Group (ed) (2005) *Advanced paediatric life support. The practical approach,* 4th edition. Oxford: BMJ Books/Blackwell's.

9   Macnab A, Alexander SM, Macrae D, Green G (2001) Interfacility transport. In: Macnab A, Macrae D, Henning R (eds) *Care of the critically ill child,* 4th edition. London: Churchill Livingstone, 36–44.

10  Davies J, Tibby SM, Murdoch IA (2005) Should parents accompany children during inter-hospital transport? *Archives of Disease in Children.* **90**: 1270–1273.

11  Hanson C, Strawser D (1992) Family presence during cardiopulmonary resuscitation: Foote Hospital emergency department's nine year perspective. *Journal of Emergency Medicine* **18**(2): 104–106.

12  Stokoski LA (2005) Ensuring safety for infants undergoing magnetic resonance imaging. *Advances in Neonatal Care* **5**(1): 14–27.

13  Maalouf EF, Counsell SJ (2002) Imaging the preterm infant: practical issues. In: Rutherford MA (ed) *MRI of the neonatal brain.* London: WB Saunders, 17–21.

14  Advanced Life Support Group (ed.) (2008) *Paediatric and neonatal safe transfer and retrieval. The practical approach,* 1st edition. Oxford: Wiley Blackwell.

15  Weller BF (1997) *Bailliere's nurses' dictionary,* 22nd edition. London: Ballière Tindall.

## FURTHER READING

Aylott M (1997) Inter-professional telephone communication on transport. *Journal of Neonatal Nursing.* (July) 24–28.

Davies J (2001) Paediatric retrieval – aiming for the gold standard. *Care of the Critically Ill* **17**(3): 94–98.

Doyle YG, Orr FE (2002) Interhospital transport to paediatric intensive care by specialised staff: Experience of South Thames combined transport service 1998–2000. *Archives of Disease in Childhood.* **87**(3): 245–247.

Hallworth D, McIntyre A (2003) The transport of critically ill children. *Current Paediatrics* **13**: 2–17.

Handy JM, Van Zwanenburgg G (2006) Secondary transfer of the critically ill patient. *Current Anaesthesia and critical care* **11**(3): 1–8.

Heward Y (2003) Transfer from ward to PICU: a standard. *Paediatric Nursing* **15**(1): 11–13.

Leslie A, Middleton D (1995) Give and take in neonatal transport: communication hazards in handover. *Journal of Neonatal Nursing* (October) 27–31.

Lewis MM, Holditch-Davis D, Brunssen S (1997) Parents as passengers during pediatric transport. *Air Medical Journal* (April–June) 38–42.

Melville M, Print M (1996) Legal issues surrounding neonatal emergency transport: Minimising the risk of litigation. *Journal of Neonatal Nursing* (October) 18–22.

Morrison G (2000) Transportation of the critically ill child. In Williams C, Asquith J (eds) *Paediatric Intensive Care Nursing.* London. Churchill Livingstone, 51–58.

Neill C, Hughes U (2004) Improving interhospital transfer. *Paediatric Nursing* **16**(7): 24–27.

Stack CG (1997) Stabilization and transport of the critically ill child. *Current Anaesthesia and Critical Care* **8**: 25–30.

# Neonatal care

Sandie Skinner

## LEARNING OUTCOMES

*Upon completion of this chapter, the reader should be able to accomplish the following:*

1 Provide basic nursing care for a sick or preterm infant
2 Understand how to provide a thermoneutral environment for a newborn infant
3 Discuss the principles of feeding in newborn care
4 Discuss the care of an infant undergoing phototherapy
5 Perform a heel lance
6 Describe the principles of developmental care
7 Discuss the attachment process

## CHAPTER OVERVIEW

Newborn infants provide a different challenge to nurses from older infants and young children. This chapter aims to highlight the principles of care that are important when caring for this vulnerable group of patients. More detailed reading is required for nurses wishing to specialise in the area.

Approximately 10 per cent of all births require additional support for the newborn infant. These infants are usually admitted to a neonatal unit.

There are three levels of care that may be provided in neonatal units: Level 1, special care; Level 2, high-dependency care; and Level 3, intensive care. Special care describes additional input to that required by a healthy newborn. High-

dependency care describes the care that a more poorly infant requires – this infant may be having convulsions, weigh below 1000 g or require respiratory support in the form of nasal continuous positive airways pressure. Intensive care is provided for infants with complex needs – respiratory support via an endotracheal tube, major surgery or complex clinical procedures such as an exchange transfusion.

Neonatal nurses are challenged with providing the necessary care an infant requires while also balancing the principles of minimal handling and supporting the attachment process with parents. Communication and support of parents is a vital role of the neonatal nurse.

## KEY WORDS

Neonate development care
Attachment thermoneutral environment    Jaundice
Phototherapy    Comfort measures

## TEMPERATURE MEASUREMENT IN TERM AND PRETERM NEONATES

We measure temperature because good health is associated with a normal temperature range. We also measure body temperature in the newborn to track the thermal effect of environmental exposure – hypothermia and hyperthermia.

## Normal body temperature

Throughout the body, thermoregulatory systems serve to keep the body within a range that is best for bodily functions to take place. According to Leick-Rude and Bloom,[1] what constitutes normal temperature in term and preterm infants is unclear. However, maintenance of core body temperature between 36.5°C and 37.5°C is considered desirable to achieve a state in which heat loss and heat production are in balance.

## Thermoregulation

The capacity to balance heat loss and gain is known as thermoregulation. This capacity to regulate temperature is limited in the newborn, especially if they are born prematurely.

Several factors predispose preterm infants to temperature instability, in particular their decreased subcutaneous fat and glycogen stores, large surface area to weight ratio, lack of muscle tone and flaccid posture, underdeveloped hypothalamus leading to poor vascular control and increased transepidermal loses.

## Heat production

Non-shivering thermogenesis, the production of heat by metabolism, is the primary source of heat production in the neonate. The fuel is the infant's supply of brown fat (deposited after 28 weeks' gestation principally around the scapulae, kidneys, adrenals, neck and axilla). This increased metabolic activity can result in respiratory distress, anaerobic metabolism and metabolic acidosis. In small for gestational age and preterm infants, these consequences may be devastating and may increase both mortality and morbidity rates.[2]

## Heat loss

Body heat is dynamic, always changing, always moving across tissue boundaries. Heat transfers when there is a difference in heat between adjacent areas, i.e. energy in motion in search of equilibrium from warmer to cooler. Heat transfers in four ways:

1 *Radiation*: through space without contact
   Action: Do not place cot near cool external walls, avoid direct sunlight.
2 *Convection*: through air or liquid as contact medium
   Action: Maintain room temperature at 24–26°C.

Close incubator doors as soon as possible.
3 *Conduction*: through objects by direct contact
   Action: Place a sheet on cold weighing scales, pre warm towels.
4 *Evaporation*: through liquid then air.
   Action: Dry quickly following delivery or bath.

## Temperature measurement

There is no best place to measure temperature, because each body site has a temperature that is different from that of any other body site. The aim when taking a temperature is to record core temperature. A variety of sites can be used, for example thermistors placed in the bladder or oesophagus record temperatures that closely correspond to pulmonary artery temperatures. However, these sites are impractical for daily monitoring.

We try to capture temperature at a moment in time, although the next moment it may be slightly different. If it is necessary to keep track of temperature on an ongoing basis, for a very small or sick baby an abdominal skin temperature is used, often in conjunction with a peripheral temperature by a probe attached to the foot. A widening temperature difference between these sites serves as an early warning of hypovolaemia or increasing cold stress.

Recording the axilla temperature has become the accepted method for temperature measurement for the neonate.[2] Although temperatures measured from the axilla or abdomen are slightly lower than actual core temperature, they reflect increases and decreases in temperature consistent with differences in core temperature.

To obtain an accurate measurement the thermometer is placed deep within the axilla, midway between the anterior and posterior margins. The baby's arm may require flexing across the chest and to be held in place to ensure that the thermometer remains in contact with the skin. The length of time required for the measurement will depend on the individual instrument used.

The measurement is repeated 3–4 hourly. Frequency of recording depends on the result obtained, bearing in mind the principles of minimal handling, which is a cornerstone of good neonatal care. Frequent disturbance may lead to hypoxia and health deterioration.

## Signs of hypothermia

- Mottled, pale skin
- Cold extremities (>1°C from central temperature)
- Apnoeic spells
- Bradycardia
- Lethargy
- Hypotonia
- Weak cry
- Increased gastric residuals, abdominal distension or emesis.

## Signs of hyperthermia

- Warm to touch
- Sweating on forehead in infants <36 weeks
- Increased respiratory/heart rate
- Flushed, bright pink skin
- Irritable/lethargic.

## Thermal neutral environment

The thermal neutral environment (TNE) is the environmental temperature in which an infant can maintain normal body temperature while consuming the least amount of oxygen. Within a carefully maintained TNE, an infant minimises oxygen and calorie consumption and is able to use energy and nutrition for growth.[3]

## Thermoregulatory devices

Heated mattresses, radiant overhead heaters and incubators are used in neonatal nurseries to help maintain the TNE. Enclosed and heated, an incubator provides a heated stable thermal environment, with the added advantage of being able to administer humidity (Figure 29.1).

Transepidermal water loss is one of the greatest factors in thermal balance. Keratin, which helps the skin retain water, is not developed in infants born at 30 weeks or less and is not established until 2 or 3 weeks after birth.

In general, incubators are set to maintain an initial temperature of 36.5°C. The incubator temperature set point can be increased or decreased according to axilla temperature measurements.

Incubators work in air servo mode or skin servo control mode. In servo mode the heat output automatically changes according to the changes in either the ambient temperature or abdominal skin

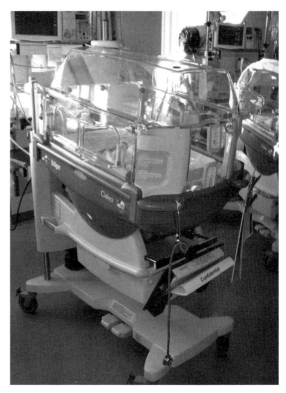

**Figure 29.1** Incubator.

temperature set point. The ambient incubator temperature should be recorded as well as the axilla measurement to guide future adjustments.

## Nursing interventions

- Determine cause of hypothermia, e.g. excessive handling/exposure.
- Temperature instability can be a sign of infection or other conditions.
- Monitor blood sugars.
- Monitor for complications, observe vital signs and report findings.

## Conclusion

It is important to remember that infants are unable to communicate their thermal needs and they cannot react appropriately, for example by increasing their incubator temperature, removing a hat or vest, or by replacing a cover. Maintaining a baby's temperature and reacting to their needs ensures their growth, comfort and safety and is a fundamental aspect of neonatal care.

# FEEDING OF THE NEONATE

An essential part of caring for small or sick neonates is to provide them with the best possible nutrition in order to optimise their health status and promote growth.

For the term healthy infant, breastfeeding on demand, started soon after birth and continued for a minimum of 6 months, is upheld by the World Health Organization[4] as the best feeding choice for mothers and babies in both developed and developing countries. This is not a possibility for most premature infants, who are often born unable to feed themselves. This can be due to many reasons.

- They are born with significantly reduced energy reserves and a poorly developed sucking reflex.
- Intubation and ventilation leave the infant unable to take food by mouth.
- Immaturity of the gastrointestinal system, hence the inability to tolerate milk in sufficient quantity to meet their nutritional requirement.
- Inability to coordinate sucking, swallowing and breathing.
- The presence of congenital abnormalities awaiting surgical repairs such as cleft palate, abdominal wall defects, gastrointestinal atresias or fistulae.

Different approaches are available to manage these problems.

First it is necessary to understand fluid volume and caloric requirements of the premature neonate. To mimic uterine growth, weight gain should equate to 15–20 g/kg/day, and for this to be achieved an intake of 120–130 kcal/kg/day is required. Well-established feeding guides such as shown below are in place in neonatal units to achieve this.

### Example of fluid volume required by a well preterm neonate

Day 1: 60 mL/kg/day
Day 2: 90 mL/kg/day
Day 3: 120 mL/kg/day
Day 4: 140 mL/kg/day
Day 5: 150 mL/kg/day
Day 6 and beyond: increase gradually to 180 mL/kg/day if required

Initially, maintenance of homeostasis alone can be challenging, as it is heavily affected by the degree of prematurity and/or specific conditions of the infant. Blood glucose stability, fluid balance and normal serum electrolytes all require close and regular monitoring.

The ultimate aim of all feeding strategies is to achieve, by the time of discharge, successful infant oral feeding using whichever method is favoured by the mother. Crucially, this should be attained with full parental involvement as a means to promote parent–infant bonding and socialisation of the neonate.

## Ways of feeding the premature neonate

### Oral and enteral feeding

1 *Choice of milk*: human milk or artificial formula

- Expressed breast milk (EBM) obtained from the infant's own mother is the feed of choice for any neonate, especially the vulnerable preterm. It is better tolerated with increased fat and nutrient absorption; it contains specific antibodies and helps reduce the risk of sepsis and lowers the incidence of necrotising enterocolitis. It is thought to improve the infant's long-term neurological outcome.[5] It promotes mother–infant bonding by putting emphasis on the mother's role. Regular supply, however, depends on the mother's ability to express adequate volumes over a prolonged time. The caloric content may not be sufficient for optimal growth requiring the need for fortification. This will usually stop once the infant's weight is >2 kg.
- Donor expressed breast milk (DEBM) carries the benefits of human milk but the pasteurising and freezing destroys some of the immunological properties.[5] The storing process is complex and expensive and is therefore not available in all centres.
- Low birthweight infant formulae is specifically developed to meet the additional nutritional needs of the low birthweight infant. They are unable to provide the immunological component of human milk.
- Supplements are given routinely to all babies born at 2.5 kg and under. The most common are iron supplements and multivitamins.

## 2 *Choice of feeding method*

- Breast: successful breastfeeding technique requires time to develop and establish over days and often weeks and is rarely mastered before 35 weeks' gestation. The nurse must have an understanding of the anatomy and physiology of lactation to be able to give knowledgeable and consistent advice on milk expression. Nursing interventions to support mothers over that period include help and advice about positioning and fixing the baby to the breast and interpretation of the infant's hunger cues.
- Bottle: not usually introduced until 34 weeks of gestation due to poorly developed suck/swallow reflex.
- Nasogastric or orogastric tube: the most common way of feeding the well preterm infant, sometimes referred to as gavage feeding. It allows the administration of enteral feeds while minimising energy expenditure by the neonate, thus promoting growth. Placement and care of the tube used is one of the basic neonatal nursing skills and is detailed in Chapter 13.
- Trophic feeding: also referred to as minimal enteral feeding consists of small volumes of human milk given in order to stimulate gut hormone production, promote intestinal maturation and motility and prevent gut atrophy. It is thought to reduce the time taken to achieve full enteral feeding.

Controversy still exists as to the optimum time to commence enteral feeding in the preterm. The main concern remains that the low birthweight infant is unable to cope with gut stimulation and is therefore exposed to the risk of necrotising enterocolitis.

### Parenteral feeding

Total parenteral nutrition (TPN) allows the complete provision of nutrients to be delivered to the neonate by intravenous means when oral feeding is not possible or been established. It is usually delivered via a central venous line. The nursing care of an infant receiving TPN involves monitoring intake and output, weight, blood glucose and electrolytes.[6] Observation of the insertion site, amount of fluid delivered and line patency is required. Strict aseptic technique is employed when breaking into the line. The neonatal nurse must have an awareness of the possible complications. Some of these include:

- risk of sepsis from central indwelling intravenous lines;
- metabolic acidosis due to amino acid load: acetate is added to counteract this complication;
- hyperglycaemia due to increased insulin resistance;
- hypoglycaemia due to low energy stores combined with increased metabolic rate or direct problem in delivery of infusion such as leakage around site or connection;
- hyperlipidaemia due to lipid intolerance.

## Summary

The preterm infant requires significant nutritional input to achieve growth similar to that of the fetus. Any deficiency can be harmful and create long-term health problems. Nutritional needs must be met by enteral or parenteral measures or a combination of both. The best option is using the mother's milk or artificial milk specially formulated for low birthweight infants.

## PERFORMING A HEEL LANCE

Heel lance is a technique that is commonly used in neonatal units to obtain small blood samples. Samples that are frequently collected by this route include blood glucose testing, blood gas analysis, newborn blood spot testing and serum bilirubin. If other samples are required venepuncture may be the preferred route as it is less painful. It is important to coordinate tests in this vulnerable group.

### Equipment

Gloves
Paper towel
Sterile cotton wool
Sterile water
Lancet device
Warming device
Capillary tube, newborn blood spot card or glucose meter
Sucrose for pain relief
Sterile gauze swabs or sterile cotton wool

## PROCEDURE:  Performing a heel lance

| Procedural steps | Evidence-based rationale |
| --- | --- |
| **1** Consider timing and necessity of procedure | It may be more appropriate to combine a heel prick with some other handling to allow the infant longer periods of rest. Always consider whether the procedure has to be performed or if it could wait until a venous or arterial sample is being collected to save the infant unnecessary discomfort[7] |
| **2** Explain procedure to parents if present | Clear explanations will help the parents understand the reason for the procedure. This will also promote the partnership between parents and staff |
| **3** Collect necessary equipment | To allow the procedure to be undertaken without delays or interruptions |
| **4** Wash hands prior to handling infant | Essential infection control measure to reduce risk of cross-infection |
| **5** Speak to infant prior to handling and gently move infant into a supine or semi-lateral position. The cot or incubator should be tilted slightly. Encourage a neutral flexed position. The procedure can be performed on the parent's or nurse's knee. This allows the infant to be held securely and gently rocked after the procedure | This facilitates self-regulatory behaviour and minimises the discomfort of the procedure |
| **6** Inspect the heel checking that there are no cuts or excessive bruising. Ideally, the heel should be pink and warm. If both heels are very bruised, poorly perfused or scarred from previous sampling it may be appropriate to consider venous sampling by a senior nurse or doctor | To prevent further damage. A warm, pink heel will bleed more easily than a cold cyanotic heel |
| **7** Consider warming the heel, e.g. if it is cold, by using a glove filled with warm water (<42°C) or a commercially available warming device | Warming the heel may increase blood flow and will reduce haemolysis and potential bruising. There is some evidence to suggest that this is not necessary |
| **8** Administer sucrose as per unit policy associated | Sucrose has been used to ease neonatal pain with heel lancing[7] |
| **9** Identify the area to sample from on the plantar surface of the foot medial to a line drawn posteriorly from the middle of the large toe to the heel or lateral to a line drawn posteriorly from between the fourth and fifth toes to the heel (Figure 29.2, page 509). The puncture site must not be on the curvature of the heel[7] | There is a risk of osteomyelitis if the bone is punctured. In a preterm infant the calcaneous bone may be as little as 2.4 mm below the skin surface on the plantar (bottom) area of the heel. At the posterior curvature (back) of the heel it can be 1.2 mm below the skin surface[7] |
| **10** Put gloves on. Clean area with sterile cotton wool and sterile water. Allow to dry for about 30 seconds | Essential infection control measure to reduce risk of cross-infection |
| **11** Following cleaning ensure that the cleaned area contaminated by touching and surfaces | To maintain a clean area and reduce risk of is not cross-infection |
| **12** Ensure the blood sampling device is also kept sterile and does not come into contact with any surfaces | Minimise risk of cross-infection. |

## PROCEDURE:  Performing a heel lance (continued)

| | |
|---|---|
| **13** Encircle the foot with your non-dominant hand, using the index finger wrapped around the foot and the thumb around the ankle below the site to be used for lancing. This positioning is very important for the success of the procedure (Figure 29.3, page 509) | Reduce the chance of the infant moving and this could lead to inadvertent puncture of the wrong area or needle stick injury to operator |
| **14** Remember the safe area for sampling. Place the puncturing device against the heel so that it is correctly aligned with the desired puncture site. When certain that positioning is correct and the device is flush with the skin, gently depress the trigger. Immediately, remove the device from the infant's heel | To perform a safe procedure |
| **15** Safely dispose of puncture device in a sharps container | To prevent inadvertent needlestick injury |
| **16** With the heel in a lowered position wait for the blood to flow. Try to avoid squeezing the heel | Gravity will assist blood flow |
| **17** Carefully collect the required volume of blood avoiding direct contact with the puncture site. If insufficient blood obtained do not repeat procedure without seeking advice from senior colleague | To minimise risk of cross-infection |
| **18** When the blood is collected raise the foot and apply a sterile gauze pad or sterile cotton wool | To reduce blood loss and prevent a haematoma from forming |
| **19** Provide comfort measures to the infant: swaddle or positioning appropriately in cot or incubator | To promote developmental care and comfort infant following an invasive procedure |
| **20** Ensure that bleeding has stopped. If not inform a senior nurse or medical practitioner | To ensure patient safety. Prolonged clotting times may require further investigation |
| **21** Correctly label the specimen or record the result of the test as appropriate | To maintain patient safety |
| **22** Dispose of all used materials according to hospital policy | To prevent cross-infection |

## CARE OF INFANT UNDERGOING PHOTOTHERAPY FOR JAUNDICE

### What is jaundice?

Jaundice is a yellow discolouration of the skin and sclera caused by raised serum bilirubin levels. Over half of healthy newborns develop clinical jaundice around day 3 to day 10 of life, known as physiological jaundice. Pathological jaundice occurs within 24 hours of birth or after 2 weeks of life. There are two forms of bilirubin in the blood, unconjugated/indirect/fat-soluble bilirubin and conjugated/direct/water-soluble bilirubin. Kernicterus results from high levels of free-floating unconjugated bilirubin in the blood which is lipid soluble, and in this form can cross the blood–brain barrier. The blood–brain barrier is more permeable in preterm babies, systemic illness, hypoxia and acidosis. When this happens the basal ganglia in the brain is stained yellow, leading to cell death. This could result in encephalopathy and deafness. Early detection and treatment assists in preventing this irreversible neurological sequel; therefore, educating healthcare providers in early detection

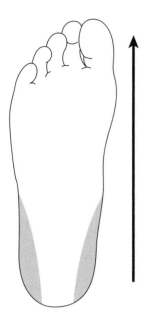

**Figure 29.2** Identifying the sampling area. The shaded areas represents the sampling area.

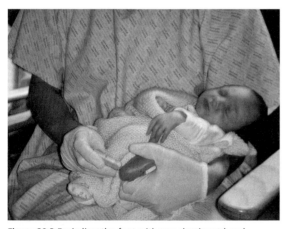

**Figure 29.3** Encircling the foot with non-dominant hand.

and treatment of jaundice is paramount to reduce the risk of kernicterus. In recent years a change has occurred with caring for the newborn predominantly in the hospital environment during the first week of life to community-led midwifery care; therefore, educating parents to recognise the signs of jaundice is important to lower the incidence of kernicterus.

## Bilirubin production, metabolism and excretion

Bilirubin results from the breaking down of haemoglobin, which is stored in subcutaneous tissue. Red blood cells in the newborn have a shorter lifespan than adults, causing production of bilirubin at higher rates. Bilirubin produced by the fetus is transported across the placenta and excreted by the maternal circulation. After birth the liver is responsible for the metabolism of bilirubin. For bilirubin to be transported to the liver it has to bind to a molecule know as albumin. Bound unconjugated bilirubin is converted in the liver by the enzyme uridine diphosphate glucuronyl transferase to conjugated bilirubin. The liver can now excrete the water-soluble bilirubin into the biliary tree, which travels to the intestine. Here, it is converted to urobilinogen by bacteria, the majority is excreted in faeces after conversion to stercobilinogen, which contributes to the stools having a yellow/brown colour. In the intestine conjugated bilirubin may become unconjugated bilirubin again by the action of an enzyme beta-glucuronidase and be reabsorbed to return to the liver for reconjugation. In the newborn this mechanism may not be fully developed hence many newborns develop jaundice.

## Risk factors for jaundice

Jaundice in the newborn is mostly benign and may resolve without treatment, but it may indicate serious underlying disease which could result in brain cell damage. Babies who are at the greatest risk include

1   preterm babies;
2   babies jaundiced within the first 24 hours of birth; blood group incompatibility; sick babies; babies with prolonged jaundice; breastfed babies.

Other causes of jaundice include
1   physiological
2   increased haemoglobin load (e.g. bruising, cephalhaematoma)
3   congenital spherocytosis (abnormal red cell shape)
4   infection
5   metabolic disorder.

### Preterm babies

Rationale includes:
- immature liver
- increased red cell breakdown
- lower levels of albumin for bilirubin binding
- increased risk of acidosis, resulting in decreased bilirubin binding which may facilitate entry of free bilirubin into brain cells.

Hypoxia and hypoglycaemia cause increased free fatty acid levels which may in turn displace bilirubin from binding sites such as albumin, thus preterm babies are at increased risk of kernicterus.

### Babies jaundiced within the first 24 hours of birth; blood group incompatibility

*ABO incompatibility:* More common than rhesus disease, and is possibly less severe than rhesus incompatibility. The mother is often blood group O and the baby group A or B. The mother has naturally occurring anti-A or anti-B antibodies in her blood, which destroy fetal red cells leading to jaundice and possibly anaemia.

Rhesus isoimmunisation: 15 per cent of women are rhesus negative (D antigen). Father must be rhesus positive and mother rhesus negative. With the introduction of anti-D the numbers of affected babies has considerably dropped. Rhesus antigens (c, E) can also lead to haemolysis of the red cells.

Tests should include:
1 total bilirubin
2 full blood count and film
3 baby's blood group and Coombs test
4 mother's blood group and establish her antibody status from case notes
5 full infection screen in ill babies
6 glucose-6-phosphate dehydrogenase (G6PD) concentration depending on ethnic origin, e.g. Mediterranean, Middle Eastern and South East Asian.

### Sick babies

Babies who are jaundiced and clinically unwell should be screened for sepsis with a full septic screen work-up. Also include 1–4 of the above tests. Acidosis will reduce binding sites for bilirubin and increases the uptake of free bilirubin in cerebral cells.

### Babies with prolonged jaundice

Generally can be defined as jaundice that is apparent in a preterm baby at around 3 weeks of age and around 2 weeks in a term baby. According to Hadzic,[8] clinical examination is not complete unless the following question is asked: Does the baby have pale stools and yellow urine? This can indicate liver disease.

Tests include:
- total and conjugated bilirubin (split bilirubin)
- urine microscopy and culture and sensitivity
- stool colour documented.

Unconjugated persistent jaundice test for:
- G6PD screen in African, Asian or Mediterranean patients;
- thyroid function;
- blood galactose-1-phosphate;
- congenital infection screen, e.g. toxoplasmosis, rubella, cytomegalovirus and herpes;
- metabolic investigations, e.g. urine for reducing substances.

Split bilirubin levels may assist in diagnosing liver disease such as biliary atresia, which is not always easy to diagnose. Urine should be tested for reducing substances, particularly for the presence of sugar. If urine tests positive to sugar, a sample should be obtained and sent to the laboratory for chromatogram studies.

## Management of jaundice

Assessing whether jaundice is significant or not can be difficult as over 50 per cent of term babies and up to 80 per cent of preterm babies develop jaundice in the first week of life. Jaundice usually becomes visible when the serum bilirubin level rises above 85–100 µmol/L. Jaundice can be made more apparent by blanching the nose lightly with a finger. Visual detection of jaundice is unreliable and newborns who are less than 38 weeks' gestation, especially when they are breastfed, are at a greater risk of developing hyperbilirubinaemia. However, in non-Caucasian babies detection of jaundice can be more difficult; in this group examination of the sclera and the gums is recommended. Any baby who develops jaundice should have their serum bilirubin level measured and plotted correctly, taking into consideration the gestational age and hours of age of each baby.

Treatment for jaundice is phototherapy, occasionally in conjunction with an exchange transfusion. Phototherapy works by detoxifying bilirubin and changing it to lumirubin, which is water soluble and can be excreted by the body.

There are a number of various ways for delivering phototherapy, depending on the baby's total serum bilirubin levels; the most commonly used are overhead blue lights with varying strengths, and the BiliBlanket, which the baby lies on.[9] The level of bilirubin, age of onset and history will be taken into account when deciding which method of treatment is best. Each baby should receive individualised care depending on their history and clinical picture. Jaundice presenting in the first 24 hours can result in levels rising rapidly; the levels generally do not elevate as rapidly when jaundice presents on day 3. Appropriate nursing care will boost the effectiveness of phototherapy thereby reducing complications.

## Nursing care of baby receiving phototherapy

*Serum bilirubin levels:* The frequency of blood samples will depend on the severity of the jaundice and age of presentation. The blood sample is usually taken from the heel, or venous sampling is used when exchange transfusion is to be considered. The blood should not be exposed to the phototherapy light, and the result should be recorded correctly on the appropriate chart.

*Parents:* Parents may feel distressed when they see that their baby is naked and wearing eye protection pads. They should be given accurate information about jaundice and phototherapy.

*Rationale:* To reduce anxiety, stress and assist them in understanding why their baby is jaundiced.

## Assure effective irradiance

The phototherapy lamps or mattresses should be positioned to provide the most complete skin exposure.[10] The lamps should be placed 16–18 inches (40.5–45.5 cm) from the baby as an optimal distance or follow manufacturer's instructions. It is recommended to turn the baby frequently, as this will allow for maximal exposure to the phototherapy lamp. The baby should have as much skin exposed as possible. In some cases it may be recommended to use the overhead lamp and the bili-bed together to increase the surface area covered and the effectiveness of the phototherapy.9 If using the BiliBlanket alone, this is usually wrapped directly around the baby leaving only the nappy in situ.

## Eye care

The eyes should be covered by a correctly fitting a protective shield, which should be removed at regular intervals. Commercially coloured Plexiglas shields are available, which are placed over the baby's head; however, for maximum exposure the eye pad is recommended. Check that infections or abrasions are not occurring.

*Rationale:* To prevent retinal damage.

Parents can see their baby without this shield in situ.

## Fluid therapy

Each baby should be assessed individually with regards to hydration, sodium levels, urine output, weight and electrolyte balance before extra fluids are given. Breastfeeding where possible should be promoted; it may be necessary to provide top-ups with either expressed breast milk or formula milk after assessing the baby with regards to hydration.

Phototherapy can increase insensible water loss via the skin and loose stools, and some units may consider giving extra fluid to counteract this water loss. If exchange transfusion is required then intravenous fluids are recommended and the baby should be nil by mouth prior to the exchange.

*Rationale:* Exchange transfusion increases risk of necrotising enterocolitis in the bowel. Keeping the infant nil by mouth reduces this potential risk.

## Thermoregulation

Temperature should be monitored closely while the baby is nursed naked under the overhead light. It may be necessary to reduce the incubator temperature as the lights generate heat. This is done on an individual basis.

*Rationale:* To prevent hyper/hypothermia and maintain temperature within the neutral thermal environment.

*Rashes:* May occur as a side-effect to the phototherapy.

## Exchange transfusion

This procedure has become less common with improved phototherapy and the introduction of anti-D immunoglobulin to prevent rhesus isoimmunisation. The level of serum bilirubin that requires an exchange transfusion will vary from unit to unit. The rate that bilirubin increases and age of the baby need to be considered. The procedure is often performed through the umbilical vein and involves removing blood from the circulation in 5- to 20-mL aliquots, and transfusing the same volume of donor blood. A double volume exchange may be required to remove the high level of bilirubin. Refer to unit guidelines for the procedure.

*Rationale:* To reduce the risk of kernicterus.

## ATTACHMENT AND NEONATAL INTENSIVE CARE

The last 20 years have seen much progress in the area of neonatology, and sick neonates who would have previously died are now surviving. This progress is largely due to technological advances in the field and includes improved techniques for artificial ventilation, the use of medications such as exogenous surfactant to minimise ventilatory requirements and maternal steroids, which improve lung maturity in the fetus. Extremely preterm infants are now surviving, but they may require long-term intensive care in the first months of life, which can have an adverse affect on the relationship between parents and infant and, indeed, reduce their ability to bond and form an attachment. These parents may be deprived of the opportunity for early postnatal contact that is experienced by mothers of full-term infants.

An infant born at 24 weeks' gestation may spend the first 4 months of his or her life in the neonatal unit. It is essential not to lose sight of the consequences that long-term separation may have on the parents and infant. Many units have modified the neonatal environment and endeavour to offer developmental care which supports the process of attachment in this high-risk group.

A loving and secure attachment between parents and child is associated with optimal growth and emotional development of the infant. In addition, there is also evidence to suggest that strong attachments between parents and child can help prevent negligence and abuse. Nurses and other healthcare professionals involved in the care of sick and preterm infants should be aware of the importance of attachment and how to promote this during the newborn period, thus helping these infants achieve an optimal outcome. The ability to enhance attachment is linked to an understanding of the attachment process. The concept of attachment

is not clearly defined; Muller[11,p.130] described it as

*... the unique, affectionate relationship that develops between a woman and her infant and persists over time.*

Buus-Frank[12,p.122] stated that

*Nurses have a dual obligation both to understand the pathophysiology of a disease and the human response to that disease. In the critical care environment, it is all too easy, and often socially acceptable, to focus solely on disease management.*

The importance of involving parents in their infant's care can be forgotten, especially in the first days of life when an infant may be critically ill. At this stage the mother may also be unable to visit due to physical problems after delivery. Minimal handling of the infant is a priority and this can extend to excluding maternal touch which could hinder the attachment process.

The unexpected preterm delivery and admission to the neonatal unit of their infant is an extremely stressful time for mothers. They are concerned about the survival of their infant, the fragile appearance, separation, the neonatal intensive care environment and loss of the anticipated maternal role. Mulsow *et al.*[13] noted that mothers who are stressed report less secure attachment with their infants. It therefore seems relevant to explore maternal feelings when interested in learning how to support attachment in the neonatal unit.

Early studies in the 1970s suggested that the first hours and days were crucial to the developing relationship between mother and baby. Separation at this time may interfere with the new mother's feelings towards her baby and she may never achieve a loving closeness with him/her and may even abuse him/her.[14] This critical period for 'bonding' was highly regarded for many years, but it is now disputed that a critical period exists: bonding is a process which can begin at a later stage and develop into successful attachment. However, it seems inadvisable to totally dismiss the importance of earlier research which beneficially influenced clinical practice in maternity units by encouraging maternal infant contact in the early days of life. Bialoskurski[15] explored the nature of attachment in a neonatal intensive care unit and concluded that attachment is not automatic – it may be immediate, delayed or problematic.

Delayed or problematic attachment was more

likely with preterm infants and this was due to many factors, including lack of physical contact and as a coping strategy to limit grief if the infant did not survive. An interesting factor research has identified is that the appearance of a very preterm infant may not conform to the anticipated appearance of a healthy newborn and this can cause problematic attachment.

Staff in neonatal units are very familiar with the appearance of very preterm infants but they should be aware that mothers of these infants do not always find their appearance attractive.

The staff on the neonatal unit can influence the care practices and assist with maternal attachment by improving communication with the mother, facilitating skin-to-skin holding and positive touch when appropriate and engaging with the mother as a partner in her infant's care. Breastfeeding may help with the attachment process and should therefore be encouraged and supported even more than usual in this vulnerable group. Diaries have been successfully used by one Scottish neonatal unit to further include parents in their infants' lives. Neonatal staff should be aware that mothers may be distressed by procedures which are routine to them, for example testing equipment which is beside their infant or moving their infant from an incubator to a cot. Parents are normally informed if their infant has had to move space in the unit but occasionally, in an emergency, this happens without notification and can be very upsetting. This practice should be avoided.

Nurses have a pivotal role in supporting maternal attachment because of their prolonged contact with infant and mother. A loving and secure attachment is important if each preterm infant is to achieve their full potential. Promoting attachment must be an aim of all staff.

# DEVELOPMENTAL CARE

## Introduction

Preterm birth brings about a sudden interruption from the warm protective environment of the womb to the cold, bright and noisy environment of the neonatal unit, thus disrupting the natural development of the brain and sensory systems.[16,17] For many years it was thought that preterm infants were unaware of their environment; however, it is now known that they are in fact very sensitive to stimuli, which can result in long-lasting negative effects.

Developmental care is a philosophy of care which aims to minimise the harmful stimuli, recreating an environment that is closer to that of the womb and so optimising neurological development and leading to a more physiologically stable infant.[17]

## Concept of developmental care

The concept of developmental care is based on the infant being the central recipient of care provided by the family and other healthcare professionals.[17] It incorporates the macro- and micro-environments as well as the relationships between the infant, the family and caregivers.[17] This approach provides individualised care to the infant and is reliant on the caregiver interpreting the infants' physiological and behavioural cues. A well-organised infant will maintain stable saturations, heart rate, respiratory rate, temperature and colour, demonstrating clear sleeping patterns and maintaining good flexion and muscle tone.[17] Whereas an infant who is stressed and over-stimulated will display unstable physiological parameters, motor responses such as finger splaying, facial grimacing and frowning and arm extension.[16] Therefore developmental care should support the infant to maintain stable physiological and emotional behaviour leading to positive growth and development.[16]

## Implementation of developmental care

In order for developmental care to be implemented effectively, all healthcare professionals involved with preterm infants need to have accurate knowledge of their development.[17] Through this knowledge professionals will be better able to read the infant's cues and teach parents, allowing them to be active participants in the developmental care of their infant.[17] The Newborn Individualized Developmental Care and Assessment Program (NIDCAP) is a tool which can be used as an aid in the assessment of the infant's cues and behaviours when implementing developmental care; however, specialist training is required to use it effectively.[17]

In practical terms there is much that can be done to provide an environment that is developmentally supportive, minimising the iatrogenic effects of the neonatal unit.[18] Such developmental care strategies include management of the following:

- light
- noise
- handling/clustering of care
- non-nutritive sucking
- involvement of the family
- positioning.

### Light

For the preterm neonate the retina and visual cortex are the last of the senses to develop and over-stimulation may interfere with the development of the central visual system. The constant bright lights of the neonatal unit also interfere with the development of circadian rhythms, and in order to minimise these effects the amount of light the infant is exposed to can be reduced by covering the incubator with a blanket or specially designed incubator covers which allow staff adequate visualisation of the infant and dimming lights to simulate night and day. While using phototherapy lights, eyes must be covered and the establishment of 'quiet time' when all but essential procedures are ceased and the lights are dimmed will allow the infant time for an afternoon nap.

### Noise

In utero the fetus is exposed to continuous noise of 40–60 decibels (dB), whereas the noise levels in the neonatal unit often exceed 60–90 dB, with an IV pump alarm recording 60–78 dB, closing a porthole 80–111 dB and a pulse oximeter alarm 86 dB. These noise levels can cause hearing loss, as levels above 100 dB may damage cells in the ear and stress induced by noise can lead to apnoea, bradycardia, desaturations and changes in blood pressure resulting in intracranial haemorrhage. Noise levels can be reduced by closing incubator doors quietly, attending to alarms promptly and, as with light reduction, covering the incubator.

### Handling/clustering of care

Handling of the preterm infant can cause stress leading to tachycardia, bradycardia, apnoea, desaturations and aversion behaviour such as crying, squirming and recoiling of limbs. It is therefore important to minimise stress by limiting tactile stimuli, which can be achieved by practising minimal handling and clustering of care and invasive procedures. It is also helpful to arouse the infant to a more awake state by talking to them gently prior to handling, handling gently and avoiding sudden changes of position, thus ensuring that any intervention is better tolerated. If the infant appears to be getting distressed, containment holding can be provided by placing a hand over the infants' trunk, containing limbs until the infant is more relaxed. Parental involvement in providing positive touch should be encouraged and private space for breastfeeding and kangaroo care should be provided.

### Non-nutritive sucking

Non-nutritive sucking on a pacifier has been demonstrated to decrease the time to full oral feeding and to relieve stress during painful procedures such as heel lancing. In a systematic review by Symington and Pinelli[8] positive outcomes were associated with the use of non-nutritive sucking and no negative outcomes were identified.

### Involvement of the family

Involvement of the family is one of most essential parts of developmental care. Communication, and frank, open sharing of information with parents not only helps to reduce the stress and anxiety they may be feeling but also helps them to feel that they are active partners in their infant's care.[17] It is part of the neonatal nurse's role to teach parents how to recognise their infant's cues and behaviours, how to provide appropriate support and aid the establishment of their parental role.[17]

### Positioning

Because preterm infants lack muscle control they are unable to place themselves in a well-flexed position. If left for long periods with limbs extended this can lead to abnormal tone and motor developmental delay; it is important therefore that support measures are used to assist the neonate maintain a curled up, flexed position. The subject of positioning is too wide to be covered here and further reading is recommended.

## Conclusion

Developmental care is a philosophy of care which provides support for positive growth and development of the preterm infant and their family. The care provided should be individualised to the stage of development and should include the macro- and micro-environments. Each healthcare professional should strive to provide developmental care that is evidence based or based on their professional judgement and infants' responses. Developmental care therefore aims to promote and support holistic development of the preterm infant and their family in the neonatal unit and beyond.

# NEONATAL PAIN

Nurses who work in neonatal intensive care units (NICUs) will have to perform many procedures that will cause pain and distress to the baby. Many years of research has helped us to understand how we can manage this pain and distress, and so protect the emotional, psychological and physiological needs of the baby.

Neonates can experience acute pain from brief interventions, such as suctioning, heel lancing or venepuncture, established pain from damage to tissues at sites of heel lancing or extravasation injuries and postoperative pain. They may also experience prolonged pain from inflammatory damage to heels, burns from extravasation injuries, necrotising enterocolitis, meningitis.

Neonates are exposed to this pain and distress by the inevitable repeated procedures, for example:

- ventilation, intubation, continuous positive airways pressure (CPAP);
- insertion of chest drains;
- X-ray;
- lumbar puncture;
- delivery trauma, e.g. cephalhaematoma;
- suprabupic aspiration;
- heel lancing: for blood sugar monitoring, blood gases;
- venepuncture: for intravenous fluids, routine blood assessment;
- arterial stabs: for accurate assessment of blood chemistry;
- endotracheal and nasopharyngeal suctioning;
- nasogastric tube insertion;
- sore bottom;
- routine nursing care in a sick neonate.

Effective measures to help reduce this pain can be easily provided by those caring for neonates.

The more intensive care a baby requires the more it will be repeatedly exposed to these procedures.

## Pain tools

The level of pain experienced is very individual to each neonate, and the unpleasant and emotional experience was defined by Mersky (cited in Ref. 19).

Research of levels of pain and the use of pain tools may assist us in how to recognise this pain, and have been in use for many years.

When a pain tool is chosen it must be suitable for the NICU in which it is to be used, taking into account the level of intensity of the NICU, it must be user friendly, validated from appropriate tools and suitable for nursing and medical staff.[20]

Observing and listening to the baby are our only cues when assessing the level of pain a neonate is experiencing.

The baby's response to pain and distress can be assessed by observing their cry, facial expression, body movement, finger splaying and hand fisting.

If a baby is being monitored, the heart rate, blood pressure saturation monitoring and respiratory changes can be observed as an indication of the level of pain or distress a baby is experiencing. Importance should also be given to how we can console the baby post procedure and how long a baby takes to reorganise itself to a quiet state.

However, the responses we see must be observed in context to the baby's condition, and may not only indicate pain.

### How and what to observe

The sleep and awake state of a baby can influence the level of pain felt by a baby.

### Body movement

By observing motor responses and behavioural reactions in neonates and the movement of their arms, legs, head and torso we can assess how much discomfort a baby is experiencing. By assessing whether a baby is relaxed, restless or showing exaggerated movement, with arching of the back or rigidity, we can question the level of pain, from little discomfort to severe pain. Recently, evidence of finger splaying and hand fisting has been observed as an indication of pain, described by Holsti and Grunau[21] using the Behavioural Indicators of Infant Pain.

## Crying

Crying is a communication to us that a baby wants something or they want something to stop happening. This cry can be heard as a whimper, a vigorous cry or a shrill, moaning or demanding cry. The Neonatal Infant Pain Score, and CRIES (Children's Revised Impact of Event Scale), used to measure neonatal response to postoperative pain, validated by Krechal and Bildner in 1995 (cited in Ref. 22), have been used to aid our assessments of a baby's cry.

Babies who are nursed on neonatal units and ventilated are the babies exposed to the highest levels of pain.

The Distress Scale for Ventilated Newborn Infants (DSVNI) was based upon existing tools. It provides illustrations to help in our assessment of the ventilated infant, and recognising 'the silent cry'.

## Facial expression

Crying can be simultaneously observed with facial expression.[23] We can observe whether the babies have taut tongues and open, stretched mouths or quivering chins and pursed lips, each indicating the level of pain being experienced; observation of the eyes squeezing together, bulging, with furrowing and brow movement all help us to understand babies' pain.

## Vital signs

If a baby is attached to monitors, the heart rate, respiratory rate blood pressure and saturation monitoring will show deviations to baseline observations,[23] which can be due to many factors and prove difficult to assess.

# Managing pain and distress

How we can manage this pain and distress remains a challenge; many drugs are unlicensed for neonatal use, and recent research challenges the use these drugs and the effectiveness of morphine.

There are many ways nurses can comfort babies while procedures are being performed. Careful planning and organisation before and after the procedure, taking into account feed times and rest periods of the baby where possible, will help to minimise their discomfort.

## Comfort measures

Non-pharmacological interventions can be very effective for the relief of pain and distress caused to neonates. There is much evidence to support ways we can provide this comfort. Positioning of the baby, swaddling and containment, and facilitated tucking alongside non-nutritive sucking provided by a dummy can greatly reduce the pain and distress felt by babies. The analgesic effect is thought to be activated via non-opioid pathways and can be combined with sucrose.

Kangaroo care can be provided by parents; this can encourage parents to be involved with their babies.

## Sucrose

The use of sucrose has been well researched and found to be effective in relieving brief episodes of painful procedure. The age at which neonates are administered sucrose is discussed by Johnson et al.[24] A 24 per cent sucrose solution is given prior to a procedure; the administering of sucrose will be variable and set by local policy. The calming and pain-relieving effect as discussed by Stevens et al.[25] is thought to be mediated from endogenous opioid pathways activated by the sweet taste of the sucrose. Small amounts (0.05–0.5 mL) given frequently with a maximum daily amount allows us to use it more effectively. The optimum effect is thought to be at 2 minutes.[25]

# Conclusion

We recognise that despite many years of research neonatal pain is under-managed. As the neonate develops, the neonatal brain remains very vulnerable. The possibility of damage from early repetitive pain experience, and our management of this pain, remains to be researched, if we are to succeed in our management of neonatal pain and prevent the long-term consequences to vulnerable newborn infants.[26]

---

 Go to the website to find the **PowerPoint** presentation for this chapter and MCQs to test your knowledge. **www.hodderplus.com/childnursingskills**

# REFERENCES

1  Leick-Rude M, Bloom L (1998) A comparison of temperature taking methods in neonates. *Neonatal Network* **17**: 21–37.

2  Bailey J, Rose P (2000) Temperature measurement in the preterm infant: a literature review. *Journal of Neonatal Nursing* **6**: 28–33.

3  Hey E (1994) Thermoregulation. In: Avery G, Fletcher M, McDonald M (eds) *Neonatology, path physiology and management of the newborn*, 4th edition. Philadelphia: Lippincot-Raven, pp. 395–406.

4  World Health Organization/UNICEF (2003) *Global strategy for infant and young child feeding*. Geneva: WHO.

5  Heinman H, Schanler RJ (2006) Benefits of maternal and donor human milk for premature infants. *Early Human Development* **82**: 781–787.

6  Spence K (2000) Nutritional management of the infant in the NICU. In: Boxwell G (ed.) *Neonatal intensive care nursing*. London: Routledge, pp. 234–258.

7  Folk L (2007) Guide to capillary heelstick blood sampling in infants. *Advances in Neonatal Care* **7**: 171–178.

8  Hadzic D (2008) Early detection of liver disease in neonates. *Infant* **4**(2): 44–49.

9  Maisels MJ, Watchko JF (2003) Treatment of jaundice in low birthweight infants, *Archives of Disease in Childhood, Fetal and Neonatal Edition* **88**(6): 459–463.

10  Stokowski LA (2006) Fundamentals of phototherapy for neonatal jaundice. *Advances in Neonatal Care* **6**(6): 303–312.

11  Muller ME (1994) A questionnaire to measure mother-to-infant attachment. *Journal of Nursing Measurement* **2**: 129–141.

12  Buus-Frank ME (2004) Everyday inspiration. *Advances in Neonatal Care* **3**: 121–123.

13  Mulsow M, Caldera Y, Pursley M, Reifman A, Huston A (2002) Multilevel factors influencing maternal stress during the first three years. *Journal of Marriage and Family* **64**: 944–956.

14  Klaus MH, Kennell JH (1976) *Maternal–infant bonding*. St Louis: Mosby.

15  Bialoskurski M, Cox CL, Hayes JA (1999) The nature of attachment in a neonatal intensive care unit. *Journal of Perinatal and Neonatal Nursing* **13**: 66–75.

16  Vandenberg KA (2007) Individualized developmental care for high risk newborns in the NICU: a practice guideline. *Early Human Development* **83**: 433–432.

17  Aita M, Snider L (2003) The art of developmental care in the NICU: a concept analysis. *Journal of Advanced Nursing* **41**(3): 223–232.

18  Symington A, Pinelli J (2006) Developmental care for promoting development and preventing morbidity in preterm infants. *The Cochrane Database of Systematic Reviews* **2**: CD00181.

19  Sparshott M (1996) The development of a clinical distress scale for ventilated newborn infants: identification of pain and distress based on validated behavioural scores. *Journal of Neonatal Nursing* **12**:5–11.

20  Halima S (2003) Pain management in nursing procedures on premature babies. *Journal of Advanced Nursing* **42**: 587–597.

21  Holsti L, Grunau R, (2007) Initial validation of the Behavioural Indicators of Infant Pain (BIIP). *Pain* **132**(3): 264–272.

22  Franck LS, Miaskowski C (1997) Measurement of neonatal responses to painful stimuli: a research review. *Journal of Pain and Symptom Management.* **14**(6): 343–378.

23  Stevens B, Johnston C, Petryshen P, Taddio A (1996) Premature infant pain profile: development and initial validation. *Clinical Journal of Pain* **12**(1): 13–22.

24  Johnston *et al.* (2002) Routine sucrose analgesia during the first week of life in neonates younger than 31 weeks post conceptual age. *Pediatrics* **110**:523–528.

25  Stevens B, Gibbins S (2001) Mechanisms of sucrose and non-nutritive sucking in procedural pain management in infants. Pain Research & Management: *The Journal of the Canadian Pain Society* **6**(1): 2.

26  Grunau RVE, Tu MT (2007) Long term consequences of pain in human neonates. In: Anand KJS, Stevens BJ, McGrath PJ (eds) *Pain in neonates and infants*, 3rd edition, *Pain Research and Clinical Management*, London: Elsevier, pp. 45–55.

# FURTHER READING

Jones E, King C (2005) *Feeding and nutrition in the preterm infant*. Edinburgh: Elsevier.

Lang S (2002) *Breastfeeding special care babies*, London: Bailliere Tindall.

Young J (1996) *Developmental care of the premature baby*. London: Baillière Tindall.

## CHAPTER 30

# Managing children and young people with mental health problems

Colman Noctor

## LEARNING OUTCOMES

*Upon completion of this chapter, the reader should be able to accomplish the following:*

1 Understand the complexity of mental health and mental illness
2 Understand the different approaches and understanding of mental health
3 Appreciate the communication and emotional needs of children with mental health problems
4 Understand the different mental health disorders that may present in the paediatric hospital

## CHAPTER OVERVIEW

When one thinks about mental health and mental illness we are sometimes automatically drawn to our preconceived assumptions as to what these terms mean. Perhaps we think of someone who is talking to themselves in the street or perhaps a high-profile celebrity who is reported to be in rehab for alcohol dependence or an eating disorder. Although these are aspects of mental 'disorder', the concept of 'mental health' is somewhat different. It is perhaps helpful to consider that mental health, mental health problems and mental illness exist on a spectrum, each not mutually exclusive to the other. One's degree of mental health oscillates on a constant basis and therefore there may be periods

of our lives where our mental health may move along a continuum towards mental health problems or in some cases mental illness. This is not only possible but probable with young people as the statistics show that one in five young people suffer from mental health problems.[1]

It is worthwhile therefore investing some time attempting to understand the concept of mental health, even if one is not directly involved in the Child & Adolescent Mental Health Services. This chapter is aimed at children's nurses and much of the material will surround issues that may arise within the specific clinical area of paediatrics. First, we must define a differentiation between the terms mental health, mental health problems and mental illness.

## FACTORS AFFECTING MENTAL HEALTH

There are many questions and theories about why mental health problems exist in some people and not in others. The biological, social and psychological schools all differ somewhat in their views on this discussion. Much of a person's degree of mental health can be judged on their ability to cope with life stressors. There are some schools of thought, e.g. attachment theory, that believe the experiences of our formative years greatly influence our ability to cope, form relationships and function in later life. Theorists who subscribe to attachment

## Definitions

**Attachment theory:** Refers to the study of the affectionate bonds that infants form with their caregivers that endure across time and situations.[3]

**Mental health:** A state of wellbeing in which the individual realises his or her own abilities, can cope with the stresses of daily life, can work productively and fruitfully, and is able to make a contribution to his or her community.

**Mental health problems:** A situational or developmental condition which causes short-term distress and impaired functioning.

**Mental illness:** A condition that causes alterations in thinking, mood or behaviour that leads to more severe and long-term distress and impaired functioning or disability.[2]

**Somatoform disorders:** Involves the conversion of anxiety symptoms into physical symptoms.

theories feel this is a major influence on one's long-term mental functioning.[4] Other schools are more concerned with the influence of the social contexts and suggest that it is one's environment and psychosocial circumstances that are central to predicting later coping styles and mental health. Furthermore, the medical or biological theorists argue that the influence of genetics and neurobiology contain the most accurate explanations for mental illness. Perhaps it is worth considering that a combination of the above suggestions might form an eclectic criteria of factors that serve to protect or increase the risk of mental illness, and it is this combined view that will form the basis for this chapter (Table 30.1).

## MENTAL HEALTH PRESENTATIONS IN THE PAEDIATRIC SETTING

In describing the nursing care of mental health disorders it is desirable that these treatments take

> **KEY POINTS**
>
> Mental health problems can exist in all ages across the young person's lifespan. This can manifest in sleeping, feeding and behavioural problems in infants to actual psychological pathology such as eating disorders, depression and suicidal behaviours presenting in adolescence.

place in a purpose-built child and adolescent mental health service with fully trained personnel and all of the required resources. Unfortunately, this is not always the case and, much of the time, young people with these difficulties will present to paediatric hospitals or children's units in adult hospitals, making it necessary for their treatment and management to be carried out in these environments. For the purpose of this chapter we will draw on the author's experience of working as a clinical nurse specialist in a paediatric setting and attempt to describe various clinical skills and observations that are both important and possible within such settings.

**Table 30.1** Factors affecting mental health and illness

| | |
|---|---|
| Protective factors against mental illness | Emotional resilience<br>A sense of hopefulness about the future<br>Feeling respected, valued and supported<br>Having strong networks and social inclusion |
| Risk factors for mental illness | Poverty<br>Emotional abuse or neglect<br>Parents with mental health problems<br>Chronic illness or disability |

Health Education Authority[5]

# MOOD DISORDERS

## Depression

Affective disorders are characterised by distortions of a person's mood. The most common of these disorders is depression. Depression becomes a pathological disorder when the symptoms persist for longer than a 2-week period, being experienced every day.[6] Often the adolescent will complain of a disturbed sleep pattern, eating pattern and/or a lack of enjoyment in previously enjoyed activities. Depressed or lowered mood can lead to self-harm and suicidal behaviours, although these presentations can exist in the absence of a depressive disorder also.

### Diagnostic and statistical manual IV criteria for depression

- Five or more of the following symptoms being present for a 2-week period being experienced nearly every day and representing a change in functioning.
- At least one of the symptoms must be either depressed mood or a loss of interest or pleasure in previously enjoyed activities.
  - Depressed mood: in children and adolescents can be irritable mood.
  - Markedly diminished interest in almost all daily activities.
  - Significant weight loss or gain or decrease or increase in appetite.
  - Insomnia or hypersomnia.
  - Psychomotor agitation or retardation.
  - Fatigue or loss of energy.
  - Feelings of worthlessness or excessive guilt.
  - Poor concentration.
  - Suicidal ideation or recurrent thoughts of death.[6]

### Treatment

Initial psychological treatment (either cognitive behavioural therapy, family therapy or interpersonal psychotherapy) should be offered for up to 3 months and should be the first line of treatment.

If the psychological symptoms have not improved within 6 weeks then antidepressant medication should be considered cautiously, especially in the younger age groups.

Clinical follow-up and 'booster sessions' of therapy may be helpful to prevent relapse.[7]

## Suicide and deliberate self-harm

Deliberate self-harm (DSH) includes two separate concepts:

1 deliberate self-poisoning (including overdoses);
2 deliberate self-injury: described as intentional self-injury, irrespective of the apparent purpose of the act. It may include scratching, punching, kicking, head-banging and cutting.

A recent Irish study showed that a lifetime history of DSH was reported by 9.1 per cent of adolescents. DSH was more common among females (13.9 per cent) than males (4.3 per cent) and self-cutting (66.0 per cent) and overdose (35.2 per cent) were the most common methods used.[9] These descriptions might cause you to ask why someone would take part in this behaviour?

Possible reasons or motivators for this behaviour include:

- a coping strategy for emotional pain or distress;
- a limited or primitive expression of distress;
- to feel real;
- to express anger, relieve tension or punish self or others;
- to feel in control;
- a cry for help or need for attention;
- as self-preservation/suicide prevention.[8]

Observable features of suicidal children include:
- marked changes in personality;
- sudden changes in sleeping or eating patterns;
- marked decline in school performance;
- loss of interest in activities;
- poor concentration;
- unusually disruptive or rebellious behaviour;
- inability to tolerate praise;
- social withdrawal;
- lack of concern about their appearance;
- death or suicide themes dominate written, artistic or creative work;
- impulsivity.[8]

### Treatment

Following any suicide attempt by a child, brief therapeutic interventions involving families should be considered.

Children who have self-harmed need to be assessed for any mental health problems and if any are identified they need to be treated as appropriate.

For young people who repeatedly self-harm, they should be given the additional intervention of group psychotherapy.

In assessing a young person presenting with self-harm, seriousness of intent needs to be assessed whatever the degree of self-harm.[7]

Nursing someone who is depressed can be an anxiety-provoking task. Some nurses verbalise being afraid of saying something wrong. It is important to remember the value of 'being with' as opposed to 'doing for' when it comes to caring for young people with mental health problems. Often young people will identify a time when a nurse sat with them and chatted with them as being really useful in distracting them from their sadness. When this acknowledgement for this intervention was given back to the nurse she replied 'Why? I did nothing'. However, there are also some practical clinical needs that need to be identified in order to care for a young person with a depressive disorder and suicidal behaviour.

### Clinical skills: depression and suicidal behaviour

- Providing a safe environment. This implies that the young person feels contained in your care. Where impulsivity and perhaps suicidal impulses are present it is important for the nurse to impart a sense of safety for the young person by removing any possible routes of harm from the immediate environment and being available to support them from their own thoughts.
- Organise a system of regular close observation.
- Be aware of the young person's activities at all tim, especially during unstructured times. Sometimes if there is considered to be a significant risk, some young people will be placed on one-to-one observations. However, even if this is not the case, close supervision is essential. This must continue even after the young person's mood begins to lift as this is also a potential time for suicide or self-injury.[10]
- Encourage the young person to mix with peers of a similar age on the unit milieu and discourage long periods of withdrawal or isolation.
- Try to maintain sleep hygiene by promoting sleeping and waking times akin to someone of the young person's age.
- Encourage the young person to attend to their physical needs and monitor and record these. Low mood can cause apathy towards self-care

and it is important the young person is supported with this issue.
- Spend time with the young person exploring different activities to assist in distracting them from rumination.
- Encourage healthy activities and reinforce any sense of acomplishment or positivity.
- Use a moderate tone of voice and try to avoid being overly cheerful.[10] Use silence and active listening and convey concern and interest in the young person's feelings.
- Avoid asking too many questions and try not to press the young person for information. Allow the young person to cry and try not to limit this behaviour for the sake of your own sense of feeling comfortable.
- Do not belittle the young person's feelings and give support to expressions of emotion.
- Help the young person examine problem-solving and possible options looking at the consequences of each alternative.
- Help the young person to find some confidence in their abilities and try to instil hope for the future.[10]
- Involve the young person's family where deemed appropriate and remember that families may not always be part of the problem but more often than not they are always part of the solution.
- Encourage the young person to have a voice in their care plan and advocate their views regarding their treatment plans and medication, etc., to multidisciplinary colleagues.
- Respect each young person as an individual in their own right.
- Encourage the young person to pursue personal interests.
- Explore activities according to their own world and points of interest.
- Validate their individuality and examine their priorities as opposed to just what you might think is best

## ANXIETY DISORDERS

Anxiety is a core problem in both children and adolescents. Anxiety can take many forms and manifests in a number of disorders.
- *Generalised anxiety disorder* (GAD): This presentation features free-floating states of

anxiety in social situations. GAD may also feature the presence of panic attacks or avoidance behaviours.

- *Phobia*: Here there is a specific situation or object where fear is located. This could be a fear of specific social situations or leaving home, e.g. social phobia or school phobia.
- *Conversion disorders*: Here the anxiety is manifested in a physical symptom such as abdominal pain, headache or hysterical paralysis.
- *Obsessive–compulsive disorders*: Here the child feels compelled to carry out rituals in order to manage their anxiety. These rituals include repetitive behaviours which can surround themes of safety, germs, contamination or sexual disturbance. Here the child experiences intrusive thoughts and must act out the ritual in order to cope with these disturbing cognitions.
- *Tourette's syndrome*: Although sometimes portrayed for comedic value in the media, Tourette's syndrome is a serious disorder characterised by a series of motor and vocal tics. These tics are characterised by involuntary movements and/or verbal outbursts that are disturbing for the sufferer and make the task of socialisation very difficult for the young person. There are varying degrees of severity of Tourette's syndrome and many mild cases go undetected.[11]

### Treatment

Behaviour therapy and cognitive behaviour therapy (CBT) (individual or group) should be the first line of treatment for phobias, GADs and obsessive–compulsive disorders.

Parents need to be actively involved in these therapeutic interventions especially in children under 11 years of age.[7]

Educational support is also recommended in children with anxiety problems.[12]

### Clinical skills and interventions: anxiety disorders

- Try to ensure that the environment is predictable and inform the young person of any changes to routine. When panic attacks occur, sit with the young person and reassure them that this episode will pass.
- Provide external control by being firm but caring where necessary.

- Maintain a quiet, safe environment for the patient to reduce external stimuli.[13]
- Monitor sleeping patterns, eating patterns and mood changes. Record any alterations in these aspects of the young person's presentation that may be due to anxiety levels.
- Inform the young person of what is happening where possible (much anxiety is caused by the unknown).
- Provide the young person with timetables if they find visual aids helpful.
- Meet with the young person at the beginning of the day to plan activities.
- Set small, surmountable weekly and daily goals that the young person must aim to achieve and reward effort as opposed to just achievement.
- Encourage the use of a reflective journal indicating the frequency and severity of anxiety thoroughout the day, therefore allowing you to investigate any patterns to their anxiety and possible triggers in their environment.
- Be with the young person when they are anxious.
- Provide regular reassurance and support that they are doing well.
- Help them to identify triggers for their anxiety and commend them when they successfully manage to self-soothe themselves.
- Teach the young person strategies to manage their anxiety like relaxation, deep breathing and relaxation tapes.
- Inform the young person of changes in their treatment plan.
- Allow the young person to identify potential stressors and support a gradual desensitisation programme to overcome the feared scenario.
- Appreciate the young person's individual perception of the anxiety-provoking situations.
- Acknowledge that this fear is real to them and do not dismiss this on account of your own perceptions.
- Encourage the young person to challenge negative thoughts about themselves and concentrate on their individual strengths as well as difficulties.[13]

## AUTISTIC SPECTRUM DISORDERS

Collectively known as pervasive developmental disorders, these disorders exist on a spectrum varying from autism and Asperger's syndrome to pervasive developmental delay. These disorders are characterised by significant social, communication and behavioural problems[14] the most severe being autism. Early identification is essential.[14] Autism is suggested to be a lifelong neurodevelopmental disorder in which about 60 per cent of sufferers are unable to lead an independent life. Autism occurs in 2–5 per 10 000 children and occurs three times more in males.[14] These children can have sensitivities in the areas of noise, crowds and have many specific sensory-motor needs. These symptoms persist in less severe forms across the spectrum of pervasive developmental disorders.

Diagnostic and statistical manual (DSM) IV criteria for autism includes

- impairment in social interaction characterised by poor eye contact, facial expressions, ability to form friendships with peers of a similar age, lack of a spontaeity in seeking to share an activity and lack of emotional reciprocity;
- impairment in communication by delay or lack of spoken language or inability to sustain conversations with others, with repetitive or idiosyncratic use of language and lack of imaginative play;
- restricted repetitive patterns of behaviour, preoccupation with restricted patterns of interest which appears abnormal in intensity or focus, inflexible adherence to fixed routines, repetitive motor actions (like finger flapping) and persistant preoccupation with parts of objects onset prior to 3 years of age.[6]

### Treatment

Intensive behavioural interventions need to be considered to improve the adaptive functioning of children with autism.

Medication is not indicated in the treatment of autism but may help alleviate some of the behaviours associated with autism.[7]

### Clinical skills and interventions: autistic spectrum disorders

- Provide as safe and predicable an environment as possible minimising noise and any posibilities of over-stimulus.
- Closely observe for any triggers of discomfort for the young person.

- Limit the number of individuals communicating with the young person and always communicate with someone familiar where possible.
- Observe for distress and manage any outbursts using only professional clinical holding procedures.
- Observe sleeping, eating and encourage the young person's self-care.
- Adhere to the young person's structure as much as possible.
- Avoid last minute changes to plans. Give the young person sufficent notice of any activities or interventions.
- Spend time with the young person and role model good social interaction.
- Communicate in an age-appropriate manner.
- Give praise to progress noted and minimise any mistakes.
- Engage the young person in activities that they are willing to take part in.
- Establish an understanding of any symbolic speech.
- Be congruent between body language, tone of voice and demeanour when communicating with this young person.
- Appreciate the limited ability of the young person's communication style.
- Speak clearly and ascertain whether the young person is attending to you.
- Never shout or raise your voice around the young person.
- Encourage a variety of interests and respect the young person's views, opinions and individuality.

## ATTENTION DEFICIT HYPERACTIVITY DISORDER

Attention deficit hyperactivity disorder (ADHD) is a condition in which a child has difficulty controlling some aspects of his/her behaviour leading to three major symptoms: inattention, hyperactivity and impulsivity.

Children who present as predominantly inattentive find it hard to keep their mind on tasks and they can get bored or distracted easily. These children also appear to not listen and have difficulty following through with instructions. They may struggle to finish tasks and be disorganised. However, these children can give effortless attention to something they enjoy, such as computer games.

Children who present as predominantly hyperactive tend to be moving all the time, they may struggle to sit still and squirm and fidget while sitting. They can often be over-talkative and often cannot play quietly.

Children who present as predominantly impulsive tend to do things without thinking, for example blurt out inappropriate answers, interrupt other people and find it hard to take turns.[16]

There are four different types of ADHD; these are

1 predominantly inattentive
2 predominantly hyperactive–impulsive
3 combined type
4 ADHD not otherwise specified.

(In order to diagnose ADHD there needs to be an exclusion of a psychosis or Asperger's syndrome diagnosis.)[16]

*DSM IV criteria* include:

- predominantly inattentive or hyperactive–impulsive;
- combined features;
- age less than 7 years;
- minimum of 6-month history of disturbance and in more that two settings;
- disturbance in social, academic and occupational functioning.[2]

### Treatment

If diagnostic criteria for ADHD are met following a comprehensive assessment by a suitably qualified professional, and other reasons for the behaviour have been excluded, then a trial of stimulant medication is indicated as the first line of intervention.

If there is insufficient response with the medication then individual behavioural therapy both in school and at home should be added.

Effective monitoring of children given medication is needed to minimise adverse side-effects and optimise treatment benefit.[6]

### Clinical skills and interventions: attention deficit hyperactivity disorder

- Many young people with ADHD will benefit from clear rules and direction.

- A firm and understanding approach will establish a good therapeutic relationship where the young person will feel understood and therefore safer.
- Managing the environment by reducing stimulus and redirecting the young person before things get too excitable are often the most effective strategies.
- Discuss with the young person how they are feeling and monitor their mood as it is common that young people with ADHD can have low self-esteem and may feel very negative towards themselves.
- Monitor their behaviour and supervise them closely as sometimes hyperactive behaviour can result in accidental injury to the young person or others.
- Young people with ADHD need structure. Ensure that activities are of short duration and varied. The tendency to be easily distracted will work against the young person and therefore the management of their time and their environment is essential to effective functioning.
- Look for the young person behind the difficult behaviour and attempt to draw them out.
- The more that the positive aspects of the child are recognised the more they will be noticeable. Often it is easy to fall into a pattern of constant limit setting and sanctions with these young people and it is important to avoid this where possible.
- Give the young person small goals and responsibilities and reward good behaviour.
- Acknowledge when they appear to be managing well and praise wherever possible.
- Reassure and support the young person to stop and think.
- Teach them the skills of problem solving and encourage them to see things from others' perspective.

Contrary to what some will think, not all young people with ADHD are naughty. Many young people who are diagnosed with ADHD convey a real sense of sadness when they are discussing how they feel. Many are remorseful about the consequences of their behaviour and feel they cannot control their impulses, and so tend to get into a lot of trouble. When caring for someone with ADHD one needs to understand the young person's predicament and try to form an alliance with them so as to improve behaviours as opposed to commencing a series of battles.

# EATING DISORDERS

As we all use food in Western society as a form of emotional currency, i.e. for reward, punishment and bribery, it is not surprising that this association can get entangled with mental health problems and underlying unhappiness. Food can become the vehicle for powerful emotional transactions and so this is sometimes reflected in a power struggle of a more serious nature in the form of anorexia nervosa. The onset of adolescence coupled with additional stressors such as conflict in the family, separation problems or tense relationships can contribute to the development of anorexia nervosa.[17] Invariably these children are perfectionistic, highly self-critical, with a drive to please others.[17] There are a number of different types of eating disorders but perhaps the most likely to be encountered in the role of a sick children's nurse is anorexia nervosa.

The *DSM IV criteria* defines anorexia nervosa as follows:

- refusal to maintain body weight at or above a normal weight for height (e.g. weight leading to maintenance less than 85 per cent of that expected);
- intense fear of gaining weight or becoming fat, even though underweight;
- disturbance in the way one's body or shape is experienced, undue influence of body weight on self-evaluation, or denial of the seriousness of current low body weight;
- in post-menarche females, amenorrhoea, i.e. the absence of at least three consecutive menstrual cycles.[6]

### Treatment

Therapies to be considered for the psychological treatment of anorexia nervosa include cognitive analytic therapy (CAT), CBT, interpersonal psychotherapy (IPT) and family interventions focused explicitly on eating disorders. Patient and, where appropriate, carer preference should be taken into account in deciding which psychological treatment is to be offered. The aims of psychological treatment should be to reduce risk, to encourage weight gain and healthy eating, to reduce other symptoms related to an eating disorder and to facilitate psychological and physical recovery.

Family therapy is recognised as the treatment of choice for anorexia nervosa as an outpatient or after inpatient treatment.

Behavioural treatment should be considered in hospital to increase weight.

Early identification of anorexia is recommended with refeeding where necessary.[7]

## NICE guidelines for the inpatient care of children and adolescents with anorexia nervosa

Most children with anorexia nervosa can be treated effectively on an outpatient basis. However, the condition of some children deteriorates significantly to warrant an inpatient admission. The goal of inpatient treatment is to manage the immediate threat to the young person's physical and mental health, weight restoration and providing a context for the first stage of family-based treatment.[15,18]

For inpatients with anorexia nervosa, a structured symptom-focused treatment regimen with the expectation of weight gain should be provided in order to achieve weight restoration. It is important to carefully monitor the patient's physical status during refeeding. Psychological treatment should be provided which has a focus both on eating behaviour and attitudes to weight and shape, and on wider psychosocial issues with the expectation of weight gain. Rigid inpatient behaviour modification programmes should not be used in the management of anorexia nervosa.[18]

Family interventions that directly address the eating disorder should be offered to children and adolescents with anorexia nervosa. Children and adolescents with anorexia nervosa should be offered individual appointments with a healthcare professional separate from those with their family members or carers. The therapeutic involvement of siblings and other family members should be considered in all cases because of the effects of anorexia nervosa on other family members. In children and adolescents with anorexia nervosa, the need for inpatient treatment and the need for urgent weight restoration should be balanced alongside the educational and social needs of the young person.[18]

In most patients with anorexia nervosa, an average weekly weight gain of 0.5–1 kg in inpatient settings and 0.5 kg in outpatient settings should be an aim of treatment. This requires about 3500–7000 extra calories a week. Regular physical monitoring, and in some cases treatment with a multivitamin/multimineral supplement in oral form, is recommended for people with anorexia nervosa during both inpatient and outpatient weight restoration. Total parenteral nutrition should not be used for people with anorexia nervosa, unless there is significant gastrointestinal dysfunction.[18]

Feeding against the will of the patient should be an intervention of last resort in the care and management of anorexia nervosa. Feeding against the will of the patient is a highly specialised procedure requiring expertise in the care and management of those with severe eating disorders and the physical complications associated with it. This should only be done in the context of the Mental Health Act 1983 or Children Act 1989. When making the decision to feed against the will of the patient, the legal basis for any such action must be clear.[18]

### Clinical skills and interventions

- In order to work effectively with a young person with anorexia nervosa one must establish a model of understanding for the illness. Remember, anorexia nervosa is about feelings and not just about food. It is believed that the actions of the anorexic adolescent and the pursuit of thinness is a measure of their need for control rather than an act of misguided vanity. In order to effectively engage with the young person and form the therapeutic alliance so as to assist in the recovery of the young person, a model of understanding this psychological dimension of the disorder needs to be achieved.
- Meals and snacks are major sources of anxiety for the young person; therefore, the arrival and organisation of these periods need to be both punctual and respectful. A goal of recovery from anorexia is to have a healthy attitude towards food, so some element of variety and less structured menu plans may be required. Weigh-ins need to be carried out at the same time and under the same conditions. There must be clarity about the meal plan so as to prevent the anorexic ambivilance to corrupt any pre-agreed plans.
- This should be gradual as the young person improves and gains the ability to manage more choice and responsibility. Restrictions on food choices, supervision and exersise can be gradually handed back to the young person at a rate which he or she can manage. Involve the family in the recovery process and eduacte them to assist in this journey.
- Respect the young person for their individual history and attempt to establish the role of anorexia in his or her life. Anorexia serves the role of both friend and foe and therefore each young person will have a unique relationship with their symptoms. Explore the rationale for this need and examine alternative ways of achieving these goals.
- This is essential to the psychological progress that the young person should make in tandem with the concurrent weight gain. The nurse must provide pre- and post-meal support to the young person in whatever way is deemed helpful. Some young people respond well to discussing the task ahead or gone by, where others will benefit from distraction techniques instead. Supporting a young person to eat, gain weight and hand over the control of his or her anorectic symptom is incredibly difficult for them; therefore copious amounts of support may be necessary.

**KEY POINTS**

Owing to the ambivalence and control worries displayed by the young person with anorexia they may attempt to split their team of carers so as to preserve their desire for thinness and weight loss. This has the potential to cause considerable interpersonal dynamics in the team; therefore, an open and high level of inter-team communication and clinical supervision is essential if these dynamics are to be managed effectively.

## SOMATOFORM DISORDERS

Some young people have difficulty expressing emotions and dealing with interpersonal conflict in a direct manner. This difficulty may manifest in various physical symptoms that are related to emotional or psychiatric problems.[10] Although there is no explainable organic cause for the pain or distress, the discomfort, pain or symptoms are experienced as very real to the sufferer. Prevalence rates vary between 2 and 10 per cent of children.[15] These pains typically occur in the gastrointestinal area or headaches and/or tiredness. The most notable somatoform presentation in children is recurrent abdominal pain.

This disorder is characterised by numerous complaints of severe tummy pain that proves benign on all physical investigations. It is believed that this pain, although real to the child, has origins in a psychological disturbance or anxiety and therefore the intervention needs to address this psychological difficulty in order to be effective. Other somatoform disorders include irritable bowel syndrome, cyclical vomiting syndrome and pains in the limbs.[15]

### Treatment

Cognitive behavioural therapy should be considered for recurrent abdominal pain.

If attention to diet has not covered, a high-fibre diet is also recommended for recurrent abdominal pain.[7]

### Clinical skills and interventions

- The child may be anxious that they are suffering from an undetected serious physical illness so in order to contain this anxiety you must supportively communicate that a number of tests have been done and despite their pain they are in no danger of serious illness or death.
- Assess the child's current range of activity and establish pre-morbid activity levels and sources of enjoyment.
- Gradually introduce small tasks to increase the child's range of activity.
- Allow certain time periods for the child to discuss their symptoms as opposed to total prohibition of the discussion.
- Ask the child about their perception of their symptoms. Do not argue or overly challenge their statements.
- Try to make links between possible stressors in the child's life and the onset or trigger of symptoms.

- Give positive feedback when the young person focuses on emotional and interpersonal issues as opposed to physical symptoms.
- Teach the young person relaxation techniques and problem-solving skills in order to manage and name stress.
- Acknowledge that the young person's experience of the symptom is real to them without colluding with their beliefs surrounding its origins.
- Involve family members in creating a framework for understanding the young person's difficulties.
- Generally build up a repertoire of acomplishments that the young person has managed with support.
- Encourage that they have influence over their symptoms in relation to reducing stress and a concurrent reduction in symptoms and increasing stress and a coresponding exacerbation of symptoms.
- Try and get the child to name and discuss the stressors in their life so that their difficulties can be verbalised through language as opposed to enacted via the symptom.[10]

# CORE SKILLS IN CHILD AND ADOLESCENT MENTAL HEALTH

## Assessment

A comprehensive assessment is vital in assessing the needs of the child and their family. Because mental state is constantly changing and rarely static, assessments can be momentary and change dramatically very quickly. It is therefore important to revisit assessments and reassess throughout your contact with a child or adolescent with mental health difficulties. Consideration should be given to interviewing the young person alone without their parents (especially in the case of adolescents). However, when you are interviewing an adolescent, it is important to explain the considerations of confidentiality and your obligation to report to their parents any information that is potentially harmful to the young person or other people. Collateral histories from parents and schools are also important in obtaining a comprehensive view of the young person but should only be sought with their permission.[8]

### Information required for a comprehensive mental health assessment of a young person presenting with mental health difficulties

#### Demographic data

Name, address, parents' names and occupations, who lives at home, general practitioner or referrer details.

#### Family structure/genogram (family tree)

How many people are in the family? Ages of each person? Biological parents/step-parents? Are there any extended family members living at home?

It is important that the beginning of the interview does not begin with immediate attention to the problems the young person is experiencing. This can often involve a considerable amount of blame and can set the interaction off to a negative beginning and negatively effect subsequent interactions.

#### Family history

Any history of mental illness in the family? Does the child remind parents of any other family members?

Any events or triggers in the family context preceding the onset of the young person's difficulties, i.e. bereavement, house move, separation, divorce.

#### Child's developmental history

Were there any problems during pregnancy? What type of birth or delivery occurred? What was the young person's sleeping patterns like as an infant? Were there any weaning/feeding problems? What time did the child begin crawling, walking, talking, mastering toileting, motor skills? What was the child's sociability history like? Were there any notable issues around attachment or separation in the child's formative years?

Given the importance of attachment disruption and its effects on coping and mental health and the importance of the first 2 years of life, these questions will establish any early concerns or abnormal behaviours and also track the developmental history of the child and highlight any developmental delays that are so pertinent in suggesting a multitude of children's mental health difficulties.

#### Medical history

Has the child any allergies or chronic illnesses? Has the child ever been sick of hospitalised?

Has the child been treated for mental health problems in the past? If so, what treatment was prescribed and what were the effects of it?

#### Presenting problems

Why has the child attended this service? When did the identified behaviour or concern begin? How long has it been occurring? What are the frequency, intensity and severity of the young person's difficulties? Has anything that has been tried to help to manage these problems worked? How do the parents and young person understand these issues?

#### School performance and history

When did the young person begin school/nursery? How did they settle in? How has school been since then? Are there any recent changes in the young person's performance, application or willingness to attend school? Is there a history of bullying, expulsion or behavioural concerns?

#### Other professional involvement

Has there been any other professional involvement, e.g. social worker, educational officer, juvenile liaison officer or therapist?

#### Family's hopes and expectations of the service

What are the priorities for the family and young person? What would they like to happen? Does the young person share their concerns? Do they recognise that there are any changes needed? Are the family and young person motivated to work to improve the situation?[8]

## Risk assessment

In order to assess the possible risk to the young person or other people it is important to be cognisant of the following:

- What is the quality of the young person's network of support?
- What is this young person's coping strategies and self-regulatory ability?
- Is there any stress at home?
- Is there possible communication with a responsible other and does the young person have access to that support?
- Is there any immediate risk to their safety?[8]

## Observation

Alongside the information gathered by the comprehensive assessment, there are also the observational data that the nurse must take heed of during their interaction with the young person and their family. The following is a useful schema designed by Cooper *et al.*[8] for assessment of a parent–child relationship.

### Aspects to consider

- The parent's confidence in their own parenting skills.
- Their ability to set limits.
- Their consistency of approach.

### General attitude of the parents

- Are they warm/hostile to the child?
- Does the parent 'cue' in to the child?
- Is the parent 'child-centred'?
- How do the parents gain cooperation or are they coercive?
- Does the parent understand the developmental stage of the child?
- How would you best describe the parent's emotional health?

### The child

- Are they physically well, appropriate height/weight? Happy or sad?

- What kind of temperament does the child have? Active/passive? Emotionally labile or easy?
- What is the child's concentration level? Attention? Speech and language? Comprehension? Use of gesture? Vocabulary? Pronunciation?
- Can the child cope with frustration?
- Can they distinguish reality from fantasy?
- Assess the child's motor movement. Are they clumsy?

### Assess

- Fine motor control
- Play skills/ hobbies
- Ability to engage in creative play
- Whether the play/hobbies are appropriate to their developmental level
- Whether they persevere at play/hobbies
- Interaction with parents, siblings, staff, other children
- Ability to follow rules
- Waiting
- Turn taking
- Acceptance of losing
- Acceptance of criticism or praise
- Separation from their parents
- Listening or following instructions
- What the eye contact is from parent to child? Child to parent? With staff?
- Whether they have the skills to negotiate with their parents and whether it works.[8]

 Go to the website to find the PowerPoint presentation for this chapter and MCQs to test your knowledge. **www.hodderplus.com/childnursingskills**

## REFERENCES

1 Mental Health Foundation UK (1999) *Bright futures*. London: Mental Health Foundation.
2 World Health Organization (2001) *Mental health: strengthening mental health promotion*. WHO: Geneva.
3 Ainsworth M, Blehar M, Waters E, Wall S (1978). *Patterns of attachment*. Hillsdale, NJ: Erlbaum.
4 Liekiman M, Urban E (1999) The roots of child and adolescent psychotherapy in psychoanalysis. In:

Lanyado M, Horne A (eds) *The handbook of child and adolescent psychotherapy: psychoanalytic approaches*. London: Routledge, pp. 19–31.
5 Health Education Authority (1997) *Mental health promotion: a quality framework*. London: HEA.
6 American Psychiatric Association (2000) *Diagnostic and statistical manual of mental disorders* (DSM-IV-TR), 4th edition (text revision). Washington DC: APA.

7   Wolpert M, Fuggle P, Cottrell D (2006) *Drawing from the evidence, advice for professionals working with children and adolescents*, 2nd edition. London: CAMHS Publications.

8   Cooper M, Hooper C, Thompson M (2005) *Child and adolescent mental health theory and practice*. London: Oxford University Press.

9   Morey C, Corcoran P, Arensman E, Perry I (2008) The prevalence of self-reported deliberate self-harm in Irish adolescents. *BioMed Central Public Health* 8:79.

10  Schultz JM, Videbeck SL (2005) *Lippincott's manual of psychiatric nursing care plans*, 7th edition. Philadelphia: Lippincott.

11  Lynch G (2008) In: Morrisey J, Keogh B, Doyle L (2008) *Childhood and adolescent mental health problems. Psychiatric/mental health nursing an Irish perspective*. Dublin: Gill & McMillan.

12  Barker P (2003) *Psychiatric and mental health nursing*. The craft of caring. London: Arnold.

13  Shives LR (2005) *Basic concepts of psychiatric: mental health nursing,* 6th edition. Philadelphia: Lippincott.

14  Cohen D, Volkmar F (1997) *Handbook of autism and pervasive developmental disorders*, 2nd edition. New York: Wiley.

15  Carr A (1999) *The handbook of child and adolescent clinical psychology*, a contextual approach. London: Routledge.

16  Noctor C (2005) ADHD Early assessment is vital. *World of Irish Nursing* 13: 4.

17  Lask B, Bryant-Waugh R (2000) *Anorexia and related eating disorders in childhood and adolescence*, 2nd edition. London: Taylor & Francis.

18  National Institute for Clinical Excellence (2004) *Eating disorders, core intervention in the treatment and management of anorexia nervosa, bulimia nervosa and other related eating disorders*. Clinical Guideline 9. National Collaborating Centre for Mental Health. www.nice.org.uk/CG009quickrefguide.

## CHAPTER 31

# Developing child oncology skills

Michelle Wright and Caroline Langford

## LEARNING OUTCOMES

*Upon completion of this chapter, the reader should be able to accomplish the following:*

- Gain a basic understanding about paediatric oncological conditions and their treatments/side-effects

- Be able to care for a child receiving chemotherapy safely, being aware of potential complications and their management and have the knowledge to write an individualised care plan for a child receiving chemotherapy

- Be able to care for a child with febrile / neutropenia, being able to recognise clinical signs of deterioration and potential complications and able to write a nursing care plan

- Be able to care for a child with a central venous line and discuss how to perform a central venous line dressing and line flush, being aware of potential complications and risk factors

- Understand the importance of mouth care in the prevention of infection and in the treatment of mucositis. Capable of producing a care plan for the child with mucositis and assessing a child's mouth using an assessment tool

- Be able to care for a child receiving radiotherapy, being able to assess skin integrity and provide appropriate care

## CHAPTER OVERVIEW

Generally cancer occurs when cells within the body become out of control and multiply. The cells are unable to function effectively. When cancer cells break away from their original location and spread to other parts of the body they may produce secondary tumours known as metastases.[1] Cancer is the leading cause of death from disease in the paediatric population.[2] Childhood cancer is, however, rare, with only 1 in 600 children under the age of 15 years developing the disease, with approximately 1700 new cases annually in the United Kingdom.[1] Treatment of childhood cancers has progressed dramatically over recent years, with the development of clinical trials and 7 in 10 children are now cured following treatment.[1] Treatment includes chemotherapy, radiotherapy, surgery, stem cell/bone marrow transplantation and novel therapies such as molecular-targeted therapy, given individually or as combination therapy.

There is no clear evidence as to what causes cancer,[3] although many theories have been suggested. Certain conditions, however, increase a child's risk of developing cancers, for example children with Beckwith–Wiedemann syndrome have an increased risk of developing Wilms' tumour, hepatoblastoma and rhabdomyosarcoma, and have routine imaging to detect such malignancies.[4]

In order to clinically care for a child with a malignancy, it is important to have a basic understanding of the underlying condition.[5]

# TYPES OF CHILDHOOD CANCER

## Non-Hodgkin's lymphoma

Non-Hodgkin's lymphoma (NHL) is a malignancy of the lymphoid cells and can be classified into four different categories:

- anaplastic large cell lymphoma (10 per cent);
- Burkitt's lymphoma (40 per cent);
- large B-cell lymphoma (20 per cent);
- lymphoblastic lymphoma (30 per cent).

The incidence of NHL seems to be increasing over recent years, with a peak incidence in children aged 7–10 years.[6] There are different stagings for NHL, ranging from stage 1 to stage 4, dependent on the site or sites of disease at diagnosis, with the most common site being the abdomen. With recent developments in treatment, usually chemotherapy followed by surgery of any residual mass, survival rates have dramatically increased.[7]

## Hodgkin's disease

Hodgkin's disease or Hodgkin's lymphoma is a malignancy of the lymphatic system and commonly affects children over the age of 5 years. Hodgkin's disease is characterised by the presence of Reed–Sternberg cells. Treatment is dependent upon staging of the disease and consists of chemotherapy and in some cases radiotherapy. Prognosis for children and young adults with Hodgkin's disease is a 95–100 per cent cure rate at 5 years.[8]

## Wilms' tumour

Wilms' tumour is defined as a malignant tumour of the kidney. Most children are under the age of 7 years at diagnosis and overall survival rates are as high as 90 per cent, dependent upon the staging of the disease.[9] Staging for Wilms' tumour is dependent upon the histopathology of the resected tumour at surgery. Treatment includes a combination of chemotherapy, surgery and occasionally radiotherapy.[5]

## Leukaemia

Leukaemia represents around 30 per cent of all childhood cancers and is the most common of all paediatric cancers.[10] Leukaemia is a cancer of the blood-forming or haematopoietic tissues[11] and is categorised in terms of the type of cells affected and whether the disease is chronic or acute.[5] Acute lymphoblastic leukaemia (ALL) is the most common of all childhood leukaemias, accounting for approximately 75 per cent of childhood leukaemia, with acute myeloid/myeloblastic (AML) leukaemia accounting for approximately 15–20 per cent and chronic forms of the disease being much less common.[12] The prognosis for leukaemia has increased dramatically over recent years, with event-free survival for ALL patients at 80 per cent and for AML at 60 per cent. Chemotherapy is the treatment of choice for leukaemia; however, regimens are dependent upon the type of leukaemia and clinical trials.[13]

## Central nervous system tumours

Central nervous system tumours represent 20 per cent of all paediatric cancers, and represent the highest percentage of significant morbidity and cancer-related death. There are approximately 100 different types of central nervous system tumours, generally named after the area they have grown in or the type of cell affected.[14] Treatment may consist of radiotherapy, chemotherapy, surgery or a combination of the three.[5]

## Hepatoblastoma

Hepatoblastoma is a malignant tumour of the liver accounting for only 2–5 per cent of all paediatric cancers. Treatment consists of chemotherapy and surgery, with prognosis as high as 80 per cent in children who have complete surgical resection. The majority of children with hepatoblastoma are under the age of 5 years because of the embryological origin of the tumour.[4]

## Neuroblastoma

Neuroblastoma is a tumour derived from nerve cells, initially developing in the adrenal glands, but often spreading throughout the abdomen and the rest of the body. Neuroblastoma represents around 10 per cent of solid malignancies in early childhood and is associated with high levels of mortality. Treatment consists of a combination of radiotherapy, chemotherapy, surgery and stem cell transplant in children with stage 4 disease.[15]

## Retinoblastoma

Retinoblastoma is a malignant tumour of the retina and is commonly diagnosed in infancy following observation of a white pupil. Sixty per cent of children with retinoblastoma have the non-inherited form, with 40 per cent of children having an inherited retinoblastoma. Treatment is dependent on the extent of disease and may consist of enucleation, chemotherapy, radiotherapy, laser therapy, cryotherapy or thermotherapy.[16]

## Bone tumours

Ninety per cent of bone tumours in childhood and adolescents are Ewing's sarcoma and osteosarcoma.[17] Treatment consists of intensive chemotherapy, and reconstructive limb salvage surgery or in some cases amputation and radiotherapy for children with Ewing's sarcoma. Prognosis is dependent upon metastatic involvement and histology of the removed tumour.[17]

## Soft-tissue sarcomas

Soft-tissue sarcomas are a group of malignancies involving many tissues within the body, including contractile tissue, connective tissue and supportive tissue.[18] Soft-tissue sarcomas are grouped into rhabdomyosarcoma and non-rhabdomyosarcoma. Rhabdomyosarcoma constitutes approximately 50 per cent of all soft-tissue sarcomas in children and young adults. Rhabdomyosarcomas arise from primitive muscle cells and can develop anywhere in the body. Treatment involves chemotherapy and local therapy, consisting of radiotherapy and/or surgery.[19] Prognosis is very much dependent on the extent of disease. Non-rhabdomyosarcoma is a group of tumours including extra-osseous Ewing's sarcoma, malignant peripheral nerve sheath tumours, fibrosarcoma and synovial sarcomas. Treatment varies dependent on the histology of the tumour.[5,18]

# CARING FOR A CHILD RECEIVING CHEMOTHERAPY

Cancer in children is rare, with around 1500 new cases diagnosed each year in the United Kingdom.[20] The ultimate aims of treatment are cure and quality of life. Chemotherapy was first used in the 1950s; prior to this surgery and radiotherapy were the only treatment options.[21] Chemotherapy refers to any drug/chemical used to treat a disease. Cytotoxic chemotherapy agents are used to treat cancer; these are drugs which have cytotoxic or cell-killing properties. Chemotherapy can be given by nearly all accepted drug routes. The most common routes used in paediatrics include intravenous, intrathecal, oral or intramuscular/subcutaneous, depending upon the child's diagnosis and treatment protocol. Chemotherapy is used to kill or control the growth of cancer cells in the body and in doing so has a systemic effect on all cells in the body, resulting in many side-effects, some life threatening. To provide care for a child receiving chemotherapy a basic understanding of how chemotherapy, works is important. In order to understand the principles of chemotherapy it is vital to have an understanding of the cell cycle, which describes the series of events that take place in a cell leading to its replication.

Chemotherapeutic agents have the same cytotoxic effect on both normal and malignant cells. Normal cells need to have the opportunity for recovery between treatments to avoid life-threatening toxicities or unacceptable effects on quality of life. Hence chemotherapy cycles are generally given following blood count recovery. Cytotoxic chemotherapy is extremely toxic with many unwanted side-effects. Some are unpleasant but reversible and non life-threatening. The areas most affected by short-term toxicity are where normal cells rapidly divide and grow, namely the bone marrow, mouth, digestive system, hair follicles and skin. However, there are also potentially life-threatening side-effects that can damage organs irreversibly.

The care of a child receiving chemotherapy requires comprehensive monitoring and interventions. An overview of these follows.

## Administration

Chemotherapy administration must be undertaken by highly trained professionals. Those administering chemotherapy need to be aware of issues related to handling such toxic agents as there is a very small margin between a therapeutic effect and a toxic effect. The potential dangers associated with errors in chemotherapy administration have necessitated the development of national standards.[22] The manual of cancer services standards[23] states that all staff who administer chemotherapy should receive appropriate training and be assessed as competent.

## Safety

Principles of safe practice are to minimise exposure by educating staff, patients and carers, which in turn will minimise hazards, side-effects, toxicity complications and distress. Most cytotoxic agents are potentially hazardous, as they are mutagenic, teratogenic, carcinogenic and irritant. Exposure can occur from absorption, inhalation and ingestion. Documents such as The Health and Safety at Work Act[24] and the Management of Health and Safety at Work Regulations[25] clearly state the legal duty to protect both employees and the public. The Health and Safety at Work guidelines outline procedures for the safe handling of cytotoxic drugs.[26] COSSH (The Control of Substances Hazardous to Health)[27] regulations define cytotoxic chemotherapy as hazardous substances that should be subject to a risk assessment. The Oncology Nursing Society[28] recommends work practices to reduce risk of contamination. Nurses have a duty of care to others and therefore are responsible in ensuring a safe environment, protecting themselves, colleagues, patients and carers. It is not only administering cytotoxic treatment that poses danger; disposal of waste is another potential source of drug exposure which must be guided by policy.

## Nausea and vomiting

A commonly associated side-effect of chemotherapy is nausea and/or vomiting. The emetogenicity will vary according to the drug or drug combination the child receives. Although this is not a long-term damaging side-effect such as cardiotoxicity/nephrotoxicity, it is often very distressing for both the child and family. It is as a result of stimulation of the vomiting centre, which is located in the brain in the medulla oblongata near the respiratory centre. Management needs to start with prevention. All professionals should ideally follow an antiemetic protocol, designed with consideration to individual chemotherapy agents/protocols as this may prevent nausea and/or vomiting. Antiemetics need to be given regularly and their effects monitored. There are also non-medical/non-pharmacological interventions that should be considered, particularly in the situation of anticipatory vomiting. These may include distraction, guided imagery, hypnosis and acupressure, and will commonly involve the play specialist/clinical psychologist.

Medical problems associated with nausea and vomiting include issues such as dehydration, metabolic abnormalities and weight loss. Therefore, within the nursing management of a patient receiving chemotherapy, nursing staff must ensure they assess their patient's hydration status by maintaining a strict fluid balance record that includes daily weights to monitor for signs of fluid loss/retention. Patients must be referred for a dietetic assessment and then monitored throughout their treatment course.

Chemotherapy administration as an outpatient via a day unit is increasing with the advent of protocols and development of nursing roles including nurse-led assessment.[29] For such interventions to be successful, effective management of nausea and vomiting is even more crucial.

## Extravasation

Extravasation is defined as the inadvertent infiltration/leakage of intravenous fluids from the vein into the surrounding tissues.[30] Varying degrees of tissue damage, from mild skin reactions to severe necrosis, can occur if vesicant chemotherapy extravasations are left untreated.[31,32] The true incidence of vesicant chemotherapy extravasations is not known; however, it is estimated to occur in <1–6 per cent of vesicant administrations.[33] This may not seem like a large percentage, but it means a large number of patients are at risk because of the vast proportion of patients receiving this type of chemotherapy treatment. Generally extravasation will occur in situations when cytotoxic drugs are administered via a peripheral cannula/long line as opposed to a central venous device, which is the preferred/safer route of administration

The amount, type and concentration of the vesicant, plus the location of the extravasation, all influence the severity of an extravasation injury. Vesicants that bind to the DNA in healthy tissue, such as the anthracyclines, are not metabolised in the tissue and consequently cause a greater degree of tissue destruction.[31,34] Signs and symptoms of an extravasation injury are not always immediately visible and it may take hours or days to detect any adverse reactions. First signs are usually erythema, swelling and tenderness/pain. It is therefore essential to educate parents/carers/patients on the signs to observe the skin for, particularly if they are receiving this treatment during an outpatient visit. Forming local policies to standardise procedures for administration, management, and appropriate training for all staff will provide precautionary steps to help prevent risk of extravasation (Table 31.1).

| KEY POINT |
|---|
| In practice, corticosteroids are often given to treat inflammation following extravasation; however there is little evidence to support their use.[31] |

Table 31.1 Initial management of vesicant chemotherapy extravasation

Stop administering the vesicant
Leave cannula in place, attempt to aspirate the vesicant
Mark and measure the extravasation area
Remove cannula
Apply topical heat/cooling
Notify medical staff
Administer analgesics as needed
Complete documentation
Photograph the area

| Localise and neutralise (apply cold pack ± antidote according to drug) | Disperse and dilute (warm compress, subcutaneous hyaluronidase) |
|---|---|
| Amsacrine | Vinblastine |
| Actinomycin D | Vincristine |
| Carmustine | Vindesine |
| Dacarbazine | Vinorelbine |
| Daunorubicin | |
| Doxorubicin | |
| Epirubicin | |
| Idarubicin | |
| Mitomycin-C | |
| Mustine | |
| Streptozotocin | |

Adapted from EONS (2007).[32]

## PROCEDURE: Care plan for a child receiving chemotherapy

| Problem | Goal | Intervention |
|---|---|---|
| Patient requires chemotherapy | Patient will receive prescribed treatment safely. Side-effects will be minimised | Ensure checklist completed<br>Baseline observations including weight/height<br>Administer medication as prescribed, in accordance with protocol<br>Monitor effects and for any side-effects<br>Follow trust policy for administration<br>Always wear gloves when handling cytotoxic drugs and body fluids<br>Educate family about safety<br>Maintain strict fluid balance chart<br>Regular observations (i.e. 4-hourly pulse/blood pressure, temperature) |

| | | |
|---|---|---|
| | | Chemotherapy side-effects: actions to be taken with specific drugs, e.g. urine testing<br>4-hourly observations |
| Patient has a central line | Central venous line (CVL) will remain patent and free from infection. Entry site will remain clean and dry. Line will be well secured | Use aseptic technique when accessing line<br>Access as infrequently as possible to reduce risk of introducing infection<br>Change IV giving sets as per trust policy<br>IV fluids: record volume infused and pressures hourly<br>Observe central line exit site for leak age/redness<br>Central line dressing: clean and dress according to policy. Ensure line is secure and looped at exit site<br>Discharge planning: central line care for discharge, community referrals for weekly flushes and dressings |
| Patient may experience nausea/vomiting | Patient's nausea and vomiting will be controlled | Regular antiemetics including prior to chemotherapy<br>Liaise with prescriber if not effective<br>Monitor fluid balance<br>Daily weight<br>Dietetic referral<br>Change in condition: inform senior nurse/medics |
| Patient and child may experience anxiety | To reduce anxiety of the patient/and family and promote effective coping | Assess levels of anxiety<br>Assist patient/carer to identify specific stressors and strategies for coping<br>Keep patient/carer fully informed re care and check understanding<br>Encourage questions<br>Provide relevant literature<br>Refer/liaise with play specialist/psychological services as necessary |

## NURSING CARE OF THE CHILD WITH FEBRILE NEUTROPENIA

Chemotherapy drugs aim to kill or control the growth of cancer cells. Chemotherapy drugs not only have an effect on cancer cells, but also have a systemic effect on all cells within the body, including white cells, red cells and platelets. The systemic effects of chemotherapy on the bone marrow usually takes place 7–10 days following administration of the chemotherapy; however, all children react to chemotherapy in different ways. The effects of chemotherapy on the bone marrow usually begin to recover 21 days after

> **KEY POINTS**
>
> Children febrile and neutropenic are at high risk of developing septic shock. IV antibiotics should be commenced within 30–60 minutes.[38]

administration of treatment, dependent upon the individual child and the dose and type of chemotherapy given.

Children with neutropenia are immuno-suppressed and at high risk of infection. Children with febrile neutropenia are the second most common oncology-related admissions to hospital,

| Definitions | |
|---|---|
| **Neutropenic:** neutrophil count of <0.5 × 109/L (dependent upon local policy) | **Thrombocytopenia:** a reduction in the amount of circulating platelets within the blood stream[36] |
| **Anaemia:** reduction of circulating red blood cells or haemoglobin leading to a reduction in the oxygen-carrying capacity of blood[35] | |

second only to chemotherapy admissions.[37] Children who are febrile and neutropenic may initially be at home or be an inpatient for another reason. Nurses need to be aware of the dangers of febrile neutropenia and the risk of severe sepsis or death in order to give the appropriate phone advice to patients or parents and to recognise any changes in the child's condition.

It is important to remember that septic shock in patients with febrile neutropenia is the commonest cause of mortality in childhood cancer.[39] The majority of children, however, who attend with febrile neutropenia are generally well. Recent work carried out by CCLG/PONF (Paediatric Oncology Nursing Forum) supportive care group has highlighted the inconsistencies in paediatric care of children with febrile neutropenia.[40] Inconsistencies were not only found in the treatment of these children, but also in the definitions of febrile neutropenia. The majority of oncology centres within the United Kingdom define fever as a single temperature of 38.5°C or prolonged temperature of 38°C. The definition of neutropenia is again inconsistent; however, for the purpose of this chapter neutropenia is classified as a neutrophil count of 0.5 or below in accordance with Alder Hey Children's NHS Foundation Trust Oncology guidelines. This definition is, however, not set in stone, and if a child is admitted clinically unwell with a neutrophil count of 0.8 and falling, clinical judgement would be used and febrile neutropenic treatment would commence. There are inconsistencies in practice within the UK for treating febrile neutropenic episodes. Individual paediatric oncology centres appear to use differing protocols for supportive care.[41] Large-scale randomised trials are required to ensure evidence-based protocols can be employed.

When a child attends hospital with a fever of 38.5°C or a prolonged fever of 38°C there is a series of investigations that need take place. A full blood count (FBC) would initially be taken to establish the neutrophil count in order to determine treatment; an FBC also gives information regarding whether blood or platelet transfusions are required. Urea and electrolytes (U&E) would be taken as well as liver function tests (LFTs), in order to ascertain liver and kidney function and to assess the hydration status. Other investigations are to try and establish a focus for infection. Blood cultures should be taken to assess for a central line infection, a urine sample should always be taken even if the child has no symptoms, as a neutropenic child may not display normal responses to infection. Swabs should be taken according to local policy and, if a child has any external devices, they should be swabbed as a potential source of infection. Other investigations such as chest X-ray and nasopharyngeal aspirate may be needed, dependent on the individual child's clinical symptoms and condition.

> **KEY POINT**
>
> When a child is febrile, blood cultures from the central line need to be taken as soon as possible. At the same time FBC, U&Es and LFTs can be taken. If a child has two or three lumens blood cultures need to be taken from each lumen, to establish cause of infection

When a child is found to be febrile and neutropenic following FBC results, prompt treatment is essential. If a child develops septic shock as a result of febrile neutropenia, then early recognition and quick intervention with administration of antibiotic therapy is critical to a good outcome.[41]

## PROCEDURE: Investigations that need to be taken when a child presents with fever after chemotherapy

| Procedural steps | Evidence-based rationale |
|---|---|
| 1 FBC | To establish general condition of the bone marrow and whether blood products required |
| 2 U&E and LFTs | To establish renal and liver function and hydration status |
| 3 Blood cultures from all lumens (if no CVL, peripheral blood cultures) | To establish focus of infection |
| 4 Urine sample (dependent on local policy) | Dipstick urine to establish any focus for infection |
| 5 Imaging of any problematic site (e.g. chest X-ray if symptomatic) | To establish focus of infection and any complications |
| 6 Surveillance swabs (dependent on local policy) | To establish focus of infection and any resistance |
| 7 Stool sample if symptomatic | To establish focus of infection |
| 8 Gastrostomy site if present | To establish focus of infection |
| 9 Central line swab if looks clinically infected (dependent on local policy) | To establish focus of infection |
| 10 Nasopharyngeal aspirate (NPA) (dependent on local policy) | To establish focus of infection: looking in particular for respiratory viruses |

**KEY POINT**

If a child is unwell or is known to be around 7–10 days after administration of chemotherapy, then intravenous antibiotics should be started straight away, without waiting for FBC results.

Antibiotic therapy is very much dependent on local policy and particularly related to local drug resistance patterns.[42] Antibiotic therapy always consists of broad-spectrum antibiotics until a specific isolate has been identified. Treatment tends to consist of a broad-spectrum beta-lactam monotherapy or broad-spectrum beta-lactam with aminoglycoside combination antibiotic therapy, such as pipericillin/tazabactam with gentamicin. There is no difference between using a single beta-lactam and using a beta-lactam with an aminoglycoside.[43] The majority of patients with febrile neutropenic sepsis are caused by an endogenous infection due to gut translocation or exogenous infection caused by contamination of the central venous catheter by micro-organisms.[44] Gram-negative infections commonly cause life-threatening septicaemia;[44] however, Gram-positive infections can occasionally cause sepsis and mortality in the neutropenic patient and are common with the increasing usage of central venous catheters. A Cochrane review[46] in 2004 identified that there are a group of 'low-risk' patients who could safely be treated with oral antibiotics as opposed to intravenous. However, this tends not to be current practice in paediatric oncology units. There are limitations in this review and it requires updating with randomised controlled trials including home administration of oral antibiotics.

Nursing observation of the febrile and neutropenic child is critical in detecting any deterioration in the child's condition and any signs of sepsis and shock. Vital signs should be regularly monitored, such as blood pressure, respiratory rate, pulse, temperature and monitoring the overall condition of the child, including oxygen saturations and capillary refill if the condition dictates. Children who are febrile and neutropenic are at risk of sepsis not only on admission but throughout their neutropenic episode, emphasising the importance of regular observations.[42] An accurate fluid balance chart should always be started for children with febrile neutropenia to establish the overall condition, nutritional status and renal function. It is important to consider all routes of fluid loss associated with febrile neutropenic episodes; these may include perspiration due to fever, hyperventilation and haemorrhage. Families should be educated prior to discharge on the importance and monitoring of adequate dietary and fluid intake to maintain hydration and growth.

Antibiotic therapy continues until the child has been afebrile for a total of 48 hours; however, local policies may differ. Antibiotic therapy such as teicoplanin may be added if a child has a positive infection isolated from a blood culture sample.[42] Microbiology results must be checked regularly during the hospital admission to ensure antibiotics are adjusted appropriately if any culture sensitivities are obtained. Children with continuing fevers after 72 hours or who have recognised symptoms of fungal infection will have an antifungal agent added to their treatment regime, for example liposomal amphotericin.

Other side-effects affecting the bone marrow following chemotherapy associated with the febrile and neutropenic patient include thrombocytopenia and anaemia. Thrombocytopenia is defined as a reduction in the amount of circulating platelets within the blood stream.[36] Clinical features of thrombocytopenia include bleeding (often in the gums, nose and menorrhagia), petechiae, bruising and purpura.[42] Platelet transfusion can be given to children; however, criteria for requiring a transfusion is dependent on hospital policy. Generally platelet transfusions are given only to children who are bleeding, are febrile with a low platelet count or have a platelet count of less than 10.[42] Platelet and blood transfusion reactions are common in oncology patients.

Other care plans needed for this child relate to mouth care, possible need for blood products and central venous line care.

**VIGNETTE**

**Problem:** 'Sarah' is a 9-year-old girl with a rhabdomyosarcoma of her forearm. She presented to the paediatric oncology unit, 9 days post chemotherapy, complaining of fever, lethargy and a sore throat. On examination she was found to be pale – blood results identified anaemia. She had an ulcerated mouth, and low white cell count.

**Discussion:** 'Sarah' was admitted to the unit, commenced broad-spectrum antibiotics and morphine patient-controlled analgesia. She was cross-matched for 2 units of packed red cells.

## PROCEDURE: Care plan for the care of a child admitted with febrile neutropenia (for example a relatively well child who is currently eating and drinking)

| Problem | Goal | Intervention |
| --- | --- | --- |
| Patient has a fever and is neutropenic | For patient to become afebrile and to reduce the risk of further infection | Monitor temperature, blood pressure, pulse and respiratory rate 4 hourly to assess for signs of deterioration and sepsis<br>To administer paracetamol as appropriate if uncomfortable<br>To carry out full septic screen looking for any signs of infection<br>To administer broad spectrum intravenous antibiotics safely<br>When accessing central line use aseptic technique in accordance with local policy<br>Nurse child in accordance with local infection control policies |

## PROCEDURE: Care plan for the care of a child admitted with febrile neutropenia (for example a relatively well child who is currently eating and drinking)

| Problem | Goal | Intervention |
|---|---|---|
| Patient has a fever and is neutropenic, therefore at risk of decreased fluid and dietary intake | For patient to remain well hydrated and able to tolerate adequate diet and fluid | To keep medical staff up to date with any new issues<br>To educate and inform child and family of ongoing treatment plan<br><br>If there is a fever spike of 38 or above after 48 hours take further blood cultures<br>If there is a further fever spike after 72 hours liaise with medical staff as to what further investigations need to be carried out, e.g. ultrasound, CT scan (looking for other signs of infections causing the ongoing fever)<br><br>To keep accurate fluid balance chart, documenting all oral and IV intake including accurate documentation of output, i.e. bowels and urine output<br>To be aware of adequate oral intake and establish hydration statues<br>To liaise closely with medical staff to establish whether intravenous fluids are required and report any changes<br>To liaise closely with the dietician to assess dietary intake (some children admitted febrile and neutropenic may require parental nutrition to support them during these episodes, particularly if they are receiving intensive chemotherapy regimens)<br>To offer the child oral fluids and diet and give encouragement<br>To educate the child and family on the importance of diet and fluid intake and following negotiation with family encourage parents or child to be involved in the fluid balance chart if appropriate<br>Assess child for any signs of clinical dehydration, i.e. dry skin, poor skin turgor, dry lips, reduced urine output, lethargy |

# CENTRAL VENOUS LINES

## Overview

A CVL is a device widely used in paediatric oncology for its comfort and practicality. The device has many benefits in the management of children with malignancies: for the administration of cytotoxic drugs, antibiotics, blood products and nutritional products (TPN). A central venous line also reduces the frequency of unpleasant procedures such as cannulation and phlebotomy.[45]

## Types

There are two types of central venous devices commonly used: external and internal systems. An external system, such as the Hickman/broviac line is a central venous catheter that is surgically tunnelled with only the end of the catheter brought through the skin. An internal system, for instance a portacath, is also surgically tunnelled but is a completely implantable catheter consisting of a stainless steel chamber with a silicone membrane placed under the skin. Both devices are commonly inserted into subclavian veins, preferably low within the superior vena cava or the right atrium, as these locations are associated with fewer complications, for example clots.[46] A PICC (peripherally inserted central venous catheter) is a line inserted into a vein in the arm; such devices are less commonly used in paediatric oncology patients because of their limited length of duration.

## Complications associated with central venous lines

Although there are many benefits of using a long-term indwelling catheter, there are potential problems to be aware of, namely pneumothorax, infection, and thrombosis. Regular flushing with heparinised saline is recommended to reduce the likelihood of central venous line-related thrombus formation, and consequently the risk of catheter infection. Many clots are not symptomatic, such as intraluminal thrombosis, and are commonly only identified from failure to withdraw blood from the catheter. Risk factors for thrombosis include the type of malignancy and chemotherapeutic agents being used to treat this, plus type and insertion site of the central venous catheter.[46] Thrombosis is a major risk factor for infection.[47] Sterile technique is highly important, as a line may serve as a portal of entry for pathogenic organisms, and the line itself may become infected with organisms. A risk factor for children receiving treatment for a malignancy is their immunocompromised state. Evidence suggests neutropenia is a contributing risk factor for infections related to central venous lines and sepsis.[45]

Further possible problems arising from a central venous line include displacement, extravasation and exit site infections.[47]

A systematic review in 2003[48] concluded there is insufficient evidence around the superiority of dressings for central venous line exit sites. Different centres tend to offer dressings based on patient preference and cost. As with many aspects of central venous line care, national guidelines have not yet been formulated; therefore, local policies must be developed within each treatment centre.[49] Department of Health guidelines recommend cleaning and changing exit site dressings every 7 days.

## Central venous line dressing (step-by-step guide)

### Equipment required

Chlorhexidine cleansing solution for (washing hands)
Triclosan antibacterial hand rub to (resterilise hands)
Chlorhexidine gluconate solution (to clean exit site)
Dressing pack
Sterile gloves
Sterile mepore/IV3000 dressing
Skin-fix loop

**KEY POINT** If the central venous line fails to sample blood, check exit site dressing to ensure lumen is not kinked, and encourage patient to change position, including raising arm, and turning neck, to encourage blood flow.

## PROCEDURE: Central vendous line dressing

| Procedural steps | Evidence-based rationale |
|---|---|
| **1** Changing exit site dressing requires aseptic technique | To minimise potential introduction of infection |
| **2** Explain procedure to child and family | Informed consent, reduce anxiety |
| **3** Remove old dressing and inspect exit site | To check for signs of infection and 'pulling' |
| **4** Clean exit site with chlorhexidine using aseptic technique | Antibacterial and anti-fungal properties[64] |
| **5** Redress exit site with appropriate dressing | To keep site clean and dry (choice of dressing may be based on patient preference and/or cost)[48] |
| **6** Secure central venous line with skin fix holder | To increase security and reduce risk of accidental displacement |

### Definitions

**Mucositis:** painful inflammation and/or ulceration of the mucous membranes[50]

**Candidiasis:** yeast infection commonly caused by *Candida albicans*, usually limited to skin and mouth

**Xerostomia:** dryness in the mouth

**Herpes simplex virus (HSV):** Virus causing pain and blistering (cold sore lesions)

## MOUTH CARE

The oral mucous membranes within the mouth and digestive tract as a whole are highly susceptible to the effects of chemotherapy, as rapidly dividing cells are in abundance within these areas and are therefore sensitive to the damaging effects of cytotoxic chemotherapy.[50] Mucositis is a common side-effect of chemotherapy and can be very debilitating.[51,52] Patients' quality of life can be affected by pain, infection, altered nutrition and impaired oral function.[53,54] Chemotherapeutic agents inhibit the growth and maturation of oral mucosal cells and disrupt the primary mucosal barrier in the mouth and throat.[55] The direct effects on the oral mucosa from chemotherapy can begin as early as 2 or 3 days after the administration and generally peak in severity 7–10 days later, with resolution occurring within 2 weeks[56] on average; however, it may take longer in some cases.

Nurses play a central role in the prevention and management of children with mucositis.

Nurses have three main nursing responsibilities relating to mouth care of children: (1) effective assessment and monitoring of oral cavity; (2) the use of appropriate oral care interventions; (3) patient education.[57]

Mucositis can be extremely painful and it is not uncommon for children to require opioid infusions such as morphine or fentanyl. Children with severe cases of mucositis can require infusions of an opioid, ketamine and a sedative such as midazolam.

The clinical features of mucositis are swelling, pain, xerostomia, ulceration, inflammation, desquamation of mucosa, dry and cracked lips and bleeding mouth (Table 31.2, page 543).

There is no research suggesting any recommended successful treatment for mucositis and its associated pain relief. Nutritional support (often including total parental nutrition), regular assessment and pain management should be the focus of nursing care.[50] If opportunistic infections are present, such as the herpes simplex virus or candidiasis, then appropriate treatment to treat such infection is needed.

**KEY POINT**

It is important to remember that mucositis can be extremely painful and an appropriate pain tool is essential for pain management.

**Table 31.2** Chemotherapeutic agents causing mucositis

| Alkylating agents | Anti-metabolites | Nitrosureas | Anthracyclines | Antineoplastic antibiotics | Plant alkaloids |
|---|---|---|---|---|---|
| Busulfan | Cytarabine | Carmustine | Daunorubicin | Bleomycin | Etoposide |
| Cyclophosphamide | 5-Fluorouracil | Lomustine | Doxorubicin | Dactinomycin | Vinblastine |
| Ifosfamide | Hydroxyurea | | Idarubicin | | Vincristine |
| Melphalan | Mercaptopurine | | Mitozantrone | | |
| Procarbazine | Methotrexate | | | | |
| Temozolamide | Thioguanine | | | | |

## Prevention of mucositis

Standards for oral care for the prevention of mucositis and prevention of oral candidiasis are not consistently implemented and advice often varies.

The evidenced-based RCN guidelines for mouth care in children and young people with cancer have made various recommendations for the prevention of mucositis.[50]

- All children diagnosed with a malignancy should have a dental review at diagnosis and at regular intervals during treatment.
- Oral hygiene advice and education should be given to the child and family prior to commencement of chemotherapy and throughout treatment (oral hygiene and mouth care should be an important aspect of the nursing assessment).
- Advice should include brushing teeth twice a day with fluoride toothpaste.
- Toothbrush should be changed every 3 months

**KEY POINT**

There is no evidence to suggest that nystatin prevents oral candidiasis in paediatric oncology patients.

or following an infection and should be for the sole use of the child.
- If a child is beginning to develop a sore mouth a soft brush with a smaller head should be used.
- If it is not possible for children to use a brush, instructions should be given to clean the mouth with oral sponges temporarily, with water or a antimicrobial agent, for example diluted chlorhexidine.
- Advice should be given regarding restricting sugary food and drink at meal times.

The care plan for a child with mucositis will need to be adjusted to take into account any opioid infusions, IV fluids, TPN, etc.

## PROCEDURE: Treatment of mucositis

| Problem | Goal | Intervention |
|---|---|---|
| Patient has mucositis resulting in pain | For patient to remain as pain free as possible while mucositis heals | To assess the child's mouth regularly using an appropriate mouth care tool Encourage appropriate mouth care and educate child and family (see above) To administer prescribed pain relief and assess its effectiveness using an appropriate pain assessment tool Liaise closely with medical staff/pain team regarding effectiveness of pain relief |

## PROCEDURE: Treatment of mucositis (continued)

| | | |
|---|---|---|
| Patient has mucositis resulting in reduced oral intake | To ensure adequate oral intake and to reduce the risk of infection | Keep an accurate fluid balance chart including all intake and output (it is common for children with mucositis to require total parental nutrition) Liaise closely with dietician and all members of the multidisciplinary team |

## RADIOTHERAPY

Many childhood cancers will be treated using radiotherapy. Radiotherapy has had a recognised therapeutic potential in treating cancer since the late nineteenth century.[58] This may be as an adjunct to surgery/chemotherapy or used alone. Radiotherapy uses targeted high energy rays to kill cancer cells by damaging the cells' internal molecules.[59] Radiotherapy, however, has a similar effect on the body as chemotherapy, in that it will damage healthy cells also. The side-effects experienced by children receiving radiotherapy treatment may be short or long term and will vary depending on the area/organ radiated and type of radiotherapy.

Healthy non-cancerous cells are able to repair their chromosomal tissue far more effectively than malignant cells, although they do have a maximum tolerance dose.

Both healthy and malignant cells attempt to repair themselves within 6 hours after exposure to radiation.[60] However, malignant cells may be far less effective in their attempt to recover.[61]

Fractionation is the process of giving radiation in smaller doses. This means that the patient receives the same total dose but as it is given in smaller doses fewer damaging effects are generated.[62]

Radiotherapy can serve various functions for treating paediatric cancers:

- to improve control of tumour growth, e.g. brain tumours
- to cure
- to manage symptoms, e.g. palliative care/end of life
- to deal with emergencies, e.g. spinal cord compression.

An obvious initial side-effect of radiotherapy is seen on the patient's skin. Radiotherapy affects the integrity of the upper dermis layer of skin (Table 31.3).[63]

Nursing care must focus on good skin care to promote healing, reduce the risk of infection and relieve pain/discomfort. There is little available research to support national skin care guidelines; practice tends to be based on a growing knowledge base gathered through experience. The Radiation Therapy Oncology Group (RTOG) has devised a formal assessment tool for assessing skin integrity. This is adult based, but provides a tool for assessment and recommended interventions and is available online (www.rtog.org/members/toxicity/acute.html).

Aside from the unwanted effects on the skin, dependent on which area of the body is being treated, the patient may experience a multitude of side-effects as illustrated in the Table 31.4, (page 545).

**Table 31.3** Clinical signs of radiotherapy damage to skin

| Signs | Cause | Note |
|---|---|---|
| Erythema | Dilation of capillaries | Within 7 days |
| Dry desquamation | Cell death in upper layers of skin Damage to sweat/sebaceous glands | Within 2–4 weeks |
| Moist desquamation | Extreme damage to epidermis Serous fluid leaks from tissue | Risk of infection |

**Table 31.4** Side-effects

| Area | Effects | Nursing support |
| --- | --- | --- |
| Brain/spine | Headaches/nausea/vomiting/ cerebral oedema/alopecia/ somnolence/fatigue | Analgesia/education/ psychological support and preparation/antiemetics |
| Eye | Conjunctivitis/reduced tear production | Eye care: artificial tears |
| Chest | Pneumonitis/oesophagitis | Antacids/ nutritional support |
| Head/neck | Stomatitis/ taste alterations/ reduced saliva production | Analgesia/ oral assessment/ nutrition |
| Pelvis | Pain/diarrhoea/cystitis/ proctitis | Antispasmodics/ analgesia |
| Abdomen | Pain/abdominal cramping/ diarrhoea/nausea/vomiting/ anorexia/infertility | Analgesia/antispasmodics/ antidiarrhoea medication/ antiemetics/nutrition |
| Bone marrow | Anaemia/neutropenia/ thrombocytopenia | Monitor bloods/ blood products/education |
| Hair follicles | Hair loss: permanent at >55-Gy dose Temporary: up to 30-Gy dose | Support wig referral |
| Bone | Pain/impaired mobility/ fracture | Physiotherapy/ education |

Other effects from radiotherapy treatment which nurses will be involved in monitoring and managing are discussed.

### Nutrition

The ability and desire to consume adequate calorific intake may be affected by factors such as pain, decreased salivary production, stomatitis, nausea/vomiting. It is therefore crucial that the child's nutritional state is assessed prior to treatment and monitored throughout. Proactive as opposed to reactive strategies are beneficial. The insertion of a PEG (percutaneous endoscopic gastrostomy) or nasogastric tube prior to side-effects being experienced can prevent a significant weight loss and reduce anxiety/pressure to maintain sufficient oral intake.

There is supporting evidence that good nutrition is vital for cell repair, resistance to infection and thus maximising a child's ability to tolerate therapy.[58] A weight loss above 10 per cent is not acceptable and requires dietetic input.

### Pain

The child receiving radiotherapy may experience pain from many of the side-effects highlighted in Table 30.4. Preparation and regular pain assessment are necessary to ensure the child is supported and able to tolerate his/her prescribed treatment. Pain relief will usually require opiates; however, topical preparations can be beneficial as an adjunct.

### Fatigue

During radiotherapy treatment, fatigue is often attributed to other causes such as pain, somnolence and malnourishment. There is little paediatric literature available to support the extent of fatigue caused by radiotherapy alone.

### Psychosocial

The impact radiotherapy may have on the child and family from issues ranging from radiation damage to the skin to fears for the future because of late effects cannot be underestimated.

Nurses have a central role in prompt identification of these symptoms and also in facilitating adequate preparation of the child and family. It is essential that the child and family are well prepared for treatment and the role of the play specialist cannot be undervalued in this process.

Go to the website to find the PowerPoint presentation for this chapter and MCQs to test your knowledge. **www.hodderplus.com/childnursingskills**

## REFERENCES

1 Children's Cancer and Leukaemia Group (CCLG) (2007) www.cclg.org.uk (accessed 14 October 2008).

2 National Cancer Institute (2007) www.cancer.gov/cancertopics/types/ childhoodcancers (accessed 20 October 2007).

3 Plon SE, Peterson LE (1997) Childhood cancer, heredity, and the environment. In: Pizzo PA, Poplact DG (eds) *Priniciples and practice of pediatric oncology*, 3rd edition. Philadelphia: Lippincott Raven Publishers.

4 Shafford EA, Pritchard J (2004) Liver tumours. In: Pinkerton R, Plowman PN, Pieters R (eds) *Paediatric oncology*, 3rd edition. London: Arnold.

5 Selwood K, Wright M, Crawford D (2009) Care of the child with haematological and oncological conditions. In: Dixon M, Crawford D, Teasdale D, Murphy J (eds) *Nursing the highly dependent child or infant*. Oxford: Blackwell Publishing.

6 Lymphoma Information Network (2007) www.lymphomainfo.net/childhood/nhl.html (accessed 4 January 2009).

7 Patte C (2004) Non-Hodgkin's lymphoma. In: Pinkerton R, Ploughman PN, Pieters R (eds) *Paediatric oncology*, 3rd edition. London: Arnold.

8 McDowell HP, Messahel B, Berlin O (2004) Hodgkins disease. In: Pinkerton R, Ploughman PN, Pieters R. *Paediatric oncology*, 3rd edition. London: Arnold, pp. 267–286.

9 Metzger ML, Dome JS (2005) Current therapy for Wilm's tumor. *Oncologist* **10**(10): 815–26.

10 Smith OP, Hann I (2004) Pathology of leukaemia. In: Pinkerton R, Plowman PN, Pieters R (eds) *Paediatric oncology*, 3rd edition. London: Arnold,.

11 Colby-Graham MF, Chordas C (2003) The childhood leukemias. *Journal of Pediatric Nursing* **18**(2): 87–95.

12 Altman AJ, Fu C (2006) Chronic leukaemias of childhood. In: Pizzo PA, Poplack DG (eds) *Principles and practice of pediatric oncology*, 5th edition. Philadelphia: Lippincott Williams & Wilkins, 645–673.

13 Smith OP, Hann I (2004) Pathology of leukaemia. In: Pinkerton R, Plowman PN, Pieters R. *Paediatric oncology*, 3rd edition. Arnold: London,.

14 Hargrave DR, Messahel B, Plowman PN (2004) Tumours of the central nervous system. In: Pinkerton P, Plowman PN, Pieters R. *Paediatric Oncology*, 3rd edition. London: Arnold, 287–322.

15 Pearson ADJ, Pinkerton R (2004) Neuroblastoma. In: Pinkerton R, Ploughman PN, Pieters R. *Paediatric oncology*, 3rd edition. London: Arnold,.

16 Melamud M, Palekar R, Singh A (2006) Retinoblastoma. *American Family Physician* **73**(6): 1039–44.

17 Whelan J, Morland B (2004) Bone tumours. In: Pinkerton R, Ploughman PN, Pieters R. *Paediatric oncology*, 3rd edition. London: Arnold,.

18 Carli M, Cecchetto G, Sotti G, et al. (2004) Soft tissue sarcomas. In: Pinkerton R, Plowman PN, Pieters R (eds) *Paediatric oncology*, 3rd edition. London: Arnold, pp. 339–371.

19 Breitfield PP, Meyer WH (2005) Rhabdomyosarcoma: new windows of opportunity. *Oncologist* **10**: 518–527.

20 UK Childhood Cancer Research Group (2004) National registry of childhood tumours www.info.cancerresearchuk.org/cancerstats/ childhoodcancer/incidence (accessed 23 December 2008).

21 Hollis R, Denton S, Chapman G (2008) General surgery. In: Gibson F, Soanes L (eds) *Cancer in children and young people*. Chichester: John Wiley and Sons, p. 187.

22 Lomath A (2008) Quality Assurance In: Gibson F, Soanes L (eds) *Cancer in children and young people*, 2nd edition, Chichester: John Wiley & Sons, p. 21.

23 Department of Health (2004) *Manual of cancer service standards*. London: DH.

24 Health and Safety at Work Act 1994. London: The Stationery Office.

25 Health and Safety at Work Regulations 1999. London: The Stationery Office.

26 Health and Safety Executive (2003) *Safe handling of cytotoxic drugs*. London: Department of Health.

27 Control of substances Hazardous to Health Regulations 2002. London: HSE

28 Oncology Nursing Society (2008) Safe handling of hazardous drugs. In: Gibson F, Soanes L (eds) *Cancer in children and young people*, 2nd edition. Chichester: John Wiley & Sons Ltd, p. 23.

29 Boyer H, Whiles L (2004) Nurse led assessment of children receiving chemotherapy. *Paediatric Nursing* **16**(5): 26–27.

30  Holmes S (2008) Cancer chemotherapy: a guide for practice. In: Gibson F, Soanes L (eds) *Cancer in children and young people acute nursing care.* Chichester: John Wiley and Sons, Ltd, p. 322.

31  European Oncology Nursing Society (EONS) 2007 Extravasation Guidelines www.cancerworld.org/CancerWorld/moduleStaticPage.aspx?id=3891&id_sito=2&id_state=1 2007 (accessed 3 January 2009).

32  Schulmeister L (2007) Extravasation management. *Seminars in Oncology Nursing* 23: 184–190.

33  Langstein HN, Duman H, Seelig D, et al. (2002) Retrospective study of management of chemotherapeutic extravasation injury. *Annals of Plastic Surgery* 49: 369–374.

34  Sauerland C, Engelking, C, Wickham R (2006) Vesicant extravasation, Part 1: Mechanisms, pathogenesis and nursing care to reduce risk. *Oncology Nursing Forum* 33: 1134–1141.

35  Hastings CA, Lubin BH, Feusner J. Hematologic supportive care for children with cancer. In: Pizzo PA, Poplack DG (eds) (2006) *Principles and practice of pediatric oncology*, 5th edition. Philadelphia: Lippincott Williams & Wilkins, 1231–1268.

36  Lowis SP, Goulden N, Oakhill A. Acute complications In: Pinkerton R, Plowman PN, Pieters R (eds) *Paediatric oncology*, 3rd edition. London: Arnold, 2004.

37  Chisholm JC, Dommett R (2006) The evolution towards ambulatory and day-case management of febrile neutropenia. *British Journal of Haematology* 135(1): 3–16.

38  Pizzo PA (1999) Current concepts: fever in immunocompromised patients. *New England Journal of Medicine* 34(12): 893–900.

39  Tan SJ (2002) Recognition and treatment of oncologic emergencies. *Journal of Infusion Nursing* 25(3): 182–188.

40  Phillips B, Selwood K, Lane SM, et al. (2007) Variations in policies for the management of febrile neutropenia in United Kingdom Children's Cancer Study Group centres. *Archives of Diseases in childhood* 92(6): 495–498.

41  Larche J, Azoulay E, Fieux F, et al. (2003) Improved survival of critically ill cancer patients with septic shock. *Intensive Care Medicine* 29: 1688–1695.

42  Selwood K (2008) Side-effects of Chemotherapy. In: Gibson F, Soanes L (eds) *Cancer in children and young people*, 2nd edition. Chichester: John Wiley & Sons Ltd,

43  Paul M, Soares-Weiser K, Grozinsky S, Leibovici L. Beta-lactam versus beta-lactam-aminoglycoside combination therapy in cancer patients with neutropenia. *The Cochrane Database of Systematic Reviews 2*: CD003038.

44  Paulus SC, van Saene HKF, Hemsworth S, *et al.* (2005) A prospective study of septicaemia on a paediatric oncology unit: A three-year experience at The Royal Liverpool Children's Hospital, Alder Hey, UK. *European Journal of Cancer* 41: 2132–2140.

45  McLean TW, Fisher CJ, Snively BM, Chauvenet AR (2005) Central venous lines in children with lesser risk acute lymphoblastic leukemia: optimal type and timing of placement. *Journal of Clinical Oncology* 23(13): 3024–3029.

46  Kuter DJ (2004) Thrombotic complications of central venous catheters in cancer patients. *The Oncologist* 9(2): 207–216.

47  Bagnall-Reeb H, Perry S (2008) In: Gibson, F. and Soanes, L (eds) *Cancer in children and young people. Acute Nursing Care.* Chichester: John Wiley and Sons, p. 211.

48  Gillies D, Carr D, Frost J, et al. (2003) Gauze and tape and transparent polyurethane dressings for central venous catheters. *The Cochrane Database of Systematic Reviews 2*: CD003827.

49  Pratt RS, Pellowe CM, Loveday HP, et al. and the EPIC guideline development team (2001) The epic project: developing national evidence based guidelines for preventing healthcare associated infections. *Journal Hospital Infections* 47(S1): 82.

50  Glenny A (2006) *Mouth care for children and young people with cancer: evidence-based guidelines*. London: UKCCSG-PONF Mouth Care Group.

51  Stiff P (2008) Mucositis associated with stem cell transplantation: current status and innovative approaches to management. *Cited in European Journal of Oncology Nursing* 12(4): 291.

52  Bellm LA, Epsetin JB, Rose-Ped A, et al. (2008) 2000 Patient reports of complications of bone marrow transplantation. Cited in *European Journal of Oncology Nursing* 12(4): 291.

53  Sonis ST, Oster G, Fuchs H, *et al.* (2008) Oral mucositis and the clinical and economic outcomes of hematopoietic stem-cell transplantation. Cited in *European Journal of Oncology Nursing* 12(4): 291.

54  Vera-Llonch M, Oster G, Ford C, *et al.* (2008) Oral mucositis and outcomes of allogeneic hematopoietic stem-cell transplantation in patients with hematologic malignancies. *Cited in European Journal of Oncology Nursing* 12(4): 291.

55  Larson P, Miaskowski C, MacPhail L, *et al.* (2004) The pro-self mouth aware program: An effective approach for reducing chemotherapy induced mucositis. Cited in Wohlschlaeger A. (ed.) Prevention and treatment of mucositis: a guide for nurses. *Journal of Paediatric Oncology Nursing* 21(5): 281.

56  Wilkes JD (2004) Prevention and treatment of oral mucositis following cancer chemotherapy. Cited in Wohlschlaeger A (ed.) Prevention and treatment of mucositis: A guide for nurses. *Journal of Paediatric Oncology Nursing* **21**(5): 281.

57  Stone R, Fliedner MC, Smiet AC (2005) Management of oral mucositis in patients with cancer. *European Journal of Oncology Nursing* **9**(1): S24–S32.

58  Iwamoto R (2008) Radiation therapy. In: Gibson F, Soanes L (eds) *Cancer in children and young people acute nursing care*. Chichester: John Wiley and Sons, pp. 282, 331.

59  Hopkins M (1999) The nature of radiotherapy. In: Gibson F, Evans M (eds) *Paediatric oncology. Acute nursing care*. London: Whurr Publishers, pp. 395–404.

60  Tarbell NT, York T, Kooy H (2008) Principles of radiation oncology. In: Gibson F, Soanes L (eds) *Cancer in children and young people acute nursing care*. Chichester: John Wiley and Sons, p. 321.

61  Hilderley L (2008) Radiation oncology: historical background and principles of teletherapy. In: Gibson F, Soanes L (eds) *Cancer in children and young people acute nursing care*. Chichester: John Wiley and Sons, p. 321.

62  Adamson D (2003) The radiological basis of radiation side-effects. In: Gibson F, Soanes L (eds) *Cancer in children and young people acute nursing care*. Chichester: John Wiley and Sons, p. 285.

63  Hopewell J (2008) The skin, its structure and response to ionising radiation. In: Gibson F, Soanes L (eds) *Cancer in children and young people acute nursing care*. Chichester: John Wiley and Sons, p. 322.

64  Maki DG, Ringer M, Alvarado CJ (1991) Prospective, randomised trial of povidone-iodine, alcohol and chlorhexidine for prevention of infection associated with central venous and arterial catheters. *Lancet* **338**: 339–343.

## CHAPTER 32

# Orthopaedic skills

Alan Glasper and Jane McConochie

## LEARNING OUTCOMES

*Upon completion of this chapter, the reader should be able to accomplish the following:*

1 Describe the anatomy of bones and muscles
2 Describe the sequence of bone healing
3 Discuss with rationale the importance of neurovascular assessment to prevent the development of life-long disability
4 Identify the equipment required to apply skin and or skeletal traction
5 Discuss the nursing care of a child on traction including the potential complications
6 Discuss the care of a child in plaster casts
7 Discuss with rationale recommended pin-site care

## CHAPTER OVERVIEW

Nurses care for infants, children and young people with a variety of orthopaedic conditions and bone injuries. This can involve both long-term and short-term care. This chapter will focus on clinical orthopaedic care skills.

Orthopaedic care can be a complex nursing activity with potential life-long complications. The cardinal rule of the children's orthopaedic nurse is the prevention of infection and the preservation of function.

The impact of modern society on children despite improvements is still manifest through an increasing range of bone or muscle injuries sustained by them though road traffic accidents involving motor vehicles or cycles. In addition, the risk-taking behaviour of young people is often linked to bone and other injuries caused through contact sports or activities taken under the influence of drugs or alcohol.

Children's nurses are likely to see a wide variety of such children in hospital settings, where in modern terms treatment can still be lengthy and protracted. Not all children can be successfully cared for in their own homes and therefore many will have to endure admission for appreciable periods of time, which can adversely impact on their development and education.

Although the prime focus of this chapter revolves around the skills of caring for sick or injured children with orthopaedic conditions, other aspects of management need to be explored within the context of family centred care. In particular the chapters on play and hygiene are fundamental to this.

## OVERVIEW OF THE ANATOMY AND PHYSIOLOGY OF BONE

Tortora and Derrickson[1] describe one of the prime functions of bone and the whole skeletal system as one of support and protection.

## Bone types

The skeleton is made up of a variety of bone types to fulfil this function:

- long bones, typically dealing with movement and support;
- short bones, typically dealing with complex movements in the hand and foot;
- flat bones typically providing protection in, for example, the head and pelvis;
- irregular bones which have complex shapes and are used typically in, for example, the spinal vertebrae.

## Bone structure

All bones have an outer hard cortex and an inner softer medulla where, for example in flat bones, the majority of blood cells such as erythrocytes are manufactured. (This explains why in certain haematological diseases such as thalassaemia, a haemoglobinopathy, or bone marrow hypertrophy can cause facial abnormalities, although in the less severe form, thalassaemia minor, the elevated check bones give the face an attractive heart shape.)

## Anatomical features of long bones

The features of bones can best be understood by examining a typical long bone such as the femur. The shaft of the bone is known as the diaphysis. The diaphysis is separated from the epiphysis or the ends of the bone by the metaphysis, which contains a layer of cartilage that allows the diaphysis to grow in length. The ends of the bone, as in the head of femur for example, are covered in articular cartilage, which allows it to move easily within the hip joint with another articular surface.

The remaining bone surface is covered by a carpet-like casing rich in blood, called the periosteum. This rich blood supply provides nutrients to the living bone made up of osteocytes. Additionally, the periosteum contains bone-forming cells known as osteoblasts which are crucial to fracture repair. The medulla of the bone within the diaphysis of the long bones contains yellow marrow. The ends of the bone and the medulla of flat and irregular bones contain red bone marrow, which is responsible for blood cell production.

## Bone healing

When the bone of a child is fractured a number of configurations are possible.[2]

- transverse fractures, where the line of the break lies across the shaft of the bone usually as a result of a direct blow;
- oblique fractures, where the line of the break is diagonal and usually the result of a bending and twisting injury;
- spiral fractures, where the line of the fracture spirals around the shaft of the bone frequently the result of a twisting injury;
- comminuted fractures, where the bone is broken into several fragments often the result of a severe force;
- greenstick fractures are unique to childhood, where the blow to the bone bends it, like a green stick, and the periostium on the obtuse angle prevents the break from being fully completed;
- crush fractures are normally found in adults but sometimes seen in children with bone disease such as osteogenesis imperfecta, where vertebral bodies might be crushed. (Crush fractures in children can be caused by falls from heights and also from crush-inducing trauma.)

During a fracture the periosteum is torn and bleeding occurs. In large long bones such as the femur the bleeding might be very severe, leading to significant swelling of the limb. Once the bleeding has ceased a clot forms around the fracture, which commences the healing process. As the phagocytic macrophages (the body's housekeeping cells) remove the debris of the clot, the strands of the clot become infiltrated with osteoblasts, the bone-building cells, which are released by the periosteum. Soon the clot is replaced by soft fracture callus, which over time hardens to form new bone. This process will create a structurally sound but weak bone between 4 and 6 weeks after the break (depending on the child's age and also the type of bone involved). Great care is needed at this stage as the child's bone can easily be rebroken or damaged if weight bearing or use of the limb is started too early. Strengthening of the bone fracture site continues for 6–12 weeks as the fracture callus hardens. This strengthening process continues up to 26 weeks. The new bone is eventually remodelled by bone cells known as osteoclasts, and in children unlike adults this remodelling is so efficient that normal bone shape can be fully restored. This remodelling process can continue for up to 2 years after the original fracture. The younger the child the more rapid the process.

## Complications of fractures

Fracture complications[3] can be observed immediately at the point of the injury, during the early days or weeks or later in the healing process. The immediate complications might include damage to the surrounding soft tissue. This is often seen in road traffic accidents involving a bicycle or motor cycle in a young person. In this situation, especially if there has been a compound fracture where the bone fragment has pierced the skin and muscle, road debris may have excoriated the tissues. These dirty and contaminated fracture sites require 'debridement' under anaesthetic, where the wound is literally scrubbed clean or debrided. Other complications that may occur at the time of the fracture include nerve damage or haemorrhage, which is sometimes sufficiently severe to warrant transfusion.

Early complications of fractures in children include infection, compartment syndrome and fat embolism, where fat from yellow bone marrow at the site of the fracture can enter the blood stream causing, among other things, a potential pulmonary embolism. Later complications include malunion, where the fracture heals in the wrong position; delayed union, where the healing of the fracture is slower than anticipated; non-union, where the fracture fails to heal; and vascular necrosis, where a poor blood supply prevents optimum healing.

Many of these complications can be avoided by good fracture management and careful and comprehensive observation of the child.

## TRACTION

Traction simply means the application of a pulling force to a part of the body, usually a limb, along a horizontal direction. However, in order to apply a pulling force in one direction to treat the pain of the disease or to achieve and maintain the reduction of a fracture, there must be an equal pulling in the opposite direction. This is called counter-traction and is achieved in one of two ways: fixed and sliding.

### Methods of traction

#### Fixed traction

This is the term used when the traction or pulling force is conducted between two fixed points. Classically this is seen in cases where a Thomas splint is used. Although not used so often in children, in contemporary practice it is still used as a temporary measure to maintain alignment until another method of management has been adopted. The two fixed points in this case are the U bend at the end of the splint and the ischial tuberosity of the pelvis. The traction and counter-traction are entirely maintained between these two points. This is because force is applied via the pull of the skin extensions and the cords which are tied to the U-bend end of the splint, and the counter-traction force that is transmitted along the parallel bars of the splint pushing against the ischial tuberosity (Figure 32.1).

#### Sliding traction

This is commonly known as balanced traction. This is because in sliding traction there must be two opposing forces equally balanced to provide both traction and counter-traction. The child's own body

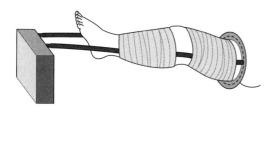

**Figure 32.1** Fixed traction. (Redrawn with permission from *A Textbook of Children's and Young People's Nursing*. Glasper and Richardson, (Oxford: Elsevier)

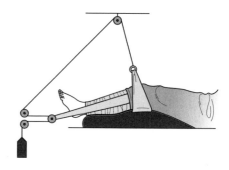

**Figure 32.2** Sliding traction. (Redrawn with permission from *A Textbook of Children's and Young People's Nursing*. Glasper and Richardson, (Oxford: Elsevier)

weight is used in balanced traction to provide the counter-traction force. This is usually achieved by elevating the foot of the child's bed so the child actually moves in the opposite direction to the line of traction. It is important that this arrangement is balanced and each of the components of comparable pull weight. Failure to get this right will reduce the effectiveness of the traction, and too little elevation of the bed or too much applied weight will drag the child to the foot of the bed with the traction weights no longer suspended but lying on the floor. In this situation the traction will be ineffective and could potentially adversely affect bone alignment or increase muscle spasm and pain in other conditions. Simply put, balanced traction is the balance achieved from the traction forces along the length of a limb through skin extensions via suspended weights, and the counter-traction provided by the child's own body weight sliding in the opposite direction (Figure 32.2).

## Types of traction used in childhood disorders[2]

- *Thomas splint traction:* This splint was invented in the late nineteenth century by Hugh Owen Thomas, a Liverpool bone setter and the uncle of Sir Robert Jones, who went onto become a world famous orthopaedic surgeon. Originally used to

treat hip disorders it is now universally used to initially treat fractures of the femoral shaft. Although rarely used for the entirety of the treatment for a fracture in children, the Thomas splint can use either a fixed traction method or a sliding traction method as a temporary measure prior to the use of internal or external fixation. In times past, children's wards were full of children in Thomas splints while they languished for weeks waiting for the fracture to heal. In the modern health service it is unacceptable for social, emotional, fiscal and educational reasons to keep a child in hospital for longer than is strictly necessary, and because of this other methods of treating fractured femurs have been developed to allow earlier discharge.

- *Gallows traction:* This is a unique variation of fixed traction which is appropriate for very young children under 16 kg* (Some authorities specify 12 kg) with fractured femurs and which uses the child's own body weight to maintain counter-traction with the legs suspended and attached by skin extensions to a Balkan beam and pulley system fixed to the child's cot.[4,5] It is important to check the specified maximum weight against local policy before placing a child in Gallows traction.) The traction is therefore achieved because the child's bottom is raised off the bed surface allowing the fracture alignment to be maintained between the fixed points of the Balkan beam and the child's gravitational pull towards the bed surface. Clearly, if the child's bottom is allowed to rest on the surface of the bed then no traction is achieved. *Always ensure that the buttocks are just off the bed surface.* Vascular impairment is the most dangerous complication of Gallows traction and the neurovascular observations must be made frequently to ascertain good integrity. As children in Gallows traction are like all young children 'confined to quarters' they are slippery customers to manage and nurses and family members need the patience of the biblical Job and the eyes of a hawk to ensure that traction is maintained. Excellent diversion therapy is mandatory and the role of the play specialist essential. To alleviate this and to promote early discharge (and) once the swelling has subsided, the child is placed in a hip spica (broomstick variety). However, this element of family-centred care will be predicated on home and personal circumstances as some parents/carers may not able to care for their child in a hip spica (Figure 32.3).

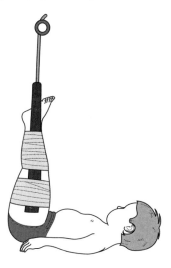

**Figure 32.3** Gallows traction. (Reproduced with permission from *A Textbook of Children's and Young People's Nursing.* Glasper and Richardson, (Oxford: Elsevier)

- *Simple skin traction (Pugh's traction):* Simple skin traction is often applied to a child's limb to reduce pain or muscle spasm. It is frequently used in children with leg or hip problems prior to surgery or more permanent fixation. With this simple traction, weights are attached to the extension tapes of either the adhesive or non-adhesive foam extension strips via a traction pulley at the end of the bed. As with all types of traction the nurse must exercise great care in ensuring that in securing the extension bandages they remain loose enough to prevent swelling and allow good circulation to the part of the limb beyond the point where the traction is applied. In a child with an irritable hip, for example, it is important to ascertain the circulatory competence of the lower leg by examining the feet. Only a moderate amount of pull can be exerted using skin traction because excessive weight applied to the skin surface via any type of extension can cause serious skin irritation, thus reducing the effectiveness of the treatment.

- *Skeletal traction:* This type of traction is now not regularly used in children as surgical interventions have improved greatly, allowing internal fixation of fractures and thus early discharge. Flynn,[6] in a comparison of the use of titanium elastic nails and traction and the subsequent application of a hip spica, found that recovery was enhanced in the group of children treated with intermedullary nails. Skeletal traction is sometimes used to treat fractures of the femur that are difficult to align or where there has been skin damage, and may be used in conjunction with a Thomas splint and Pearson's flexion knee piece. Although rare, when this is advocated a sterile metal pin is inserted through an area of strong bone such as the tibial tuberosity. Traction by means of weights is then applied to the pin via a stirrup, which is clamped to the ends of the pin. The traction cords are then allowed to run through a pulley at the foot of the elevated Balkan beam bed end where the weights hang free.

## APPLYING SKIN TRACTION

### The procedural goal is to

- reduce dislocation or fracture
- prevent movement of injured part, thus facilitating bone healing
- reduce and overcome muscle spasm
- prevent and correct deformity
- rest joints (e.g. irritable hip)
- allow healing in the optimum position.

## PROCEDURE: Applying skin traction

| Procedural steps | Evidence-based rationale |
|---|---|
| 1 Applying simple skin traction requires two people one of whom should be experienced in traction applications (Pugh's traction)[7] | Safe management. Moving and handling |
| 2 Ascertain the need for either an adhesive or non-adhesive traction kit or appropriate bandages | Skin integrity |
| 3 Prepare the bed with appropriate Balkan beam bed frame and pulleys, and weights as prescribed. Some hospitals have special beds and cots with orthopaedic frames already attached | Safe practice |
| 4 Provide appropriate information to the child and family members using a variety of methods. Involve a play specialist to provide distraction/pre-procedural play when required | Family centred care. Therapeutic play. Avoidance of psychological distress |
| 5 Ascertain the integrity of the skin. Check allergy status of the child with parent/guardian | Skin integrity |
| 6 Administer prescribed analgesia where necessary | Pain relief and comfort |
| 7 Measure the traction extensions against the unaffected limb to avoid causing pain, making sure that you have left enough space to allow the child to plantar flex the foot without restriction when the spreader bar is inserted. Cut off the excess material with scissors | Accuracy and pain avoidance |
| 8 Starting at the malleoli of the foot apply the extensions to the medial and lateral aspects of the leg. Keep the extensions straight to prevent medial or lateral rotation of the limb and to ensure that the malleoli are covered by the foam padding. If you are using adhesive extensions peel back the adhesive covering slowly to enable you to apply the material to the skin without causing wrinkles which in turn could damage the child's skin integrity | Pain minimisation and skin integrity |
| 9 Apply bandage (not too tightly) starting just above the malleoli. Leave the knee free | Skin integrity, uncompromised circulation |
| 10 Take the traction cords at the spreader and pass through the pulley at the end of the bed and attach securely to the prescribed weights | Maintenance of adequate traction, overcome muscle spasm, pain relief, correct fracture alignment. Maintain limb length |
| 11 Elevate the foot of the bed to provide the counter-traction ensuring that the child does not slide down the bed too much | Maintenance of adequate traction |
| 12 Ensure neurovascular observations are recorded | Detection of neurovascular impairment (compartment syndrome) |

# APPLYING A THOMAS SPLINT USING ADHESIVE TRACTION (SKELETAL TRACTION RARELY USED)

## Equipment required for the application of a Thomas splint

A suitable bed with Balkan beam attached and equipped with various traction pulleys

Modern splints can be used on either leg and are fully adjustable with half rings secured with Velcro

Skin preparation material as directed by your own hospital protocol

Skin extension pack (in rare circumstances a skeletal pin holder for skeletal traction will be needed, where a sterile skeletal pin is drilled through the proximal end of an adjacent long bone; this is usually performed in the operating theatre)

Ready made Velcro-fastening foam slings which come in different sizes. These are disposable for single use

Crepe bandages and adhesive strapping

Scissors

Possible Pearson knee flexion piece (rare for skin traction but usually used with skeletal traction)

Traction cord

Pulleys as required

Prescribed weights

Suspension system

## PROCEDURE: Applying a Thomas splint

| Procedural steps | Evidence-based rationale |
|---|---|
| **Pre procedure** | |
| 1 Shaving of limb hair may be required in older children | Skin integrity. Promotion of adhesion. Adhesive extensions are used with a Thomas splint |
| 2 Pain relief (femoral blocks) prior to alignment of the limb and the position of the child | This may be undertaken under general anaesthetic but if not, pain relief will be required. Use an appropriate pain measurement tool |
| 3 Skin care in the groin area where the splint will lie | The infected ring sores of the past can be avoided by initial and subsequent good hygiene. Modern slit splints allow for post-fracture swelling |
| 4 All lower clothing will have been removed to expose the affected limb but remember to protect the child's dignity | Access to the limb |
| **During procedure** | |
| 5 The splint is prepared by using the foam slings to create a cradle along the length of the Thomas splint for supporting the limb | Padding the spilt with the slings prevents undue bowing of the fractured bone and helps maintain full alignment |
| 6 Depending on the site of fracture the splint configuration may be adjusted to achieve 5° of knee flexion. This is achievable by increasing the padding around the dorsal knee area. If more than 5° of knee flexion is prescribed, a Pearson knee flexion piece may be used. This is attached to the parallel bars of the splint and allows the limb to be placed in a degree of flexion | Post-recovery knee flexion integrity |

## PROCEDURE: Applying a Thomas splint (continued)

| | |
|---|---|
| 7 After skin preparation the skin (or skeletal) extensions are then applied longitudinally and without creases and the prepared splint passed over the limb. The splint is pushed up to the groin and the tension of the slings adjusted to maintain the normal bowing of the femur. In boys it is important to prevent the testicles from being excoriated by the ring | Skin integrity |
| 8 When used with a fixed traction method at the W-shaped distal end of the splint, the skin extension cords are tied to the end of the splint with sufficient force to prevent the ring from embedding in the groin. When the splint, as is customary, is used with sliding traction, the cords are passed over a pulley on the bed frame. In this way the traction is achieved by the pull on the extension, and the foot of the bed is elevated for counter-traction. After application of the traction, the suspension system is set up to facilitate the mobility of the patient while being maintained on the Thomas splint | Maintenance of traction and mobility |
| 9 The skin traction should then be secured from thigh to the ankle using crepe bandages. Note that crepe bandages are applied above and below the knee to keep the extensions in place over the limb and are secured with adhesive strapping | The knee and therefore the fibula head are kept free from the bandage to reduce the risk of peroneal nerve compression at the fibular head. This nerve descends obliquely along the lateral side of the popliteal fossa to the head of the fibula and is prone to compression damage. This can be assessed by ensuring that the child can dorsiflex the foot |
| **Following procedure** 10 Undue pressure in the popliteal space must be prevented by ensuring that the slings are and remain crease-free and, if used as fixed traction, the pillow on which the splint rests is not hard | Prevent nerve compromise |
| 11 Although in contemporary UK practice the use of a Thomas splint is usually a temporary measure, children will still need to be taught to lift their buttocks off the bed frequently by using the overhead trapeze and their unaffected leg | Reduce risk of sacral tissue damage. Pressure area care is essential |
| 12 Ring care: check for excoriation frequently | Prevent pressure ulcers developing |
| 13 Foot exercises must be encouraged regularly to the affected foot to maintain strength. Check that the splint slings do not place pressure on the Achilles tendon | Prevent foot drop |
| 14 Exercise regime should be instigated for the duration of bed rest | Prevent muscle wastage and other complications of prolonged bed rest |

## APPLYING GALLOWS TRACTION

Gallows traction is usually used in children under 2 years of age but can be used up to the age of 3 if the child is small and, importantly, weighing usually not more than 16 kg.

Normally Gallows traction is used with adhesive extensions but in the case of skin problems a non-adhesive traction kit may be prescribed. Note that all children under 1 year of age presenting with a femoral fracture are screened under hospital safeguarding policies.

### Equipment

A suitable cot with Balkan beam attached equipped with various traction pulleys
Skin preparation material as directed by your own hospital protocol
Crepe bandages and adhesive strapping
Scissors
Pulleys as required
Prescribed weights if a pulley system is being used

## PROCEDURE: Applying Gallows traction

| Procedural steps | Evidence-based rationale |
|---|---|
| **During procedure** | |
| 1 After ascertaining the child's weight, two people are required to perform this procedure one of whom is experienced in applying traction | Child safeguarding. Moving and handling protocol |
| 2 Prepare the cot/bed with an appropriate Balkan beam bed frame and pulleys where necessary | Maintenance of traction |
| 3 Provide appropriate information using a variety of methods to the members of the family about the traction system and why it is important to keep the buttocks raised from the bed surface | Meeting national policy guidelines relating to partnership and family empowerment through enhanced information giving |
| 4 Always Involve the hospital play specialist to provide distraction/pre-procedural play when required | The role of therapeutic play is to:<br>• help children to master and cope with anxieties, feelings and pain<br>• help children to cope with hospital experiences<br>• help the child regain confidence and self-esteem<br>• normalise the environment/aids normality<br>• help children to learn in an enjoyable way<br>• promote and encourage development<br>• significantly reduce stress and anxiety<br>• facilitate communication<br>See Chapter 7 |
| 5 Ascertain the integrity of the skin. Check with the family if the child has any allergies of previous skin conditions | Maintain skin integrity |
| 6 Administer prescribed analgesia where necessary | Alleviation of pain |

## PROCEDURE: Applying Gallows traction (continued)

| | |
|---|---|
| 7 Measure the traction extensions against the unaffected limb to avoid causing the child pain. Ensure that that you have left enough space to allow the children to dorsiflex and plantar flex the foot without restriction when the spreader bar is inserted. Cut off the excess skin extension with scissors | Prevention of pain. Foot movement |
| 8 After skin preparation and starting at the malleoli of the foot, apply the extensions to the medial and lateral aspects of the leg. Keep the extensions straight to prevent medial or lateral rotation of the limb and to ensure that the malleoli are covered by the foam padding | If you are using adhesive extensions peel back the adhesive covering slowly to enable you to apply the material to the skin without causing wrinkles which in turn could damage the child's skin integrity |
| 9 Apply bandage (not too tightly) starting just above the malleoli. Leave the knee free | Nerve integrity |
| 10 Take the traction cords at the spreader and tie them to the beam above for simple gallows or thread the cords through the pulleys on the Balkan Beam bed frame and attach to the prescribed weights. In both cases ensure that you provide counter-traction in ensuring that the child's buttocks are a flat handbreadth off the surface of the mattress | Maintenance of adequate traction. Ensure that the counter-traction is only facilitated by the 'flat of the hand, principle' as too little counter-traction cause pain from muscle spasm and may result in malunion of the bone. Too much counter-traction similarly as with tight bandages may cause neurovascular impairment |
| **During procedure** | |
| 11 Ensure frequent observation of neurovascular status | Detection of early warning signs |
| 12 Provide play therapy | Most children adapt very well to being suspended in mid-air but they do initially find the experience strange and frightening. The use of the play specialist in providing distraction at the outset is crucial. Children in Gallows traction may become quite disruptive and fractious if not occupied and may become entangled in their traction cords if they try to spin around. The play specialist can proactively prevent or modify such behaviour by providing high quality play materials and visual distraction such as DVDs |
| 13 Address all the activities of daily living | These children also need considerable help in undertaking the activities of daily living.[2] In particular, skin care, elimination and nutrition are all important when nursing a child in Gallows traction |

# SPECIFIC NURSING CARE OF CHILDREN IN TRACTION

## Skin care

The extension bandages should be checked and renewed only as appropriate but 4-hourly observations of neurovascular function should be recorded.

## Nutrition

This is always difficult as children in traction are either flat in bed or in the case of Gallows traction flat with their legs in the air. After family negotiation, a suitable diet, which will involve small, frequent and easy to digest meals with plenty of fibre and fluids, will be authorised. It is important to stress that children in Gallows traction should be supervised during meal times as the danger of inhalation and choking is potentially high. Given the emphasis on fluids and nutrition a record and annotation on the fluid balance chart should be kept until the child has resumed a normal nutritional pattern.

## Elimination

Children being treated by traction will find it difficult to adapt to their limitations and in particular confinement to bed. Nurses also need to involve parents in the management of elimination as some children may be discharged home in Gallows traction, although a hip spica is usually applied.[8,9] Eaton[10] stresses the importance of involving children's community nurses when sick children are transferred from hospital to home, and all orthopaedic nurses must assess the ability of parents to manage a child in traction at home. Constipation can be avoided by encouraging fluids, fibre and fruit. If this fails, an aperient may be prescribed, and if this fails a one-off suppository or enema may be required. This may take place in hospital or with input from a community nurses if the child is being cared for at home.

# CARE OF CHILDREN IN SPLINTS

## Applying a plaster cast and cast management

Casts used to treat a variety of childhood disorders are made up of plaster of Paris bandages or synthetic materials. Plaster of Paris is less frequently used now as it has been superseded by fibreglass or lighter and sturdier materials. In many parts of the world, however, the cheapness and easy availability of plaster of Paris ensures that it retains its popularity as an easy to apply splinting material. This section will focus on the procedure of applying plaster of Paris and fibreglass or polyester casting.

### Procedural goal is to

- prevent and correct deformities
- provide support
- provide pain relief
- protect an injury
- immobilise fractures
- improve function by stabilising a joint
- facilitate early ambulation and weight bearing.

## Plaster of Paris casting

### Equipment

Equipment trolley
Plaster of Paris
Softband padding and stockinette
Plaster of Paris slabs if required and plaster strips to finish
Plastic sheeting and aprons and plastic-covered pillows
Plaster scissors
Bucket or bowl of water at 20–25°C, wash bowl for the child and towel(s)
Rubbish bag
Elbow or knee rest
Instruction leaflets
Felt padding

## PROCEDURE: Application of plaster of Paris

| Procedural steps | Evidence-based rationale |
| --- | --- |
| 1 Any jewellery and clothing on the affected limb must be removed and stored safely by the child's family or according to local policy | Swelling always accompanies fractures for example and jewellery such as rings could cause vascular damage necessitating a frightening mechanical removal |
| 2 The prescription authorizing the procedure is checked for the correct details, and in readiness for undertaking the procedure an equipment trolley for the application of the cast must be prepared | To ensure that the correct type of cast is applied (e.g. back slab, short or long arm cast) |
| 3 The child is appropriately positioned | Position the child with the body part to be plastered appropriately exposed. The limb or body (in the case of spicas) to be casted needs to be appropriately positioned). For upper-limb casting, the child is nursed in a supine position, with the shoulder abducted at 90°, elbow flexed at 90° and the digits held towards the ceiling. In lower-limb casting, the child is positioned sitting up for a below-knee plaster of Paris, and supine for a full-length or cylinder plaster. A footrest is often used to hold the ankle in a neutral position during application |
| 4 The environment of care should reflect the age group of the child | As this procedure is likely to be performed in a plaster room which is often rather stark and clinical, mobile equipment such as Starlight distraction boxes should be available to offer distraction and temporarily change the environment of the room (http://www.starlight.org) |
| 5 Family members should be given a protective disposable apron and plastic overshoes | Plaster of Paris can ruin clothing and leather shoes |
| 6 A stockinette is applied to the limb. It needs to be measured and cut a little longer than the plaster and then rolled up and applied to the limb | This is to provide comfort, and to protect the skin of the child from the sharp edges of the plaster. It is important to note that the application of stockinette may be contraindicated if there is likelihood of severe swelling. In such cases the stockinette may create a tourniquet effect and cause constriction |
| 7 Bony prominences must be padded with a layer of Softband applied smoothly and evenly over the stockinette. The width of padding is usually 10–15 cm for legs and 5–10 cm for arms but is dependent on the age of the child. The padding is applied by rolling distally to proximally, tearing it off to go around joints. Appropriate-sized plaster of Paris bandages are selected for casting: 8–10cm plaster is used for upper limb and 10–15 cm for lower limb but is also age dependent | For protection and to prevent plaster sores from developing |

## PROCEDURE:  Application of plaster of Paris (continued)

| | |
|---|---|
| 8  The plaster bandage roll is prepared by unrolling the first 5–8 cm; keep hold of the end and then immersed into the container of lukewarm water (20–25°C) until the bubbles stop. Note that cold water retards the setting process while warm water quickens it. With one end in each hand, the roll is gently squeezed to get rid of excess water | Satisfactory setting time with least mess |
| 9  Bandaging commences at one end of the limb, rolling the wet bandage away from the person applying the cast from within to without applicator. The bandage is applied evenly, covering about one-third of the previous turn. The remainders of the bandages are then applied quickly before the first bandage is set | Ease of application to provide an homogeneous finish |
| 10  During the application process the palms of the hands and palmar eminences, rather than the fingertips, are used to constantly smooth and mould the plaster to coalesce the plaster bandages into one | The cast should resemble fine china and in using the palms rather than the fingers prevents pressure points from developing under the cast |
| 11  An additional person may be required to assist and hold the limb | It is important that the limb position is maintained until the plaster dries to a firm consistency |
| 12  After application the limb is rested on a pillow to prevent the cast from denting | Plastic or rubber pillows should not be used as they trap heat under the cast, which prevents heat dissipation and prolongs cast drying |
| 13  Where necessary the edges of the cast are trimmed and the proximal and distal ends of the stockinette are turned back over the cast edges, making a neat finish | The raw edges of a plaster cast can cause skin excoriation and turning down of the stockinette is undertaken to prevent discomfort or injury |

## APPLICATION OF FIBREGLASS CAST

Casts made of polyester or fibreglass casting tape are becoming increasingly popular because they are durable, lightweight and waterproof. However, fibreglass is difficult to mould and significantly more expensive than plaster of Paris, and is therefore used less for acute injury. The new polyester casts are easier to apply; wear gloves to handle the product.[11]

The preparation of the patient is similar to that undertaken for the application of a plaster of Paris splint. The procedure is also similar to the application of plaster of Paris described, except that wearing gloves is mandatory for handling the fibreglass material.

- A nylon stockinette and padding should be used.
- The roll of casting should be opened immediately before using.
- Fibreglass material must be applied with a little more pressure than plaster of Paris, and conforms more easily if applied spirally, squaring the upper and lower ends by making horizontal turns.
- The cast needs to be applied so as to decrease the amount of trimming needed as fibreglass casts cannot be cut by a cast knife or scissors.
- After application the cast takes approximately 7 minutes to dry by the open-air drying method; weight bearing is allowed only after 20 minutes.

## PROCEDURE: Post-procedure

| Procedural steps | Evidence-based rationale |
|---|---|
| 1 Elevate the casted limb as appropriate, especially if swelling is anticipated | Elevating the limb will help prevent excessive swelling by encouraging venous return and may prevent the need for bivalving the cast |
| 2 Allow the cast to dry naturally at room temperature and leave uncovered for 48 hours but be careful not to allow the child to be become cold. At the drying stage, do not, when moving or touching the cast use excessive pressure with your fingers<br><br>Never apply direct heat to a plaster of Paris cast | This can cause indentations as the cast is still relatively soft and can result in unnecessary plaster sores subsequently developing. This is especially so for hip spicas, where the child's position has to be changed every 2 hours to prevent pressure sores<br><br>When caring for children in hip spicas and moving them prone to supine, you will need to adjust the pillows and foam blocks to accommodate the shape of the spica especially if the knee in plaster is flexed Drying times for casts varies and depends on the thickness of the plaster cast. As a rule, for regular, non-weight-bearing plaster casts the drying time is 24 hours<br>For weight-bearing plaster casts the drying time is at least 48 hours. The child is usually allowed to bear weight only after an X-ray has shown a successful reduction and immobilisation of the fracture but normally tibial fractures will require a minimum of 2 weeks non-weight bearing. In consultation with medical staff, clarify if the child is allowed to weight bear on the cast |
| 3 Ensure that joints not encased in plaster are exercised | To prevent of stiffness and muscle wasting; if cast edges become rough, cover the rough ends with tape. Wash the skin area around the cast, but take care not to wet it |
| 4 Hip spicas and other body casts especially in very young children will need to be protected from urine and excrement | Waterproof tape can be used to tape around all edges of the plaster cast. The smell of these plasters can become very unpleasant and therefore the area around the groin requires strict hygiene |
| 5 Monitor the cast regularly for cracking, denting or softening (of cast). Also observe for swelling and discoloration of limb and reports of soreness, unpleasant smells, discharges and undue or increasing pain. Ensure neurovascular observations are performed. This is especially pertinent for fractures involving the elbow such as supracondular fractures of the humerus. If the child has had an open reduction or some type of surgery before the application of the cast, blood loss should be assessed. The blood will stain the plaster and the simple measure of drawing a line around the stain will allow you to observe subsequent blood loss. All deviations should be reported and fully documented within the child's records | Plaster sores may initially be recognised only by a burning pain beneath the plaster as the superficial pain receptors are affected by the friction of the plaster. Later signs such as staining or an unpleasant smell may indicate where damage has already have been done. When a child is discharged in a cast, ensure that full care instructions are given to the family with the telephone number of someone to contact for advice. Some healthcare professionals at discharge actually adhere the instructions to the cast itself. |

## General cast rules

- Encourage exercising of finger and toes.
- Keep limbs elevated when resting.
- Do not get plasters wet as they are not waterproof.
- Caution the child and family not to put small objects down the cast – inform child and family that no pencils or knitting needles are to be used for scratching. Any of these can lead to skin damage and the development of plaster sores. If this occurs on a heel, the child's rehabilitation could be severely impaired.
- Do not ever put a child in plaster next to any direct heat such as an electric fire or radiator. Plaster will retain heat for a long time and the risk of burns is high.

### Removing a plaster cast

Although plaster casts can be removed with plaster shears it is customary to use an oscillating saw, which emits fluctuating levels of high frequency noise and can cause a vibration sensation in the bone which some children find very uncomfortable.

Children can find the whole process frightening and the nurse should take steps to prepare the family for the procedure. Anxiety reactions can be partially mitigated by the use of hearing protectors.[12]

## NEUROVASCULAR ASSESSMENT

It is vital to undertake neurovascular observations as part of a neurovascular assessment and you should monitor for numbness or pins and needles, cyanosis or discoloration of the toes or fingers. Feel the extremities with your own fingers and check for warmth or coldness, at the same time comparing both limbs. Ascertain that the child can wiggle their fingers or toes and in the case of supracondular fractures of the humerus, check the integrity of the radial pulse. Compartment syndrome is still a worrying complication of a limb fracture. Andrews[13] describes the five Ps of neurovascular assessment (Table 32.1)

### The procedural goal is to

- regularly monitor neurovascular status of the limb to ensure early detection of complications.
- prevent a child from developing a potential life-long disability.

**Table 32.1** Neurovascular assessment

| Five Ps of neurovascular assessment | Rationale |
| --- | --- |
| Pain | Early indicators of damage |
| Pallor | |
| Paraesthesia | |
| Pulselessness | Late signs of damage |
| Paralysis | |
| Document neurovascular assessment findings | Facilitates ongoing evaluation |

## PIN-SITE CARE

### External fixation and pin site care

The use of external fixation in children is well established, but the management of the skeletal pin site skin care is subject to continuing debate.[14]

The presence of a pin through a bone and skin is always a potential source of infection, and as the skin cannot heal around the pin site exit it is necessary to ensure that the infection risk is minimised.[15] Davis *et al.*, have described a

prospective study in which patients were monitored for infection rates using two pin site care methods. The pin site methods used open and closed methods of covering the exit wounds. Although not a randomised controlled trial, the study showed no significant differences in infection rates between the two groups.

Always refer to your own hospital procedure guidelines for instructions on how to undertake pin site care.

## Sample pin site protocol (Bristol children's hospital)

### The procedural goal is to

- prevent infection of the bone;
- maintain wound/skin hygiene and skin integrity.

### Equipment

One dressing pack
Extra packets of sterile sponge sticks
One sheet of Biatan softhold foam dressing
Pink chlorhexidene 0.5% or normal saline
Sterile scissors
Alcohol hand-rub

| Procedural steps | Evidence-based rationale |
|---|---|
| 1 Wash your hands as normal and use hospital alcohol hand-rub afterwards | Prevention of infection |
| 2 Open dressing pack and set out equipment using forceps | |
| 3 Pour cleaning solution into the plastic receptacle | |
| 4 Cut Biatain sheets into squares about 3 cm by 3 cm | |
| 5 Make keyhole dressings out of the squares by using the sterile scissors to make a 1.5-cm cut as if you were making shorts | |
| 6 Push the plastic clips up the wire or pin. These can be removed and cleaned and replaced over the new dressings | |
| 7 Remove the old dressings and discard in the bag provided | |
| 8 Wash your hands again with the alcohol rub | |
| 9 Clean the pin sites individually using the sponge sticks dipped into the cleaning solution remembering to clean in one direction only but using all sides of the stick | |
| 10 Make sure the skin can move freely around the pin and where necessary remove crusts with the forceps | |
| 11 Ensure all sites are dry; where necessary use dry gauze | |
| 12 Wash your hands again with alcohol rub | |
| 13 Cover pin sites with at least two layers of Biatain; with some pin sites you may need to use three or four layers. Remember to ensure that the keyhole slits in the dressings are all opposed | |
| 14 Push down the plastic clips and again make sure that the slit of the clip is in a different direction to the slit in the top layer dressing. Do not press the clips down too hard: they are to hold the dressing in place not to cause a pressure sore | |
| 15 Dispose of the dressing pack in the normal way | |

## CONCLUSION

Dressings should be changed every 7 days unless there is pain or purulent discharge from around the pin site or there are other signs of infection.

In this chapter we have explored some of the basic skills of nursing children with common orthopaedic problems.

 Go to the website to find the PowerPoint presentation for this chapter and MCQs to test your knowledge. **www.hodderplus.com/childnursingskills**

## REFERENCES

1  Tortora GJ, Derrickson B (2007) *Introduction to the human body. The essentials of anatomy and physiology*, 7th edition. Chichester: John Wiley and Sons.

2  Silverwood B (2006) Caring for children with orthopaedic disorders. In: Glasper EA, Richardson, J (eds) *A text book of children's and young people's nursing*. Edinburgh: Churchill Livingstone, Chapter 35.

3  Whiting NL (2008) Fractures: pathophysiology, treatment and nursing care. *Nursing standard* **17**(2): 49–57.

4  Glasper EA, McConochie, J, Twells S (2007) Fundamental aspects of musculoskeletal and integumentary care. In: Glasper EA, Aylott M, Prudhoe G (eds) *Fundamental aspects of children's and young people's nursing procedures*. London: Quay books.

5  Davis PD (1999) Principles of traction. *Journal of Orthopaedic Nursing* **3**: 222–237.

6  Flynn JM, Luedtke LM, Ganley TJ, *et al.* (2004) Comparison of titanium elastic nails with traction and spica cast to treat femoral fractures in children. *The Journal of Bone and Joint Surgery* **86**: 770–777.

7  Doman M (2006) Skin traction: application and care (principles). In: Glasper EA, McEwing, G, Richardson, J (eds) *Oxford handbook of children's and young people's nursing*. Oxford: Oxford University Press, Chapter 8.

8  Holmes SJK, Sedgewick DM, Scobie WG (1983) Domiciliary gallows traction for femoral shaft fractures in young children. Feasibility safety and advantages. *Journal of Bone and Joint Surgery* **65**(3): 288–290.

9  Clayton M (1997) Traction at home. The Doncaster approach. *Paediatric Nursing* **9**(2): 21–23.

10  Eaton N (2000) Children's community nursing services: models of care delivery. A review of the United Kingdom literature. *Journal of Advanced Nursing* **32**(1): 49–56.

11  Munshi P, Neale G, Maclellan G (2000) Detachable functional forearm focused rigidity cast: A one off definitive treatment for stable forearm greenstick fractures. Injury **31**(4): 239–242

12  Katz K, Fogeleman R, Attias J, et al. (2001) Anxiety reaction in children during removal of their plaster cast with a saw. *Journal of Bone and Joint Surgery* **83**: 388–390.

13  Andrews LW (1990) Neurovascular assessment. *Advanced Clinical Care* **6**(6): 5–7.

14  Williams H, Griffiths P (2004) The effectiveness of pin site care for patients with external fixators. *British Journal of Community Nursing* **9**: 206–210.

15  Davies R, Holt N, Nayagam S (2005) The care of pin sites with external fixation. *The Journal of Bone and Joint Surgery* **87-B**: 716–719.

## CHAPTER 33

# Care of the child with spinal injury

Karen O'Donnell

## LEARNING OUTCOMES

*Upon completion of this chapter the reader should be able to accomplish the following:*
- Gain a knowledge and understanding of the anatomy and physiology of spinal cord injury (SCI) and the subsequent deficit following damage at different levels
- Identify the physical, psychological, developmental and social needs of children and young people with SCI
- Describe the impact and management of SCI on the growing child
- Discuss child-centred care and working in partnership with children and families
- Illustrate the significance and value of specialist spinal paediatric services

## CHAPTER OVERVIEW

This chapter aims to introduce the complexity of the care involved in the 'lifelong' impact of spinal cord injury (SCI) on the growing child. Children with SCI have ongoing rehabilitation needs throughout their growth into adulthood. They are constantly evolving, cognitively, physically, psychologically and socially. In view of this, their needs, through the stages of development, should be reviewed by specialist services in order to monitor their existing SCI, to diminish impairment secondary to growth with SCI and to promote verbal independence and functional ability. SCI is a multisystem disorder and as such results in a dramatic disturbance of motor, sensory and autonomic function with a host of end organ effects. The impact of SCI extends beyond physical impairment of function and every aspect of the child's life can be altered.

## Definitions

**Digital stimulation:** insertion of one gloved lubricated finger into the rectum, rotate finger gently and remove/exit

**Flaccid:** flaccid paralysis is associated with a lower motor neuron lesion (LMN), where the lesion affects nerve fibres travelling from the anterior horn of the spinal cord to the relevant muscle

**Neurogenic/neuropathic:**

**Paraplegia:**

**Poikilothermia:** SCI affects a person's ability to control their body temperature. Instead, the paralysed body adopts the temp' of the local environment.

> **Definitions**
>
> **Reflex:** reflex paralysis is associated with an upper motor neuron lesion (UMN), where the lesion affects the neural pathway above the anterior horn.
>
> **Spinal shock:** period after trauma to the spinal cord which may last for up to 6 weeks during which time there is no reflex activity
>
> **Tetraplegia/tetraplegic:**

# INCIDENCE AND AETIOLOGY

Spinal cord injury is an uncommon condition among adults and is rare in children. In a European study Augutis *et al.*[1] estimated that the incidence of paediatric SCI (non-fatal injuries) varied from 0.9 to 21.2 children/million of children/year in the 0–14 years age group. The prevalence of SCI is approximately 40 000 individuals in the UK,[2] and injuries to those under 16 years of age are thought to account for only 5 per cent of these.[3] However this is likely to be an underestimate as many children are not referred to specialist units, nor is there a national database requiring registration of injured individuals.

# NEUROLOGICAL ASSESSMENT AND FUNCTIONAL CLASSIFICATION OF SCI

The American Spinal Injury Association (ASIA)[4] first published a standard system for neurological assessment and classification of SCI in 1982 (Figures 33.1 and 33.2, page 568). This involves bilateral strength testing of 10 key muscles (five upper extremity and five lower extremity) and bilateral sensory testing (sharp/dull discrimination and light touch) of 28 dermatomes. At present there is no specific assessment tool for neurological assessment and examination in children under 4 years and no published adapted tool for children under 10 years.[5] The ASIA impairment classification is therefore currently used as the international standard for neurological classification of spinal cord injury in adults and children.

The spinal cord has 31 pairs of nerves, which connect it to different parts of the body. Spinal nerves contain motor fibres innervating certain

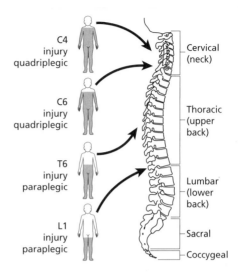

**Figure 33.1** Extent of injury after damage to specific spinal segments. A - Complete: No motor or sensory function is preserved in the sacral segments S4-S5. B – Incomplete: Sensory but no motor function is preserved below the neurological level and includes S4-S5. C – Incomplete: Motor function is preserved below the level and more than half the key muscles below the level have a grade less than 3. D – Incomplete: As C but grade of 3 or more. E – Normal: Motor and sensory function are normal with permission from American Spinal Injury Association: International Standards for Neurological Classification of Spinal Cord Injury, revised 2000; Atlanta, Georgia, reprinted 2008.

muscles (myotomes) and sensory fibres innervating certain areas of skin (dermatomes). Although slight variations do exist, dermatome and myotome patterns of distribution are relatively consistent from person to person.

Knowledge of the classification scale of SCI provides the rational for expectations of the functional outcomes at the different levels of spinal cord injury

Anatomical differences in children include:

- increased mortality and morbidity at any age;
- the larger head size in the smaller child, in relation to their body size, creating greater force on the neck when the head is jolted;

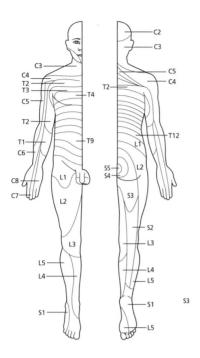

**Figure 33.2** ASIA sensory key points by spinal dermatomes. Reproduced from American Spinal Injury Association: International Standards for Neurological Classification of Spinal Cord Injury, revised 2000; Atlanta, Georgia, reprinted 2008.

- greater flexibility of the spine and its supporting structures (Their ligaments and joints are elastic and can withstand considerable stretching without tearing. This allows additional stretching of the spinal cord when force is applied, damaging the spinal cord without bony injury. This is described as spinal cord injury without radiological abnormality. [SCIWORA];[6]
- craniocervical disruption and/or atlantoaxial dislocation, which is almost unique to children and difficult to diagnose;
- growth plates present in the developing spine so that injury and compression of the vertebrae can cause bone damage;
- ossification centres present at birth and fusion occurring as the child grows; prior to fusion children are predisposed to subluxation and distraction resulting in spinal injury.[7]

# ACUTE MANAGEMENT/SPINAL STABILISATION

Despite the incident or mechanism of SCI it is both primary and secondary damage that leads to the spinal cord lesion. Nursing care is directed at preservation of functional ability and prevention of secondary complications.

Each injury has to be assessed for instability and the decision to treat operatively or non-operatively taken on an individual basis by the treating medical team.

## Traumatic injury

The implications of the same traumatic force on a child compared with an adult will be a massive difference in the extent of trauma sustained. The injury mechanism for SCI in most cases is that of severe flexion and extension, which may result in physical tearing of the spinal cord. The instability, laxity and range of movement of the immature cervical spine, combined with the disproportionate size of the child's head compared with the body means that cervical lesions predominate in very young children.[7] In addition, complete motor and sensory paralysis is more likely due to the less stable vertebral column.

## Non-traumatic injury

This may include:

- vascular incidents: haemorrhaging or thrombosis;
- inflammatory conditions: transverse myelitis;
- infections: meningitis and tuberculosis;
- spinal cord compression: tumours.

## Maintain spinal alignment

Damage to the cord does not stop at the time of injury but continues for a period of time following. Prevention of further cord damage can be achieved by immobilisation of the spine.

**KEY POINTS**
- Inspect the injury and identify the level of cord damage
- Immobilise the spine
- Maintain and preserve function
- Prevent complications

## PROCEDURE: Acute management/spinal stabilisation

| Procedural steps | Nursing skill | Evidence-based rationale |
|---|---|---|
| **1 Immobilisation**<br>Suspected injury: spinal immobilisation[8] | Avoid neck flexion due to the larger head of the younger child as this can lead to further trauma | To prevent further damage to the spinal cord and preserve neurological recovery |
| Identify the level of spinal cord damage | Use appropriate immobilisation for head size | To prevent secondary complications |
| Internal fixation is not usually recommended in the very young child as it may affect future growth and development | The Pegasus atlas bed is used for the older child (age and weight dependent, using a foam pressure relieving mattress) | Air mattresses are not recommended due to the alternating air pressures causing instability.[8] Refer to SCI centre for specialist advice |
| Halo brace or traction may be used as medically directed | The younger child should be nursed on a static bed<br>Use pillows or sandbags to hold and maintain spinal alignment and limb position<br>Log roll every 24 hours<br>Wear a backless gown or night shirt | To inspect skin condition, perform hygiene needs and bowel care<br>To avoid unnecessary movement of the spine, minimise the risk of skin damage<br><br>To maintain dignity |
| **2 Respiration**<br>Respiratory function may be compromised due to nerve damage affecting the diaphragm, intracostal, accessory and abdominal muscles | Observe child's colour<br>Commence oxygen-saturation monitoring | Pale or blue tinge with poor capillary refill may indicate the need for oxygen therapy<br>Blood gas monitoring as indicated |
| The child may therefore fatigue and depression of adequate ventilation is likely | Record respiratory rate and listen for equal air entry<br>Record functional vital capacity (FVC) | Shallow breathing may be an indication of neurological damage to the spinal cord<br>Reduced FVC may indicate respiratory deterioration[9]<br>Regular use of incentive spirometers can maintain and improve functional vital capacity |
| An increase in intra-abdominal pressure may also decrease respiratory function | Consider insertion of a nasogastric tube | Prevents the splinting effect on the diaphragm caused by paralytic ileus or air swallowing which can occur in the distressed child |
| The child's cough may be poor leading to secretion retention, atelectasis and chest infection.[9] | Chest toilet<br>Regular chest physiotherapy, assistive cough techniques and use of mechanical insufflator–exsufflator | Mobilise chest secretions and assist expectoration and prevention of chest infection and pneumonia<br>Consider nebulised saline,[9] acetylcysteine or bronchodilators |
| If the child has a tracheostomy, performing tracheal suction can stimulate bradycardia due to autonomic alterations with high vagal tone<br>Early autonomic nervous | Observe child during tracheal suction | Monitor pulse and oxygen using pulse oximetry |

## PROCEDURE: Acute management/spinal stabilisation (continued)

| | | |
|---|---|---|
| system changes can also result in nasal congestion | | |
| **3 Cardiovascular**<br>Bradycardia and hypotension are common in cervical lesions | Record baseline observations | To prevent venous pooling |
| Disruption of descending sympathetic pathways results in loss of vasomotor tone and hypotension | Apply anti-embolism stockings<br>Administer anticoagulation therapy<br>This should be followed for a 12-week period post injury or until discharge as per advice[10] | To prevent venous pooling<br>To prevent risk of thrombosis<br><br>To minimise the risk of pulmonary embolism |
| Unopposed parasympathetic activity may result in bradycardia | | |
| **4 Elimination**<br>*Bladder*<br>Urinary incontinence and/or retention | Explain the procedure to the child and family<br>Obtain consent<br>Insert a urethral foley catheter size appropriate to the age/size of the child<br>Perform at least daily catheter toilet | To prevent urinary retention<br>Preservation of kidney function<br>To reduce risk of infection and inspect urethral area for signs of excoriation and trauma |
| Note that bladder training must *not* be commenced until reflex activity returns and the child is haemodynamically stable. | Record observations and temperature<br>Monitor and record urine output<br>Observe for any signs of urinary tract infections (colour, smell)<br>Excess debris or frequent blocking of the catheter may indicate hypercalcaemia (management described later in the chapter)<br>The child is kept nil by mouth<br>Insert a nasogastric tube until spinal shock subsides and peristaltic function returns | To ensure monitoring of kidney function and early detection of infection<br>To reduce risk of paralytic ileus, abdominal distention and prevention of aspiration<br>To prevent deterioration of bowel function<br>Follow national guidelines for the management of this intimate procedure[11,12]<br>To stimulate the gut to start working<br>To reduce any further complications |
| *Bowel*<br>Paralytic ileus is a temporary arrest of intestinal peristalsis and is an autonomic dysfunction response to spinal shock[3,8]<br>Establish a predictable bowel routine (the insertion of lubricated suppositories, whether or not the child is eating, will stimulate the gut to start working again)[13,14] | Record abdominal girth measurements at least daily<br>Establish feeding aspiration cycle to assess absorption<br>Listen for active bowel sounds or the passing of flatus and/ or stool<br>Explain the procedure to the child and family<br>Document consent for insertion of suppositories and digital rectal stimulation | from a distended abdomen<br>To initiate bowel routine<br>To prevent early-onset complications from constipation, paralytic ileus and autonomic dysreflexia |
| Establish early-onset control of bowel continence | Establish a daily bowel routine using a combination of rectal | |

## PROCEDURE: Acute management/spinal stabilisation (continued)

|  |  |  |
|---|---|---|
|  | stimulants such as glycerine suppositories and oral laxatives Monitor stool output using the Bristol stool scale[15] Mild oral laxatives such as movicol, sennekot or lactulose are used to stimulate the gut to work The child with an unstable spine should to be log rolled (usually on to left side for insertion of suppositories and digital stimulation if required) Intravenous fluids may be prescribed and a strict fluid balance recorded Dietetic referral may be required with consideration to supplemental nutrition | Adequate hydration and nutrition of the child |
| **5 Skin** Causes of pressure ulcer development: pressure; friction; shearing forces | Gap the bony prominences (especially the occiput, sacrum and heels) Log roll the child at least daily | To prevent tissue damage or ulcerations of the pressure areas Pressure area care, pressure relief and skin inspection |
| Post injury there will be reduced vasomotor control leading to a decrease in vascular tone and pressure | Reposition the child every 3 hours with alternating turning positions (i.e. rotating from side positions) to lying on their back) |  |
| The occiput is very vulnerable to breakdown | A non-adhesive polyurethane foam dressing, i.e. Lyofoam or Allevyn can be used as a protective measure under the occiput |  |
| **6 Pain** The child and family need to be supported throughout all medical procedures and investigations such as plain X-ray, computerised tomography (CT), magnetic resonance imaging, venepuncture | Adequate preparation of the child and family prior to any procedures is essential | Give clear explanations to promote child- and family-centred care |
|  | Use distraction techniques and the play specialist services Assessment of pain using recognised pain tool and administer prescribed analgesia as appropriate | Reduction of pain and distress Maximise the potential of all joints |
| **7 Postural care and passive range of movement** Start immediately | Collaboration with the physiotherapist | This is their only means of future function and will affect |

### PROCEDURE: Acute management/spinal stabilisation (continued)

| | | |
|---|---|---|
| | | respiratory effort. This can improve on mobilisation (because of the effect of gravity on the shoulders) |
| Performed daily and more often if contracture or increased tone is present<br><br>Areas of common deformity associated with typical levels of SCI: | | |
| • the neck of the cervical injury | The high level of cord injury with the trapeziums innervated but nothing else at the shoulder will generally contract in this area and lose the length of the neck | To prevent functional limitations during the rehabilitation phase Tightening of the biceps impacts on the child's potential to prop. Additionally wheelchair propulsion/ transfers/lifts may be impeded |
| • the shoulder and elbow of the tetraplegic | Full range of motion is required to the shoulder | Hand to mouth activities will also be affected |
| • the hip joint | 90 degrees of hip flexion will be required for sitting out of bed/wheelchair | A hip flexor that is not accompanied by a hip extensor will always shorten. This in time will impact on their spinal alignment and future potential to ambulate whether this is in callipers or without if the child is more incomplete |
| • the foot and knee | An ankle that is left to contract will lead to a foot that cannot fully weight bear on the floor | The foot position will in turn impact on the knees, hips, pelvis and spine |
| **8 Hand management of the tetraplegic**<br>Maintain and preserve hand position and function | Collaboration with the occupational therapist Application of appropriate splints and maintain prescribed splint regimen<br><br>Inspect skin integrity and report any marking caused by poor fitting splints | Appropriate splinting for the child's level of tetraplegia<br><br>Those with wrist extension will be splinted to encourage a tenodesis grip for future function<br><br>Resting/paddle splints maintain tendon length, reduce risk of contractures and promote function in the child without high tone C1–C6 SCI<br><br>In the child with C7–C8 SCI short paddle splints will be used to allow active wrist extension |

## REHABILITATION OF SPINAL CORD INJURY

The rehabilitation of the SCI paediatric patient demands a holistic long-term approach by a team composed of staff with specialised combined paediatric and spinal knowledge and skills.

Paediatric spinal cord rehabilitation should be designed to optimise functional ability, participation, independence and growth throughout their childhood.

In 1991 The National Spinal Injuries Centre developed a 'child needs assessment checklist', referred to as the CLNAC. It is a comprehensive tool to assess children's needs, plan rehabilitation and measure outcomes. It consists of 12 sections covering the main areas that are included in the child's rehabilitation programme. This checklist provides a way to monitor the child's acquisition of age-appropriate functional skills at each stage of development.

## Nursing outcomes and rehabilitation goals

- Preserve neurological recovery.
- Aid development of compensatory strategies for neurological loss.
- Provide a comprehensive and interdisciplinary rehabilitation programme in the context of the child's developmental needs.
- Educate the child, and their family, to be expert patients.
- Work in partnership with families and communities to produce the best possible outcome for each child.
- Work in partnership with schools and external agencies to maximise educational, social and vocational opportunities for each child.

### Potential for independence

*High cervical injuries*: verbal independence with full assistance in care, powered mobility (orthosis for limb positioning) and standing via tilt table.
*Lower cervical injuries*: basic functional independence with assistance/supervision in care needs. Standing in mobile standing frames with calliper, powered or manual mobility.
*Paraplegia*: manual mobility, advanced functional independence, mobile standing frame, calliper training.
*Incompletes*: all of the above, possible ambulation.

## AUTONOMIC DYSREFLEXIA

Autonomic dysreflexia (AD) occurs after the spinal shock phase.[8]

Individuals with traumatic upper thoracic and cervical spinal cord injuries are at increased risk for the development of both thermoregulatory dysfunction and autonomic dysreflexia. It is an exaggerated sympathetic nervous response to pain/stimuli below the level of spinal cord damage. The condition results from a lack of supraspinal control of the major splanchnic outflow in people with spinal cord injury at or above the 6th thoracic vertebral level (T6).

When the autonomic nervous system is stimulated, creating a hypertensive response, peripheral vasodilation, which would normally have relieved the hypertension, does not occur because stimuli cannot pass distally through the injured cord. AD is a medical emergency and requires immediate intervention to reduce the possibility of a cerebral vascular accident.[16]

### Presentation

Children may have one or more of the signs and symptoms when experiencing an episode of autonomic dysreflexia. There is usually an increase in the systolic measurement of more than 15–20 mmHg (2–2.7 kPa) above the baseline in those over 13 years, or more than 15 mmHg (2 kPa) in children and young people with cervical SCI and upper thoracic SCI. Upper thoracic and cervical lesions have a lower baseline blood pressure than the general population; therefore, it is important to document the child's resting blood pressure.

Chronic causes of AD may require longer acting medication such as a GTN patch or consider advice from anaesthetic services.

If an invasive or surgical procedure is to be considered in those injured above T6 AD should be considered within the treatment plan.

Following an episode of AD the patient is hypersensitive to painful stimuli and has an increased vulnerability to have further attacks of dysreflexia. An alert bracelet or an emergency medical card identifying the risks is recommended for children or young people prone to this condition.

Parents, carers, schools and youth organisations should be aware of AD and how to manage it.

### Emergency pack

- Spare urethral/suprapubic/intermittent catheters (size currently used by the child)
- Catheter pack
- Gloves 10-mL syringe
- Instilagel: lignocaine-based lubricating jelly
- Baby wipes
- Nifedipine/GTN

## PROCEDURE: Nursing AD

| Common signs | Nursing skills | Evidence-based rationale |
|---|---|---|
| Profuse sweating and blotching/flushing of the skin above the level of the injury which may include piloerection and goose pimples<br>Visual disturbances and complaints, e.g. blurred vision, unequal pupil size<br>Child or young person becomes flustered, agitated, apprehensive and irritable<br>A sudden-onset frontal headache | Elevate the child's head and lower the feet<br>Identify and remove the source of painful stimulus<br>Record blood pressure during acute episode every 5 minutes until episode is resolved<br>If the hypertension is severe or if the cause can not be identified treat initially with nifedipine or GTN (sublingual or spray) | To reduce the blood pressure<br>To reduce pain<br>An elevated blood pressure with bradycardia or tachycardia (often with arrhythmias) |

Approximately 80 per cent of AD is caused by bladder issues. It is estimated that 10 per cent is caused by bowel issues and 10 per cent by any other sources of pain.

## PROCEDURE: Nursing AD

| Common causes | Nursing skills | Evidence-based rationale |
|---|---|---|
| **1 Urinary tract**<br>Bladder distention/retention, blocked or kinked urinary catheter, urinary tract infection, bladder stones | Check method of bladder management<br>*Intermittent:* an intermittent catheter is inserted usually every 3–4 hours depending on fluid intake and activity<br>If child has a distended lower abdomen then insert an intermittent catheter using a lubricated single use catheter<br>*Urethral*<br>Check that the catheter is not kinked, that the child is not sat on it or that it is not tangled in underpants/pads<br>Check urine output in leg bag<br>A bladder washout can be done to check if the catheter is blocked; however, if the child is really distressed, in pain with elevated blood pressure, then it is best to change the catheter using a lignocaine based lubricating gel<br>*Suprapubic catheter*<br>Follow the same guidelines as | To empty the bladder<br>To reduce painful stimulus<br>Remove and monitor urine flow<br>To prevent retention of urine<br><br><br><br>This will increase pain |

| | | |
|---|---|---|
| | for the urethral catheter<br>If the child or carer is unable to change a suprapubic catheter then either an intermittent or urethral can be inserted<br>Ensure that with the indwelling catheters the child is on continuous drainage until the pain is resolved<br>**Do not try to manually express the bladder**<br>Education of the child, family and carers to safely manage method of emptying the bladder in emergency situations<br>**Carry emergency pack at all times** | To empower the child and family to safely manage bladder<br><br>To reduce blood pressure and manage the pain |
| **2 Distended rectum:**<br>flatus, impacted bowel or constipated stool | Insert lignocaine-based gel into the rectum<br>Perform digital rectal examination<br>Check for impaction, an anal tear, fissure or haemorrhoids<br>If impacted attempt to gently remove faeces manually.<br>Consider nifedipine or GTN medication prior to evacuation of stool if blood pressure continues to increase | To numb and lubricate the rectum<br><br>To identify any source of pain<br><br>To relieve blood pressure |
| **3 Skin**<br>Pressure ulcers | Loosen any tight clothing, splints or orthosis<br>Check for skin insults/trauma<br>Check for pressure ulcers, burns (including sunburn and frostbite), ingrowing toenails.<br>Also observe for insect bites, cellulitis | |
| **4 Orthopaedic issues**<br>Fractures and trauma<br>Joint subluxation or dislocation<br>Heterotopic ossification | Immobilise suspected limb<br>Seek specialist medical advice on the management of a fractured limb | To avoid further damage<br>If injured above T6 may have symptoms of AD |
| **5 Reproduction and sexual issues**<br>Scrotal compression, epididymitis/vaginitis,<br>Menstruation, pregnancy, labour<br><br><br>Sexual intercourse and ejaculation | Early-warning signs, increased spasm<br>Remove pressure from testicles (avoid sitting on scrotum)<br>Education of the female child to manage referred menstrual pain and possible alterations in bladder and bowel management<br>Seek specialist medical advice for the management of pregnancy and labour in the young person injured above T6 | To reduce pain to avoid further problems<br>Clear explanation will enhance confidence and competence in managing personal care needs<br><br>To provide specialist advice |

**KEY POINTS**

- AD is a medical emergency and requires immediate intervention to reduce the possibility of a cerebral vascular accident
- Elevate the head and lower the feet
- Identify and remove the source of painful stimulus
- Reduce the blood pressure to within the normal limits
- If necessary give prescribed medication

**VIGNETTE**

**Problem**: parent reports that the child has become increasingly blotchy on the upper chest and is blotchy and flushed in the face.

**Discussion**: on investigation it is noted that there has been no urine output for the last 4 hours; on investigation the urethral catheter is found to be kinked; this is relieved and the urine is able to flow and symptoms gradually resolve.

## TEMPERATURE CONTROL

Because of vasomotor paralysis with loss of sympathetic response the SCI child has the inability to sweat and shiver below the level of injury and cannot maintain adequate body temperature, also defined as poikilothermia. Therefore, because of SCI the poikilothermic child has a limited protective response to adjust to external environmental temperatures.

Heat is lost from the body chiefly through the

**KEY POINTS**

- Heat is lost through the skin
- Child or young person must be nursed in a consistent environmental temperature

**VIGNETTE**

**Problem**: cervical injured child attends hydrotherapy and returns to the ward complaining of feeling cold and tired

**Discussion**: check temperature, apply several layers of clothes and encourage to have a warm drink

skin and the child and family need to develop an awareness of the effects of extreme temperature changes and take the necessary precautions such as:

- provide appropriate clothing for the child's immediate environmental temperature;
- keep child/young person in a consistent environmental temperature;
- avoid excessive exposure, especially during procedures;
- ensure the child is dried quickly and thoroughly following shower or attend to hygiene needs, otherwise they will become cold very quickly;
- consider using antipyretic medication if indicated.

## SKIN

Post injury there will be reduced vasomotor control leading to a decrease in vascular tone and pressure. Therefore minimum effort is required to occlude the blood vessels of children with SCI.

### Objectives

- Develop awareness of the specific issues in skin management.
- Knowledge of age-appropriate risk factors.
- Age-appropriate education plan for the child, young person or carer.

### Causes of pressure ulcers

- Prolonged pressure
- Friction
- Shearing

### Physiology predisposing to skin problems

- Sensation is impaired or lost dependent on level of spinal cord damage.
- Unaware of pain associated with local tissue ischaemia.
- Impaired blood supply resulting in delayed healing.
- Reduced physical activity and immobility.
- Poor circulation may result in oedema in lower limbs causing increased vulnerability due to thinning of the skin (apply anti-embolism stockings, elevation of limbs overnight).
- Increased tone resulting in excessive muscle

spasm in upper motor neurone injuries.
- Decreased muscle tone in lower motor neurone injuries. Muscle wastage results in bony prominences becoming more prone to skin damage.
- Malnutrition and dehydration.
- Obesity.
- Ill-health and pyrexia.
- Unmanaged incontinence and nappy rash.
- Ingrowing toenails.

Table 33.1 shows the common causes of pressure ulcers.

Prevention by regular skin checking is the best treatment of pressure areas (Figure 33.3).

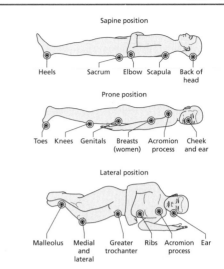

Figure 33.3 Bony prominence prone to ulder development.

**Table 33.1** Common causes of pressure ulcers in SCI

| Cause | Action |
| --- | --- |
| Hot water bottles, hot drinks, radiators, car heaters, heated car seats, and electric blankets | Teach awareness of the dangers of hot liquids and heating |
| Sun burn | Reduce exposure to direct heat, long periods in the shade, use sun cream |
| Tight fitting shoes | Recommend shoe size bigger to avoid marking |
| Clothing: consider the location and appropriateness of fastenings, i.e. buckles, buttons and zips | |
| Splints and outgrown orthosis | REview orthosis throughout growth |
| Skin conditions, e.g. dry skin, eczema, psoriasis, fungal infections | Education of daily checking of skin |
| Crawling on the floor (carpet burns) | |
| Cuts, bumps and bruises may develop into pressure ulcers | |
| Theatre: careful postural management during theatre procedures | Ensure risk assessment is completed and theatre staff are aware of how to handle patient |
| Poor manual handling techniques | |
| Weight increase or decrease | |
| Play equipment | |

## Prevention is the best treatment for pressure ulcers

Specialist services will provide regular posture and seating clinic assessments. This will include pressure mapping and recommendations for suitable cushions and seating systems. They will also be able to recommend the most appropriate method of pressure relief for that child and level of cord damage.

It is recommended that children with SCI attend an annual posture and seating assessment to monitor posture and seating alongside their growth and development to ensure the equipment is adequate to meet their growing needs.

Development and subsequent treatment of pressure ulcers can cause further hospitalisation, extended absence from school, decreased play/leisure time and separation from friends.

Pressure ulcers can also delay achievement and long-term rehabilitation goals.

Also they can delay achievement of rehabilitation goals and can result in secondary complications such as contractures, scarring and occasionally further disfigurement from the scarring. The long-term effects of scarring may require treatment with skin or muscle grafting later in life.

## Recommendations for management

- Check skin twice daily for early detection of damage to the skin and teach self-sufficiency in task (Figure 33.4). Education of self inspection promotes compliance with skin management.

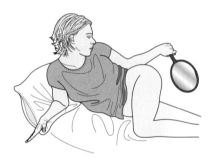

**Figure 33.4** The patient may need to use a mirror to inspect areas that are difficult to see.

- Use appropriate pressure-relieving cushions and mattresses. Pressure-relieving equipment should not be relied upon as a substitute for manual positional changes (see postural management and respiratory care, page 579). Some pressure-relieving equipment (for example air mattresses) may also reduce independence, i.e. dressing, transfers, turning.
- Maintain high standard of hygiene and skin health. Using non-perfumed soaps and moisturisers will help to reduce dryness and cracking of the skin.
- Assess the nutritional status to ensure adequate intake.
- Avoid limbs rubbing against bedding, clothing, orthosis and equipment. Muscle spasms can be aggressive and forceful which can result in skin damage. This occurs either by increased shearing forces and friction or through trauma. If spasms

affect functional ability or cause damage to skin then it must be medically reviewed to determine whether or not antispasmodic medication is required.
- Be aware of manual handling techniques by using pat slides, sliding sheets to avoid/minimise friction or shearing of the skin.
- Ensure that bed sheets are applied with no wrinkles
- Beds and pockets need to be regularly checked to ensure there are no toys, keys, coins, etc that may cause pressure ulcers
- Staff should not wear any jewellery with stones or watches and must have short nails to avoid scratching patient.

## Nursing intervention

If any redness or non-blanching erythema is present:
- Relieve/remove pressure.
- Do not apply any further pressure.
- Identify possible cause and eliminate or re-evaluate management.
- Grade skin damage (as local policy) and document findings.
- Pyrexia needs to be monitored and managed.
- Turn patient more frequently (2–3 hourly) and check skin at each position change.
- Re-assess pressure relieving mattress and/or cushion.

Continued pressure on any damaged area of skin will cause further tissue necrosis, breakdown and possible further management in hospital.

If the child is unwell or has a raised temperature the skin will be more vulnerable to marking and the effects of pressure.

## LIMB FRACTURES

Additional care and considerations are needed of a paralysed limb that is fractured and treated using a cast. Lack of sensation and movement below the level of injury puts the child at significant risk of developing a pressure sore. Extra padding is required over bony prominences and a lightweight cast should be applied where possible. Heels, malleoli, first metatarsal phalange joints, tibial tuberosities, wrists, elbows and knuckles are all particularly vulnerable. Elevating the limb on pillows will reduce the impact of swelling. The cast should be bi-valved after 24–48 hours after application and removed daily to allow the skin to be inspected for signs of pressure ulcers. Compromised skin should be treated, and cutting a window in the cast should be considered to relieve direct pressure. Once bi-valved the cast may be secured with bandages to maintain cast stability and limb immobility.

Early preventative treatment and management for contractures and spasticity need to be considered. A comprehensive plan for 24-hour positioning and postural care should be devised with the occupational therapist and physiotherapist.

Upper motor neurone injuries have increased tone resulting in excessive muscle spasm.

Lower motor neurone injuries have decreased muscle tone. Muscle wastage results in bony prominences becoming more prone to skin damage.

**KEY POINTS**

- Reduced or loss of sensation due to paralysis
- Prevention is the best treatment
- Check skin at least daily for any signs of deterioration or marking
- Use of pressure-relieving mattresses and cushions appropriate to needs
- If any redness occurs identify cause and remove the source of pressure
- Do not apply any further pressure
- Always check bed for toys, remote controls, mobile phones, etc.
- No jewellery, wrist watches or long nails

**VIGNETTE**

**Problem:** young person complains of shoulder pain to parent; parent applies hot water bottle

**Discussion:** the hot water bottle does not have a protective cover and as the child becomes distracted playing, it slips below the level of temperature sensation and causes a burn

## 24-HOUR POSTURAL MANAGEMENT

Poor postural management can impact on the quality of life of the child (family and carers). It may also have a detrimental effect on many body systems and affects functional ability, independence and body image (Table 33.2).

### Recommendations for management

- Adopt a supported 24-hour postural management

**Table 33.2** Effects of poor posture

| | | |
|---|---|---|
| Musculoskeletal | Contractures, loss of joint integrity (dislocation, subluxation), reduced bone density, pain, reduced range of joint movement and deformity, loss of function. | Recommend daily passive movement Bone density review Annual assessment Regular assessment of range of movement |
| Neurological | Spasticity, increased muscle tone, pain | Monitor spasticity Prescribe antispasmodic medication |
| Respiratory | Reduced lung function due to spinal deformity (scoliosis) | Lung function tests Vital capacity Peak flow |
| Renal | Spinal deformity could result in inadequate bladder emptying and/ or management option | Ultrasound and regular review by spinal/urology specialists |
| Gastric | Poor swallowing (caused by poor head to neck posture), aspiration | Regular spinal X-rays for early detection of deterioration. Review by spinal/orthopaedic specialists |
| Skin | Risk of development of pressure ulcers at sites of contractures or deformity Poor hygiene | Annual review posture and seating Educate skin checking Ensure adequate hygiene |

approach for the child in the lying, sitting and standing positions.

- Seating: prescribe pressure-relieving cushions and back support through appropriate posture and seating assessment or clinic.
- Standing in an appropriate standing device with supportive orthosis (also promotes growth and bone density).
- Orthosis (e.g. callipers, body brace, splints).
- Physiotherapy (including FES).
- Lying prone.
- Exercise and sport.
- Night positioning: neutral, ideally mid-range and symmetrical. (Lycra suits, Sleep systems, resting splints.)

---

**KEY POINTS**

- 24-hour postural care incorporates lying (sleeping), sitting and standing
- The younger the age at injury the higher the incidence of scoliosis, hip subluxation and secondary disabilities
- Poor postural management can have a detrimental effect on many of the body systems. The consequences will impact on functional ability, independence, body image and on the quality of life

---

## PERSONAL HYGIENE AND DRESSING

- Develop a knowledge of the functional ability at differing levels of SCI and relating that to the developmental stage of the child.
- Develop awareness of the specific implications with competence in washing, dressing and undressing the paralysed patient.
- Be aware of the consequences of choice in clothing.
- Assist with all aspects of grooming.

In the early stage of rehabilitation the child needs to be actively encouraged to initially instruct the carer to assist with their washing and dressing needs and then to be actively involved if functional ability permits. An occupational therapist can initially make minor alterations or recommend slight modifications to clothing or adaptive clothing can be used to maximise their functional ability and independence e.g. applying loops to socks. You must ensure that the clothing is not too tight, there are no harsh seams, and encourage the patient to be aware of pockets and zips. Also it is recommended that shoes are one size bigger and a family member is encouraged to wear the new shoe to help with "softening" or "breaking in" the shoe.

The child's functional ability is regularly monitored to ensure that the functional ability is in accordance or within normal expectations with the age or stage of development of the child or young person. This is updated as the child's needs and functional ability changes with growth.

Often when a child is first injured the parent is very actively involved in learning the child's care needs. As the child returns for regular follow up post injury discussions need to take place as to how actively involved the parents are and whether or not this is still appropriate with regard to age, sex and functional ability of the child or young person.

This needs to be managed sensitively. At times fears and frustations exist on both sides, parents may be afraid of "letting go" and don't want to see their child or young person struggle. On the other hand the child may be frustrated because the parent is not adjusting to their age and stage of development.

---

**VIGNETTE**

**Problem:** Both parents are actively involved in intimate care needs of their 15-year-old daughter.

**Discussion:** Discuss with the young person, assess how they feel about this and negotiate alternatives.

---

**KEY POINT**

Encourage verbal and functional independence skills at age appropriate stage of development

---

## ELIMINATION

### Bladder management (Table 33.3)

- Demonstrate understanding of the altered functioning post SCI.
- Identify different methods of bladder management.
- Describe the signs and symptoms, prevention and treatment of urinary tract infections.
- Identify the long-term complications of bladder.

**Table 33.3** Altered functioning post spinal cord injury

| Level | Impact |
|---|---|
| Injuries usually at or above T12 generally present as a reflex bladder | Sacral reflex arc is intact<br>Conscious control lost or altered<br>Detrusor overactivity<br>Detrusor sphincter dyssynergia |
| Injuries usually at T12–L1 generally present as an areflexic or flaccid bladder | Sacral reflex arc is lost<br>Conscious control lost or altered<br>Detrusor underactivity<br>Retention/overflow |

### The procedural goal is to

- establish a low pressure regular pattern of bladder emptying which is both socially accepted by the child (and parent) and prevents complications such as: kidney damage, urinary tract infection and stone formation.

Factors affecting management include compliance, family lifestyle, peer group, school, support networks (or lack of).

## PROCEDURE: Basic principles of catheterisation applied to urethral/supapubic/intermittent and Mitrofanoff catheters

| Procedural steps | Nursing skills | Evidence-based rationale |
|---|---|---|
| Equipment required:<br>• Catheter pack<br>• Saline<br>• 10 ml syringe<br>• Lubricating or lignocaine gel<br>• Catheter to be inserted | Prepare the patient and the surroundings. (If another catheter in situ, deflate the balloon using the 10ml syringe, discard catheter and gloves) | Clear explanations reduces fear |
| | Apply principles of aseptic technique: wash hands,<br>open pack<br>open other equipment required, apply gloves<br>clean urethra using gauze and saline, apply lubricating gel to the catheter to be inserted<br>if applicable | To reduce risk of infection |

## PROCEDURE: Methods of management

| Procedural steps | Nursing skills | Evidence-based rationale |
| --- | --- | --- |
| **Indwelling urethral catheter** Usually short term management whilst child is in the acute stage | The catheter is connected to a leg bag during the day and a night bag at night | To prevent urinary retention |
| | Monitor urinary output by checking the bag regularly | To ensure it does not become too full and cause problems with drainage |
| | The bag needs to be placed lower than the catheter to encourage urine to flow | |
| | Never pull or stretch or catheter | To reduce risk of trauma and autonomic dysreflexia |
| | Encourage fluid intake appropriate to the weight of the child | To prevent urinary tract infection and maintain long-term kidney and bladder health |
| Indwelling catheters can cause urinary tract infections (UTI), bladder stones and occasionlly sores | Daily catheter toilet | |
| | Check skin around catheter to ensure no inflammation or sores | |
| | Change catheter as per prescription or at least every 4 weeks | |
| | Report any problems | |
| **Suprapubic catheter** Rare in children and more common in the older child | Same principles as above | |
| | Daily checking of stoma stie | |
| | A flip-flo valve can be used | To maintain or increase bladder capacity prior to teaching intermittent catheters |
| **Intermittent catheter** Mimics normal bladder emptying | Adhere to hygiene as per urethral/suprapubic catheterisation | To reduce risk of infection and maintain long term bladder and kidney health |
| Child/young person requires urodynamic assessment to ensure bladder is suitable for this method of management | Child/carer/parent/professional is taught to empty bladder using intermittent catheter | To ensure low pressure bladder To prevent risk of reflux into kidneys |
| | Bladder emptied usually every 3–4 horus depending on fluid intake | Mimics normal bladder emptying |
| | Child taught to insert on the bed, toilet and wheelchair | To ensure independence outside the home environment |
| | Wide variety of catheters to suit user | |
| | Benefits include no need to wear legs bags/night bags | |
| | Reduced risk of infection | |

## PROCEDURE:  Methods of management (continued)

| | | |
|---|---|---|
| Leakage in between catheterisation indicates urinary tract infection or need for increase in anti-choloingeric medication | Send samples of urine for culture and sensitivity to rule out urine infection<br>Refer for medical advice | |
| **Miranoff**<br>Bladder augmentation to increase bladder capacity | Principles of catheterisation are the same as for intermittend catheters | To reduce risk of infection |
| Creation of a stoma on the abdomen or through the umbililcus | Benefits: enabling catheter independence in the young certivcal injured female as it facilitates easier access and reduces time spent transferring on/off bed | To facilitate independence in catheter management |
| **Sheath drainage**<br>A sheath (urinary condom) is applied to the penis to maintain continence | Measure penis as per manufacture guidelines specific to the sheath going to be used | To ensure adequate fit |
| | Ensure penis is clean and dry prior to application | |
| | Do not use excessive soaps or moisturisers | It will reduce effectivess of adherence of the sheath |
| | Do not put sheath on too tightly | The penis will become swollen and sore and will not allow for erections |
| | Attach sheath to leg bag during the day and night bag overnight | |
| | Encourage child or young person to check sheath regularly | |
| | Change sheath every 24 hours | To ensure it has not become kinked, twisted or fallen off especially after transfers |
| | Check penile skin regularly to ensure there are no sores<br>If sore present, depending on the severity, an appropriate barrier application or second skin dressing can be used; otherwise do not apply sheath until skin is healed | Ensure early detection of any adverse reactions to sheath, glue or sores |
| | Observe for any adverse reaction to sheath<br>If any adverse reactions to the sheath, use another brand | |

## PROCEDURE: Dealing with long-term complications

| Procedural steps | Nursing skills | Evidence-based rationale |
| --- | --- | --- |
| **Urinary tract infections**<br>Early warning signs:<br>• Colour – dark, concentrated, cloudy<br>• Smell – strong odour<br>• Consistency – thick sediment<br>• Fever | Obtain a clean specimen of urine and send for culture and sensitivity<br><br>Encourage increase in fluid intake (weight dependent)<br><br>Monitor fluid intake<br>Check and record vital signs regularly | To determine sensitivity of infection<br><br>To flush bladder<br><br><br>Early detection of the unwell child |
| Wet in between catheters | If doing intermittent catheters and is consistently wet<br>Refer to medical advice | Recommend inserting a urethral catheter |
| Increase in spasm<br>Increase in pain/dysreflexia | Ensure no other additional problems contributing to spasm or pain | |
| **Stone formation**<br>Stones form in the bladder when waste products crystalise mostly made up of calcium<br>Risk factors include:<br>• poor fluid intake – stones can block catheters<br>• incomplete emptying of the bladder<br>• irritation and incontinence caused by recurrent UTIs | Encourage fluid intake (weight dependent)<br><br>Ensure safe and adequate method of bladder emptying<br>Regular monitoring of urine output | To flush the bladder<br><br>To prevent stone formation<br><br>Early detection of any problems |

**KEY POINTS**

• Avoid retention
• Low pressure method of emptying
• Achieve continence

## Bowel Management

- Develop an understanding of the altered functioning following SCI.
- Develop knowledge of the different methods of bowel emptying 'reflex' and 'flaccid'.
- Identify goals of bowel management programme (routine, location, time, interventions).
- Demonstrate awareness of the factors affecting bowel management (functional ability, developmental stage or age, size, weight).

### Altered functioning following spinal cord injury

Complete spinal cord damage results in loss of sensation of the urge to defecate and the loss of voluntary control. Peristaltic action resumes after the period of spinal shock. This is due to the enteric nervous system, which lies within the walls of the colon, remaining intact. However, without coordination from the brain and the spinal cord an increase in colonic transit time will occur. This implication results in the neurogenic bowel with a drier stool and constipation (Table 33.4, page 585).

### Aim

The aim of bowel training is to enable the child to achieve continence, either independently or aided by a parent or carer appropriate to their age and stage of development. The child or young person

Table 33.4

| Level of injury | Impact |
|---|---|
| Injuries to the 12th thoracic vertebra (T12) and above generally result in 'reflex' bowel<br><br>Implications for management | The intact reflex arc activity can be used for effective bowel management. Stimulation of the anal sphincter and rectum can produce a reflex contraction which may excrete faeces |
| Injuries to the first lumbar vertebra (L1) and below generally result in a 'flaccid' bowel.<br><br>Implications for management | Reflex arc activity is lost resulting in a flaccid bowel with a lax anal sphincter and pelvic floor |

requiring assistance must give individual consent for this invasive and intimate aspect of their care and treatment. Also when planning the bowel routine consideration may need to be given to previous bowel habits as this can impact on a successful outcome to continence.

- Achieve regular, predictable and safe bowel emptying methods at a socially acceptable time and place.
- Avoid and prevent constipation, anal tears, faecal incontinence and autonomic dysreflexia.

Bowel management and recording of bowel motions tends to be inconsistent and haphazard. This can be very distressing for the child who has achieved toilet training. The child will feel more in control of this if it is predictive as opposed to haphazard

### Nursing intervention

- Document consent, explain the procedure to the child and family.
- Assess pre-injury bowel habit (i.e. frequency of bowel opening, time of day) and based on this information negotiate an appropriate time to suit their lifestyle and social demands.
- Ensure a private environment. Ideally bowel care should be performed while the child is sitting on the toilet (with padded toilet seat) or on a padded shower chair.
- Insert lubricated glycerine suppository to stimulate the bowel to empty. The act of suppository insertion may be stimulant enough to produce defecation and digital stimulation (REF) may be adequate to empty the rectum. The glycerine suppository also lubricates the stool allowing it to be passed with reduced effort or trauma.

- Overstimulation of the anal sphincter (more than two or three times) may cause an episode of autonomic dysreflexia or bowel accident as it will cause delayed reflect activity.
- Care should be taken when removing the stool to avoid damage to the rectal mucosa and the anal sphincter. Do not use hooked finger to remove large pieces of hard stool, which may graze or scratch the bowel mucosa.
- If the stool is hard and impacted then the child may require an increase in laxatives until this is resolved. Long-term complications of prolonged periods of constipation will cause anal tears and haemorrhoids.
- If the patient suffers local discomfort or autonomic dysreflexia during the procedure then a lignocaine gel 1 per cent should be used. This usually requires 5–10 minutes to take effect and lasts for approximately 30 minutes.
- Ensure dignity of the child is maintained while performing the procedure.
- Provide facilities and care to meet the child's hygiene needs following toileting.
- Record outcome using the Bristol stool scale.
- Educate the parents and the child about the procedure. They must be assessed as competent with supervised clinical practice.

The child or young person will require an individual assessment of equipment needs appropriate to their functional ability. Occupational therapist assessments will also need to take into account equipment suitability within the home environment.

### Equipment

- accessible toilet
- padded toilet seat
- grab rails

or

- padded shower chair or flamingo chair (R82)
- commode facility if showerchair unable to wheel over toilet facility.

## SEXUALITY AND FERTILITY

The aims here are to:

- understand the psychosocial stages of development and the formation of sexual identity.
- demonstrate awareness of the impact of SCI on body image.

The *Tanner stages* (also known as the *Tanner scale*) are stages of physical development in children, adolescents and adults. The stages define physical measurements of development based on external primary and secondary sex characteristics, such as the size of the breasts, genitalia and development of pubic hair. Owing to natural variation, individuals pass through the Tanner stages at different rates, depending in particular on the timing of puberty.

The impact of a SCI on sexual functioning depends on the degree of the injury and its location on the spinal cord. Sexual dysfunction in people with SCI may have both physiological and psychological (e.g. body image, self-esteem) elements that can be distressing regardless of the person's gender, age or culture.

Adolescents with disabilities are reported to have similar rates of sexual activity as those without disability. Therefore teaching and education on 'safe sex' sexual health issues should be the same for as able-bodied young people. The young person with SCI should receive age appropriate information about sexual function and how that has altered following their level of cord damage.

Alterations in sexual desire, response and function will be dependent on the level and extent of spinal cord damage. For example, psychogenic erections may be absent but reflex erections may still be present in those with SCI above T12–L1.

## Menstruation and pregnancy

It is important that sanitary pads are changed regularly and that the genitalia is kept clean to prevent any infections or any excoriation of skin. If tampons are used patients must remember to check and replace regularly. We recommend that some sort of alarm or timer is used, e.g. mobile phones, to remind them to attend to hygiene needs or to insert a catheter.

Female fertility is unchanged by SCI. Therefore advice regarding the use of contraception should be sought if a sexual relationship is planned. Also if a family is planned, it is recommended that they seek specialist advice about preparing for and keeping healthy throughout the pregnancy. Those injured above the T6 and vulnerable to autonomic dyreflexia need to be reviewed by specialist spinal centres for dual management with obstetrics.

### Male fertility

Male fertility is often affected following SCI with altered body image (poor self image), depression, denial and neglect.

For any further information visit www.sexual health.com or www.spinalnet.co.uk

## PSYCHOLOGY

Support the child and parent with the 'sense of overwhelming grief' and through the stages of grief, i.e. denial, anger, bargaining, depression and acceptance.

Assist the child, young person and parents to cope with this catastrophic event which results in a high sense of loss, loss of control, loss of independence, loss of normal bodily function, and a change to their whole way of life.

- Adaptation to injury
- The healing process
- Individual, different pace and progression through the stage of grieving
- Dealing with the reaction of other people towards the spinal cord injury

- Children will ask lots of questions so be prepared to answer truthfully and age appropriately
- Assessment screen for pre-existing problems or adjustment difficulties
- Support with effective coping strategies
- Goal planning programme named keyworker, ChNAC assessment
- Normalise: both normalise how the family is reacting and their experiences of the situation, encourage familiar things and activities, routines.

The consequences of SCI are wide ranging and cause long-term changes physically, emotionally and socially. Often the perception is that the main problem is not being able to walk, but families quickly find out that that's the tip of the iceberg and this is very overwhelming.

- Assessment screen for pre-existing or adjustment difficulties
- Support the child and family with effective coping strategies
- Commence a goal planning programme using the Child Needs Assessment Checklist (ChNAC)

### Aims

- Create a sense of normality
- Provide a feeling of safety
- Make SCI manageable

### Procedural steps

- Engage the child/young person in a goal plan process at a pace which is safe, achievable and manageable for them.
- Familiarise with the environment, equipment

and the rehabilitation routines.
- Contact with friends, family, school and wireless internet are all ways to promote reintegration and coping ability.
- Studies of post-traumatic stress syndrome show it is not just the event causing the injury but also the emergency and ongoing medical care, rehabilitation and reactions of other people that can be traumatising.

### Transition into the adult service

Investing time, from early-onset SCI, promoting development into 'a healthy adult' enhances transition (DOH 2008) into the adult SCI service.

The ultimate goal is that the young person enters the adult population as a healthy, well-adjusted functioning individual. In the years prior to transition the focus will be on assessing and educating the young person to take responsibility for themselves and integrating them into the adult service.

Use adults as role models throughout rehabilitation: adult SCI mentors such as from the SIA or backup trust.

Being regularly reviewed throughout their growth and development by a spinal cord injury unit initially ensures continuity of care throughout the child's life.

### Continuity of hospital professionals

Children and young people who are disabled or who have complex health needs receive coordinated, high-quality child and family-centred services which are based on assessed needs, promote social inclusion and where possible, enable them and their families to live ordinary lives.

 Go to the website to find the PowerPoint presentation for this chapter and MCQs to test your knowledge. **www.hodderplus.com/childnursingskills**

# REFERENCES

1  Augutis M, Abel R, Levi R (2006) Pediatric spinal cord injury in a subset of European countries. *Spinal Cord* **44**: 106–112.

2  Kennedy P, Gorsuch N, Marsh N (1995) Childhood onset of spinal cord injury: self esteem and self perception. *British Journal of Clinical Psychology* **34**: 581–588.

3  Grundy D, Swain A (2002) *ABC of spinal cord injury*, 4th edition. London: BMJ Books.

4  American Spinal Injury Association (1982) *Standards for classification of spinal injured patients.* Chicago: American Spinal Injury Association.

5  Mulcahey MJ, Gaughan J, Betz RR, Johansen KJ (2007) The international standards for neurological

classification of spinal cord injury: reliability of data when applied to children and youths. *Spinal Cord* **45**: 452–459.

6  Pang D, Wilberger JE Jr (1982)Spinal cord injury without radiographic abnormalities in children. *Journal of Neurosurgery* **57**: 114–129.

7  Hayes J, Arriola T (2005) Pediatric spinal injuries. *Pediatric Nursing* **31**: 464–467.

8  Harrison P, Graham A, Hancock S (2007) Managing spinal cord injury: the first 48 hours. In: *SCI in children*. Oxford: Wiley Blackwell pp. 80–82.

9  Consortium for Spinal Cord Injury Medicine (2005) *Respiratory management following spinal cord injury*. Washington DC: Paraylzed Veterans of America.

10  Consortium for Spinal Cord Medicine (2005) *Prevention of thromboembolism in spinal cord injury*. 2nd edition. Washington DC: Paralysed Veterans of America.

11  Royal College of Nursing (2003) *Digital rectal examination: guidance for nurses working with children and young people*. London: RCN.

12  Royal College of Nursing (2003a) *Digital rectal examination and manual removal of faeces: the role of the nurse*, 3rd edition. London: RCN.

13  Goetez L, Hurvitz E, Nelson V, Warding W (1998) Bowel management in children and adolescents with spinal cord injury. *Journal of Spinal Cord Medicine* **21**(4): 331–341.

14  Coggrave M, Wiesel P H, Norton C (2006) Management of faecal incontinence and constipation in adults with neurological diseases. *Cochrane Database of Systemic Reviews* 2006, **2**. Art. N.: CD002115.

15  Heaton, K (1999) The Bristol stool form scale. In: *Understanding your bowels. Family Doctor Series*. London: BMA.

16  Gleeson R (1990) Bowel continence for the child with a neurogenic bowel. *Rehabilitation Nursing* **15**: 319–321.

17  Webster G, Kennedy P (2007). Addressing children's needs and evaluating rehabilitation outcome after spinal cord injury: the child needs assessment checklist and goal planning program. *Journal of Spinal Cord Medicine* **30**: 63–68.

18  Short DJ, Frankel HL, Bergstrom EMK (1992). Injuries of the spinal cord in children. *Handbook of Clinical Neurology* **17**(61): 233–251.

20  Department of Health (2004) National Service Framework for Children, Young People and Maternity Services. *Change for children – every child matters, Standard 4 'Growing up into adulthood'*.

London: Department of Health.

21  Department of Health (2004) National Service Framework for Children, Young People and Maternity Services *Change for children – every child matters, Standard 8, 'Disabled children and young people and those with complex health needs'*. London: Department of Health.

22  Vogel LC, Hickey KJ, Klass SJ, Anderson CJ (2004) Unique issues in pediatric spinal cord injury. *Orthopaedic Nursing* **23**: 300–307.

23  Department of Health (2000) *Good practice in continence services*. London: The Stationery Office.

24  Department of Health (2003) *Good practice in paediatric continence services: benchmarking in action*. London: NHS Modernisation Agency.

25  Assessment checklist and goal-planning program. *Journal of Spinal Cord Medicine* **30**(1): S140–145.

26  Gorman C, Kennedy P, Hamilton LR (1998) Alterations in self-perception following childhood onset of spinal cord injury. *Spinal Cord* **36**: 181–185.

27  Consortium for Spinal Cord Injury Medicine (2001) *Acute management of autonomic dysreflexia: individuals with spinal cord injury presenting to health care facilities*, 2nd edition. Jackson Heights: Eastern Paralyzed Veterans Association.

# FURTHER READING

Betz R, Mulcahey M (eds) (1996). *The child with a spinal cord injury*. Rosemont: American Academy of Orthopaedic Surgeons.

Hickey KJ, Vogel LC (2002) Autonomic dysreflexia in pediatric spinal cord injury. *SCI Nursing, Pediatric Perspectives* **19**(2): 82–84.

Hickey KJ, Hickey EM (2004) Educating children, adolescents and their families following spinal cord injury. SCI *Nursing* 21(3): 168–171.

Martin BW, Dykes E, Lecky FE (2004) Patterns and risks in spinal trauma. *Archives of the Disabled Child* **89**: 860–865.

Punchard, L (1999). *Wheelie power: a book for young people about growing up with a spinal cord injury*. London: Spinal Injuries Association.

Vogel LC, Hickey KJ, Klass SJ, Anderson CJ (2004) Unique issues in pediatric spinal cord injury. *Orthopaedic Nursing* **23**: 5.

Vogel L, Mulcahy MJ, Betz R (1997) The child with spinal cord injury. *Developmental Medicine and Child Neurology* **39**: 202–207.

# APPENDIX

## Bristol stool chart

| | | |
|---|---|---|
| **Type 1** | | Separate hard lumps, like nuts (hard to pass) |
| **Type 2** | | Sausage-shaped but lumpy |
| **Type 3** | | Like a sausage but with cracks on its surface |
| **Type 4** | | Like a sausage or snake, smooth and soft |
| **Type 5** | | Soft blobs with clear-cut edges (passed easily) |
| **Type 6** | | Fluffy pieces with ragged edges, a mushy stool |
| **Type 7** | | Watery, no solid pieces **Entirely liquid** |

## CHAPTER 34

# Venesection, cannulation and the care of children requiring intravenous infusions

Sarah Chalk, Joanne Harvey, Naomi Watson and Janet Kelsey

## LEARNING OUTCOMES

*Upon completion of the chapter, the reader should be able to accomplish the following:*

1. Identify veins suitable for cannulation and venesection
2. Choose the appropriate size cannula for the required therapy or appropriate blood-taking device for venesection
3. Understand the importance of asepsis
4. Appreciate the need to adequately prepare and reassure the child
5. List complications that may arise
6. Assist in the safe insertion of peripheral intravenous cannula
7. Successfully care for the cannula once in situ and aftercare for venesection
8. Effectively carry out the procedure
9. Understand the role of the nurse in cannulation and venesection in relation to the scope of professional practice. This incorporates the need for regular updates to practise the skill regularly, good documentation and to always work within your own limitations
10. Manage the care of a child with an intravenous cannula
11. Recognise and manage the potential complications of an intravenous cannula
12. Choose an appropriate infusion device
13. Calculate infusion flow rate using a gravity

flow device
14. Assist in the safe insertion of peripheral intravenous cannula
15. Manage the care of a child with an intravenous cannula
16. Recognise and manage the potential complications of an intravenous cannula
17. Choose an appropriate infusion device
18. Calculate infusion flow rate using a gravity flow device

## CANNULATION AND VENESECTION

*Sarah Chalk, Joanne Harvey and Naomi Watson*

## OVERVIEW

In line with *The Code*[1] nurses are increasingly performing tasks that were previously considered to be the responsibility of doctors. Cannulation and venesection are such skills. The code places an emphasis on knowledge, skills, responsibility and accountability, permitting nurses to perform enhanced roles as long as they are appropriately skilled, trained and competent to do so and it is in the best interests of the patient.

Intravenous cannulation involves inserting a small plastic tube directly into a vein for the purpose of administering intravenous fluids or medicines either continuously or intermittently.

Venesection is the procedure of entering a vein with a needle, normally for the purposes of obtaining a blood sample for laboratory analysis.

These procedures are not without risk of complication. The potential for introducing infection at varying stages of the procedure is high and therefore careful consideration must be applied before, during and after insertion to reduce the risk. Furthermore, venepuncture and cannulation impacts psychologically on children and therefore requires adequate preparation to minimise any distress to the child and family. Topical anaesthetics should also be a consideration for peripheral access in paediatric or needle phobic patients.

> ### KEY WORDS
>
> Intravenous   Venepuncture   Cannulation
> Visual infusion   Phlebitis   Score   Asepsis   Non-touch technique

## KEY CONSIDERATIONS

- Vein choice: for cannulation consider what you are going to be infusing and the length of use required. For both venesection and cannulation consider previous sites used, infection, bruising and phlebitis
- Palpation will help determine location and condition of vein
- Asepsis
- Knowledge of own limitations and ability: seek advice/refer on when appropriate
- Preparation: yourself and the patient
- Patient's condition

- Patient choice
- Own experience and preferences
- Follow policy
- Disposal of equipment, sharps
- Documentation

## EXTENDED ROLE

Performing venesection and cannulation are seen as extended roles and this can be defined as 'A role, not included in basic nurse training and comprises tasks, normally performed by a doctor, which a nurse may undertake: who has received appropriate training and is assessed as competent.'[2]

There are legal requirements pertaining to extended roles, for the nurse and the employing authority:

- training needs to be specific and adequate for the nurse;
- nurses have agreed to take on this extended role;
- training is recognised as satisfactory by the employing authority;
- a training programme must be provided by the employing authority;
- competency must be assessed;
- there is policy and procedure documentation in place.

## LOCAL PROCEDURAL POLICIES

In order to perform procedures such as venepuncture and cannulation safely, local policies and procedures must be adhered to at all times. It is rare for a policy to be used in total isolation, for example when performing venepuncture other policies and guidance should be adhered to including ANTT, hand hygiene, infection control, waste disposal, sharps policy, handling of bodily fluids, etc.

> ### Definitions
>
> **Intravenous:** provides a direct access to the circulatory system.
>
> **Venepuncture:** the process of obtaining a sample of venous blood.
>
> **Cannulation:** a plastic tube that, when inserted into a vein, facilitates the delivery or removal of fluids.
>
> **Asepsis:** free from infection or infectious material.
>
> **VIP score:** visual infusion phlebitis, scoring system to support the monitoring of cannula sites.
>
> **Aseptic non-touch technique:** this is the foundation for all aseptic procedures including venepuncture and cannulation

Policies and guidelines are designed to direct practice and achieve rational outcomes. Please see the website for an example of a policy document.

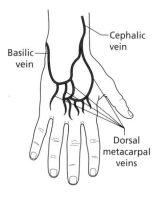

Superficial veins are selected for peripheral cannulation.[3] In children the most common sites include basilic, cephalic, median cubital veins in the antecubital fossa and the dorsal veins of the hands and feet. The child should be carefully assessed and where possible their opinion sought and considered in order to determine the most suitable vein (Figure 34.1).

## Considerations for site selection

- Age of the patient
- The patient's previous experience
- Vein accessibility
- Clinical condition and hydration status
- Treatment plan and other procedures required
- The device to be used along with the condition and location of the vein.

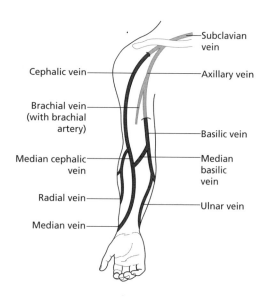

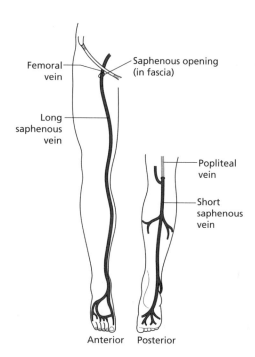

**Figure 34.1** Superficial veins of (a) the hand, (b) the upper limb, (c) the leg (reproduced with permission from Ingram and Lavery [2007]).

## ANATOMICAL ASPECTS OF CANNULATION

It is important to have some anatomical knowledge in order to perform cannulation successfully and avoid structures such as arteries, nerves, bone, etc.

## Good veins

- Move from distal to proximal sites
- Avoid previous sites
- Visible, ideally straight
- Large lumen

- Well supported by surrounding structures
- Easy to palpate
- Bouncy and soft
- Refills when depressed
- Feels round
- Non-dominant side where possible

## Sites and veins to avoid

- Overlying bony prominences
- Ideally only use veins in feet up to age child can walk
- Veins in close proximity to arteries
- Fibrosed, sclerosed or thrombosed veins
- Tortuous/mobile
- Thin/fragile
- Areas of flexion
- Bruised, painful or inflamed sites
- Veins affected by regular use
- Infected sites or broken skin
- Free of valves

## Valves

Valves prevent the backflow of blood in the vein. They are found in the majority of veins but not in the head, neck and thoracic area. Valves in veins should be avoided where possible as, if they are punctured, they can cause pain to the patient and damage to the valve, causing backflow of blood making a blood sample difficult to obtain. Valves can sometimes be located by a visible small bulge, and are always present at vein bifurcations (where the vein branches).

## Improving venous access

- Application of tourniquet 7–8 cm above site of access (disposable as per hospital policy)
- Lowering limb below level of the heart
- Immersing the limb in warm water or applying a warm compress
- Opening and closing the fist: encourages distention (blood to the vein)
- Gentle tapping
- Relaxing the patient to reduce anxiety

## Choosing your device

In children the commonest range of cannula is 26–22 gauge (26 gauge for a neonate and 22 gauge for the older child).

For venesection it is normally a 21 or 23 gauge whether a winged device or neonatal needle. The ideal device is the smallest possible size that will accommodate all the prescribed therapy. Allowing blood flow around the cannula reduces the likelihood of phlebitis.

# ANALGESICS

When you are undertaking venesection or cannulation topical anaesthetics should always be considered but not always used. Topical anaesthetics should be used unless there are contraindications that dictate otherwise, such as allergic reactions, prolonged anxiety due to prior knowledge or complications with procedure, etc.

The analgesics that are available are discussed below.

## EMLA: lignocaine and prilocaine

- Local anaesthetic
- Licensed in UK for use with children over 1 year of age
- Examine all sites before applying
- Apply 1 hour prior to needle procedure
- Lasts 5 hours only if occlusive dressing left in place
- Once dressing is removed it lasts 30–60 minutes
- Works in 5–10 minutes when applied to mucosa.

### Side-effects of EMLA

EMLA sometimes causes initial vasoconstriction, then dilatation. In rare cases there may be transient paleness, erythema or oedema. It should not be used on open eczematous skin.

## Ametop

- Local anaesthetic
- Licensed in UK for use with children over 1 month
- Examine all sites before applying cream
- Apply 30 minutes for venesection, 45 minutes for cannulation
- Remove occlusive dressing after time
- Anaesthetic effects last 4–6 hours after removal of occlusive dressing.

### Side-effects of Ametop

- Slight erythema: vasodilator action
- Slight oedema: common over adipose tissue sites, especially on toddlers

Note that this does not indicate allergy, but may make vein difficult to see. If irritation occurs – obvious oedema, erythema and itching – remove the dressing and wipe off remaining gel.

### Ethyl chloride

Ethyl chloride is a vapocoolant (skin refrigerant) intended for topical application to control pain associated with injections, venesection or cannulation.

Spray the target area with ethyl chloride continuously for 3–7 seconds from a distance of 3–9 inches (8–23 cm).

Spray the area until the skin just turns white; do not frost the skin. Swab the target area with antiseptic and quickly introduce the needle with the skin taut.

## CHILDREN WITH DEBILITATING FEARS SUCH AS NEEDLE PHOBIA

Increasingly some children have a morbid fear of needles and cannulation. See Chapter 7 related to play for ways of distracting children.

## COMPLICATIONS OF CANNULATION AND VENESECTION

- Pain
- Cellulitis
- Infiltration
- Extravasation
- Phlebitis
- Thrombosis
- Transfixation
- Infection

### VIP 'visual infusion phlebitis'

Phlebitis is caused by irritation to the wall of the vein; it is characterised by redness, inflammation, swelling and pain around the vein. Phlebitis is most commonly caused by the cannula itself rubbing against the wall of the vein but it can also occur because of irritation by the medication or fluids that are being infused. VIP scoring is a standardised tool; the RCN advocate that all infusion sites are monitored by this method as it determines when it is appropriate to remove and replace the cannula.

In children it is recommended that VIP scoring is

assessed and recorded hourly if an infusion is running. If the cannula is being used intermittently, the VIP score should be assessed at each time of use. Please see the website for an example of a paediatric cannula care form.

### Infiltration

Accidental administration of a non-vesicant solution or medication into surrounding tissues is a result of dislodgement of a cannula. It is recognised by increasing oedema at or near the venepuncture site.

#### *Action*

- Assessment: swelling, blanching, stretched skin, firm tissues and/or coolness.
- Compare with other limb.
- Pressure application at 2 inches above tip of cannula will stop infusion if still in vein.
- Blood return check unreliable as small veins may not permit blood flow around cannula.
- Remember VIP score!

### Extravasation (cannulation)

Inadvertent administration of a vesicant solution and/or medication into the surrounding tissues. Early identification is vital! If in doubt stop the infusion.

#### *Action*

- Never increase flow rate to confirm.
- Never confirm by blood return.
- Indications: pain or burning at site with progression to erythema and oedema.
- If suspected, *stop*!
- Act in accordance with local policies and prescriptions.

### Phlebitis

- A condition in which inflammation of the intima of the vein occurs.
- Characterised by pain, tenderness along course of vein, erythema and inflammatory swelling with a feeling of warmth at site.
- Chemical: response of the vein intima to certain chemicals infused.
- Mechanical: associated with the placement of the cannula, e.g. flexion
- Bacterial: associated with bacterial infection.

### Action

- Remove device
- The severity of infection needs to be assessed and treated accordingly

## Thrombosis (cannulation)

- The formation of a blood clot within a blood vessel.
- Caused by any injury that breaks the integrity of the endothelial cells causing platelets to adhere to the injured wall.
- Infusion stops: red, tender area.
- Thrombophlebitis: presence of a thrombus and the occurrence of inflammation.

### Action

- Discontinue infusion immediately.
- Relocate site to opposite extremity.
- Notify doctor to determine need for further action.

## Transfixation

Transfixation is when either the blood-taking device or cannula penetrates through one side of the vein wall or out through the other side; this will often result in a failed procedure and discomfort. It may also cause permanent damage.

### Action

Remove device and apply direct pressure; provide appropriate after care consisting of an applied dressing and observation and document all actions correctly.

## Needlestick injuries or sharps injuries

### Action in the event of a sharps injury

1 Bleed it.
   Encourage bleeding, but do not massage the site.
2 Wash it.
   Wash the injury, under hot running water.
3 Report it.
   Inform your line manager and contact the appropriate occupational health department (out

of hours, contact the Emergency Department).
4 Complete an incident form.
5 Further blood samples are required from the patient, so consent needs to be obtained. Follow-up treatment can then be planned where required, and counselling is available where necessary; this is normally organised by the occupational health department.

### Preventative measures

1 Select veins with ample blood volume when infusing irritating substances.
2 Avoid veins in areas of flexion.
3 Anchor cannula securely to prevent movement.
4 Thoroughly prepare skin and use aseptic technique.
5 Inspect site for pain, erythema, oedema, necrosis.

## PREPARATION PRIOR TO PROCEDURE

It is important to prepare all parties who are involved prior to the procedure. (Please see Chapter 1A).

Here are a few points to remember:

- ensure the child/family understand
- acquire informal verbal consent
- involve the play specialist
- confirm any allergies
- use topical anaesthesia
- review treatment plan
- confirm past experience
- assess availability of suitable veins
- ensure all equipment selected.

As mentioned earlier in this chapter the following policies should be used in accordance with other policies and guidance to minimise the risk of introducing infection or harm to the patient. Both venepuncture and cannulation are invasive procedures that involve breaking the integrity of skin; skin is one of the body's natural defences against infection. Such procedures increase the patient's risk to both local and systemic infections and should therefore be performed as aseptically as possible. ANTT is the core technique for both venepuncture and cannulation (for more information (see Chapter 1B).

## Venesection

This is based on Southampton University Hospitals NHS Trust policy. As procedures vary in different healthcare institutions, you are strongly advised to review local policy before implementing a specific skill detailed within this chapter.

## Intravenous cannulation

This is based on Southampton University Hospitals NHS Trust policy. As procedures vary in different healthcare institutions, you are strongly advised to review local policy before implementing a specific skill detailed within this chapter.

## PROCEDURE: Venesection

| Procedural steps | Evidence-based rationale |
|---|---|
| 1 Assess and prepare the child and family, using a play specialist if required | To allay anxiety and assist in obtaining the samples required |
| 2 Consult the child and family regarding any preferences and problems that may have been experienced at previous venepunctures | To involve the patient in the treatment. To acquaint the nurse fully with the patient's previous venous history and identify any changes in clinical status which may influence vein choice |
| 3 Check the identity of the patient matches the details on the requisition form | To ensure that the sample is taken from the correct patient |
| 4 The member of staff carrying out the procedure washes hands using soap and water, and alcohol hand gel – ensure hands are dry before commencement. Check hands are free of broken areas and cover with waterproof dressing if required | Minimises risk of cross-infection |
| 5 Find an appropriate vein or veins. Apply topical anaesthetic cream, if required, for the appropriate amount of time or consider using ethyl chloride spray (see manufacturer's instructions) the analgesic) | To ensure patient comfort and successful sampling |
| 6 Ensure adequate lighting | To ensure limb can be seen properly |
| 7 Ensure privacy for patient | |
| 8 Assemble the appropriate equipment in accordance with ANTT before the patient is brought into the room | To ensure that time is not wasted and that the procedure goes smoothly without unnecessary interruptions |
| 9 Recommend order of draw, prioritising samples for that patient | Sometimes not sufficient blood obtainable for all tests requested |
| 10 Remove occlusive dressing, wipe then wash off the remaining cream and select site | To remove cream and select optimal vein for venepuncture |
| 11 Ensure that the hand/arm is warm – placing the hand in a bowl of warm water will promote vasodilatation and relaxation | To ensure patient comfort, safety and access to the vein |
| 12 Put on non-sterile gloves – use non-latex and consider protective clothing | Minimises risk of cross-infection to staff and child |
| 13 Assistant fully supports the limb and support and squeeze appropriate limb or apply tourniquet if for an older child | Dilates veins by obstructing venous return |
| 14 Encourage patient if appropriate to open and close fist. Maintain limb in extensor position | Encourages prominence of veins |

## PROCEDURE:  Venesection (continued)

| | |
|---|---|
| 15  Vein may be tapped lightly or gently stroked | Promotes blood flow and therefore distends veins |
| 16  Prepare patient's skin by rubbing skin with Chloraprep® applicator for 30 seconds according to manufacturer's instructions or 70 per cent alcohol solution (Alcowipe or 0.5 per cent chlorhexidine cleaning solution). Allow to dry for 30 seconds | Promotes skin disinfection and helps to distend the vein |
| 17  If using anaesthetic spray, this should be applied immediately prior to insertion of needle (see manufacturer's instructions) | To ensure maximum analgesic effect |
| 18  Anchor the vein by applying traction on the skin a few centimetres below proposed insertion site | Immobilises the vein. Provides counter-traction, which will facilitate smooth needle entry |
| 19  Insert device with a steady smooth motion with bevel uppermost, keeping the skin taut | To ensure successful venepuncture causing least the discomfort to patient |
| 20  As soon as the wall of the vein is punctured, blood will be seen to flow. The needle should not be advanced any further and should be held in this position | Ensures successful venepuncture and minimises complications such as inadvertently puncturing small, delicate veins |
| 21  Gently draw back on syringe plunger. Do not exert pressure. | To prevent collapse or puncture of the vein |
| 22  Relax pressure around the limb or release tourniquet once all blood required is obtained | |
| 23  Place sterile gauze swab gently over needle. Do not press | To stop leakage and haematoma formation. |
| 24  Remove needle carefully. Apply digital pressure directly over puncture point. Do not apply pressure until needle has been fully removed | To prevent pain on removal |
| 25  Inspect puncture site before applying sterile dressing | Check puncture site is sealed |
| 26  Blood bottle should be filled straight from the syringe via a blood transfer device or green needle, not via the butterfly<br>Bottles should be filled in order of importance leaving any clotted samples till last | To reduce the risk of damaging blood cells<br>To ensure appropriate samples obtained |
| 27  Gently invert if specimen bottle contains chemical | To ensure blood is properly mixed. Vigorous mixing will damage blood cells |
| 28  On completion of procedure, ensure patient is left comfortable and recheck puncture site | Assess for excessive bruising |
| 29  Do not resheath needles; dispose of needle and syringe as 'whole' item directly into a sharps bin or use safety device to remove needle from barrel | Minimises risk of needlestick injury |
| 30  Label specimens carefully before leaving patient, match with request cards and place in specimen bag ready for delivery to laboratory | To ensure specimens from correct patient are delivered to the laboratory<br>To ensure requested tests have been performed |
| 31  Remove gloves. Dispose of all equipment appropriately following the sharps policy and the disposal of waste policy. Wash hands | To ensure safe disposal and avoid laceration or injury to staff |

## PROCEDURE: Intravenous cannulation

| Procedural steps | Evidence-based rationale |
| --- | --- |
| 1 Assess and prepare the child and family, giving a full explanation of the procedure. Use a play specialist if appropriate for preparation and distraction therapy. Prepare child for using Entonox if required | To identify any previous problems and allay anxiety<br>To maintain effective anxiety/pain management through the procedure |
| 2 Prepare the appropriate equipment | To carry out the cannulation |
| 3 Wash hands using soap and water, ensure they are dry | To prevent cross-infection |
| 4 Draw up 5 ml of 0.9 per cent saline into a syringe and prime T piece and smartsite /interlink bung | To enable flushing of the cannula prior to connecting IV infusion or giving medication |
| 5 Obtain verbal consent and involve the parent and informationchild in his/her treatment | To alert to potential problems and provide |
| 6 Ensure adequate lighting | To enable limb to be properly observed |
| 7 Ensure privacy for the patient | |
| 8 Identify an appropriate vein or veins that may be used | |
| 9 If using topical anaesthetic cream, apply according to the manufacturer's instructions and the appropriate PGD (Patient Group Direction) for application and length of time to be applied for | To ensure patient comfort and safety |
| 10 Warm hands if veins not visible: the hand may be placed in a bowl of warm water | This promotes vasodilatation and relaxation |
| 11 The member of staff who will carry out the procedure will wash their hands thoroughly and apply alcohol gel. Ensure they are dry | To minimise risk of cross-infection to staff and child |
| 12 Request assistance of another member of staff. Fully support limb with a pillow or hold child securely, supporting the limb but ensure that the arm is below the level of the heart. Support parent/carer if they wish to hold the child | To ensure patient comfort and reduce risk of injury by movement<br>To maximise venous drainage to the dependent limb |
| 13 Put on non-sterile gloves. Protective clothing should be worn if appropriate | For staff protection |
| 14 Squeeze or request assistant to squeeze identified limb or apply disposable tourniquet if required (older child only). Vein may be rubbed lightly | To ensure patient comfort and reduce risk of injury by movement |
| 15 Prepare patient's skin: clean with Chloraprep® applicator for 30 seconds according to manufacturer's instructions.<br>Allow to dry for 30 seconds | To promotes skin disinfection |
| 16 If ethyl chloride spray is chosen for topical anaesthesia, it should be applied now (see Manufacturer's instructions) | To minimise pain |
| 17 Remove needle guard and inspect the device for any faults | To detect faulty equipment and discard needle in the sharp's box if fault is seen. If fault noted then complete incident form |

## PROCEDURE:  Intravenous cannulation (continued)

| | |
|---|---|
| 18 Anchor the vein by applying traction on the skin a few centimetres below proposed insertion site (Do not touch the insertion site once cleaned) | To prevent vein moving during procedure and provide counter traction, facilitating smooth needle entry |
| 19 Insert device with bevel uppermost at selected angle, according to the depth of the vein. Using a steady, smooth motion, keep the skin taut until flashback of blood is seen or when puncture of wall is felt | To ensures successful venepuncture and minimises complications |
| 20 When flashback is seen, gently advance cannula off the needle. Advance the plastic cannula off the needle until it is inserted up to the hub. Keep traction on the vein with the other hand. Do not re-introduce the needle into the cannula | To ensure bevel of needle and end of cannula is in vein before advancing cannula |
| 21 Relax pressure around the limb. Loosen tourniquet if used/cannula and insertion care form (see website). | To reduce pressure in vein |
| 22 Secure cannula as per securing guidelines (attached). Ensure the insertion point is covered with a sterile dressing. | To secure cannula and prevent movement. |
| 23 Apply digital pressure to vein above cannula whilst removing needle | To avoid blood spillage |
| 24 If blood is required, attach T piece with syringe to end of cannula and withdraw blood required, using tourniquet if necessary. Clamp T piece and release tourniquet | To take blood. |
| 25 Instil 5 mL (or appropriate smaller amount) of 0.9 per cent saline via T piece, observing for signs of infiltration and then close the clamp | To ensure patency of vein and correct positioning |
| 26 If blood sample is not required, T piece and bung should be primed with 0.9 per cent sodium chloride prior to attaching and flushing the cannula. Observe for extravasation and clamp T piece | To prevent blood flow while connecting the T piece |
| 27 Observe the site for signs of swelling or leakage, and ascertain if the patient is in any discomfort or if pain is felt | To check the device is positioned correctly |
| 28 Attach the giving set to the bung on the end of the T piece | To reduce risk of infection through the cannula |
| 29 Apply splint and cover with bandage | To protect cannula from being dislodged and to promote comfort of the patient |
| 30 Ensure the patient is comfortable and safe, explaining any restrictions of movement to the child | To ensure child is not distressed by the device being left in situ |
| 31 Remove gloves and wash hands. Dispose of all equipment appropriately, following the sharps policy and waste policy | To prevent infection and sharps injury |
| 32 Document insertion by completing DH peripheral cannulation record card | For accountability and reference |

## CONCLUSION

The Royal College of Nursing have compiled a competency document which encompasses an education and training framework for capillary blood sampling and venepuncture in children and young people.[5] This document covers guidance for programme development, competencies, learning outcomes and four essential domains:

- Domain 1 Professional and legal issues
- Domain 2 Preparing self/child and family
- Domain 3 Performing capillary blood sampling and venepuncture
- Domain 4 Risks and hazards.

This competency document forms a basis for all local and national policies. Each individual trust or organisation will adapt and develop their own document relevant to subject area.

This document is useful for understanding what is required and expected in order to undertake venepuncture correctly.

All staff should ensure that they have undergone training and education to ensure competence.[5]Training should be ongoing with regular updates and assessment when necessary. The knowledge and the assessed skill will enable you to fulfil the learning outcomes as stated at the beginning of this chapter.

> Practitioners should strive not only to provide skill and dexterity. Specific knowledge and technical expertise, but also concern for all patients as individuals.[2]

## REFERENCES

1 Nursing and Midwifery Council (2008) *The Code. Standards of conduct, performance and ethics for nurses and midwives.* London: NMC

2 Lavery I, Ingham P (2005) Venepuncture: best practice. *Nursing Standard* 19(49): 55–65.

3 Dougherty L, Lister S (2006) *The Royal Marsden Hospital manual of clinical nursing procedures* (Chapter 45), 6th edition. Oxford: Blackwell Science

4 Royal College of Nursing (2005) *An educational and training competency framework for peripheral cannulation in children and young people.* London: RCN.

5 Nursing and Midwifery Council (2005) *Code of professional conduct*, London: NMC.

## FURTHER READING

Action for Sick Children (2003) *Helping children cope with needles.* www.actionforsickchildren.org (accessed 26 June 2009).

Broome ME (1990) Preparation of children for painful procedures. *Pediatric Nursing* 16: 537–541.

Campbell J (1995) Making sense of the technique of venepuncture. *Nursing Times* 91(31): 29–31.

Caws L, Pfund R (1999) Venepuncture and cannulation on infants and children. *Journal of Child Health Care.* 3(2): 11–16.

Dougherty L, Lamb J (2008) *Intravenous therapy in nursing practice*, 2nd edition. Oxford: Blackwell Publishing.

Duff A (2003) Incorporating psychological approaches into routine paediatric venepuncture. *Archives of Disease in Childhood* 88: 931–937.

Franklin L (1998) Skin cleansing and infection control in peripheral venepuncture and cannulation. *Paediatric Nursing* 10(9): 33–34.

Hadaway L (1995) *Anatomy and physiology related iv therapy, intravenous therapy: clinical principles and practice.* Philadelphia: WB Saunders.

Ingram P, Lavery I (2007) Peripheral intravenous cannulation: safe insertion and removal technique. *Nursing Standard* 22(1): 44–48.

Jackson A (1997) A battle in vein: infusion phlebitis. *Nursing Times* 94(4): 68–71.

*Longman family dictionary* (2000) London: Chancellor Press

Mallett J, Bailey C (eds) (1996) Intravenous management. In: *the Royal Marsden manual of clinical nursing procedures*, 3rd edition. London: Blackwell Science.

McCann M (2003) Securing peripheral cannulae: evaluation of a new dressing. *Paediatric Nursing* 15(5): 23–26.

Nursing and Midwifery Council (2008) *A–Z advice sheet.* London: NMC.

Royal College of Nursing (2003) *Standards for infusion therapy.* London: RCN.

Royal College of Nursing (2003a) *The recognition and assessment of acute pain in children.* London: RCN.

Royal College of Nursing (2005) *An educational and training competency framework for peripheral venepuncture in children and young people.* London: RCN.

Royal College of Nursing (2005) *Good practice in infection control; guidance for nursing staff.* London: RCN.

Sclare I, Waring M (1995) Routine venepuncture: improving services. *Paediatric Nursing* 7(4): 23–7.

Thurgate C, Heppell S (2005) Needle phobia – changing venepuncture practice in ambulatory care. *Paediatric Nursing* 17(9): 15–18.

Willock J, Richardson J, Brazier A, et al. (2004) Peripheral venepuncture in infants and children. *Nursing Standard* 18(27) pp 43–50.

## PERIPHERAL INTRAVENOUS THERAPY

*Janet Kelsey*

## OVERVIEW

The aim of this section is to support nurses in developing the necessary knowledge and skills required to assess venous access for the insertion of a peripheral cannula or blood taking device and how to appropriately care for them.

Intravenous (IV) therapy is integral to the care management of many children in every healthcare setting from critical care to the community. It is the process by which an infusion device is used to deliver fluids or drugs in solution to the patient by the intravenous route. However, it is not without risk, ranging from phlebitis to death,[1] hence the IV route should only be used when no other route is available. Training and development in the use of IV therapy is vital to ensure consistent standards of care.[2] The NMC's code of professional conduct reflects this ideal stating that individual nurses have a responsibility to deliver evidence-based care. Patients have the right to receive a uniformly high standard of care, regardless of whom they are and where they are treated.[3]

## INSERTION OF VASCULAR ACCESS DEVICE

IV therapy is administered via a vascular access device (VAD) of which the four main groups are

- peripheral cannulae
- midline catheters
- central venous catheters
- subcutaneous ports.

The type of VAD used will depend on the type of intravenous (IV) therapy and proposed duration, whether additional therapies may be necessary, the child's clinical condition and the safest method of inserting the VAD. The type of VAD should therefore be the most appropriate to meet the demands of the individual's requirements.

The indications for peripheral venous access are that it is either a short- or mid-term intervention (3–5 or 5–21 days) for IV therapy requiring fluid replacement, blood products, antibiotics, analgesia and insulin, or a mid-term intervention requiring, for example, parenteral nutrition.[4]

Cannulae are placed into a peripheral vein,[5] usually in a small vein in the back of the hand, lower arm or foot; scalp veins may also be used in small infants. The child's condition, age and diagnosis, vascular condition, infusion device history, and the type and duration of the therapy as well as the potential complications associated with VADs are all factors to be taken into consideration before placing cannulae.[6-9] Unless in an emergency it is advisable to avoid areas of flexion, for example the wrist and antecubital fossa, as movement of these joints when fluids and/or medicines are administered may cause the device to puncture the wall of the vein, resulting in damage to the surrounding tissues as a consequence of infiltration or extravasation.[5,10]

Prior to insertion consideration should be given to:

- informed consent from the child;
- preparation for the procedure and distraction therapy;
- the use of a topical local anaesthetic;
- hand hygiene and universal precautions during device placement;
- skin cleansing with 2 per cent chlorhexidine in 70 per cent alcohol, unless the child is known to have an allergy to chlorhexidine, in which case 70 per cent alcohol may be used. Local policy should be consulted for infants less than 8 weeks of age as recommendations may be in place that 70 per cent alcohol alone is used. Skin should not be repalpated after cleansing and should be allowed to dry completely before cannula insertion.

> **KEY POINT**
>
> It is essential that hand hygiene, universal precautions and skin cleansing are carried out when placing a cannula.

## MANAGEMENT OF VAD

After insertion of the cannula, documentation of the procedure should include evidence of consent, type, length and gauge of vascular access device, date and time of insertion,[11] number and location of attempts, identification of the site, type of dressing, patient's tolerance and understanding of the insertion, and the name of the person placing the device.

Care of the site must be performed using aseptic technique and observing universal precautions.[12] The peripheral IV site should be covered with a dressing that is sterile[5] and semi-permeable to enable the site to be regularly inspected.[13] IV sites should be treated as a surgical wound and the dressing changed if it is wet, bloodstained or has haemoserous fluid collecting around the site. The infusion site should be checked regularly, at least daily, and each time an intravenous drug is administered, for signs of phlebitis, infiltration and extravasation and the observations documented to comply with the guidelines for records and record keeping.[14] In addition the child's response to therapy, relevant observations of vital signs should be recorded.

When accessing lines to administer fluids or injections, aseptic technique should be used and ports or hubs cleaned with alcohol.

In infants and young children catheter security may be a problem; catheters may therefore be secured with sterile tape or wound closures. The use of non-sterile tape is not recommended.[15] Bandaging of the IV site may inhibit the moisture permeability of transparent dressings and increase the temperature of the area, providing warmth, which may encourage bacterial growth.[16] However, children may prefer the site bandaged preventing them from seeing it and reducing the possibility of it catching on clothing or bed linen. If a bandage is applied it should be a light cling bandage and it must be removed every time a drug is administered and at regular intervals to allow visual inspection of the site.[17] Movement of limbs may be minimised by splinting; however, this should only be carried out using suitable manufactured devices or locally made thermoplastic splints. Limbs must be splinted correctly to reduce the risk of trauma, nerve or circulatory damage and infection. Using wooden tongue depressors is contraindicated.[18]

Peripheral cannulae in adults are replaced every 72–96 hours depending on cannula type and therapy; however, in children cannulae are not replaced unless it is clinically indicated or the cannula has not been placed aseptically.[5,19] Administration sets and connections for non-blood products should be replaced every 72 hours unless a cannula-related infection is suspected.[13] Administration sets for blood or blood products and lipid feeds should be changed every 24 hours or after completion of the infusion. All add-on devices should be changed at the same time as the administration set.

> **KEY POINT**
>
> Observation and documentation of the continuing care of an intravenous cannula is essential.

Removal of the cannula should be carried out following explanation to the child, using universal precautions and an aseptic technique. The IV dressing is removed, a piece of sterile gauze held over the insertion site and the cannula removed carefully, using a slow steady movement, keeping the hub parallel to the skin. Gentle pressure is applied for at least 1 minute or as long as necessary, elevating the arm if bleeding persists. A sterile dressing is applied to the puncture site. If the site appears infected with a phlebitis score of 3 or more then the tip of the cannula is sent for culture and sensitivity. The used cannula and unused intravenous fluid is disposed of according to local clinical waste disposal guidelines and the removal of the device documented in the clinical record.

## INFUSION DEVICE SELECTION

The Medicines and Healthcare Products Regulaory Agency (MHRA) classifies infusion devices into three categories according to the potential risks involved, enabling users to make an appropriate choice of device for the therapy and patient. The pattern of delivery of fluid from an infusion pump is dependent on the type of pump used, e.g. some have the capacity for variable pressure, maximum flow rate and flow rate increments. It is therefore essential that the pump is chosen in accordance with MHRA categories to enable suitable accuracy of the infusion rate (measured over 60 minutes) and satisfy short-term minute-to-minute requirements which determine smoothness and consistency of flow. They should also meet the requirements for pressure occlusion, alarm delay time and size of bolus. Hospitals are required to label pumps to enable the correct pump to be chosen for the chosen therapy. You should follow the link to the MHRA website and familiarise yourself with the information on the suitability of different devices; this can be obtained from www.mhra.gov.uk. The MHRA also provide recommendations for safety checks to be carried out when using infusion or syringe pumps. All staff should be educated and competent in the use of infusion devices and have regular updates when new devices are introduced.[20]

## Gravity flow devices

These are dependent on gravity to drive the infusion and are influenced by a number of variables including patient movement and height of infusion container; the optimun height is 1 metre above the child to overcome venous pressure. Alterations in the child's position may alter the flow rate and necessitate changing the speed of the infusion.[20,21] The gravity system consists of an administration set containing a drip chamber and a roller clamp to control the flow of fluid, the roller clamp should be placed on the upper third of the of the infusion tubing away from the patient and the clamp should be repositioned to prevent 'cold creep', which is when the tubing tries to retain its round shape pushing the clamp open, but pinched tubing does not apply the same pressure thus potentially affecting flow rate.[20,21] Inclusion of other in-line devices, e.g. filters, may also affect the flow rate.[21]

The appropriate administration set is chosen according to need. Neonates should always be infused via a category A infusion pump;[22] children normally require the use of either an infusion pump or an administration set with a burette. Specific administration sets are required for the transfusion of blood or blood products. Administration sets will deliver different numbers

of drops per millilitre. This has to be taken into consideration when you are calculating the drip rate of infusions delivered without an infusion device. The drip rate should be checked on the packaging prior to administration to ensure an accurate calculation of flow rate.

### Calculating intravenous infusion flow rates

number of mL per hour (mL/h) =
total volume/duration
For example, 500 mL of fluid transfused over 12 hours: mL/h = 500/12
= 41.6 mL
The prescribed rate is 41.6 mL/h

In this example the burette is filled with at least 41.6 mL of infusion fluid or the infusion pump is programmed to deliver the nearest whole equivalent to 41.6 mL depending on local policy as to whether it is rounded up or down.

To calculate the drip flow rate for the same fluid prescription of 500 mL over 12 hours using an administration set with a drip rate of 20 drops per mL, use the following algorithm.

volume of fluid in mL × drops per mL of administration set ÷
duration of infusion in minutes
(500 × 20 drops/mL) ÷
= 720
13.8 drops per minute (round up or down according to local policy)

## Complications of IV therapy

Infiltration and extravasation are complications that can occur during IV therapy; both can result in problems with the siting of future devices, nerve damage, infection and tissue necrosis.[22] Infiltration is the leakage of non-vesicant medication or solution into the surrounding tissue instead of the intended vascular pathway. It occurs when the cannula moves out of the vein and may be complete (when the cannula moves out of the vein or is forced through the wall of the vein) or incomplete (where either only the tip of the cannula remains in the vein or the vessel wall does not seal around the cannula, allowing leakage into subcutaneous tissues)[23,24] The clinical symptoms of infiltration are coolness, leakage at the site, swelling, tenderness, change in flow of infusion or injection, and stretched skin. Infiltration should be identified, assessed and care planned to minimise the effect of the infiltration. Infiltration should result in immediate discontinuation of the infusion.[23] Accurate and immediate documentation is vital.[25]

Extravasation is the leakage of vesicant medication or solution into the surrounding tissue instead of the intended vascular pathway.[26] Vesicant drugs are those that cause blister formation with subsequent tissue necrosis. The clinical symptoms of extravasation are therefore redness, burning, stinging, tissue necrosis and ulceration as well as those for infiltration. Extravasation requires immediate assessment and discontinuation of the infusion by the nurse. Again accurate and immediate documentation is vital.[25] The incident should be documented in the patient's medical and nursing notes and on a clinical incident form.

Children at risk from infiltration and extravasation include:

- those with small, fragile or thrombosed veins;
- those with chronic disease including cancer;
- those with impaired circulation;
- those unable to communicate;
- those who have had repeated IV cannulations or venepunctures.

In addition, patients taking anticoagulants and obese patients are also at risk.[27–29] In neonates the incidence of extravasation is reported to be 38 per 1000.[30]

Phlebitis is the inflammation of the wall of the vein. It can be caused by chemical factors where the infusate may irritate the vein, mechanical factors such as irritation of the venous endothelium by the catheter, e.g. if the dressing is not secure and the cannula moves in the vein, and physical factors such as bacteria, causing irritation to the vein wall following poor insertion technique. Signs and symptoms of phlebitis are pain, swelling, erythema, tenderness, itching and warmth. Evaluation of the site for signs of phlebitis should be documented using a standard scale (Table 34.1) and action taken accordingly. Panadero et al.[32] report that 20–80 per cent of patients receiving peripheral IV therapy will develop phlebitis.

> **KEY POINT**
>
> Always document observations of cannula site referring to a recognised phlebitis scale.

**Table 34.1** Phlebitis evaluation scale (from Jackson[33])

| | | |
|---|---|---|
| *IV site appears healthy* | 0 | No signs of phlebitis |
| *One of the following is evident:* | | |
| • Slight pain near IV site | 1 | Possibly first signs of phlebitis |
| *or* | | |
| • Slight redness near IV site | | |
| *Two of the following are evident:* | | |
| • Pain at IV site | 2 | Early stages of phlebitis |
| • Erythema | | Resite cannula |
| • Swelling | | |
| *All of the following signs are evident:* | | Medium stage of phlebitis |
| • Pain along path of cannula | 3 | Resite cannula |
| • Erythema | | Consider treatment |
| • Induration | | |
| *All of the following signs are evident and exensive:* | 4 | Advanced stage of phlebitis or the start of thrombophlebitis |
| • Pain along path of cannula | | Resite cannula |
| • Erythema | | Consider reatment |
| • Induration | | |
| • Palpable venous cord | | |
| *All of the folllowing signs are evident and extensive:* | | Advanced stage of thrombophlebitis |
| • Pain along path of cannula | 5 | Initiate treatment |
| • Erythema | | Resite cannula |
| • Induration | | |
| • Palpable venous cord | | |
| • Pyrexia | | |

## PROCEDURE: Priming and connecting the administration set (from Kelsey and Bloxham[34])

| Procedural steps | Evidence-based rationale |
|---|---|
| **1** Decontaminate hands | Maintain universal precautions |
| **2** Check intravenous fluid by two registered nurses (as per local policy) against the prescription | According to local policy |
| **3** Check the outer wrapper is not damaged | All medical equipment, dressings and solutions usd during invasive proceedures must be sterile[5] |
| **4** Open the outer wrapper and remove the bag | |
| **5** Check the IV fluid bag for<br>• expiry date<br>• leakage<br>• particles<br>• cloudiness<br>• batch number | Medications, products and equipment must not be used beyond their expirydate[5] |
| **6** Check the outer wrapper of the administration set is not damaged and that the contents are sterile | |
| **7** Check the expiry date or date of sterilisation | |
| **8** Open the wrapper and remove administration set | |
| **9** Close the roller clamps on administration set | |
| **10** Remove the protective cap from the insertion port on the IV fluid bag maintaining sterility | |
| **11** Remove protective cover from administration set spike maintaining sterility. Note the ridge at the base of the spike. The spike should always be inserted into IV fluid up to this ridge | To prevent contamination of giving set |
| **12** Maintaining sterility insert the spike into the IV fluid insertion port pushing and twist until fully inserted | |
| **13** Hang IV fluid on IV stand | |
| **14** Release upper roller clamp and half fill the on line bubble of the admistration set by squeezing | |
| **15** Slowly open lower roller clamp and allow fluid to run into administration set expelling remaining air | |
| **16** When all air has been expelled close the lower roller clamp | |
| **17** When using administration set with burette release upper roller clamp and fill burette with 20–30 mL of fluid close clamp then half fill the on line bubble of the admistration set by squeezing. Fill burette to prescribed fluid dose prior to infusion | |
| **18** When using infusion pump place the adminstration set in the pump as per manufacturer's instructions | |
| **19** Maintaining sterility remove protective cap from administration set and IV cannula | |

## PROCEDURE: Priming and connecting the administration set (from Kelsey and Bloxham[34]) (continued)

| | |
|---|---|
| **20** Put on disposable gloves. Put on disposable plastic apron | To reduce the risk from cross-contamination to both patients and staff of organic matter, micro-organisms and toxic substances (DH 20001b)<br>To prevent contamination of clothing by blood or body fluids[5,35] |
| **21** Connect admistration set to IV cannula | |
| **22** Secure IV infusion suitable to child's age and activity level | Dressing should be sterile and allow visual inspection of the site[5,35]<br>Securing of the infusion should not interfere with the assessment or monitoring of the site or impede the infusion[5] |
| **23** Set the rate of infusion as prescribed | |
| **24** Open lower roller clamp and commence infusion | |
| **25** Document expiry date and batch number of IV fluid, time infusion commenced, names of people checking prescripion and commencing IV infusion | |
| **26** Document serial number of pump used | |
| **27** If not already in place commence fluid balance observations | |

## CONCLUSION

As the NMC code makes clear, all nurses are responsible for ensuring their competency. All healthcare staff have a duty to maintain peripheral intravenous devices safety, including patency of lines and prevention of complications during insertion and maintenance. Training and development in the use if IV therapy is vital to ensure consistent standards of care.

Go to the website to find the PowerPoint presentation for this chapter and MCQs to test your knowledge. **www.hodderplus.com/childnursingskills**

## REFERENCES

1 Gabriel (2008) Infusion therapy part one: minimising the risks. *Nursing Standard* **22**(31): 51–56.

2 Royal College of Nursing and British Medical Association (1993) *Intravenous therapy: a statement.* RCN/BMW: London

3 Department of Health (2000). *The NHS plan.* London: DH.

4 Hamilton (2000) selecting the correct intravenous device: nursing assessment. *British Journal of Nursing* 9: 15.

5 Royal College of Nursing (2005) *Standards for infusion therapy.* London: RCN.

6 Hamilton H, Fermo K (1998) Assessment of patients requiring IV therapy via a central venous route. *British Journal of Nursing* 7: 451–460.

7 Sansivero GE (1998) Venous anatomy and physiology. Considerations for vascular access device placement and function. *Journal of Intravenous Nursing* **21**(5)(Suppl): 107–114.

8   Gabriel J (1999) Long-term central venous access. In: Dougherty L, Lamb J (eds) *Intravenous therapy in nursing practice*. London: Harcourt, Chapter 11.

9   Wise M, Richardson D, Lum P (2001) Catheter tip position: a sign of things to come. *Journal of Vascular Access Devices* **6**(2): 18–27.

10  Hadaway L (2006) Technology of flushing vascular access devices. *Journal of Intravenous Nursing* **29**(3): 137–145.

11  Department of Health (2003) Winning ways. *Working together to reduce healthcare associated infection in England*. London: DH

12  National Institute for Clinical Excellence (2003) *Infection control prevention of heralthcare-associated infections in primary and community care* (clinical Guidelines 2) London: NICE.

13  Healthcare Infection Control Practices Advisory Committee (HICPAC) (2002) Guidelines for the prevention of intravascular catheter-related infections. *American Journal of Infection Control* **30**(8): 476–489.

14  NMC (2005) *Guidelines for records and record-keeping*. London: NMC.

15  Oldman P (1991) A sticky situation: a microbiological study of adhesive tape used to secure IV cannulae. *Professional Nurse* February: 265–269.

16  Nicol M (1999) Safe administration and management of peripheral intravenous therapy. In: Dougherty L, Lamb J (eds) *Intravenous therapy in nursing practice*. Edinburgh: Churchill Livingstone.

17  Dougherty L (2004) *Central venous access devices. Care and management*. Oxford: Blackwell Publishing

18  Medical Device Agency (1996) *Hazard notice* MDA. HN 9604. London: DH.

19  Centers for Disease Control and Prevention (2002) Guidelines for the prevention of intravascular catheter-related infections. *Morbidity and Mortality Weekly Report* **51** (RR-10), S35–S63. CDC. London: RCN/BMA,

20  Medical Devices Agency (2003) *Infusion systems device bulletin*. DB 9503. London: MDA.

21  Perucca R (2001) Types of infusion therapy eqipment. In: Hankin J, *et al.* (eds) *Infusion therapy in clinical practice*. Philadelphia: W.B. Saunders.

22  Medicines and Healthcare products Regulatory Agency (2007) www.mhra.gov.uk (accessed 16 April 2009).

23  Lamb J (1999) Local and systemic complications of intravenous therapy. In: Dougherty L, Lamb J (eds) *Intravenous therapy in nursing practice*. Edinburgh: Churchill Livingstone, pp. 163–194.

24  Perdue MB (2001) Intravenous complications. In: Hankin J, *et al.* (eds) *Infusion therapy in clinical practice*, 2nd edition. Pennsylvania: WB Saunders, pp. 418–445.

25  Royal College of Nursing (2008) *Standards for infusion therapy*. London: RCN.

26  Stanley A (2002) Managing complications of chemotherapy administration. In: Allwood M, *et al.* (eds) *The cytotoxic handbook*, 4th edition. Oxford: Radcliffe Medical Press, pp. 119–194.

27  Polovich M, White JM, Kelleher LO (eds) (2005) *Chemotherapy and biotherapy guidelines and recommendations for practice*, 2nd edition. Pittsburgh: Oncology Nursing Society.

28  Sauerland C, Engelking C, Wickham R, Corbi D (2006) Vesicant extravasation part 1: mechanisms, pathogenesis and nursing care to reduce risks. *Oncology Nurse Forum* **33**: 1134–41

29  European Oncology Nursing Society (EONS) (2007) *Extravasation guidelines*. Belgium: EONS

30  Wilkins CE, Emmerson AJ (2004) Extravasation injuries on regional neonatal units. *Archives of Disease in Childhood Fetal and Neonatal Edition* **89**(3): 274–275.

31  Panadero A, Iohom G, Taj J, *et al.* (2002) A dedicated intravenous cannula for postoperative use: effect on incidence and severity of phlebitis. *Anaesthesia* **57**: 921–925.

33  Jackson A (1998) Infection control: a battle in vein infusion phlebitis. *Nursing Times* **94**(4): 68–71.

34  Kelsey J, Bloxham N (2008) Peripheral intravenous therapy. In Kelsey J, McEwing G (eds) *Clinical skills in child health practice*. Edinburgh: Elsevier.

35  Department of Health (2001) Standard principles for preventing hospital-acquired infecion. *Journal of Hospital Infection* **74**(Suppl.), S21–37.

## FURTHER READING

Dougherty (2008) IV therapy; recognizing the differences between infiltration and extravasation. *British Journal of Nursing* **17**: 14.

Hadaway L (2001) Anatomy and physiology in infusion therapy. In: Hankin J, *et al.* (eds) *Infusion therapy in clinical practice*, 2nd edition. Pennsylvania: WB Saunders.

Medical Devices Agency (2003) *Infusion systems device bulletin*. DB 9503. London: Medical devices agency.

NMC (2004) *The NMC code of professional conduct: standards for conduct, performance and ethics*. London: NMC.

## CHAPTER 35

# Caring for children with life-threatening and life-limiting conditions

Helen Bennett and Liz Hopper

## LEARNING OUTCOMES

*Upon completion of this chapter the reader should be able to accomplish the following:*

1  Have a greater knowledge of the development of children's palliative care
2  Define concepts surrounding children's palliative care practice
3  Determine the criteria for classifying palliative care in children
4  Acknowledge the skills inherent in children's palliative care practice
5  Discuss best practice in relation to the use of palliative care pathways and understand the importance of choice for children and families in regards to accessing services

## CHAPTER OVERVIEW

In discussing palliative care many will focus on the care of adults and think of care at the end of life. It is also too readily assumed that palliative care is for patients with cancer. Yet in the last 20 years key professionals and palliative care organisations have driven practice and developed an approach to care that is available to all people with malignant and non-malignant disease, including children.

Although at the beginning of the twenty-first century we do not expect children to die (6 per 100 000 population 0–19 year olds),[1] there remain a number of childhood illnesses where there is no cure or where further treatment is not appropriate. Life-threatening and life-limiting illness in children present a diverse range of conditions from cancers to neurodegenerative and metabolic disorders. For these children and families (if unsupported) the burden of living with a life-threatening illness can be great. The need for guidance and support is essential to improve their quality of life. This is possible for all children if families have access to appropriate quality services.[2] Such services provide care that supports the ongoing needs of children and families as well as offering help to face the continuing challenges that arise.

This chapter describes the development of children's palliative care and outlines a number of definitions and concepts surrounding palliative care in general. The criteria used to classify palliative care in children are explored. The underpinning principles for children's palliative care are explained in order to facilitate an understanding of models of service delivery and promote the use of palliative care pathways.

Current discussions and recommendations highlight the importance of choice for children and their families in accessing services. This extends throughout the illness journey from diagnosis to the end of life and support in bereavement.

# DEVELOPMENT OF CHILDREN'S PALLIATIVE CARE

Palliative care for adults is recognised as an approach to care which grew from the pioneering work of Dame Cicely Saunders and the first adult Hospice, St Christopher's in London, in 1968. The palliative care movement and speciality of palliative medicine has developed to become a recognised worldwide approach for the care of dying patients.

Children's palliative care is a relatively recent development with the acknowledgement of the specific needs of children and young people that are different from the services offered to adults (see below). This was recognised in the early 1980s with the first children's hospice, Helen House, and the first children's palliative care consultant at Great Ormond Street.

However, there is an increasing emphasis for children's palliative care services to be more organised and delivered to meet the needs of children and their families throughout the UK.

Recommendations are driven by recent policy from the Department of Health[3] emphasising collaborative partnerships and accessibility of palliative care services for children and young people.

## Aspects of palliative care needs specific to children

- Illnesses in children are diverse and often rare.
- Many illnesses are genetic requiring family support for genetic counselling.
- Illnesses in children can extend over a number of years.
- Additional attention is paid to child development, cognitive ability.
- Educational requirements continue until 19 years
- Childhood illnesses tend to demonstrate complex needs.
- The child's experience of symptoms is important.
- The ability of children to communicate either verbally or non-verbally differs.
- The support of the family, including siblings and grandparents is integral to all care.
- The introduction of palliative care is not always clearly defined.

# THE NEED FOR CHILDREN'S PALLIATIVE CARE

The causes and nature of childhood deaths have changed over the years; in addition to advances in medical science, the course of a child's illness trajectory continues to change (e.g. cystic fibrosis, Duchenne's muscular dystrophy, Rett's syndrome). Many children are living longer with far more complex needs and long-term ventilation being increasingly common. The need for a quality sustainable service is essential to meet the ongoing palliative care needs of children and young people with a life-threatening illness.

# DEFINITIONS OF CHILDREN'S PALLIATIVE CARE

Children's palliative care is an approach to care that can be applicable from the moment of diagnosis throughout the child's life, extending through death and beyond into bereavement. It is concerned with the symptom management and quality of life but most importantly it is about supporting the individual child, young person and family to live life to its fullest.

> You matter because you are you.
> You matter to the last moment of
> your life, and we will do all we can,
> not only to help you die peacefully,
> but also to live until you die.
>
> Dame Cicely Saunders,
> founder of the modern hospice movement

A widely agreed definition highlights the multidimensional nature of children's palliative care:

> Palliative care for children and young people with life
> limiting conditions is an active and total approach to
> care embracing physical, emotional, social and spiritual
> elements. It focuses on enhancement of quality of life for
> the child and support for the family and includes the
> management of distressing symptoms, provision of respite
> and care through death and bereavement.[4]

Children's palliative care is offered primarily to support those children and young people with a life-threatening or life-limiting illness. However, defining those children and young people requiring

## Definitions

**Life-limiting conditions** are those where there is no reasonable hope of cure and from which children and young people will die. Some of these conditions cause a slow progressive deterioration and the child becomes increasingly dependent.

**Life-threatening conditions** are those where curative treatment may be an option but can fail or is deemed inappropriate because of the risks involved, for example childhood cancers.

**Complex healthcare needs** is a term used to describe childhood conditions that sometimes require intense ongoing care from health services (and social services) over a significant period of time. Many of these children require continuing care packages that support the child and family in what might be considered over and above the core universal health services.

**Palliative care** encompasses all aspects of holistic care to support the child and family from the moment a life-threatening illness is diagnosed.

**Supportive care** is an umbrella term for all services and based on the assumption that support and care are required before a diagnosis is reached.

**End of life care** recognises the end of life phase of a child's illness and provides care during, around the time of death and into bereavement. It focuses on symptom management, as well as psychological and spiritual support to ensure a sensitive, individualised approach.

---

palliative care is not easy. The prognosis of certain illnesses can be uncertain. In addition, the overlap of children with a disability and complex care needs are increasingly observed. The criteria for referring children to different services are becoming significantly blurred. The following definitions are given as a guide to aid understanding in determining the nature of childhood illness and the need for palliative care.

Given the strong overlap in complex care needs within children's conditions, referring children to palliative care services can be challenging. Many services including children's hospices recognise the ACT criteria for classification of childhood palliative care. Life-threatening and life-limiting conditions are classified into four groups (Box 35.1).

## CARING FOR CHILDREN WITH PALLIATIVE CARE NEEDS

Caring for a child and their family is unique and is an opportunity for care professionals to enable families to make the most of time left and enrich experiences with their child. It offers an opening to work with the child, parents and siblings to meet the individual needs of the family.

Children requiring palliative care have distinctive needs. Guidelines addressing the core principles for children's palliative care practice

> **Box 35.1 Criteria for life-threatening and life-limiting conditions classified into four groups[4]**
> - Group 1: life-threatening conditions for which curative treatment may be feasible but can fail. Where access to palliative care services may be necessary when treatment fails or is no longer appropriate.
> - Group 2: conditions where premature death is inevitable, where there may be long periods of intensive treatment aimed at prolonging life and allowing participation in normal activities, e.g. cystic fibrosis.
> - Group 3: progressive conditions without curative treatment options, where treatment is exclusively palliative and may commonly extend over many years, e.g. Batten's disease, mucopolysaccharide conditions, muscular dystrophy.
> - Group 4: irreversible but non-progressive conditions causing severe disability leading to susceptibility to health complications and likelihood of premature death, e.g. severe cerebral palsy, multiple disability such as brain or spinal cord injury.

(Box 35.2) have been established to underpin all services and care delivery. Established initially in the UK, the following principles and standards are recognised worldwide, strengthening care for all children with a life-limiting or life-threatening illness.

## Box 35.2 Principles of children's palliative care[5]

1 Every child should expect individualised, culturally and age appropriate palliative care.

2 Palliative care for the child and family shall begin at diagnosis and continue alongside any curative treatments throughout the child's illness, during death and in bereavement.

3 The child's parents or legal guardians shall be acknowledged as the primary care givers and recognised as full partners in all care and decisions involving their child.

4 Every child shall be encouraged to participate in decisions affecting his or her own care, according to age and understanding.

5 A sensitive but honest approach will be the basis of all communication with the child and the child's family. They shall be treated with dignity and given privacy irrespective of physical or intellectual ability.

6 Every child or young person shall have access to education and wherever possible be provided with opportunities to play, access leisure opportunities, interact with siblings and friends and participate in normal childhood activities.

7 Wherever possible, the child and the family should be given the opportunity to consult with a paediatric specialist with particular knowledge of the child's condition and should remain under the care of the paediatrician or a doctor with knowledge and experience.

8 The child and family shall be entitled to a named and accessible key worker whose task it is to build, coordinate and maintain appropriate support systems which should include a multi-disciplinary care team and appropriate community resources.

9 The child's home shall remain the centre of care wherever possible. Treatment outside of this home shall be in a child-centred environment by staff and volunteers, trained in palliative care of children.

10 Every child and family member, including siblings, shall receive culturally appropriate, clinical, emotional, psychosocial and spiritual support in order to meet their particular needs. Bereavement support for the child's family shall be available for as long as it is required.

# CHILDREN'S PALLIATIVE CARE APPROACH

Palliative care is therefore an approach and philosophy of care, which encompasses physical, social emotional, cultural and spiritual dimensions. It is underpinned by a number of principles that shape delivery. It is about being alongside the child and their family throughout the illness journey. It is not just about treating the disease or managing symptoms but providing emotional and spiritual support that is meaningful to the family.

For a nurse there are many areas besides clinical care where they can engage with the child and family and provide support. From the point of diagnosis, which requires sensitive management in the breaking of bad news (Box 35.3), all that you do will shape the care delivered and the experience for the child and family.

## Box 35.3 A six-step protocol for breaking bad news adapted from Buckman[6]

1 *Getting started*
The physical setting ought to be private, with both doctor, nurse and parents comfortably seated. You should ask the parents who else ought to be present, and let them decide: studies show that different patients have widely varying views on what they would want. It needs to be a two-way conversation.

2 *Finding out how much the family knows*
By asking a question such as, 'What have you already been told about your child's illness?' you can begin to understand what they already know, what they have understood and how they feel.

3 *Finding out how much the parents want to know*
It is useful to ask the parents what level of detail should be covered. For instance, how much medical detail to cover, or an outline of the big picture. It is important to establish what they would prefer now. They may ask for something different during the next conversation.

4 *Sharing the information*
Decide on the agenda before you sit down so that you have the relevant information at hand. The topics to consider in planning an agenda are diagnosis, treatment, prognosis and support or coping. However, an appropriate agenda will usually focus on one or two topics. Give the information in small chunks, and be sure to stop

**Box 35.3 (continued)**

between each chunk to ask the parents if they understand. Long lectures are overwhelming and confusing. Remember to translate medical terms into English.

5 *Responding to the parent's feelings*

If you don't understand and respond to the parent's reaction, you will leave a lot of unfinished business, and you will miss an opportunity to support. Learning to identify and acknowledge a person's reaction is something that definitely improves with experience, if you're attentive, but you can also simply ask 'Could you tell me a bit about what you are feeling?'

6 *Planning and follow-through*

At this point you need to synthesise the parents concerns and the medical issues into a concrete plan that can be carried out. Be explicit about support available. Give a phone number or a way to contact the relevant people if something arises before the next planned contact.

---

**KEY POINTS**

- Palliative care is an approach to care and can be offered from point of diagnosis.throughout the child's illness to end of life and support in bereavement.
- Children requiring palliative care have distinct needs different from those of adults.

## SKILLS REQUIRED IN CARING FOR CHILDREN WITH PALLIATIVE CARE NEEDS

The importance of a skilled workforce to meet the ongoing needs of children and their families and to provide a high-quality service is recognised throughout numerous professional bodies and documents including *Better care better lives*.[3] A number of core skills are highlighted to guide standards for palliative care practitioners including, communication, clinical skills and care management, assessment skills, role development and leadership.

### Communication

Good communication skills are essential in supporting children and families. The unique aspect of communicating with children and engaging with children about their illness in a sensitive manner on their terms is crucial. Listening to the child and family and recognising what is important to them cannot be underestimated.

There are many ways of truly listening to the needs of a child, including being alert to the possibility that what is being said and expressed may not be the whole story. For a variety of reasons a child may not be able to find words or means to express themselves.

The role of the person caring is to listen with a 'third ear', in other words to be open to what may not be so obvious. For example, the child who says to a member of staff 'I wonder what it would be like if I didn't come here (a hospice) anymore …' may be looking for more than a reassuring, 'You are always welcome here at anytime'. In this case the child concerned was trying to find a way to talk about how others might feel after she had died.

Communicating in children's palliative care is about providing opportunities and demonstrating a willingness to talk about issues related to death and dying. For example, children may have very direct questions about the dying process whereas families may want to discuss arrangements for the funeral.

We can never assume we know what another person is meaning and therefore it is best to check, possibly by asking a question. In this case by asking: What do you mean by 'not coming here anymore'? The child could clarify by saying they are about to move house, and would not be coming to the hospice again, or, as in this case, they are daring to begin to look at the fact of nearing death.

Additional questions may focus on coping with deterioration in condition and, at such a time, what is important to the child and family. These important questions cannot usually be asked directly, although this can be possible if a firm relationship has been established. What is helpful is for the staff member to be aware of such questions.

### Clinical skills

Nursing skills focus on an holistic approach to care. It concerns understanding the principles of palliative care and being able to make sound clinical judgement. Children with a life-threatening illness increasingly have complex and clinical needs from intravenous administration to ventilation and management of seizures. The clinical situation can change significantly and suddenly. Ongoing review, evaluation of care and appropriate alternatives to the management of care are essential in meeting the best outcome for the child and family. If children have the capacity they should be encouraged to enter into discussions about decisions relating to their care.

## Emotional and spiritual support

For a child who is used to having a large amount of attention to clinical need, there can be a temptation, both for the medical and nursing staff, and sometimes even for the family, to focus solely on that. It is essential that clinical aspects of care be attended to carefully, yet, alongside this, there is a need to be prepared to enter into dialogue about the emotional and spiritual needs of the child.

## The needs of parents, siblings and relatives

Each family is unique, and finding ways to relate to the wider family will demand flexibility and imagination at times. Families are continually coping with the emotions, responsibilities and adjustments associated with living with a child with a life-threatening illness and within one family there is likely to be a wide range of responses to the deteriorating condition of the child. Those caring for the child will need to find ways of engaging with the child, the parents and the wider family. It is important to offer the range of support that families require. More junior staff will benefit from a mentor to refer to and learn from.

If there are other children in the family, often parents will be concerned about their needs or behaviour. Siblings can be overlooked, and often feel the burden of having a brother or sister with a life-limiting condition. There may be activities and support offered to them through the nearest children's hospice or other children's charity. For the health professional caring for the family, involving siblings in conversation and play where possible will benefit everyone.

Parents themselves will need time to adjust to new information and changes in their child's condition. Offering specific time with a dedicated member of the team, such as a family support worker, may be what the parents are looking for. Assessment can then be made about the most appropriate sources of support, whether from friends and family, or health professionals.

Grandparents can be the forgotten carers in the family, and their particular needs can easily be marginalised. Occasionally there may be offers of support via the local hospice. On the whole it is helpful to remember their role in the family, and include them as appropriate.

As it is both understandable, and not uncommon for there to be tensions and sometimes splits in a family going through a trauma, it is important to remember that nurses are required to care, listen and possibly refer to another service for further more specialised support.

## Staff support and supervision

Such intense and sometimes emotional engagement requires self-awareness and a requirement to look after oneself – particularly in the field of palliative care. There is much evidence surrounding the need for staff support and supervision. A well-managed team with good morale will naturally provide good support to all team members; however, there may on occasion be need for more specific support. Good effective supervision means that a member of staff can not only feel supported, but is also enabled through reflection to extend his or her knowledge and skills and gain confidence in caring for children who must face their own mortality.

## The importance of professional boundaries

The challenge to staff is that in being open to new learning, there will always be emotional demands placed on them. In particular, the development of self-awareness is essential to ensure their own pain or distress related to loss does not interfere with the focus of care, which should centre on the needs of the child and family. The recognition of professional boundaries here is crucial and for staff not to become over-involved. There can be high expectations on staff to provide a safe emotional space for families to be able to offload their distressing feelings and it is important that this is enabled. More senior staff must be available to support those less experienced, and all must be alert to the dangers of crossing professional boundaries. It can be very tempting to agree to give personal contact details to a family where there has been particularly close involvement. The family will be better supported if the professional boundaries are clear, as it is not possible to be a friend and health professional.

This does not mean that involvement with families will not be intimate at times, and good supervision will offer clear guidelines as well as solid support for staff working at the frontline in palliative care.

## Role development and leadership

The field of practice enables team members at all levels to contribute to the knowledge and provision of children's palliative care, promoting and enhancing expert knowledge and skill from specialist practitioners. There are increasing opportunities for career development in children's palliative care. Expert leadership can develop individual skill but also contribute to organisational and national developments in the field.

| KEY POINTS |
| --- |
| • Nursing skills focus on an holistic approach to care. |
| • The clinical situation can change significantly and suddenly. |
| • Ongoing review, evaluation of care and appropriate alternatives to the management of care are essential. |
| • Children and the family should be supported in decision-making. |

## MODELS OF PALLIATIVE CARE DELIVERY

Most children with palliative care needs are cared for by their families in the community; however, support of other services (hospices) and occasional visits to hospital require all nurses to understand and develop a knowledge base of palliative care. All children's palliative care services, generalist (universal) or specialist promote a holistic approach to supporting children and their families. The aim for all nurses is to assist children in achieving their potential and to live their lives to the full, alongside helping them face complex medical needs and uncertainty within the illness journey.

This is achieved through a multiprofessional, multiservice approach. By recognising an approach to care that can be delivered in and across a variety of settings, children and families are given choice. Not all services are required at the same time but children and families should be able to access the services they need according to different stages of the child's condition.

Figure 35.1 (page 615) demonstrates palliative care delivery across all services from universal to specialist delivery.

## CHILDREN'S PALLIATIVE CARE PATHWAYS

To support families within the challenge of negotiating a number of services and be able to access provision of care appropriate to the child's needs, the children's palliative care pathway has proved an essential framework for support.[7]

The integrated care pathway is not just about specific clinical aspects of care but promotes continuing, ongoing care throughout the child and young person's illness journey. It helps to support and manage care across a variety of settings, involving multi-agency input and resource.

This specific multi-agency pathway for children has provided a benchmark for locally adapted pathways to meet the individual needs of children and families in their own regions.

## CONCLUSION

Children's palliative care aims to provide an holistic family-centred approach to care, enhancing the fullness of life. It requires sensitive meaningful care from diagnosis throughout the child's illness journey to care at the end of life and support through bereavement. It is about offering choice to families that is both accessible and offers high-quality care that supports the ongoing and ever changing needs of the child with a life-threatening illness.

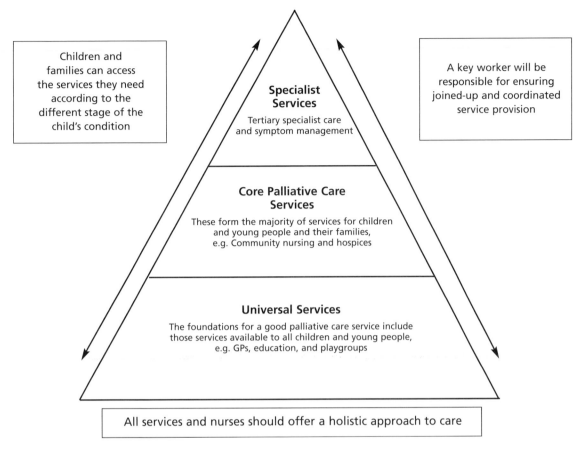

**Figure 35.1** Integrated multi-agency service delivery (adapted from Dott[3])

 Go to the website to find the PowerPoint presentation for this chapter and questions to test your knowledge. **www.hodderplus.com/childnursingskills**

# REFERENCES

1   Department of Health (2006) *Palliative care statistics for children and young people*. London: DH.
2   Craft A, Killen S (2007) *Palliative care services for children and young people in England*. London: DH.
3   Department of Health (2008) *Better care, better lives: improving outcomes and experiences for children and young people and their families with life threatening and life limiting conditions*. London: DH.
4   Association for Children's Palliative Care and Royal College of Paediatrics and Child Health (2003) *A guide to the development of children's palliative care services*. Bristol: ACT.
5   ICPCN (2008) International Children's Palliative Care Network (www.icpcn.org.uk).
6   Buckman R (1992) *How to break bad news: a guide for health care professionals*. Baltimore: The John Hopkins University Press.
7   Association of Children's Palliative Care (2004) *Integrated care pathways for children with life threatening and life limiting conditions*. Bristol: ACT.

## FURTHER READING

Goldman A, Hain R, Liben S (2005) *Oxford textbook of paediatric palliative care*. Oxford: Oxford University Press.
Watson M, Lucas C, Hoy A and Black I (eds) (2005) Paediatric palliative care. In: *Oxford handbook of palliative care*. Oxford: Oxford University Press, Chapter 7.

## USEFUL WEBSITES

Association of Children with life threatening Illness: www.act.co.uk.
Children's Hospice UK: www.childhospice.co.uk.
International Children's Palliative Care Network: www.icpcn.org.uk.

## CHAPTER 36

# End of life care

Helen Bennett and Liz Hopper

*But I have promises to keep and miles to go before I sleep.*
Robert Frost

## LEARNING OUTCOMES

*Upon completion of this chapter the reader should be able to accomplish the following:*
1  To recognise impending death and assessment of death
2  To understand the importance of supporting the family alongside the practical tasks when a child has died
3  To acknowledge the importance of information and choice for families
4  To develop a greater understanding of ongoing support following the death of a child

## CHAPTER OVERVIEW

Caring for a child at the end of life requires a sense of being and sensitivity that is not often called upon in our professional careers. It can be an intensely draining time for the family. It is important to recognise that the emotional and spiritual support for families are as essential as the practical tasks that need to be completed.

This chapter describes the care and support for the child and family at the end of life and offers guidance of a practical nature in recognising and confirming death. Wider aspects of care in supporting the whole family after death and in the planning of the funeral are also addressed.

It is also recognised to be a highly emotive time for staff and the need for staff support is acknowledged.

## CARING FOR A CHILD BEFORE DEATH

### Assessment

A child or young person at the end of life requires a comprehensive holistic assessment. Whether they are known to you within the community or are being admitted to hospital or a hospice, care planning is essential. This will enable individualised care planning and care delivery incorporating the child's and family's needs and wishes. All care provided should be inclusive of a culturally sensitive approach encompassing spiritual and emotional aspects of care.

It is helpful for the family to meet the nursing team at this time and the key member of staff who will coordinate their care. At such a critical time the professional relationship shared can provide immense support.

### Continuing review

Symptom management for children and young people at the end of life can be complex and challenging. A multiprofessional holistic approach should be delivered throughout and all care must be continually reviewed and evaluated. Any changes need to be recorded, and care altered accordingly to ensure quality care is constantly provided. The *Basic symptom control guidelines for paediatric palliative care*[1] is a useful resource and can be downloaded from the internet (www.act.co.uk). There are a number of other documents, guidelines and books providing support for symptom management, available as a further resource. Please see the website for further information.

## Care of the family

The care and support of parents and siblings and possibly the wider family is fundamental at this time. Families require relevant and appropriate information to make choices and the opportunity to be involved in decision-making.

If parents have been faced with the information that there is no further active treatment possible, they will need time to adjust to the fact that this is now nearing the time they have been dreading – the death of their child. At a time when they may feel they have little or no control, being included and involved in making plans is vital. The choice of where their child will die may be a difficult conversation, but crucial if the child/young person and the parents are to receive the best possible care.

If the child/young person and/or parents choose to be at home for end of life care, the identified key worker will need to ensure all available support services are known to the family, as well as how they may be accessed. The family may already have links with the local children's hospice; if not, the health worker can inform them, and refer as and when necessary. The parents need to know that they may use the hospice facilities even after their child dies, as he or she can be transferred to the cold room within a special suite designed so that the child may remain there until the funeral, along with separate accommodation for the parents.

Sometimes a child is treated in hospital right up until the time of death. In this case, again parents need to know what their options are so that they can make an informed choice. Some children's hospices will accept a child who has not been known to them previously so that their specialist facilities and staff can be used to support a family.

## Care of siblings

Talking with siblings about their dying brother or sister may be very difficult and may be equally challenging for parents. Siblings are often good at noticing things but may be mistaken in their interpretation of what they mean. Honest and meaningful communication is therefore important. Letting siblings know what is going on and actively involving them in what is happening can be very supportive and help them cope better, even if there are no definitive answers or solutions to their questions.

Any conversations should recognise the individual needs of each child, at the same time acknowledging their developmental stage and cognitive understanding and always with the knowledge of the parents' wishes for disclosure of information.

Wherever possible, open and sensitive communication should be encouraged with the whole family, and parents supported to talk with their children. Parents may need guidance and support, before, during and after the conversation.

There are a number of resources and further information available on support for siblings and how to help parents. Guidance also includes explaining death to children and a child's understanding of death. Please see the website for further information.

Several children's hospices now have a sibling support worker who can be a valuable source of information, and may be able to signpost local support services for children and young people.

## Play

Play is an extremely valuable means of communication with children and adults. There are a number of books, games and specific activities that can be used for the ill child, their siblings and parents. The play therapist can be involved as appropriate at all stages within the pathway to support the child and family.

## AT THE TIME OF DEATH

To predict the time of death when a child is dying is remarkably uncertain and is never recommended. Each case is unique and all children present with varying approaches at the end of life. In the days or hours prior to death it is likely that they will become more sleepy and uninterested in food. They may not be able to absorb feeds or milk and are likely to have a decreased urinary output. Breathing may become more laboured and irregular and they may appear pale and grey in colour. However, it must be stressed that this is not the case for all children.

## What to do when a child/young person dies

It is not always obvious that a child/young person has died. They may appear to have stopped breathing some time before their heart has stopped beating.

It is less important to establish death than it is for the family to spend those last few moments together. What to do:

- There is no need to rush to do anything with the child.
- Be sensitive to the needs of the family. They may want to be alone or have company – just ask.
- You can check for breath by placing your cheek near to the child's mouth and sensing for breath.
- If the doctor is not present, it is helpful to confirm death by listening for a heartbeat for a full minute.
- Take a note of the approximate time of death.
- Take a note of who is present.
- The doctor will certify the death and the time of death for the death certificate.
- If the parents have not been present at the death contact them immediately.

If the death is expected:

- telephone the duty doctor, if not present at the death;
- if the death occurs at night, the doctor does not need to come in, unless the parents would like them to, but will need to visit the following day to certify the death. However, you will need to follow local protocols for your area of practice depending on whether you are nursing in the community, hospital or respite setting.

If the death is unexpected:

- call the on-call doctor immediately; it is likely the Child Death Overview Panel will need to be informed, please see the website for further information;
- if parents are not present, contact immediately.

When contacting parents by phone:

- speak calmly and tell them straight away what has happened;
- find out if they are on their own or if there is someone to support them;
- give them the facts; be clear, use the word died and not other euphemisms;
- ask them to come to the hospital;
- assure them that nothing will be done to their child until they arrive;
- encourage them to drive safely; ask if there is someone who could drive them.

Other practical things to do:

- Inform other professionals as appropriate.
- Ask the family if there is anyone they wish you to contact.
- Record details of death and document in notes, together with names of those present at death.
- The death certificate will need to be completed by a doctor.
- If the child is less than 28 days, a separate certificate for neonatal deaths needs to be completed.
- The Child Death Overview Panel and/or Health Care and Quality Commission (depending on your area of practice) will need to be notified of the death within 24 hours.
- The Cremation Form (Part 1) will need to be completed if the family request a cremation, unless they are very sure it is to be a burial. Details of death must be written as on death certificate.

---

**KEY POINTS**

- Be calm and sensitive to the needs of the child and family.
- You do not have to rush, go at the parents' pace.
- The emotional and spiritual support is as important as the practical tasks to be completed.

---

## SUPPORTING THE FAMILY

Waiting for that last breath and recognising that death has finally come can trigger an overwhelming sense of emotions. The most important thing is to be there alongside the family, be sensitive and listen to their requests for support.

## Support of staff

It is important to recognise that caring for a child at the end of life can be highly emotive, but self-awareness is essential to ensure parents do not end up supporting staff. It is important to step aside and look after yourself, taking time out as appropriate. Where possible it is helpful to share with colleagues the support of the family.

## Caring for the child after death

Don't rush to do anything with the child.

Continue to be sensitive to the needs of the parents – they may wish to be on their own, or have a member of staff to stay with them. Don't be afraid to ask which they would prefer.

Give the parent's time.
- They may need guidance on what they are able to do. Encourage them that if they wish they may:
  - cuddle their child;
  - lie on the bed with their child;
  - sleep for a while next to them;
  - pick them up (if small enough) and move them to wherever they would like within reason, i.e. into the garden;
  - wash their child;
  - change their clothes;
  - give them a bath either in the bathroom or the bedroom.
- The child/young person could have some medical equipment, which may need to be removed from their person.
  - cannulas;
  - syringe drivers;
  - nasogastric tubes (It is essential that parent's are consulted before removing a nasogastric tube – if the child/young person has had a tube for some time, it may have become part of their features (much like glasses) so removing it may take away some of their character. If you have permission to remove the nasogastric tube, you must aspirate before doing so.
  - gastrostomy: when removing a gastrostomy button, cover the site with a dressing (preferably a waterproof one), aspirate the stomach before removal. The funeral director will advise if necessary.)

At all times inform the parents what you are doing and ask their permission before doing anything.

If subject to an inquest you may not be able to remove anything at this time – always check first.

## Family support

Do not overwhelm parents with information and offer support when they are ready.

Practical areas where you can help include:

- contacting key individuals, e.g. friends, family minister, if the family wish;
- explaining that you can field calls and visitors if they wish;
- explaining they can stay for as long as they wish (as appropriate);
- explaining that hand/foot prints and other mementos can be made/taken as and when the family are ready;
- being prepared to answer questions or direct the family to further support.

## Moving the child/young person to the chapel of rest or cooled room

It is important to recognise that the child does not immediately have to be moved to the mortuary or funeral directors. Children's hospices have a special cold room for laying the body out. If the child has died in hospital, parents may choose to take the child to a hospice or home. If the parents should wish, it is fine to move the child to the chapel of rest. If the child has died at home they may wish them to be moved to the children's hospice or the funeral directors. Although a difficult conversation to have, it is essential to ask the family where they would like their child to be.

When the parents are ready the child can be moved. If light enough the child can be carried. Agree with the parents who will move their child, and how this should be done.

Every effort should be made for the parents to feel as relaxed and in control as possible.

At this stage, an important concern is cooling the body of the child/young person.

It is advisable for the child/young person's body to have minimal clothing and thin bedcovers. This is only a guideline however, and should the parents be unhappy with this, then follow the wishes of the parents. It should be noted, however, that bed covers will prevent the child/young person's body from cooling effectively; once it has cooled a sheet or light duvet cover may be added.

The time it takes for a child/young person's body to cool will be affected by a number of things, primarily their surface area and weight.

If required, cooling can be aided by placing gel packs under the body or spraying the room with water to keep the air moist.

If the child is at home he or she can stay in their own bedroom and a funeral director may be able to supply a cooling unit.

**KEY POINTS**

Parents should be encouraged to choose what they wish for their child.
- What they would like their child to wear?
- What they would like their child to lie on (bassinet, cot or a bed)?
- What bedding they would like on the bed?
- What they would like to have in the cold room to personalise it for their child (make a few suggestions such as music, some of child/young person's personal items from their bedroom, teddy, candles, etc.)?

## Sibling support

Care and sensitive communication is important for siblings and they should be included and not shielded from grief and loss felt by others. They may also need some 'time out' with another adult they know and trust, or possibly a health professional so that they can be themselves, without expectation from anyone. If they wish to see their brother or sister who has died, attention and support should be offered to managing this in the most positive way with the family.

It is important to care for the whole family, and increasingly support is extended to grandparents, friends and others who have been special in the life of the child and family.

## Further tasks the family will need to think of in the coming days

Registration of death: When a child/young person dies the death is usually registered in the district where they have died. It must be registered *within 5 days of death.*

### Guidance notes

- An appointment will need to be made with the Registrar.
- If the siblings are not going to the Registry Office,

make sure there are adequate arrangements for their care, either with relatives or friends.
- The signed death certificate must be taken to the Registrar.
- Ask the parents if they would like someone to accompany them or drive them.
- The registration process takes approximately half an hour. There are various documents that are needed and you will need to check with your local office.
- Death certificates are needed for administrative purposes.
- One death certificate is free, more can be purchased from the registrar at a cost; prices may vary.
- The registrar will issue a certificate for burial or cremation that must be passed to the funeral director in order for the funeral to take place.

## Removing the body out of England and Wales

- There is no restriction on moving bodies within England and Wales.
- However, notification to the coroner for the district in which the body is lying is required if the child is to be moved elsewhere.
- A form is obtained from the registrar or coroner. It is a form of notice to a coroner of intention to remove a body out of England and Wales.
- The coroner will acknowledge receipt of your notice and let you know when the body can be moved – this is usually 4 clear days from when your notice was received. In urgent situations, it may be possible to bring this forward.

## Cremation/burial

*The funeral cannot take place until the funeral director or celebrant has obtained the certificate for burial or cremation.*

For a burial the only form needed is the death certificate. For a cremation an additional cremation form is required:

- Part 1 should be completed by the doctor issuing the death certificate.
- Part 2 must be completed by a second doctor.

When the funeral director/celebrant has been chosen and the date of the funeral has been confirmed, arrangements should be made for the certificates to be given to the funeral director. For a cremation there is a legal obligation to deliver the cremation certificate to the crematorium, in person, at least 24 hours before the service.

## Care of the body

It is vital that the parents retain control and choice in the care of their child. The professionals caring for the child and family should do so with dignity and respect, affording them time and privacy. It is important to respect the family's spiritual, religious and cultural beliefs and that rituals are recognised and respected both before and after death.

### Changes to the body

Parents and the wider family of a dead child/young person are unlikely to be aware of the changes that may take place after the death of their child. They may need to be prompted that it is okay to ask questions about the changes that are happening to their child, for example discolouration of the skin or leakage. In the absence of information, parents and carers may become alarmed about changes they observe and believe they are abnormal and their child is the only one it has ever happened to. This can be very frightening. Appropriate information, given gently and at an early stage is required.

*Lividity* or *livor mortis* is the dark purple discolouration of the skin resulting from gravitational pooling of blood in the veins and capillary beds following cessation of circulation. This is known as livor mortis and is more noticeable in some bodies than others; it is not associated with cyanosis. In many instances you will find that the blood pools at the part of the body that is in touch with the underlying surface, i.e. if the child/young person is on their back, it will pool along the back and the back of the legs and head. However, it is generally more noticeable in the earlobes and fingernail beds.

Lividity may become apparent about 20–30 minutes after death as dull red patches or blotches which deepen in intensity and coalesce (join together) over the following hours to form large areas of reddish-purple discolouration. After about 10–12 hours, the lividity becomes 'fixed'.

*Pallor and loss of skin elasticity* is likely: moisturiser can be applied to the face to prevent the skin from becoming dry; baby lotion is good for this. Vaseline or lip balm is helpful for keeping the lips moist too. Some parent's like to take on this responsibility, as it is something they are able to do for their child during this time. The pallor of their child's skin will also change due to the cessation of blood flow.

*The eyes* may become sunken in appearance, which will be alarming for family and carers. If the child's eyes remain open after death, they cannot be closed. After discussion with the family, the undertaker can be asked to put in 'stays' to keep the eyes closed.

*Rigor mortis (muscle stiffening)*: death is usually followed immediately by muscle flaccidity. This is then followed by muscle stiffening; this is known as rigor mortis.

*Bleeding*: since the body does not have a blood flow, agents normally used to arrest bleeding will not work. The only way to arrest bleeding is to block it, e.g. by suction or packing the nose. These proposed actions should be discussed with the family first, as any changes or intrusions to their child's body can be distressing.

Some bleeding may end after suction and cleaning.

Packing may be considered if the bleeding is not easy to control and is distressing for the family. The funeral director should be consulted for advice if bleeding persists and becomes a problem.

Using dark towels and bedding will help to make the bleeding less obvious.

Remember to use precautions related to the handling of blood.

*Seepage/leakage of bodily fluids*: this can occur at any time after a child has died. Urinary and faecal leakage is common and for this reason a pad is placed on the child and checked regularly.

Leakage from any other orifice can occur, e.g. an internal bleed can cause leakage of blood from the mouth, especially on movement of the body.

Suction should be available. This can be placed unobtrusively under the bed, so as not to be noticeable by the family.

Remember to use preventative precautions when using this equipment.

Ensure a supply of pads and change as necessary – the child will need to be checked more frequently soon after death.

Clean using wet wipes or flannel as appropriate.

Change linen as necessary.

*Prosthesis*: some children may have a prosthesis in at the time of death, e.g. nasogastric tube, central lines, tracheostomy tubes.

Unless the prosthesis is the property of the NHS it does not have to be removed. Where the prosthesis does have to be removed, it is best left for discussion with the parents in the presence of the funeral director.

A prosthesis can be removed if the parents wish. However, in a situation where the parents have never known their child without the prosthesis (for example nasogastric tube) they may consider this as part of their child and not want it removed.

Both nasogastric and gastrostomy buttons can be useful for emptying stomach contents at the time of death, thus reducing seepage/leakage of bodily fluids.

Most prostheses can be left in situ for burial/cremation except those with batteries. Please check with the funeral director for specific advice.

It is a rare occurrence, but should a post mortem be requested, it is important that all prosthesis should remain in place.

## Embalming of the body

If this is required the funeral director will:

- explain what has to be done;
- inform the family of the cost;
- let the family know when he/she will remove the body and return it.

## POST MORTEM

When a child dies unexpectedly a post mortem may be necessary to establish a cause of death. There are specific cases where a post mortem is required under the consent of the coroner, including death postoperatively or within 24 hours of a hospital admission.

A post mortem involves examining body organs and tissue to investigate and establish possible conditions or illnesses and cause of death.

Careful communication and sensitivity is essential at this time. Further information on post mortems can be sought from your own hospital/trust. Please see the website for further information.

## Transferring the body into the coffin

The child/young person is usually moved into the coffin on the day before the funeral and this can be done, with support, by the parents.

Depending on the size and weight of the child/young person, the following factors should be taken into consideration:

- You are not transferring a live body, therefore a slide sheet may be used; this task will require at least three people to facilitate the move.
- For a larger child/young person a hoist would be the preferred method to transfer to the coffin.

## Funeral planning

Planning for the funeral takes considerable thought and time and there are many practical issues that a family may require support with, from the type of service, to choices around style of coffin, to where to hold the funeral, what to wear and who to invite.

- If the child/young person has expressed any wishes about their own funeral, ensure everyone is informed.
- If a funeral director is not requested, the Natural Death Centre (www.naturaldeath.org.uk) can advise on arranging a funeral without a director.
- The family should be empowered to be involved with every aspect of the planning process.
- Encourage the parents to enable their other children to express views and be fully involved.
- Staff should be mindful of all that needs to be completed in order to gently keep parents moving towards any deadlines, e.g. printing of service sheets.
- Respect the family's ethnic, cultural and spiritual beliefs at all times and ask the family of anything we need to be aware of or make arrangements for.

Other practical and helpful areas of support may include completing memory boxes.

## Preparation for support in the community

It is important to ensure an assessment of family need before the funeral. This may be through a meeting or communication by phone, depending on associated links with other professionals in the community. Relevant information should be sought from staff, family contact, bereavement service, doctor and outside professional contacts in order to:

- discuss the family's needs and ongoing support;
- identify friends, family and professionals in the community to help them;
- identify a key professional who is willing to act as a key worker with relevant professionals who continue to be involved in supporting the family;
- find out about any local community groups that might be able to offer bereavement support;
- ensure that families know who to contact should they ever need it.

## Care of siblings

Children can be involved as much as possible in the funeral arrangements and in the service on the day. There is increasing understanding of child bereavement and a wealth of literature and books providing support. Further support for parents in helping children say goodbye, what to expect at a funeral service, experiences of grief and loss and spiritual needs for children is available.

## BEREAVEMENT SUPPORT

Bereavement support can offer practical, emotional and spiritual support during the child's illness, around the time of death and afterwards. Support aims to be open and sensitive to the individual needs of family members. It may be offered in different ways by various people, and ongoing support and bereavement care for a family will often be provided by relatives and friends and the wider community. Please see the website for further information.

### Staff support

Caring for a dying child and supporting families through their child's death is a stressful and emotional time. Ssupport for staff is therefore important and the availability for supervision, reflection and debrief should be considered. There are a number of avenues available for staff to access: peer support, one-to-one support with senior colleagues, or external supervision.

## CONCLUSION

Caring for a child at the end of life can be an extremely difficult but rewarding time. Attention to the child and family throughout, concentrating on thoughtful, sensitive communication, engaging with families and encouraging them in decision-making, is essential. There are many practical tasks to be completed but it is important to remember that the emotional and spiritual elements of support are integral to all care offered.

---

 Go to the website to find the PowerPoint presentation for this chapter and questions to test your knowledge. **www.hodderplus.com/childnursingskills**

---

## ACKNOWLEDGEMENTS

To the team at Naomi House Children's Hospice for sharing their knowledge and experience in supporting children and families at the end of life.

## REFERENCE

1   Jassal S (2008) *Basic symptom control in paediatric palliative care*, 7th edition. Loughborough: The Rainbows Children's Hospice Guidelines (available from www.act.co.uk).

## USEFUL WEBSITES

Association Of Children with Life Threatening Illness: www.act.co.uk
Children's Hospice UK: www.childhospice.org.uk
The Child Bereavement Charity: www.childbereavement.org.uk
The Natural Death Centre: www.naturaldeath.org.uk
Winston's Wish is a child bereavement charity: www.winsonswish.org.uk
The Grandparent's Association: www.grandparents-association.org.uk

# CHAPTER 37

# Developing your skills as a mentor: a guide for newly qualified practitioners

Sylvia Buckingham and Alan Glasper

## CHAPTER OVERVIEW

It is a requirement of the regulator for nursing and midwifery, the Nursing and Midwifery Council (NMC) that student nurses undertaking a children's nursing programme are mentored by an appropriately qualified registrant. The NMC use the term 'due regard' to describe the process of mentoring students by someone who is from the same field of practice. This simply means that students of children's and young people's nursing should be mentored by registered children's nurses. It is part of your professional duties as a registered nurse to mentor students in practice and this is mandated through the *Knowledge and skills framework*[1] and in the NMC standards to support learning and assessment in practice.[2]

When you yourself were a student you would have been mentored by a qualified practitioner. You may remember the ones who were outstanding, supportive and taught you all that you know about your profession. You may also unfortunately have experienced mentorship from a registrant who did not seem to like students!

This introduction to developing your skills as a mentor is written with your role model in mind. Whenever you feel frustrated with your student remember how much it meant for you to be supported with patience, kindness and understanding by that mentor. Also remember that they invested time in you to guide and nurture you

and now it is your turn to do this with other neophyte practitioners.

It is important to stress that you are part of a team consisting of the commissioners of nurse education (a strategic health authority in England), a university school or department of nursing and a healthcare institution such as the hospital you work in. All three play an equal part in the training of nurses. It is, however, you as the mentor who provides the hands-on vital link between theory and practice. It is important for you to realise that 50 per cent of a student nurse's time in training is spent in practice, and the NMC give equal weighting to this dimension of the course as they are primarily concerned with the protection of the public. The NMC believe that this 50 per cent rule is essential to prepare nurses for their future role in practice. As a consequence, when you are acting as a mentor to a student nurse you are also acting on behalf of your healthcare regulator in ensuring that only those who are fit for practice and purpose progress to become a registered nurse. It is the university who decides who is fit for the award, but as all nursing awards are conjoint, i.e. linked to registration, *your role is crucial* in ensuring that students (who are fit for practice and purpose) progress to the final award, be that diploma, advanced diploma, degree or post-graduate qualification. (Student intakes in England after 2011 will exit with a minimum award of degree.)

Some would therefore argue that the whole period of children's and young people's nurse training is only as good as the mentor who delivers it. This is why the NMC and the partnerships who provide nurse training invest so much time and energy in ensuring that you the mentor are fully enabled to play your part in the process of training and educating nurses.

As a mentor you are expected to have the following attributes:[3]

- generosity of time and spirit;
- rewarding supervisee's abilities;
- openness;
- willingness to learn;
- being thoughtful and thought-provoking;
- humanity;
- sensitivity;
- uncompromising rigour and standards;
- awareness of personal supervisory style;
- adaptation of a practical focus;
- awareness of differences in orientation between supervisor and supervisee;
- maintenance of distinction between supervisory and therapeutic relationship;
- trust.

## GETTING STARTED ON YOUR ROAD TO BECOMING A MENTOR AND SIGN-OFF MENTOR

The NMC recommend that you work for a year after qualifying before completing a recognised mentorship course. In the interim you may act as a buddy mentor or associate mentor but you are not allowed to sign off assessment paperwork. Furthermore, only those mentors who have undertaken extra experience and training to become a 'sign-off mentor' are allowed to sign off NMC competencies within a student's portfolio. It might be useful at this stage to review the NMC skills escalator process of becoming a mentor, sign off mentor, practice teacher or teacher of nursing (lecturer).

### The NMC progression route

The NMC through their standards to support learning and assessment in practice[2] provide a clear and unambiguous pathway by which a nurse such as yourself can progress from registrant to mentor, to sign-off mentor to practice teacher, to teacher or

lecturer. Importantly, nurses can use the knowledge gained in, for example, becoming a mentor to access and undertake a practice teacher qualification. This is useful if you wish to mentor children's nurses undertaking specialist practice programmes, e.g. a post-qualifying oncology course. In turn the practice teacher award can enable you to access a subsequent nurse teacher programme should you wish to become a lecturer in children's and young people's nursing (Figure 37.1).

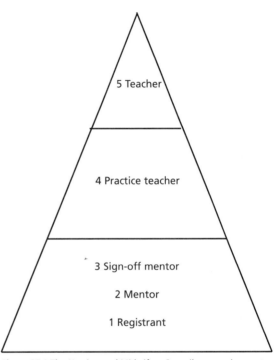

**Figure 37.1** The Nursing and Midwifery Council progression route.

### Becoming a mentor

Your first step in becoming a mentor after your first year as a staff nurse is to undergo the appropriate mentor training. It is customary for first-year staff nurses to act as buddy mentors after 6 months of being registered. Your training and development nurse on the unit you are working on will let you know when you are scheduled to attend mentorship training. If you are working in an area where there is no training and development nurse in post, then ensure that you raise this at your annual individual performance review (IPR).

Mentorship courses are organised by the NHS institution where you work in conjunction with the local university.

The mentorship course consists of 10 days' learning, of which 5 days are protected learning time often within a classroom environment. The other 5 days are made up of work-based learning in which for some of the time you will gain experience in mentoring a student under the supervision of a qualified mentor. Once you have qualified as a mentor your name will be recorded on the live database of mentors held by your institution. (A copy of this database is also held by the university.) This database is periodically checked by auditors from the NMC.

## The mentor database

The mentor database is now usually kept as an electronic spreadsheet. This is what auditing reviewers from the NMC will inspect periodically. If you meet an NMC reviewer in practice they will check that your name is appropriately entered on your hospital or healthcare institution database. In addition to the list of trained mentors and the mentorship qualification they hold, the database has a number of annotations that are a requirement of the NMC:

- the date the mentor was last updated and the method by which this was undertaken (e.g. via an online virtual learning platform such as blackboard, or via 'face-to-face' mentor updating);
- the scheduled date for triennial review (all mentors are expected to be fully updated every 3 years);
- sign-off mentors: usually a star next to the name on the database of mentors;
- practice teacher: usually a separate column on the database spreadsheet.

## Criteria for mentors

In addition to being a children's nurse and being registered for at least 1 year, aspiring mentors must demonstrate that they are able to provide a range of learning opportunities for children's and young people's nursing students and other students from across the interprofessional healthcare field. Importantly, the mentor must demonstrate that they are able to make judgements about the performance of students in practice and to be accountable for such decisions they make. Mentors especially those who achieve sign-off mentor status,

are therefore the key professionals who decide if someone is fit to be a registered children's and young people's nurse. This is an onerous role and one that the professional regulator of the profession (the NMC) scrutinises regularly through its own quality assurance and audit activities.

## Competencies expected of mentors

During your mentor training you will be enabled to achieve competency in a range of areas.

- *Establishing effective relationships:* mentors must be able to demonstrate that they are able to foster a professional relationship with students and recognise the factors which positively or negatively influence how they integrate into practice settings. It is important to stress that students need support while they become accustomed to new areas of practice and need to be helped when they move from one practice area to another.
- *Facilitation of learning:* mentors must understand the student's programme. This will change periodically as the design of the curriculum reflects contemporary healthcare. Such changes to the curriculum and practice learning outcomes will always be conveyed to mentors through a variety of mechanisms, including annual updates, mentor newsletters or mentor websites and chat rooms. Only when a mentor understands the parameters of the students programme will they be able to select and provide appropriate learning opportunities for them. Furthermore, mentors must be able to help students integrate theory with practice. Children's nursing must be delivered through the application of best evidence! Mentors should therefore help students reflect on their learning experiences to enhance their future learning in both clinical and academic settings. Creating a good learning environment for students is therefore a key role of mentors.
- *Assessment and accountability:* to achieve this, the mentor must help students to grow professionally and to become aware of their accountability to their regulatory body for upholding the principles of their profession. Therefore, mentors must be aware of how students can be assessed in practice and understand their own role as part of the overall

teaching team. To do this the mentor needs to develop the skills of providing constructive feedback to students to help them identify their future learning needs. Not all students will demonstrate either the appropriate attitude expected of a healthcare professional or prowess in clinical practice and therefore a crucial role of the mentor will be to *manage* failing students.

- *Evaluation of learning:* a major role for mentors is to contribute to the evaluation of the overall student learning experience. Universities and their partners need to provide optimum clinical learning experiences for their nursing students and rely on mentors to provide this information to enable them to modify or change learning and assessment strategies. Additionally, mentors are expected to undergo individual and peer evaluations to facilitate personal development and to contribute to the development of others.
- *Context of practice, creating a learning environment:* mentors must help students to identify and optimise learning needs and experiences commensurate with their programme level. To achieve this, the mentor should facilitate a range of learning opportunities involving children, young people and their families and members of the professional team to address the student's learning needs.

On completion of the mentor course you will become familiar with the student practice documentation, which will have been designed for students from a particular university. In practice this documentation, often in the format of a portfolio, is very similar in most parts of the country as all are designed to enable student achievement of the NMC competencies and skills clusters necessary for registration as a children's nurse. Although the outcomes are prescribed, whatever you feel a student may need to know is probably what they really do want to know about. Your particular area of practice is likely to be an exciting opportunity for them, and they will want to get as much out of the placement as possible. So in addition to the prescribed NMC outcomes, you will be able to offer students a richness of experience that is likely to be unique to your own practice area. It is the rich diversity of children's nursing that makes it attractive to potential students.

Your role as a mentor is to create and maintain a quality learning environment.

The environment that you work in will be unique in many facets. It may be in the community, in acute care or a mixture of both. The clients/patients you work with will also be familiar to you, and you will have expertise in your understanding and management of them.

However, to the student practitioner this will be a maze of new faces, disorders and situations, and the environment that they come in to is new to them and possibly a little frightening.

This is dependent largely on their stage of training; expectations of first-year students are vastly different from that of a student about to qualify. It is essential that you have an understanding of the programme of learning that the student is undertaking. Additionally, you need to understand what theoretical input they have had so that you can help them relate theory to practice situations.

The NMC[2] has an expectation that you will be conversant with the programmes that all students are studying; while this can seem quite a large task it makes sense to explore them and have some knowledge so that you can support students more fully. Also, students have a tendency to say they have not covered a subject so as to avoid being tested on it. Your knowledge of what they have already covered will enable you to further test their understanding in practice.

In order to prepare the environment it may help to take a second look at what has become all too familiar to you. The professional team you work with may have specific areas where case notes are held and clients/patents are spoken with. You may have research papers stored in files and you may have experts that enjoy sharing their knowledge with students. So how does the student get to know this?

## DESIGNING A STUDENT WELCOME PACK

One of the useful tools you can create is a welcome package for the student. The welcome pack design varies and you and your mentor colleagues can use your own flair and imagination to develop a welcome pack that uniquely encompasses your individual clinical domain. The web page electronic resource which accompanies this book and chapter features a good example of a student welcome pack for you to follow. Students really appreciate good quality welcome and learning packs, and monitoring officers from the NMC inspect these during their audit activities. In its simplest form a welcome pack will contain:

- commonly used abbreviations as these can be a minefield in some specialist areas;
- shift patterns;
- names of practitioners who work within the area, with contact numbers;
- explanations of common disorders treated in your setting;
- special phone numbers, e.g. the bleep number of the play specialist who deals with children with needle phobia;
- the procedures for calling in if an individual student cannot attend a shift or is delayed for any reason;
- list of resources held on the ward/clinical area, e.g. textbooks, journals and policies and procedures.

## DEVELOPING A PRACTICE AREA LEARNING RESOURCE CENTRE

Many mentors seek to develop a part of the clinical environment as a learning resource area for students. This can be very simple or very sophisticated, ranging from a dedicated office to a 'cubby hole' somewhere within the environment. Irrespective of the size, many mentors throughout the country use great skills in building their student resource centre. Here they will amass files of pertinent literature and policies. Additionally, they may collect audiovisual materials such as DVDs or proprietary information, for example from pharmaceutical companies. Perhaps one of the most important pieces of equipment you can provide for students is a computer with internet access, which will allow them access to electronic learning resources such as Cinahl or Medline.

### Meeting your student for the first time

Usually you will have found out in advance the name of the student you have been allocated. Additionally, the student will have been given your name and contact details from the allocation office at the university. They will have been instructed to contact you a week or so before commencing their placement.

During that first telephone conversation in which they will be nervous, you can make an appointment to see them face to face. At that first meeting the important aspect is to sit down with the student and get to know them. Remember, your role model mentor found time to do this with you so no matter how busy you are plan this occasion. It is worth hours later on!

At this stage offer them the welcome pack and show them around your ward or clinical area. You may have tried to plan the student experience around their learning needs, dependent on the level of learning required and the time they have with you. Usually this will be for a minimum of 4 weeks, as that is the minimum time specified by The NMC for signing off competencies or skills. However, some students have taster placements of 1 or 2 weeks.

If possible, all of the introductory stages can be achieved before the student commences duties. However, sitting down with them and getting to know them as a person, rather than as a second year, final year student, etc., can be very informative and will help you gauge the level at which the student can and should be working.

### Agreeing achievable outcomes with your student and facilitating learning in practice

Encouraging the 'self-management' of learning is a skill you will develop over time. At first you may rely on the student to talk about what they need to learn to complete their professional training documentation. This should be coupled with the unique experiences you have to offer in your placement. However, this will also depend on the stage that the student is at in their learning. For example, a student nurse at the beginning of training may want to explore skills above their level of training, such as taking bloods. It is up to you to both value what the student wants to do and explore what they need to know for the purposes of achieving the specified objectives and learning outcomes determined by the university. It is important to stress that this may be less attractive initially to the student, 'who may want to fly before being able to walk'.

For example, you may want the student to undertake holistic care of a child with a long-term health problem, which on the surface could appear mundane and repetitive. It is how you explore and investigate the child's and family's needs that will reveal to the student the importance of these areas of care. It is only through exploring the ordinary that you can help the student see the extraordinary in a particular child's care. The enthusiasm you impart to your student and the importance of such things as measuring and recording vital signs, performing essential hygiene, etc., can say a lot about how we value nursing care and child/family/nurse interaction.

The NMC[2] has identified the importance of a mentor's role in supervision support and guidance of students in practice; however, it is still up to the individual mentor to ensure this takes place.

## Facilitating learning in practice

Students need to be active in their own learning. However, it is important that they are supported in identifying their learning needs and making the best of the learning opportunities provided. Learning involves searching for information, selecting information and actively taking responsibility for observing practice, talking about practice and making connections about how practice evolves, using theoretical considerations of practice. If students are to engage in such activities they need guidance, someone to refer to if they get lost or confused and someone to confirm whether what they have interpreted is appropriate and valuable.

## What is the 40 per cent rule?

During the early days of mentoring you will develop an awareness of the student's capabilities and aspirations during the period of time they are with you. To foster this understanding it is a requirement of the NMC that you as a mentor facilitate the direct supervision of the student for 40 per cent of the working week.

The 40 per cent rule ensures that you are able to make accurate judgements about the performance of your individual student. This is vital if you have to make difficult decisions about a student's future.

While you may be guided by the documentation you are required to complete at the end of the placement, you will also get a sense of student

capability. If an experience is available allow the student to participate in it. The NMC now promote student participation not simply observation. This as we know underlines the practical aspects of nursing. So whenever possible allow students to take part in whatever you are doing to a particular child or young person and their family. Importantly some universities now grade clinical practice.

As part of the student learning process you may help them develop their self-awareness in certain situations. When possible, take time to reflect on events with the student. Explore the positive and the more challenging aspects of their interactions. At times it is necessary to identify shortcomings in the student approach, but even these need to be sensitively undertaken. Often students are unaware of how they come across, and they learn from open and supportive comments.

However, at times you may have a student who is less aware, a rare occurrence but it does happen. This is less likely as all students are carefully vetted before being accepted on the course. Many universities invite mentors to participate in student interviews. If you have not been invited, do ask your link teacher to arrange this.

The reasons why a student may not thrive in the clinical domain are wide and various. You may need to seek advice from other colleagues who are mentor practitioners to avoid the 'it must be me' syndrome. You may want to look at previous mentors comments if this is possible. However, it is important to address the issue. Remember your role model? How did they manage the more challenging student?

## Dealing with failing students

The NMC have established a direct link between registrants who appear before their code of conduct committee and their previous student history. It was perhaps the crimes of serial child killer nurse Beverley Allitt[4] which dramatically brought this to the attention of the world of children's nursing. Dealing with a failing student is something that will be well covered in your mentorship course but in particular the work of Duffy,[5] who was commissioned by the NMC to investigate the problems of failing students, will be fully discussed. She ascertained that it was the issue of students with inappropriate attitudes which caused mentors difficulties. Furthermore Duffy was able to indicate that the identification of failing students should be made before the student reached the final point of the clinical placement assessment. Clearly, it helps in the individual student audit trail if mentors can identify and document any concerns they may have about a particular student. Mentorship updates usually provide anonymised failing student case studies to allow you to experience future potential scenarios. It is important, however, to recognise that personality clashes between mentors and students are inevitable and universities have protocols to allow adjudication and re-allocation. Remember that the link teacher is your conduit to the university and you should always consult with them in the first instance.

## The challenging student

Many students are delightful, eager to learn and often are described as sponges eager to soak up information and experiences. Sadly not all students are seen in this light. There may be many reasons for this, including students who have a learning difference but not prepared to share this with mentors. Helping students with learning differences such as dyslexia is now a common role for some mentors. Specific advice in helping students with learning differences may be obtained via the link teacher and most universities have identified support mechanisms for these students, and as a mentor you will need to find out what they are.

There will be times when your patience is tested as a mentor. You need to develop skills of communication even in the most difficult situation. An example below gives you some insight into some issues which can arise.

> Susan is a second-year child branch student nurse and she is halfway through her second placement and staff are worried that she is not settling in and seems reluctant to communicate. Her clinical work is not up to standard, partly because of her lack of communication with staff and patients. It is coming up to her midpoint interview. June her mentor is unsure how to proceed.
> What should June do?
> Who can she seek advice from?

If a student is failing there may be many reasons for this.

Has the student got personal problems? You may ask the student but also you may need to contact the link teacher for your area.

Sometimes a sensitive encouraging talk carried out in private may be all that is needed to set the student on the right track.

Like all of us, students are human beings with outside pressures, many of which we are unaware of until there is a problem. The student may be unwell, or have personal problems, which they feel overwhelmed by, but equally cannot share with you.

It may be something about the ward or the client group of children. For example, she may have been allocated to a paediatric oncology ward and a member of her family has just been diagnosed with cancer; this happens more than we would think.

Susan is from Nigeria and has been in this country for 5 years. People from other cultures may deal with communication in different ways. We cannot be experts in understanding all these cultural differences and cannot be expected to be, but we need to be aware and accept that in some cultures people seem to us to be more reserved and quiet, or conversely more demonstrative in showing their feelings.

**ACTIVITY**

Think about all the people you work with, your patients and your friends. From within these three categories identify which group is more likely to contain people who are from white, Asian and Black ethnic minority groups. Within white ethnic groups we have a wide variety of cultures such as Greek, Polish, Spanish, and French etc.
Please don't use names

| Work colleagues | Clients/patients | Friends |
| --- | --- | --- |
| Culture | Culture | Culture |
|  |  |  |

Do those you have listed communicate in different ways/different languages/different facial expression?
Do they have mannerisms and ways of looking at you that may be different or that you are less able to interpret?
Now take a second look and think about what you have based these lists on. Was it on the person's appearance, language, religion, or behaviour or something else?
Was there a mix of cultures in all of the boxes?
We work with a diverse range of people but often we socialise with people from a small cultural group.

Some people believe that those from other parts of the UK come from different cultures. A person from Yorkshire may have their own cultural traits as does someone from Wales or Scotland. Many countries have national dress, local dishes and foods as do many parts of the UK. They may also have their own dialect or language.

Many cultural groups also have a style of communication which is slightly different. In general terms we are used to communicating with people we are more familiar with.

Do we feel or behave in the same way as we might towards someone whose culture and way of communicating we are less familiar with?

Often, if we are honest, we make assumptions about people on the way they look and present themselves in conversation: we stereotype.

**ACTIVITY**

Now think about a holiday you have had in another country. Do you expect to take a siesta, change your diet to eat the local food and drink the local water, and cover your head and limbs as some religious groups do in certain countries?

*or*

Do you still want to carry on as you do in your own country, going for a walk in the afternoon, eating at restaurants that serve English style food and bottled water and wear shorts and sleeveless tops?

If we are honest most of us still want to behave in a way that is familiar to us.

How often do we wish we could speak the language and how often can the 'locals' working in holiday resorts speak English?

Susan needs to be treated as any other student nurse is in her second year; you still need to be objective in ensuring she is able to achieve her learning outcomes and to provide the same learning opportunities as other students have, e.g. observing a child having a gastroscopy.

However, we need to be aware that cultural differences can influence the way she may present herself to us and the way we interpret this.

If there are any problems or concerns then this needs to be handled with care. It may be helpful to make contact with his/her academic tutor to see if the student is always like this. Again this needs to be non-threatening and supportive.

Many schools of nursing and midwifery employ a Cultural Support Tutor who is there to advise and support and educate if there are any problems with students from other cultural groups. Always consult with your link teacher colleague for advice if you have queries.

It may be that Susan lacks confidence and simply cannot perform to the level you are expecting. In this case you need to find out what may be helpful for her to achieve her competencies and develop her confidence.

## Suspending a student in practice

In rare situations it is sometimes necessary to suspend a student from practice. Most universities and their partners will have developed algorithms for dealing with such occurrences.

## Completing the practice assessment documentation

Occasionally students have had a difficult time in a previous placement, which undermines their confidence.

This midpoint interview is crucial so it must be halfway through the placement. If it is late, the student will have insufficient time to retrieve the situation and be empowered to be able to achieve the competencies and learning outcomes stated within the documentation. If this should happen and the student is referred, they could be entitled to take out an appeal.

If you think that the student is not performing at the correct level and you have addressed all of the issues raised above, it is important that you contact the university through the link teacher to discuss this more fully. Don't forget all of the nursing team should have some input in the process, even though the final decision is yours as the mentor.

If at the end of the placement you feel, having given the student as much input as possible and as many opportunities as you would all other students, then it is your duty to *refer* the student.

*But* please don't do this on your own; remember you are part of a partnership so contact someone for support, preferably the link or academic teacher.

There may be other issues that arise that have not been addressed in this chapter. However, the same principles apply. Ensure you talk with the student and the university link teacher as this will resolve most of the concerns as they arise.

## ASSESSING STUDENT LEARNING

### The assessment process

Assessment of ability is crucial to all learning, and the assessment of the knowledge, skills and attitude of learners is embedded in most educational programmes. The processes of the assessment can vary, dependent on the level of assessment required and the stage of educational development the student is at.

Drivers for competency-based practice come from both the regulatory bodies for nursing, the NMC, and from the expectations of the general public. Hence assessment has become a vital component of progression in practice-based vocational programmes such as nursing, which eventually lead to a registerable qualification, in effect giving that individual a licence to practise.

Think about your own experiences of learning and being assessed.

Identify all the different times you have been assessed in your life, e.g. school, driving, hobbies, swimming, dancing, your own nursing exams, etc. What learning/teaching/practice had occurred prior to the assessment? Who assessed you? What format did the assessment take? Was it practical, verbal, written, etc.? Why was that format chosen? What were the advantages/disadvantages? Was it the best way to assess that area of knowledge/skills/attitude? Why did you need to be assessed?

There are various points at which assessment can occur, often at the end of the academic year, and the assessment can either be formative or summative. Most assessments of practice are summative and students cannot progress until they have retrieved the placement. Normally nursing students have the right to a second attempt. Only in exceptional circumstances will a student be granted a third and final attempt.

### How did the assessment process make you feel?

Prior to the event were you nervous, or worried? Did you have to work hard to learn and retain the knowledge and skills?

Afterwards were you elated, disappointed, etc.? Think now about how this might relate to the students you are currently assessing.

What happened if you were not successful? Did you re-sit? Did you practise more and importantly was advice given?

By now some key principles should be emerging regarding:

- forms of assessment;
- process of assessment;
- qualifications of assessors;
- remedial action that can be taken;
- the importance of learning the art and practice of children's nursing in the clinical environment.

Assessments must be valid, fair and reliable. They must test student progress and achievement.

Actions must be clear if a problem is identified during the assessment process. Remedial action must be taken and documented.

Student and mentor must be clear of the process, who to call on for support and advice and what the possible outcomes could be.

A clear time frame should also be identified.

You will also be expected to implement the approved assessment procedures and assist with the placement evaluation.

## THE EVALUATION OF PLACEMENT LEARNING

As a mentor you should:

- understand the methods used to evaluate learning in the practice area;
- appreciate how evaluation can be used to improve opportunities for learning;
- take opportunities for self- and peer evaluation to facilitate personal professional development and the development of others.

## CONCLUSION

Your principal role in mentoring children's nursing students in practice should be to help them learn effectively instead of being exposed to inappropriate learning experiences, or given learning experiences without knowing how to use their learning strengths. The whole of a children's nursing course of study in clinical practice is really only as good as the mentor who delivers it. That person is you!

Go to the website to find the PowerPoint presentation for this chapter and MCQs to test your knowledge. **www.hodderplus.com/childnursingskills**

## REFERENCES

1 Department of Health (2004) *The NHS knowledge and skills framework (NHS KSF) and the development review process*. London: DH.

2 Nursing and Midwifery Council (2008) *Standards to support learning and assessment in practice*. London: NMC.

3 Butterworth T, Faugier J (1992) *Clinical supervision and mentorship in nursing*. London: Chapman & Hall.

4 The Allitt Inquiry (1991) *Independent inquiry relating to deaths and injuries on the children's ward at Grantham and Kesteven General Hospital during the period February to April 1991*. London: HMSO.

5 Duffy K (2003) *Failing students: a qualitative study of factors that influence the decisions regarding assessment of students' competence in practice*. Glasgow: Caledonian University.

## CHAPTER 38

# Providing and delivering information to children and their families

Alan Glasper and Cath Battrick

## LEARNING OUTCOMES

*Upon completion of this chapter, the reader should be able to accomplish the following:*

1 Appreciate the historical aspects to information giving in the NHS
2 Understand the parameters of information giving in the modern NHS
3 Design and write a child or family information leaflet following procedural guidelines
4 Recognise the role of the internet in providing health information
5 Acknowledge the deficiencies of web-based information
6 Appreciate factors that hinder the giving of information to children and their families

## CHAPTER OVERVIEW

There is growing recognition by children's nurses of the need to improve the way they communicate with children and their families. The mandate of a patient-led NHS acknowledges that written information in the form of leaflets plays a crucial role in modern healthcare, with a mission of empowering service users to optimise strategies for dealing with health and ill-health. Information communicated to clients through the format of the written word either in hard copy or via the internet must be developed with child and family users of services, and appropriate members of the inter-professional healthcare team to the highest

standards. Written communication has major advantages over verbal information, not least being the reality that verbal information stored within the brain degrades very quickly. Glasper and Burge[1] have indicated that this inability of stressed people to retain verbal information is a very good reason for communicating through different mediums such as the written word.

The families of sick children have information expectations that are now much higher than a decade ago. The type, level and depth of information requirements are increasing rapidly, especially with so much media coverage of health matters. There now exists a marketplace for health, with healthcare providers marketing their services, generating further information needs on the part of parents to enable them to make informed choices on their child's healthcare journey.

This ever-expanding desire for information requires children's nurses to adapt their roles and cater for the information needs of families.

## HISTORICAL ASPECTS

In 1992 the Patient's Charter for England and Wales was introduced. It detailed 10 'rights' to which every patient was entitled and promised patients the right to information about their healthcare. It also gave patients the opportunity to participate in decisions about their care and to be involved in decisions about their treatment if they so wished. However its impact on improving information to patients was limited, as most patients were unclear about its contents and its intentions.[2] There was a mismatch between patients' concerns and charter priorities. Patients wanted to know how they could access good-quality care and were less concerned about the charters targets on waiting times. Primarily, they wanted more clinical information to assist them to look after their own or their children's health. Because the rights of children are not enshrined in statute[3] the government subsequently issued a special version of the charter for children in hospital. This was written in child-friendly language and for the first time articulated just what children and their families should expect to receive when in hospital. Both versions of the charter weresuperseded in 2001 when the *The Patient's Charter* was replaced by *Your guide to the NHS: getting the most from your National Health Service*.[4] Additionally, the emphasis on children's rights to information have been emphasised through a range of policy documents, not least being *The national service framework for children, young people and maternity services*.[5]

In 1997, the Labour Party was elected into government with a strong manifesto setting out the basis for an extensive reform and modernisation programme of the NHS. In July 2000 *The NHS plan* was published,[6] which outlined the NHS as an organisational centrepiece of Labour's reforms. It was to be an ambitious 10-year programme designed to tackle 'systematic problems' that dated from 1948 when the NHS was formed. The plan contained 10 core principals to underpin the service and the reforms agreed by NHS staff, patients and others and formed the cornerstone of the new NHS.

Providing more information to patients was highlighted as a main feature of the government's NHS plan.[6]

*'Information is an important part of the patient journey and a key element in the overall quality of patient experience.*[6]

For the first time children and their families were to be given far greater information about how they could look after their own or their child's health and about their local health services. Importantly, they would be given the option of having much greater information about the treatment being planned for them or their child. Crucially, the NHS plan heralded the introduction of national service frameworks (NSFs) for healthcare in which health-related information giving was made a priority.

The NHS Plan was published in the wake of a number of high-profile national inquiries pertinent to children in which healthcare professionals acknowledged that the health service needed reform. It was widely agreed that the NHS had failed to meet the expectations of a better-informed population. The report of the Bristol inquiry[7] represented perhaps the most in-depth analysis of a modern health service and systems and showed how some healthcare professionals had not treated families with the proper respect due to them. It made a number of key recommendations for improving communication, and subsequently many national initiatives with information giving at their heart have emerged, e.g. NHS Direct, NHS Direct online.[8]

The Bristol Inquiry, although pertaining to children, had important ramifications for the NHS in general. If information giving is the key to empowerment,[9] then families must be given all the information they need to make crucial decisions about their children. The giving of partial, confusing or unclear information to families, as happened at Bristol, was unsatisfactory and the report recommended that all patients should be able to gain access to information about any particular hospital department. Additionally the Redfern report[10] commissioned as a result of the tragic events at Liverpool's Alder Hey Hospital, where healthcare professionals illegally retained children's body parts after post-mortem examination, was also critical of information giving to families.

Close to 200 recommendations were made following the national public 'Bristol Inquiry' and many of these relate to the means through which information is obtained and communicated to children and their families.

Key recommendations include the following:

- Families and children must be involved in decisions about their treatment and care wherever possible (recommendation 1).
- Health professionals must embrace the concept of partnership, where the child and family and healthcare professional meet as equals each bringing different expertise (3).

- Information about treatment and care should be given in a selection of media formats, be given in individual stages and be reinforced over time (4).
- Information should be customised to the individual needs, situation and wishes of the child or family (5).
- Information should be based on the best and most up-to-date evidence and importantly be offered to families as a summary of the evidence in a way which is comprehensible to them (6).
- Various modes of conveying information, whatever the format, should be regularly updated and developed and piloted with the help of family members but especially the children and young people (7).
- Families should receive guidance on those sources of information about health and healthcare on the internet and which are reliable and of good quality (9).
- Children, young people and their families must be given such information as enables them to participate in their care (12).
- Prior to any procedure, children and their families must be given an explanation of what is going to happen, and after the procedure should have the opportunity to review what has happened (13, 16).

The publication of the Bristol Inquiry and latterly Lord Carlisle's review by the Welsh Assembly,[11] in which the lack of priority given to child health services was criticised, was timely in that it accelerated the pace of development of the children's NSF in Wales and England.

A key aspect of the NSF was to address the information needs of sick children, young people and their families.

*Families need information to help them make informed decisions about the care of their children. Efforts should be made to ensure that consistent advice and information is given to parents across different care settings and agencies, and in forms that are accessible to all parents.[12]*

Compliance with NSF standards is audited by the Care Quality Commission, formerly the Healthcare Commission. An audit of compliance to these standards was published in February 2007[13] and revealed that the level of training in communicating with children was poor. Furthermore, the report is unequivocal in stating

that children (and their families) must be given information in a way that they can understand. Similarly Coles et al.[14] in a review of compliance to NSF standards showed that information giving was suboptimal

More recently, the children's strategy, *Healthy lives, brighter futures*,[15] has been published with a number of objectives to improve the lives of children and young people. This strategy recognises that parents and carers want better information about what services are available locally, with better links between the services that their children use. This report stresses the importance of information being tailored to the needs of children and their families, in a readily accessible range of formats which encompass transparency about resources, and how services work together and are commissioned.

## EMPOWERMENT

Hospitalisation during childhood is an extremely stressful experience for both the child and the family. Parents who endure the stress of a child's hospital admission may find it fraught with potential problems. Historical and contemporary work by healthcare professionals identifies that children have fears and anxieties when they are admitted to hospital that can also impact on parents and carers, not least being the development of debilitating fears such as needle phobia.[16-19]

Korsch[20] in a randomised controlled trial of parents whose children were undergoing routine day surgery concluded that by giving health information and education it enhanced patient cooperation and compliance with medical regimes. He also argued that in providing this information to parents/children it reduced their stress and anxiety, decreased or alleviated pain in their child, promoted the healing process and made it possible for the child/family to cope adequately with the procedure or experience. Caress[21] supports this stance in her review of information giving to patients by highlighting how well-informed individuals have better psychological outcomes, for example less anxiety and depression. Coulter[22] demonstrated that there are a growing number of patients requiring health information and stresses the need for health professionals to help patients access high-quality evidenced-based information.

Robertson[9] in her discussion of empowerment of parents through the giving of health information highlights how parents have specific ideas and information needs that are important for the planners of healthcare services. Some parents are able to identify how they would like to receive information about their child coming into hospital, and what specific information they need most to enable the family to function during this stressful period. Most parents' concerns are for the welfare of their child and fear of disempowerment as a parent. These concerns must be addressed so that parents can continue with parenting. She argues the key, therefore, is to identify parental concerns and address them through mechanisms that parents can efficiently use. However it must be acknowledged that families have traditionally been passive bystanders in the whole process of information giving, receiving but not contributing. This one-sided professionally led initiative of information giving mandated from a top-down policy led inevitably to an NHS that fundamentally disempowered families, for decisions about a child's welfare cannot be made without access to all the known facts. This inequality in the healthcare partnership needs to be acknowledged before true partnership can emerge.

Coulter[23] supports this view in her study examining shared decisions with patients and the quality of information given. Her evaluation of information materials gained through the use of focus groups highlighted the need for patient information needs to be sought before developing information materials and making them publicly available. Most information materials were found to be designed to educate patients or to prepare them for specific treatments or procedures. She also concluded that a didactic style of information materials was not popular with the focus group members who were more enthusiastic about materials that gave them a sense of empowerment. She also concluded patients cannot express informed preferences unless they are given sufficient and appropriate information.

Acquisition of information can provide families with the necessary knowledge to be empowered to self-care: They are able to regain control over a situation and therefore are able to request a partnership with healthcare professionals. Gann[24] has stated that information giving is the key to empowerment and if this is true, the provision of information will enhance the relationship between the professional and the family. The *National service framework for children, young people and maternity services* (NSF)[5] recognises that children should be given support and information to enable them to cope with the illness or injury and the treatment needed. This seminal policy document publication indicates that there will be greater focus on delivering better information, for children, young people and their parents on health and health services, and how to access them.

## THE GROWTH OF CONSUMER HEALTH INFORMATION AS A SPECIALISM

In 1993 the Audit Commission investigated written communication with patients, relatives and carers in the acute setting. The report lamented the poor quality of written information, concluding that patients experience difficulties with the content, amount and quality of information.[25] It also suggested that patients should not have to seek out information, as not all are in a position to do so, emotionally or intellectually. Neither should they be expected to pass uninformed through the health service during what, for many, is a bewildering and frightening life experience.

NHS Direct Online (www.nhsdirect.nhs.uk) is now considered by many to be the lead organisation in the field of consumer health information.

### Patient organisations and self-help groups

Patient organisations and self-help groups have a rich history of providing combined information services for specific target audiences. For example, people with cancer can use specialist telephone advice services provided by CancerBACUP (www.cancerbacup.org.uk) or Macmillan Cancer Relief (www.macmillan.org.uk). Through such services, users can access further information in leaflet format, or through the internet.

## Providing information to families

The exchange of information between a health professional, the child and a member of the child's family, takes place during any and almost every interaction. There are information points at each stage of the child's journey through the healthcare system. Glasper and Thompson[26] identifies four key information points in the journey for the family with a hospitalised child; pre-admission, on admission, during hospital and after discharge. The pre-admission particulars should give details of how to get to hospital; travel issues such as parking (often a significant concern to parents); how to get to the relevant department; and details of key members of hospital staff. He also highlights the need to have this information available through a dedicated hospital website. This is now mandated for all children's hospitals and units throughout England through standard [7] of the children's NSF,[5] although not all hospitals are yet compliant with this benchmarked standard.[14] The Children First for Health website, developed by Great Ormond Street Hospital and available through hypertext links on many other hospital websites, is a very good example of a kitemarked one-stop information shop for families, children and young people (www.childrenfirst.nhs.uk/).

Clearly the children's nurse has an important role in the exchange of information. This exchange takes place during almost every interaction between the nurse, the child and a member of the child's family. In relation to parents and children, the children's nurse has a critical role in ensuring that the child and their family have access to adequate, high-quality information. Whiting[27] builds upon this by arguing that children's nurses should focus their activities on the promotion of health rather than just on sickness. He stresses that there are information points at each stage of the child's journey through the healthcare system and the health professional should be aware of these, and in doing so will be in a position to provide additional information if required.

The children's nurse has a critical role in ensuring that the child and their family have access to adequate, high-quality information. Children's nurses are among the best communicators in healthcare, ideally experienced to inform, educate and advise.

Importantly, while some parents prefer not to have any information, the majority expect to have as much as can be made available.

Although pre-printed information and pre-admission visits and the like are undoubtedly helpful in informing children about what to expect in hospital, they are limited in scope. Printed information may not answer all the questions the child may have about a condition or hospital stay, particularly if they are not well designed.[1]

Giving information to some family groups can be especially challenging. These groups include:

- those with low literacy;
- young children and adolescents;
- those whose first language is not English.

Individual children with learning disabilities and special needs may require materials that have been specially developed.

## Family information services

Hospitals such as the University Hospital of Southampton provide information to a wide range of families attending with sick children. This ranges from pre-admission information to specific information related to illness.[28]

## WRITING PATIENT INFORMATION LEAFLETS*

Writing a patient information leaflet may not seem an arduous mission for well-educated children's nurses, but in reality they cannot just be written during a lunch break on a laptop computer and printed out. Although their design is made easier with commercially available desktop publishing software, their contents require rather more skill. The Write Stuff is a newsletter produced by Bruner three times per year (www.brunerbiz. com) dedicated to the art of communicating through the written word. They provide a range of pertinent rules for writing for patients which are based on much of the legacy of Robert Gunning,[29] who recognised that writers must always give

*After Lang TA. *How to write patient education handouts*. Department of Scientific Publications: The Cleveland Clinic Foundation (unpublished).

consideration to the literacy level of the client. This point is reiterated by Klare,[30] who discusses the use of readability formulae which allow writers to orientate their productions, such as information leaflets, at the right level. Additionally, some professionals have considered using formats such as comic strip characters to provide healthcare information to children. Barnes[31] discusses the development of characters such as Mr Wiggly for children with cancer.

## The Use of Readability Formulas

Readability formulas determine if documents are written at the correct reading level for their targeted audience.

The Gunnings'[29] Fog Index is one of the best known and measures the level of reading difficulty of any document. The formula for the index is as follows:

> (find the average number of words per sentence by dividing the total word count by the number of sentences) + (number of words of three syllables or more) multiplied by 0.4 = Fog index

The Fog Index level 'translates' the number of years' education a reader needs to understand the material. The 'ideal' score is 7 or 8; anything above 12 is too hard for most people to read.

The Fog Index does not determine if the writing is too basic or too advanced for a particular audience; instead, it helps you decide whether a document could benefit from editing or using 'plain language' techniques

Healthcare professionals such as children's nurses may not always be the best people to write the information leaflets and, skilled as they are, may not have the particular skills to write for differing child or family groups.

Before you start writing your information leaflet you will need to ask a number of questions to ensure that your work will be effective. Ultimately this will also save you time and money

## Before you start

- Has a need been identified?
- Are there common questions being asked by parents children or young people that could be answered by producing a leaflet?

### Who is it aimed at?

Who are you writing for? (The child or carer or both?) The key to producing accessible information is knowing who it is intended for and making the necessary adaptations. This is particularly important when considering using pictures/symbols, ensuring they are relevant and sensitive.

### Know the setting under which the target audience will read the leaflet

Will the information be given to families at a particular point in the child's or young person's healthcare journey?

### Does the NHS institution, e.g. Trust, already produce the information elsewhere?

Are you duplicating material that is already in circulation? This may be information produced in-house or by an external organisation.

### Know your purpose: ensure the information is relevant

- Make sure unnecessary detail is not included, while making sure the essential information is clear. The use of plain language is very important.
- Always consider what information you need to convey to your reader and what information will they want/need to know?

### Know your subject

Do you have the knowledge to write the material? Child and family information must be evidence based so it is imperative that someone with a direct knowledge of the procedure, condition or treatment is involved, advises on the content and checks the final draft for accuracy.

### Involve your audience

It is essential that child and family service users are involved when designing and producing information. It is important to ask if someone has any particular requirements in relation to accessing information such as colour of paper, size of print font, etc.

### Have you got the support in order to produce the leaflet?

Have you checked with your line manager that the

material is necessary and that there is a budget available for printing it?

# Writing your leaflet

The layout, tone and style of your leaflet will all influence on how effectively you communicate your information to the parents on children.

## Consider the content and style of the leaflet

- Make sure the title of the leaflet is clear.
- Use friendly, everyday language and plain English.
- Use clear and concise writing, keeping things brief and to the point.
- Use short sentences (an average of 15–20 words).
- Avoid jargon or abbreviations.
- Translate or explain essential terminology.
- Use friendly language and give the reader a sense of ownership by using words such as 'we', 'you', 'your'.
- Ensure information is accurate and up to date.
- Be evidence based where appropriate.
- To ensure a 'shelf-life' for the leaflet, avoid the use of names of staff where possible and use job titles instead.
- Be sensitive to religious, cultural, ethical and gender issues.
- Explain where the reader can obtain more information such as useful websites, organisations, PALS, etc.
- Always give contact numbers.
- Think about the questions that the reader is likely to ask. Have you answered them?
- Clearly state the date the information was produced and when it will be reviewed.

## Use the 10 principles of clear writing

1 Keep sentences short.
2 Use simple, rather than complex explanations.
3 Use familiar words where possible.
4 Avoid unnecessary words.
5 Put action into verbs used.
6 Write like you talk.
7 Use terms your reader can picture.
8 Link in with your readers' experience.
9 Use a wide variety of writing techniques.
10 Write to express, not impress (after Gunning[29]).

## Leaflets including treatment information

These should include:

- an explanation of the procedure: remember parents may be very anxious;
- an explanation of the reason for consent;
- an explanation of the risks as well as the benefits;
- an explanation of any of the alternatives including non-intervention; if there are no alternatives, which would be as effective, this should be stated;
- any areas of uncertainty surrounding the treatment;
- an explanation of the effects of treatment on the quality of life of their child;
- an invitation to ask questions about any areas of uncertainty.

## Consider the order of the information in your leaflet

The order of your information is very important. It should reflect the child's healthcare journey and will reflect events and experiences the child or young person will encounter. For example, this will include what will happen before and after a procedure.

## Test the text of your leaflet

Check the text and ask for constructive feedback from some independent readers. Draft information should be discussed with the target audience wherever possible to make sure they understand the information and message you are trying to convey. Also check for typing errors, accuracy and grammar.

## Does the leaflet comply with the Disability Discrimination Act

It is the responsibility of all NHS staff to ensure any information produced complies with Part 3 of the Disability Discrimination Act (1999), which requires public sector organisations to make their services available to people with disabilities. This includes the provision of information in appropriate formats which may include a different language, Braille, audio and large print.

# Producing your leaflet

Your leaflet should look professional and reflect a high standard of care provided. It should also be accessible to parents and children and there are a number of ways this can be achieved.

## Pay attention to the layout of your leaflet

- Use plenty of spaces so the pages look clean and uncluttered.
- Avoid large blocks of text: use short, separated blocks.
- Use headings to break up text.
- A question and answer format can help to divide up text.
- Use bullets or numbering to make important information stand out.
- Use bold type for headings and for emphasis. Use UPPER CASE letters.
- Use italics and underlining sparingly as they make the text more difficult to read.
- Align all text and sub-headings to the left (justified text is harder to read).
- Font size: minimum 12 point. Use 14 point if you are writing information for visually impaired people
- Use Arial or Frutiger font only. Times New Roman is particularly hard to read by visually impaired people and therefore should not be used.
- Do not write text over pictures or a design.

## Is the leaflet being produced an NHS leaflet?

If yes, the trust will have specific guidance or standards for producing patient information in line with the standards set for the NHS brand (see www.nhsidentity.nhs.uk)

The NHS has for some years implemented a Department of Health policy around a single identity style: NHS Identity Guidelines. This policy states the fundamental principles for all NHS Trusts to follow when designing and producing both printed and electronic information.

## Insert a logo

- All leaflets should display the logo of the originating organisation.
- You should check to see if your organisation has any specific rules relating to the use of its logo.

## Consider the size of your leaflet

- There are a number of standard sizes which you can use for information leaflets (A5, DL, A4).
- The number of words and use of images/ diagrams will determine which size is the most appropriate.
- Consider the paper quality.
- Use matt paper if possible. Avoid glossy paper, which creates glare.
- Use good quality paper.

## Using photography/pictures in a leaflet

- Pictures and photographs can be useful in supporting the text. They must be relevant and care must be taken when deciding suitability.
- Clip art should not be used on patient information leaflets when they are being professionally printed.
- If using photographs, pictures containing patients must not be used unless the patient has given written consent.
- If you are using pictures or diagrams from a third party, make sure you have obtained permission to do so. If this has been granted, please include an acknowledgement in the leaflet.

## Does the leaflet need to comply with a Trust Clinical Negligence Scheme for Trusts (CNST) 2 standard?

If so it will need to include:

- the nature of the condition;
- proposed treatment;
- benefits of the treatment;
- risks of the treatment;
- the alternatives to the treatment, including the option not to have treatment;
- information on where to get further information, for example local telephone contacts or website addresses;
- the originator;
- the date;
- the version;
- date for review.

# Reviewing your leaflet

All patient information must clearly display a published date and a review date on the back cover (usually 2 years). All information must be reviewed on a bi-annual basis to ensure it is still accurate and reflects current practice and procedures. If practice changes prior to this review date, the leaflet should be updated and reprinted to incorporate this.

## THE ROLE OF THE INTERNET IN PROVIDING HEALTH INFORMATION

In 2008, 16 million households in Great Britain (65 per cent) had internet access. This is an increase of just over 1 million households (7 per cent) over the last year and 5 million households (46 per cent) since 2002. Fifty-six per cent of all UK households had a broadband connection in 2008, up from 51 per cent in 2007. Ninety-three per cent of adults under 70 years of age who had a degree or equivalent qualification were most likely to have access to the internet in their home. Those individuals who had no formal qualifications were least likely to have an internet connection in their home.[32]

This dramatic increase in households with access to the World Wide Web will inevitably change the information-seeking behaviour of individuals. The rapid pace of change will challenge healthcare providers to seek new and innovative ways of harnessing the internet to meet the growing aspirations of healthcare consumers (Figure 38.1).

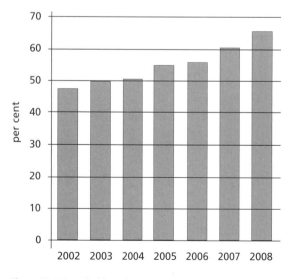

**Figure 38.1** Households with access to the internet, GB (Source: National Statistics website: www.statistics.gov.uk Crown copyright material is reproduced with permission of the Controller Office of Public Sector Information [OPSI]).

The internet has now for many but especially children and young people become a significant resource for dissemination of information. It has rapidly expanded over the last two decades with the advent of affordable personal computers and network-supporting platforms. With the advent of high bandwidth communication lines 24-hour continuous access at high speed is now available. This makes the internet most user friendly and increases the web's capacity to transfer files quickly. This expansion together with increasing affordability has led to this exponential rise in usage.

This increased access to the internet has introduced new possibilities for enhancing healthcare information sharing and communication. Lewis[33] identified that 80 per cent of the online population searches the internet for heath information and of this group half report that they use this information to help them make healthcare decisions. Importantly for children and young people's nurses, she concludes that the internet was a widely used information resource for parents of children. The majority looked to the internet for information to answer questions about their child's health, particularly at the time of diagnosis. Crucially in contemporary child health practice, parents talk to their medical carers about the information they find and generally believe their care providers such as doctors are interested in the information they retrieve. In the case of parents with children with complex disabilities, for example, many become hungry for any information, which may positively impact on their child's care and they, over time, become expert 'patients' in their own right.[34]

With the growth of home computers and increased electronic communication/information, Laporte[35] identifies the effects these changes in culture will bring in the delivery of healthcare. Until recently, it was extremely difficult for lay people to search for healthcare information, but applications such as the World Wide Web are now making it more accessible and changing the ways patients are retrieving health information. Ikemba et al.[36] identified in their study of the internet use with children requiring cardiac surgery that 80 per cent of parents who had internet access used this to obtain information relating to their child's impending cardiac surgery, with 95 per cent of families characterising the information as helpful or very helpful in furthering their understanding of their child's defect. However, Coeria[37] argues this changing nature of information distribution has important implications for healthcare: issues such as the quality of care, the validity and consistency of available information, and the effects on the doctor–patient relationship are potential major concerns to be considered. Impicciatore's[38] study supports this view: in his investigation of the reliability of health information on the World Wide Web, he concluded that parents could gain and retrieve online information about managing common health problems in their children. It is important to stress, however, that it may be difficult for them to put educational messages into practice when the information they receive can often be incomplete and partly misleading. He also argued that, because parents are often reluctant to follow advice that clashes with their beliefs and established practices, online information, to be effective, must not only be accurate but should be developed according to parents' perceived needs and draw on their skills and experience. Additionally, Johnson and Ramaprasad[39] support this view that the internet can be a good source of information on common health problems, but also stress that advice obtained through the World Wide Web should not be a substitute for routine care by a family doctor.

The internet has been demonstrated to be a useful tool in educating parents about their child's condition. Sim et al.,[40] reporting on the administration of a questionnaire to parents attending a surgical appointment at a paediatric outpatient department, found that 53 per cent of parents had accessed the internet for health information about their child's condition. He found only 25 per cent of parents discussed their findings with their surgeon, as most found the information was already covered by the surgeons or was irrelevant. He concluded the internet is a useful educational tool in teaching parents about their child's condition, especially as parents' use of the internet is widespread. Healthcare professionals such as children's nurses may need to specifically address any information gained from the internet by families during any conversations or consultations. He also advised that the best way to ensure parents have access to quality and accurate information about their child's condition on the

World Wide Web, hence providing support, is for healthcare professionals to provide the information themselves!

Effective searching of the internet by parents, children and young people seeking information is often hampered by differing uses of terminology (e.g. fits, seizures and convulsions) in different countries. Fox and Smith[41] demonstrated in his study of patients searching for information on seizures how using the word 'fit' on the Google search engine retrieved 8 360 000 web pages and a more specific search for 'febrile convulsion' retrieved almost 2500 studies. Studies of consumer habits have shown that only the first few items provided by a search engine are investigated further. Eysenback and Kohler[42] emphasise this in his study on how consumers search and appraise information on the internet, and questions the usefulness of this method of seeking quality health information

Allessandro and Kreiter[43] in a study investigating ways in which information is provided in hospitals also highlight that in using the internet in its current form it is often difficult to obtain answers to questions, as the internet provides convenient access to almost unlimited quantities of information, often unorganised and from questionable authorities. In order for families to access clear, high-quality child health information, via for example a hospital website, it is important for this information to be organised in a way that is easily accessible and understood, have its own distinct identity and be clearly differentiated from the vast array of information provided by adult services. By reorganising information in this way Allessandro has shown there is an increased usage of the internet by people accessing paediatric-related information

Swain[44] in a study of how people access information about their health and social care services highlights the need for greater attention to be paid to the design of websites intended for public use to minimise the number of false trails for information. She found websites were often difficult to navigate or failed to consider accessibility issues for those with visual impairments, low literacy or lack of experience of electronic searching techniques. She concluded all health and social care websites should include links to local voluntary groups as well as clear descriptions of the statutory services that they provide, and these links should be regularly tested to ensure they are up to date

Lewis et al,[33] however, stresses the need for caution and showed that many parents have concerns about the quality and security of internet information and most did not make treatment choices based on the internet information they found. Parents who believed that the information they found on the internet was correct were more likely to use that information and to make healthcare decisions and to trust the security of the websites they visited. This finding raises concern that parents who are less knowledgeable about internet barriers may be more likely to use inappropriate information they come across in their random unstructured searching.

Borowiztz and Ritterband[45] in a study of using the internet to teach parents and children about constipation and encopresis identified that over 25 per cent of the time available during outpatient encounters was spent educating patients, and yet patients' understanding and retention of the information provided was often marginal. He also identified that families wanted more information about their illnesses and treatments than they received during hospital visits, and less than one-third of patients received any literature about their child's condition during routine outpatient visits.

As a result, many patients seek health information from resources other than their own doctor, thus opening a Pandora's Box of misunderstanding and misconstrued evidence.

There remain, however, a series of limitations that impede access to healthcare information via the internet. Some studies have examined a number of these limitations. Aslam et al.[46] evaluated internet use by parents in a paediatric orthopaedic outpatients department and the quality of the information available. He identified a number of limitations, including quality, quantity and reliability of the information. He also highlights that the internet could not substitute for the rapport of the one-to-one basis of a consultation, but nevertheless found that the general attitude towards the internet was positive. Parents generally felt that this resource was convenient and easy to use, but it provided an excessive amount of medical information.

A number of studies have demonstrated that large numbers of parents are now using the internet as a medium for accessing health information in advance of their outpatient appointment. Tuffrey and Finlay,[47] for example, identified that over a fifth of parents attending a paediatric outpatient clinic at a district general hospital had looked for information about their child's condition on the internet prior to their hospital appointment; Aslam et al.[46] identified 65 per cent of parents used the internet for medical information prior to consultation and who found the health information sites informative, with 53 per cent saying it helped with understanding the consultation. Additionally, Aslam et al.[46] also found that 26 per cent of parents used this information to ask questions based on internet information. He also revealed that as parents become more informed about their children's conditions, an increased amount of time is required by healthcare professionals for the consultation. Informed parents consequentially expect to be more actively involved in their child's care and this may have considerable implications on the number of patients seen in for example a tertiary referral clinic.

The quality of healthcare information on the internet has been studied widely,[48,49] and the results of these studies have shown that quality of information found on the internet by patient groups is generally poor. It is important to stress that the results obtained are very much dependent on the search strategy, background knowledge and ability of the respondent to use the internet confidently. There is often found to be considerable variations in the listing of websites and their quality. The websites in these reported cases were listed based on the search engine's indexing procedure not necessarily the frequency of use, which may cause bias. The current generation internet provides a huge amount of information that is not controlled and may therefore be misleading. Despite this the Children's First health website is a beacon of excellence

## CONCLUSION

Throughout the last decade professional children's nurses have come to recognise the benefits of preparing children and their families for stressful healthcare life events wherever they occur. The role of family members throughout these components of a child's healthcare career should not be underestimated. Although families come in all shapes and sizes, all would appear to benefit from some type of preparation for stressful life events such as a hospital admission. The pre-school child is less able to cope positively with hospitalisation than his school age peers and thus preparation cannot be left to schoolroom activities. Although the school classroom is an excellent environment for teaching the skills necessary to cope with hospitalisation, other methods have to be adopted for younger children. This is highly pertinent when it is known that by the age of 5 years, 25 per cent of children will have had a stay in hospital with a third of these caused by accidents.[26] Children's nurses can continue to play an essential role as family advocates through embracing the art and science of information giving.

 Go to the website to find the PowerPoint presentation for this chapter and MCQs to test your knowledge. **www.hodderplus.com/childnursingskills**

## REFERENCES

1  Glasper A, Burge D (1992) Developing family information leaflets. *Nursing Standard* **6**(25): 24–27.
2  Coulter A (1999) Patient charters. *Health Expectations* **2**(3): 147–149.
3  Glasper A, Powell C ( 1994) The challenge of the children's charter: rhetoric vs reality. *British Journal of Nursing* **5**(1): 26–29.
4  Department of Health (2001) *Your guide to the NHS: getting the most from your National Health Service.* London: HMSO.
5  Department of Health (2004) *The national service framework for children, young people and maternity services.* London: HMSO.
6  Department of Health (DH) (2000) *The NHS plan.* London: HMSO.
7  Department of Health (DH) (2001) *Learning from Bristol: the report of the public inquiry into children's heart surgery at the Bristol Royal Infirmary 1984–1985.* Command paper CM5363. London: Stationery Office.
8  NHS Direct (2008) *NHS direct.* Available from www.nhsdirect.nhs.uk (accessed 22 September 2008).
9  Robertson L (1995) The giving of information is the key to family empowerment information from healthcare providers to children and parents. *British Journal of Nursing* **4**(12): 692. Department of Health (DH) (1992) *The patient's charter.* London: HMSO.
10  Redfern M (2001) *The Royal Liverpool children's report.* London: The Stationery Office.
11  Lord Carlisle (2000). *The Review of safeguards for children and young people treated and cared for by the NHS in Wales.* Available from

http://new.wales.gov.uk/docrepos/40382/40382313/childrenyoungpeople/403821/safeguards_text-e. pdf?lang=en (accessed 22 September 2008).
12  Department of Health (2003) *Getting the right start.* London: HMSO.
13  Healthcare Commission (2007) *Improving outcomes for children in hospital.* London: DH.
14  Coles L, Glasper EA, FitzGerald C, *et al.* (2007) Measuring compliance to the NSF for children and young people in one English strategic health authority. *Journal of Children's and Young Peoples Nursing* **1**(1): 7–15.
15  Department of Health (2009) *Healthy lives, brighter futures: the strategy for children and young people.* London: HMSO.
16  Tiedeman ME, Clatsworthy S (1990) Anxiety responses of 5 to 11-year-old children during and after hospitalisation. *Journal of Paediatric Nursing* **5**: 334–343.
17  Shirley P, Thompson N, Kenwad M, Johnson G (1998) Parental anxiety before surgery in children. *Anaesthesia* **53**: 956–959.
18  Keller F (2001) Pre-operative teaching for children. *Neonatal, Paediatric and Child Health Nursing* **4**: 4–9.
19  Weaver K, Battrick C, Glasper, A (2007) Developing a hospital play guideline and protocol for sick children with debilitating fears. *Journal of Children's and Young People's Nursing* **1**(3): 143.
20  Korsch BM (1984) What do patients and parents want to know? What do they need to know? *Pediatrics* **74**: 917–919.

21 Caress, AL (2003) Giving information to patients. *Nursing Standard* **17**(43): 47–54.

22 Coulter A (1998) Evidence-based patient information. *British Medical Journal* **317**: 225–226.

23 Coulter A (1999) Sharing decisions with patients: is the information good enough? *British Medical Journal* **318**: 318–322.

24 Gann R. (1991), Consumer health information: the growth of an information specialism. *Journal of Documentation* **47**(3): 284–308.

25 Audit Commission (1993) *What seems to be the matter: communication between hospitals and patients?* HMSO, London.

26 Glasper EA, Thompson M (1993) Preparing children for hospital. In: Glasper EA, Tucker A (eds) *Advances in child health nursing.* London: RCN, p 257–267.

27 Whiting L (1997) Health promotion: the role of the children's nurse. *Paediatric Nursing* **9**(5): 6–7.

28 Glasper EA, McWilliams R (1998) Developing a centre for health information and promotion. In: Glasper EA, Lowson S (eds) *Innovations in paediatric ambulatory care.* Basingstoke: Palgrave, pp 48—60.

29 Gunning R. (1952/1968) *The technique of clear writing.* McGraw Hill, New York.

30 Klare GR (1976) A second look at the validity of readability formulas. *Journal of Reading Behaviour* **8**(2): 129–152.

31 Barnes E (2006) Captain Chemo and Mr Wiggly: patient information for children with cancer in the late twentieth century. *Social History of Medicine* **19**: 501–519.

32 UK Office for National Statistics (2008) *Internet access.* www.statistics.gov.uk/CCI/nugget.asp?ID=8 (accessed 5 September 2008).

33 Lewis D, Gundwardena S, Saadawi G (2005) Caring connection. developing an internet resource for family caregivers of children with cancer. *Computers, Informatics Nursing* **23**(5): 265–274.

34 Coombes R. (1995) From parent to expert: information provision to parents. *Child Health* **2**: 237–240.

35 Laporte RE (1994) Global public health and the information superhighway. *British Medical Journal* **308**: 1651–1652.

36 Ikemba M, Kozinetz C, Feltes T, et al. (2002) Internet use in families with children requiring cardiac surgery for congenital heart disease. *Paediatrics* **109**:(3) 419–422.

37 Coeira E. (1996) The internet's challenge to healthcare provision. *British Medical Journal* **312**: 3–4.

38 Impicciatore P (1997) Reliability of health information for the public on the world wide web: systematic survey of advice on managing fever in children at home. *British Medical Journal* **314**: 1875.

39 Johnson L, Ramaprasad A (2000) A patient-physician relationships in the information age. *Marketing Health Services* **20**(1): 8.

40 Sim N, Kitterinham L, Spitz, L. *et al.* (2007) Information on the world wide web – how useful is it for parents. *Journal of Paediatric Surgery* **42**(2): p 305–312.

41 Fox A, Smith P (2001) Parents and the internet. *Journal of Pediatrics and Neonatology* **3**(1): 110–116.

42 Eysenbach G, Kohler, C. (2002) How do consumers search for and appraise health information on the World Wide Web? *British Medical Journal* **324**: 582–583.

43 Alesandro D, Kreiter, C (1999) Improving usage of paediatric information on the internet: the virtual children's hospital. *Paediatrics* **104**(5): 55.

44 Swain D (2007) *Accessing information about health and social care services.* Oxford: Picker Institute.

45 Borowitz S, Ritterband L (2001) Using the internet to teach parents and children about constipation and encopresis. *Medical Informatics* **26**(4): 283–295.

46 Aslam N, Bower D, Wainwright A, et al. (2005) Evaluation of internet use by paediatric orthopaedic outpatients and the quality of information available. *Journal of Paediatric Orthopaedics* **14**: 129–133.

47 Tuffrey C, Finlay F (2001) Use of the internet by parents of paediatric outpatients. *Archive of Diseases in Childhood* **87**: 534–536.

48 Plumridge G (2007) The internet as an information source for parents talking to children about genetic conditions. *Journal of Children's and Young Peoples' Nursing* **1**(5): 225–230.

49 Griffiths K, Christensen, H (2000) Quality web based information on treatment of depression: cross sectional survey. *British Medical Journal* **321**: 1511–1515.

# Index